Brief Contents

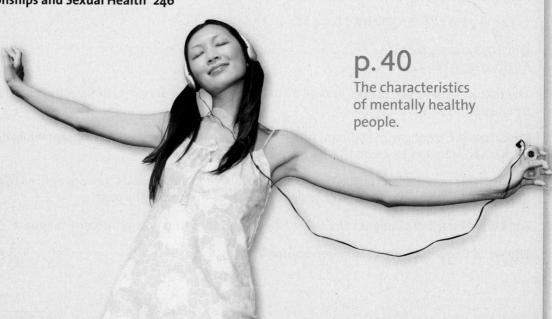

p. 40
The characteristics of mentally healthy people.

YOUR HEALTH TODAY

AUTHORS

Michael L. Teague   Sara L. C. Mackenzie   David M. Rosenthal

Vice President, Editorial   **Michael J. Ryan**
Director, Editorial   **Beth Mejia**
Executive Editor   **Christopher Johnson**
Director of Development   **Kathleen Engelberg**
Development Editors   **Kathleen Engelberg and Sarah Hill**
Editorial Coordinator   **Lydia Kim**
Marketing Manager   **Caroline McGillen**
Production Editor   **Leslie Racanelli**
Manuscript Editor   **Patricia Ohlenroth**
Art Manager   **Robin Mouat**
Designers   **Jeanne Schreiber and Amanda Kavanagh**
Cover Designer   **Jeanne Schreiber**
Photo Research Coordinator   **Alexandra Ambrose**
Photo Researcher   **Jennifer Blankenship**
Media Project Managers   **Thomas Brierly and Andrea Helmbolt**
Developmental Editor for Technology   **Sarah Hill**
Buyer   **Laura Fuller**

Published by McGraw-Hill, a business unit of The McGraw-Hill Companies, Inc., 1221 Avenue of the Americas, New York, NY 10020. Copyright © 2011, 2009, 2007 by The McGraw-Hill Companies, Inc. All rights reserved. No part of this publication may be reproduced or distributed in any form or by any means, or stored in a database or retrieval system, without the prior written consent of The McGraw-Hill Companies, Inc., including, but not limited to, any network or other electronic storage or transmission, or broadcast for distance learning. Some ancillaries, including electronic and print components, may not be available to customers outside the United States.

Printed in the United States of America

3 4 5 6 7 8 9 0 QDB/QDB 9 8 7 6 5 4 3 2

ISBN: 978-0-07-338092-6
MHID: 0-07-338092-X

The text was set in 10/12 Times Roman by Lachina Publishing Services, and printed on acid-free 45# Orion Gloss by Quad/Graphics.

Cover images: front cover: (woman) Altrendo Images/Getty Images, (leaf) Ingram Publishing/SuperStock; back cover: Harrison Eastwood/Getty Images

Because this page cannot legibly accommodate all acknowledgments for copyrighted material, credits appear at the end of the book and constitute an extension of this copyright page.

For a detailed list of changes from the previous edition, visit www.mhhe.com/teague3e.

Library of Congress Control Number: 2010938041

Contents

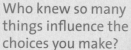

p.3
Who knew so many things influence the choices you make?

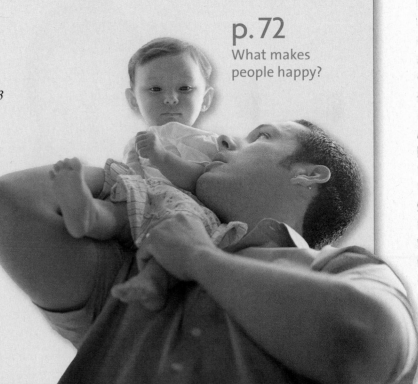

p.72
What makes
people happy?

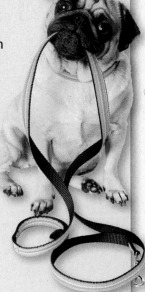

p.133
What are you waiting for? Get moving!

p. 156
Is LeBron James overweight?

p. 247
Friendship matters to your health.

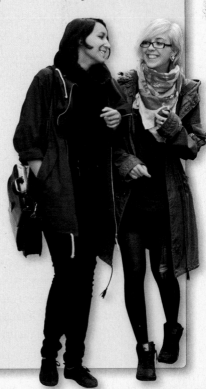

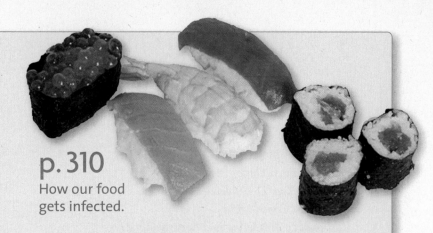

p. 310
How our food
gets infected.

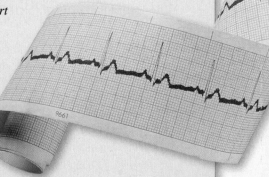

p. 350
Who's at risk
for cardiovas-
cular disease?

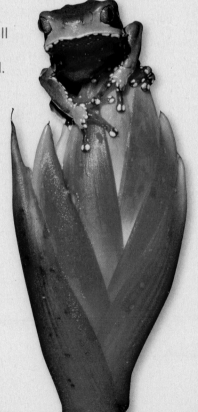

p. 444
The health of all living things is interconnected.

Health in a Changing Society

1

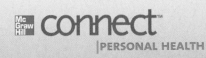

As individuals, we are all responsible for our own health. Each of us makes choices about how we live—about whether to be physically active, whether to eat a healthy diet, whether to get enough sleep, whether to see a doctor when we need to. And yet to talk about health only as a matter of individual choice assumes that we are always aware of the choices we are making and that we are always "free" to make them. The truth is that not everyone is in the same position—there are differences in how we live and the contexts in which we make decisions.

In this book we explore personal health within the context of our social and cultural environment. We recognize that individuals are ultimately responsible for their own health, but we also know that people are able to make healthier choices when their environment supports those choices and at times even provides a nudge in more positive directions.[1]

Personal Health in Context

In this section we consider the meaning of the terms *health* and *wellness*, and we explore the factors that shape and influence our personal health.

HEALTH AND WELLNESS

Traditionally, people were considered "healthy" if they did not have symptoms of disease. In 1947 the World Health Organization (WHO) broke new ground by defining **health** as a state of complete physical, mental, and social well-being, not merely the absence of disease and infirmity. Physical health referred to the biological integrity of the individual. Mental health included emotional and intellectual capabilities, or the individual's subjective sense of well-being. Social health meant the ability of people to interact effectively with other people and the social environment.[2]

More recently, a spiritual domain has been added to the WHO definition, reflecting the idea that people's value systems or beliefs can have an impact on their overall health. Spiritual health does not require participation in a particular organized religion but suggests a belief in (or a searching

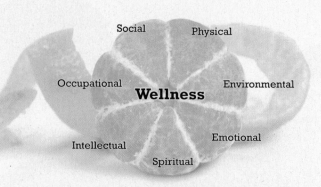

figure 1.1   **Dimensions of wellness.**

Sources: Adapted from The World Health Report 2006: Working Together for Health, *by World Health Organization, 2006, Geneva, Switzerland;* Wellness Index: A Self-Assessment for Health and Vitality, *by J.W. Travis and S.R. Ryan, 2004, Berkeley, CA: Ten Speed Press (Celestial Arts).*

for) some type of greater or higher power that gives meaning and purpose to life. Spiritual health involves a connectedness to self, to significant others, and to the community.

Wellness is a slightly different concept. It is generally defined as an active process of adopting patterns of behavior that can lead to improved health and heightened life satisfaction. Like health, wellness is seen as encompassing multiple dimensions: physical, emotional, intellectual, spiritual, interpersonal or social, environmental, and occupational (see Figure 1.1).

Wellness may also be conceptualized as a continuum. One end of the continuum represents extreme illness and premature death; the other end represents wellness and optimal health (see Figure 1.2). Historically, Western medicine has focused primarily on the illness side of the continuum, treating people with symptoms of disease. More recently, approaches to health have focused on the wellness side of the continuum, seeking ways to help people live their lives fully, as whole people, with vitality and meaning.

health
State of complete physical, mental, social, and spiritual well-being.

wellness
Process of adopting patterns of behavior that can lead to improved health and heightened life satisfaction; wellness has several domains and can be conceptualized as a continuum.

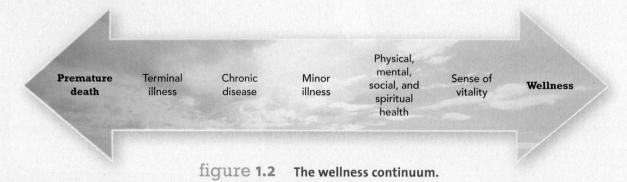

figure 1.2   **The wellness continuum.**

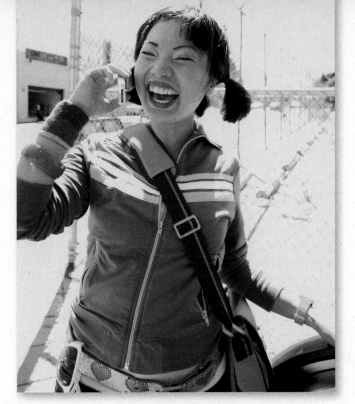

■ Qualities associated with wellness include self-confidence, optimism, a sense of humor, an active mind, vitality, and joy in life, among many others.

Although most people want to have good health, it typically is not an ultimate goal in and of itself. Usually, people desire good health in order to reach other goals—to be more productive, more attractive, more comfortable, more independent—in other words, to have a higher quality of life. In this sense, wellness and an optimal quality of life can be seen as an ultimate goal, with good health a means to attain it.

THE ECOLOGICAL MODEL OF HEALTH AND WELLNESS

How do you achieve good health and strive toward wellness? What encourages you to make healthy decisions? What makes some choices difficult?

Although there are many theories about health behavior and decision making, we focus here on the **ecological model of health and wellness**. As shown in Figure 1.3, the model is a framework that addresses the interrelationships between individuals and their environment, taking into account not just individual choices but all the factors that influence those choices. It recognizes

ecological model of health and wellness
A framework that recognizes the interrelationship between individuals and their environment; emphasizes the multiple social determinants that influence health.

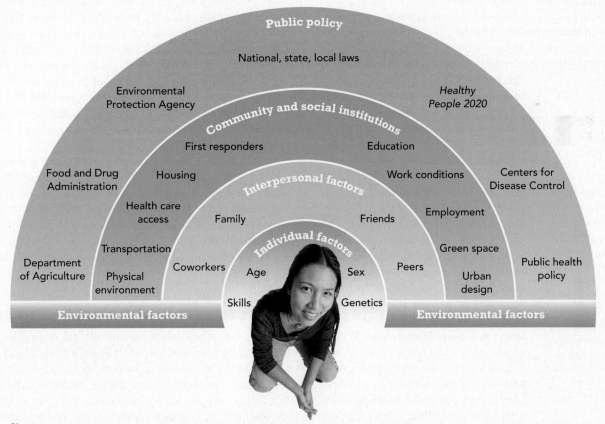

figure 1.3 **The ecological model of health and wellness.** While each of us has a unique set of individual characteristics that shape our health, our environmental factors, also called the social determinants of health, have an impact on our health and wellness as well.

that you have a unique set of characteristics—your genetics, age, and sex, along with your knowledge, beliefs, values, and skills—that guide the decisions you make about how to live your life. You also live within an environment, which in this model is defined very broadly as anything external to you. The environment encompasses your relationships with other people, your interactions with social institutions, your community affiliations, and public policies that impact each of these.

Proponents of the ecological model argue that you cannot make choices independent of friends, family, community norms, and public policy. In addition, societies can influence your health by shaping your environment in ways that increase or decrease your opportunities for making healthy or unhealthy choices. For example, in most supermarkets

what constitutes a healthy diet, attitudes toward different foods and diets, skills that enable you to prepare certain foods. In addition, depending on your genetic predispositions, age, and health conditions, you may need to pay attention to certain components of a diet, such as salt if you have high blood pressure or red meat if you have high cholesterol.

Next, your family and friends influence your eating patterns. As you were growing up, you became familiar with the foods and meals your family provided, and you may still prefer those foods and eat them when you go home. Your friends may like to eat out at fast-food restaurants and you may go with them. Or your friends may be vegetarian, so you find yourself eating more vegetarian foods. If your friends are overweight or if they gain weight, it's likely that you will find weight gain more acceptable for yourself.[5]

Worse health outcomes are associated with poorer living conditions— with poverty, unemployment, poor housing, and other negative social, economic, and physical factors.

candy is placed near the checkout counter, where you can grab it impulsively as you're getting ready to pay. The practice increases sales but encourages unhealthy choices.

These external environmental factors are also known as the **social determinants of health**. This term highlights the fact that the conditions in which you live, work, and pursue your life goals influence the options you have available and the choices you make. The social determinants of health include such factors as income, socioeconomic status, educational attainment, literacy, employment status, working conditions, housing, transportation, social support networks, and access to health care services.[3,4] Your health is also affected by your physical environment. In the *built* physical environment, you are affected by such factors as the kinds of housing, streets, schools, sanitation systems, and transportation systems that have been constructed. In the *natural* physical environment, you are affected by such factors as air and water quality, proximity to environmental hazards, and access to trees and parks.

How does the ecological model play out in a person's life? As an example, let's say you decide you want to eat a healthier diet. What influences your ability to achieve this goal, according to the ecological model? You begin with a personal history that includes knowledge, attitudes, and skills—ideas about

social determinants of health
Societal conditions that affect health and can potentially be altered by social and health policies and programs.

public health
The study and practice of health promotion and disease prevention at the population level.

health promotion
Public-health-related actions designed to maintain a current healthy state or advance to a more desirable state.

The social institutions you interact with also influence your choices. Your dining hall may have unlimited soda refills, or your church may serve donuts after services. In your community, you may have opportunities to buy fresh fruits and vegetables, or the corner store may have only candy and liquor. Finally, local, state, and national laws influence the safety of the food you eat, the nutritional labeling it features, and its cost. When all these factors are taken into account, it is clear that choosing a healthier diet is not just a matter of your individual choices—though the choices you make within the context of your environment are still critical.

Both in the United States and worldwide, worse health outcomes are associated with poorer living conditions— with poverty, unemployment, poor housing, low educational attainment, environmental pollution, and other negative social, economic, and physical factors. Addressing these inequities is one of the goals of national and international health policies; this topic is discussed in more detail later in the chapter.

PUBLIC HEALTH AND COMMUNITY HEALTH

Because the relationships among all the determinants of health are so complex, responsibilities for health and wellness extend beyond the individual to the areas of public health and community health. **Public health** is a discipline that focuses on the health of populations of people (whereas the discipline of medicine focuses on the health of individuals). Public health efforts include both health promotion and disease prevention **Health promotion** focuses on actions designed to maintain a current health state or encourage advancement to a more desirable state of health (such as campaigns to promote physical activity). **Disease prevention** focuses on defensive actions taken to ward off specific diseases and their consequences (such as food and water protections or flu shot campaigns).

Prevention efforts are designed to target different stages of disease. *Primary prevention* efforts are designed to inhibit the development of disease. *Secondary prevention* efforts are designed to detect disease before it becomes symptomatic (often called *screening*). And *tertiary prevention* involves treating people with a disease in order to reduce the problems caused by that disease. As an example, let's consider some public health approaches that may be considered if a health department wants to reduce the impact of HIV infection among young adults. Primary prevention measures—measures that would reduce the risk of contracting HIV in the first place—might include educational campaigns about how to use condoms or implementation of a needle exchange program. Secondary prevention measures—measures that would identify young adults who are infected with HIV but who are not aware of their status—might include HIV screening with mobile screening units. Tertiary prevention—ensuring that young adults with HIV receive treatment—might involve developing community clinics and securing funding for medications. If you think about your own community, can you identify other examples of public health measures? How do they affect you personally? Also, see the box "What Is Public Health?" to learn about some of the broad public health measures that affect your everyday life.

In the United States, nationwide government-sponsored public health initiatives are conducted by the Public Health Service, led by the surgeon general and the Centers for Disease Control and Prevention in Atlanta, Georgia. State, county, and city health departments are involved at the state and local levels, and many public health actions take place at the local, or community, level. *Community* implies an interdependence of people and organizations within a defined grouping. **Community health** refers to activities directed toward improving the health of those

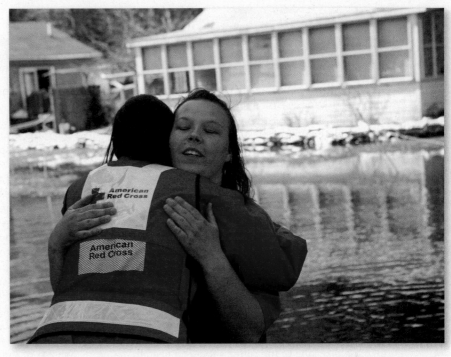

■ Heavy rains and floods periodically necessitate the evacuation of communities. Extreme weather, natural disasters, and other events that affect whole populations fall into the domain of public health.

people or activities employing resources shared by the members of the community. For example, the health department in a town (the community) with a large immigrant population may decide as part of its emergency preparedness planning that it needs to design messages in different languages in order to reach all members of the community. Community health is also supported when a community decides to create bike lanes on public streets, include parks and green spaces in development projects, and invest in neighborhood health clinics.

Health in a Diverse Society

As a nation of immigrants, the United States has always had a diverse population. As the 21st century unfolds, the U.S. population is rapidly becoming more diverse. In 2009, approximately 30 percent of people 30 and older were members of a racial or ethnic minority group and 40 percent of people 29 and younger were members of a racial or ethnic minority group.[6]

The U.S. Census Bureau identifies the primary minority groups in the United States as Black or African American, American Indian or Alaska Native, Asian, Native Hawaiian or Other Pacific Islander, and White. Hispanic origin is treated as a separate category, so people of Hispanic origin may be of any race.[7] Within each grouping there is tremendous diversity as well: Asian Americans, for example, include people from China, Japan, Korea, Vietnam, Laos, Cambodia, the Philippines, and other countries.

disease prevention
Public-health-related actions designed to ward off or protect against specific diseases.

community health
Issues, events, and activities related to the health of a whole community, as well as activities directed toward bettering the health of the public and/or activities employing resources available in common to members of the community.

Public Health in Action

What Is Public Health?

The benefits of public health are all around you, reducing your risk for disease and injury and helping you live a healthier life—even though many people aren't sure what public health is. Here are just some of the ways public health can impact your daily life:

When you get up in the morning, you brush your teeth with the water from your tap. You don't have to worry about contracting an infectious disease, because tap water in the United States is safe to drink and presents a minimal risk of infectious disease. You have had fewer cavities and dental problems in your life than people did a century ago, because the tap water you drink also contains fluoride, which strengthened your teeth when you were younger.

As you walk outside to get on your bicycle for your ride to campus, you strap on your helmet without thinking. Your state requires bicycle helmets to reduce the risk of head injuries, and wearing one has become a habit. You take the bike lane to the coffee shop—no need to dodge cars—and meet a friend for a bagel and cream cheese before class. You don't worry about eating the food, because food regulations have significantly reduced the incidence of foodborne illness.

After breakfast, you continue your ride to school, past "clean buses" that run on emissions-controlled diesel as part of your city's green energy campaign. You have to stop briefly when a road worker directs traffic around a lane closure. Although you don't notice, the road workers are wearing helmets and hearing protection while using jackhammers.

As you enter your class building, you don't think about the fact that the air you breathe is fresh and smoke-free. This is due to the fact that tobacco smoke has been recognized as a health hazard and your campus follows regulations that prohibit smoking within 25 feet of public buildings.

After class, you get back on your bike and ride to the campus health center to pick up a month's worth of contraceptive supplies. You and your partner are not ready for pregnancy; you're planning to delay starting a family until after you finish school. While at the center, you pass signs promoting HIV/AIDS awareness and a supply of free condoms. You notice that free flu shots are available as part of a campaign to get students vaccinated. You decide to get a flu shot, because you know that flu season is approaching and you want to reduce your risk of illness.

Later in the day, you go for a run on a jogging trail in a city park near your home. Many people are out walking their dogs—and following the signs to clean up after them in compliance with local ordinances. On your way home, you stop at a local grocery store, picking up some fresh fruits and vegetables as well as some packaged foods. You assume the labels on the packaged foods accurately reflect what is in them, because food labeling laws have been in place your whole life. When you get home, you know you need to wash the produce you bought, just as you know you should wash your hands frequently. The wealth of information you have about keeping yourself well and safe comes from the health education you have received in your schools and community.

Ten great public health achievements in the past century include vaccination, motor vehicle safety, safer workplaces, control of infectious diseases, safer and healthier foods, healthier mothers and babies, family planning, fluoridation of drinking water, the recognition of tobacco as a health hazard, and reduced deaths from heart attacks and stroke. Beyond these achievements, innumerable other developments and advances have contributed to your health, including health education initiatives and campaigns. In this book, you can learn more about public health from the Public Health in Action boxes that appear in each chapter and draw your attention to the different ways that public health influences your personal health. You can also learn more about public health by watching the online videos and animations at What Is Public Health (www.whatispublichealth.org) and This Is Public Health (www.thisispublic health.org).

connect ACTIVITY

Sources: "Ten Great Public Health Achievements—United States, 1900–1999," 1999, Morbidity and Mortality Weekly Reports, 48(12), *pp. 241–243;* Healthiest Nation in One Generation, *by the American Public Health Association, retrieved from www.generationpublichealth.org.*

CULTURE, ETHNICITY, AND RACE

Although diversity includes differences among individuals in many areas, including gender, age, sexual orientation, ability or disability, educational attainment, socioeconomic status, and geographical location, three important dimensions of diversity that impact groups of people are culture, ethnicity, and race. There are many different meanings of the term *culture,* but we are using the term here to mean a shared pattern of values, beliefs, language, and customs within a group. You may have a sense of belonging to a particular culture or to different subcultures, based on such factors as geographical location, socioeconomic status, religious affiliation, and so on. Your culture helps shape what you view as acceptable and unacceptable (including health-related

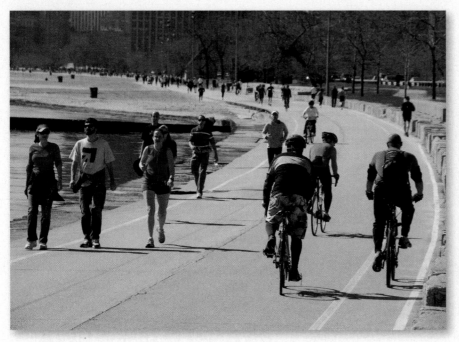

■ A healthy community provides services that support the health and wellness of community members. Community pedestrian and bike trails encourage physical activity and decrease the need for automobiles as a means of transportation.

behaviors) and may even influence how you define or view illness and wellness.[7,8]

ethnicity
The sense of identity an individual draws from a common ancestry and/or a common national, religious, tribal, language, or cultural origin.

race
Term used in the social sciences to describe ethnic groups based on physical characteristics, such as skin color or facial features; race does not exist as a biological reality.

Ethnicity refers to the sense of identity individuals draw from a common ancestry, as well as from a common national, religious, tribal, language, or cultural origin. This identity nurtures a sense of social belonging and loyalty for people of common ethnicity, helping to shape how they think, relate, feel, and behave both within and outside their group. Ethnicity is often confused with **race**, a term used to describe ethnic groups based on physical characteristics, such as skin color or facial features. Although classifying people by race has been a common societal practice, the fact is that biologically distinct and separate races do not exist within the human species. Genetic traits are inherited individually, not in clumps, groups, or "races" (as discussed further in Chapter 2). Thus, it is more accurate to view race as a social category rather than a biological one and to think of similarities or differences among people as a matter of culture or ethnicity.

HEALTH CONCERNS OF ETHNIC AND RACIAL MINORITY POPULATIONS

Over the past 100 years, advances in medical technology, lifestyle improvements, and environmental protections have produced significant health gains for the general U.S. population. These advances, however, have not produced equal health benefits for most of the country's ethnic or racial minority populations. Morbidity and mortality (rates of illness and death, respectively) for ethnic and racial minority populations are disheartening. Many have higher rates of cancer, diabetes, cardiovascular disease, infant mortality, alcoholism, drug abuse, unintentional injury, and premature death than the general population does. Most also have significantly higher lifestyle risk factors, such as high-fat diets, lack of exercise, and more exposure to carcinogens and other environmental toxins.[9]

In line with the ecological model described earlier, much of the disparity can be attributed to social and economic conditions, including poverty, discrimination, and limited access to health information and resources. Several theories have been proposed to explain how these social determinants affect health. For example, one theory suggests that minority populations are disproportionately exposed to racism, which

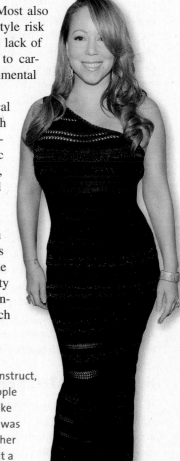

■ *Race* exists only as a social construct, not as a biological reality. People with biracial backgrounds—like Mariah Carey, whose mother was Irish American and whose father was Afro-Venezuelan—inherit a random mix of individual traits from each parent.

Biologically distinct and separate *races do not exist within the human species.*

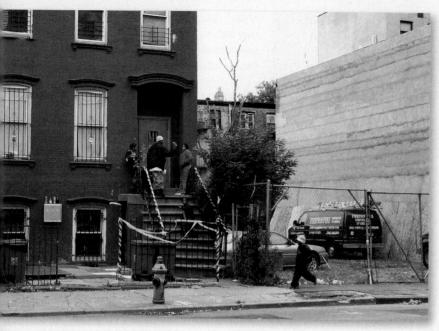

■ Health disparities between racial and ethnic groups are largely attributable to social and economic conditions. A poor neighborhood does not provide the same opportunities for a healthy life as a more affluent neighborhood.

is a source of stress. An ever-growing body of research documents the relationship between stress and health outcomes, including heart disease, breast cancer survival, chronic obstructive pulmonary disease, infant mortality, low birth weight, and depression. Reducing or eliminating health disparities is a critical challenge of the 21st century and a specific national health goal.[8,9]

Understanding Health-Related Behavior Change

The ecological model shows us that good health depends on many interacting factors, including family and friends, community resources, government policies, and even global conditions. And yet within these contexts, you still have a range of choices regarding your health-related behaviors. In this section we consider behavior choice and behavior change. How do you know if there is a behavior that you should change? When are you ready to make a change? And how can you sustain healthy changes?

HEALTH-RELATED BEHAVIOR CHOICES

A key role is played in your health and wellness by your health-related behavior choices (or lifestyle choices)—those actions you take and decisions you make that affect your own individual health (and, possibly, the health of your immediate family members). They include choices concerning your physical, mental, emotional, spiritual, and social

well-being—what you eat, how much exercise you get, whether you spend time developing meaningful relationships, and so on. For example, having an apple instead of a bag of chips is a healthy behavior choice, as is quitting smoking. Other examples are getting enough sleep, practicing safe sex, wearing a safety belt in a car, finding effective ways to manage stress, drinking alcohol in moderation if at all, and getting regular health checkups. It is in the realm of lifestyle choice that individuals have the most control over their health.

Interesting questions arise when we consider why people make choices that don't enhance their health and why they don't change behaviors they know are hurting them. Psychologists have proposed many theories about health behavior choice and change. One of the most useful is the Stages of Change model.

THE STAGES OF CHANGE MODEL

Developed in the 1990s by psychologists James Prochaska and Carlo DiClemente, the **Stages of Change Model**, or Transtheoretical Model (TTM), is a widely accepted framework for understanding individual health behavior change. The model is useful because it acknowledges that people are often ambivalent about making significant changes in their lives and because it recognizes that change happens as a process, not a one-time event. It also takes into account not just a person's knowledge but also her feelings, behaviors, relationships, and perceived **self-efficacy** (belief that one can perform a certain task). The stages are as follows:

■ *Precontemplation.* If you are in this stage, you have no motivation to change a behavior. In fact, you may not even realize or acknowledge that you have a problem. You just want people to quit bothering you about your behavior. You may be helped to see a problem by events that highlight discrepancies between your behaviors and your goals.

Stages of Change Model
Model of behavior change that focuses on stages of change.

self-efficacy
Internal state in which you feel competent to perform a specific task.

■ *Contemplation.* You realize you may have a problem behavior. You are thinking that you should make a change in the near future (usually within six months). You are trying to understand the problem and may search for solutions. Often you are weighing the pros and cons of making a change. Self-efficacy becomes important as you are more likely to prepare for change if you believe in yourself and the fact that you can make a change.

■ *Preparation.* The pros have won and you are making a plan for change. You are setting goals and have a start

Why do people make **choices** that don't enhance their health, *and why don't people change behaviors they know are hurting them?*

date. You are looking for tools to help support the change. You are building your skill set and supporting your self-efficacy.

- *Action.* You are implementing behavior change. You are committing time and energy to make it work. From this point forward, you can support your efforts to change by rewarding yourself for change, avoiding environments that trigger the unhealthy behavior, and enlisting the help of friends and family.

- *Maintenance.* You have been maintaining the new behavior for at least six months. You are working to prevent yourself from falling back into old habits. You are well on your way! This can be a long, ongoing stage—for some behaviors, lasting a lifetime.

- *Termination.* The new behavior has become such a part of your life that you have no temptation to return to the old behavior, and you have 100 percent confidence in your ability to maintain the behavior.[10]

Understanding that change is a process with different stages is important because you may need different information or different types of support, depending on where you are in the process (some are included in the list of stages). It's also important to realize that change is more like a spiral than a linear progression. You can enter and exit the process at any point, and you often cycle back through some or all of the steps (Figure 1.4). The box "Assessing Your Stage of Change" can help you determine your own readiness to make a behavior change. Most of us try several times to make changes before they really stick. **Relapse** is the rule rather than the exception. This should be seen not as failure but as a normal part of the

relapse
Backslide into a former health state.

process.[10,11] The important thing is to keep trying and not get discouraged.

Let's consider an example of how behavior impacts your health. Say you are determined to get better grades this term, especially in psychology, your major. To improve, you've been studying a lot in the afternoons, and drinking coffee and energy drinks to stay focused. Unfortunately, you keep oversleeping and missing your 8 a.m. psych class, where surprise quizzes are often given. Since you've missed several quizzes, your grade is suffering. The reason you're oversleeping is that you're having trouble falling asleep at night, which you've been attributing to stress. You don't make the connection between the caffeine you're consuming in the afternoon and your insomnia. This sort of behavior marks the precontemplation stage, in which you do not recognize that your caffeine consumption may be causing you a problem.

When a friend mentions that you might sleep better if you cut out the caffeine, your first thought is that you really enjoy those drinks in the afternoon and might not be able to study without them. But then you start to weigh the benefits of caffeine (you feel sharper, you can concentrate more easily) against the problem of insomnia (you oversleep and miss class). This thought process marks the contemplation stage, in which you weigh the pros and cons of behavior change.

You decide to try decaffeinated coffee and see what happens. You buy some decaf at the grocery store (preparation) and make a switch the following week, at the same

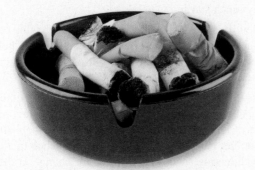

- The health effects of tobacco use are well known, yet 20 percent of Americans continue to smoke.

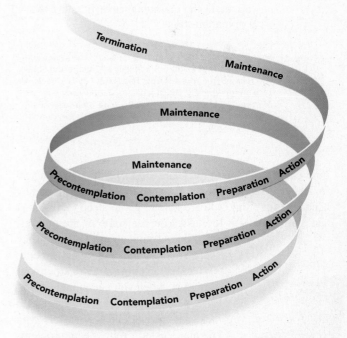

figure **1.4**   **The stages of change: A spiral model.**
Source: Adapted from "In Search of How People Change," by J.O. Prochaska, C.C. DiClemente, and J.C. Norcross, 1992, American Psychologist 47(9), pp. 1102–1114.

Challenges & Choices

Assessing Your Stage of Change

Responding to four simple statements can help determine your readiness for behavior change as well as your stage of change for a chosen health behavior. First, choose a health area in which you think there might be room for improvement or a specific health behavior that you think you might like to change. Then respond yes or no to the following statements:

_____ 1. I solved my problem more than six months ago.

_____ 2. I have taken action on my problem within the past six months.

_____ 3. I am intending to take action in the next month.

_____ 4. I am intending to take action in the next six months.

Scoring: Answering no for all four statements means you are in the precontemplation stage. If you answered yes to statement 4 and no to the other three statements, you are in the contemplation stage. If you answered yes to statements 3 and 4 and no to statements 1 and 2, you are in the action stage. If you answered yes to statement 2 and no to statement 1, you are in the action stage. A yes answer to statement 1 means you are in the maintenance or, possibly, the termination stage.

Sources: Adapted from Changing for Good: The Revolutionary Program That Exhibits Six Stages of Change and Shows You How to Free Yourself from Bad Habits, *by J.O. Prochaska, J.C. Norcross, and C.C. DiClemente, 1994, New York: William Morrow; U.S. Department of Health and Human Services (www.hhs.gov/news/2002pres/prevent.html; retrieved March 8, 2008).*

time cutting out energy drinks (action). Although you feel fuzzier and less focused at first, and you have a pounding headache for a day, you are able to get to sleep more easily and start making it to class. You ace some of the quizzes, so you know your grade will be going up. You also notice how much better you feel, and how much sharper your mind is, when you get enough sleep.

A few weeks later, you're at a friend's house and she offers you regular coffee. Your sleep problems seem to be over, so you drink it. You lie awake till 3 a.m. that night and have to force yourself out of bed in the morning. Though not a full-blown relapse, this slip reminds you of why

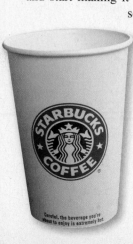

you wanted to make this behavior change. It's not as hard to get back on track, skipping the caffeine, as it was to give it up in the first place. You are on your way to the maintenance stage.

Have you ever had an experience like this one? If so, were you able to make the necessary connections and stick with the behavior change you made? Our lives are full of these "teachable moments" if we are ready to recognize them.

CREATING A BEHAVIOR CHANGE PLAN

Research has given us a great deal of information about how behavior change occurs. How can you use this information to change your own behavior? The first step is accepting responsibility for your health and making a commitment to change. Ask yourself these questions:

- *Is there a health behavior I would like to change?* It could be smoking, overeating, procrastinating, not getting enough exercise, or a host of other behaviors.

- *Why do I want to change this behavior?* There can be many reasons and motivations, but it's best if you want to change for yourself.

- *What barriers am I likely to encounter?* Having a plan to deal with barriers will increase your chances of success.

- *Am I ready to change the behavior?* Beginning a behavior change plan when you haven't fully committed to it will likely result in relapse.

Although making an initial commitment is an important step, it isn't enough to carry you through the process of change. For enduring change, you need a systematic behavior change plan. Once you have identified a behavior you would like to change, assessed your readiness to change, and made a commitment to change, follow these seven steps:

1. Set goals that are specific, measurable, attainable, realistic, and timely (SMART goals). An example of a SMART goal might be "I will increase my consumption of vegetables, especially dark green and orange vegetables, to 3 cups per day over the next four weeks, reaching my goal by October 30."

2. Develop action steps for attaining goals within a set time frame. For example, "I will include baby carrots in my lunch starting October 1."

3. Identify benefits associated with the behavior change. For example, "Eating more vegetables will help me lose weight, improve my complexion, and be healthier overall."

4. Identify positive enablers (skills, physical and emotional capabilities, resources) that will help you overcome barriers. An important capability is a sense of self-efficacy. Another capability might be the confidence that comes from having succeeded at behavior change in the past, along with skills that were used at that time. For example, "I was able to cut out caffeine last semester. I think I'll be able to improve my diet now."

5. Sign a behavior change contract to put your commitment in writing. Ask a friend or family member to witness your contract to increase your commitment. Signing a behavior change contract is one of the most effective strategies for change. An example of a behavior change contract is provided in the Personal Health Portfolio activity for Chapter 1 at the end of the book.

6. Create benchmarks to recognize and reward interim goals. Particularly when a goal is long term, it is useful to have rewards for short-term goals reached along the way. Reward yourself with something that particularly appeals to you (for example, buying a new iPhone app, going to a movie).

7. Assess your accomplishment of goals and, if necessary, revise the plan.

Many lifestyle behaviors are established early in life and have significant pleasurable aspects. Positive changes can and usually do entail losses as well, and an effective behavior change plan identifies and acknowledges both the pros and the cons of change.

Although behavior change theories offer valuable insights into the change process, they also have limitations. The major limitation of the behavior change approach is that it does not take into account health factors beyond the control of the individual,[12] primarily the kinds of social environmental factors described earlier in the chapter.

Health Challenges in a Changing Society

One of the key challenges we face in our social environment today is the glut of health-related information that inundates our daily lives, whether on TV, the Internet, or other media.

Some of this information is confusing, some is contradictory, and some is even misleading. To make good choices, you need skills that allow you to access accurate health information, to understand the evidence underlying health recommendations, and to critically evaluate important health issues in society. How do you meet the challenge of sorting through information and issues?

BEING AN INFORMED CONSUMER

Part of taking responsibility for your health is learning how to evaluate health information, sorting the reputable and credible from the disreputable and unsubstantiated—in other words, becoming an informed consumer.

Developing Health Literacy Do you read and understand the labels on foods you buy? Do you know which clinics are covered by your health insurance plan? If you learn that your dad is taking Lipitor, do you know how to find out more about it and its associated risks? These are all questions that relate to **health literacy**—the ability to read, understand, and act on health information. Health literacy includes the ability to critically evaluate health information, to understand medical instructions and directions, and to navigate the health care system. Only 12 percent of American adults are reported to have proficient health literacy skills.[13] Without these skills, people are at risk for poor health outcomes, especially as they receive more conflicting health information from a variety of sources such as Web sites and television.

A particularly perplexing concept for many consumers is **health risk**, defined as the probability of an exposure to a hazard that can result in negative consequences. Many factors contribute to an individual's health risk for a particular condition, including age, gender, family history, income, education, geographical location, and other factors that make the person unique.

Just like other skills, health literacy can be developed, and a goal throughout this book is to help you improve your health literacy. In each chapter, you will be introduced to basic health and medical

health literacy
The ability to read, understand, and act on health information.

health risk
Probability of an exposure to a hazard that can result in negative consequences.

■ Health literacy includes the ability to critically analyze health messages and distinguish credible from outlandish claims.

Consumer Clipboard

Evaluating Health Information in the Media and on the Internet

Although the media, as well as many Web sites, provide accurate health information, others contain incorrect or misleading information.

Asking yourself the following questions can help you deconstruct and evaluate health messages.

1. Who created the message?

    It can often be difficult to tell when a message is providing unbiased information and when it is selling a product. Every message has been constructed by someone, and knowing who created it can sometimes help you know if there is a hidden agenda. If you can't tell who produced the message, then you can't know the potential agenda behind the message. Reliable sources provide information about their authors and sponsors. Look for an "About Us" page on Web sites, and notice if advertisements are clearly labeled. Government organizations, educational institutions, and nonprofits tend to be sources of reliable health information.

2. What creative techniques are used to catch your attention?

    Visual imagery, creative language, and pop-up ads are frequently used to make you pay attention. If you can identify the techniques being used, you may be able to see how the designer is trying to influence you. The next time you are on a Web site or see an ad for a medicine on TV, consider the visual imagery. How is it drawing you in or influencing your thoughts and emotions?

3. What values, lifestyles, or points of view are represented in the message?

    Looking for clues about embedded (or omitted) values can help you see the purpose of the message and who it is addressed to. It may help to ask yourself how different people might view the message differently. How are the creators of the message trying to influence and appeal to you?

4. Is the information current? When was it produced?

    Information about health and medicine is always changing. Look for the date when a Web site was last updated or when information was produced. Use sources of information that are current and frequently updated.

5. What evidence is cited?

    Reliable information is based on scientific research, not opinion. Be cautious if the "evidence" consists of personal stories or testimonials, and be wary about "miracle cures." A healthy dose of skepticism is helpful when accessing health information.

Sources: "Health Literacy," National Network of Libraries of Medicine, retrieved from www.nnlm.gov/outreach/consumer/hlthlit.html; Literacy for the 21st Century (2nd ed.), 2008, Center for Media Literacy, retrieved from www.medialit.org.

language, given Internet resources where accurate information can be found, and asked to apply your critical thinking skills to health issues. For some general guidelines related to health literacy, see the box "Evaluating Health Information in the Media and on the Internet."

Understanding Medical Research Studies   Scientists use different types of research studies to explore and confirm relationships between risk factors and disease. Some types of studies—for example, *correlational studies*—suggest likely associations but do not establish cause-and-effect relationships. Other types of studies—*clinical* or *experimental studies*—are considered to establish cause-and-effect relationships. In clinical studies, researchers randomly assign matched participants to either a treatment group or a control group, apply a treatment to the first group and a *placebo* (a look-alike but ineffective treatment, such as a sugar pill) to the second, and after a period of time (usually a year or more) determine whether the treatment group has experienced

hot tip
The next time you see a shocking health headline, find out who funded the research.

a significant effect from the treatment in comparison with the control group. To be considered reliable, the same results must be obtained by other researchers replicating the study. Although they are considered to establish cause-and-effect relationships, clinical studies are often costly and time-consuming.

When you read or hear about the results of a new research study in the news, ask yourself several questions about it:

- Was it a clinical study? These studies often test one treatment against another.

- If it was a clinical study, were participants randomly assigned to groups? If not, something other than the treatment may have had an influence on the results.

- Were large enough numbers of participants used to ensure that results weren't skewed? Random change can affect results. This is less likely with large numbers.

■ Was it a *double-blind study*—that is, was researcher bias minimized by making sure the scientists were unaware of which group was receiving the treatment and which was receiving the placebo?

■ Was the study sponsored by an impartial research institute or government agency, or were there sponsors who stood to benefit from the results?

■ Has the study been replicated by other researchers?

■ Was the study published in a reputable, peer-reviewed medical or health journal?

The answers to all these questions and more affect how much credence you can put in the research results.

Keep in mind that scientists typically consider individual studies stepping-stones in an ongoing search for answers to complex questions. Members of the lay public have a tendency to regard the results of a single study as conclusive and definitive, and many times, the media are guilty of creating or fostering this impression.[14]

FACING CURRENT HEALTH CONCERNS

What are the actual health concerns faced by Americans today? To some extent, the answer depends on who you are. If you are between the ages of 15 and 24, for example, the leading cause of death for your age group is unintentional injuries (accidents) (see Figure 1.5). If you are 60 or over, the leading causes of death for your age group are heart disease and cancer. Personal health concerns also vary by race and ethnicity (see the box "Variations in Leading Causes of Death Among Americans"). If we look at the overall leading causes of death for all ages, we see that the major health concerns are chronic diseases—heart disease, cancer, stroke, diabetes, chronic respiratory diseases—and the lifestyle behaviors that contribute to them. They are the focus of both individual behavior change plans and broad public health initiatives.

The Healthy People Initiative   The Healthy People Initiative is a collaborative effort among federal, state, and territorial governments and community partners (private and public) to set health objectives for the nation. The objectives are designed to identify the significant preventable threats to health and to establish goals for improving the quality of life for all Americans.[15] The U.S. government issued the first *Healthy People* report in 1980 and has issued revised reports every 10 years since.

The initiative's most recent version, *Healthy People 2020*, was developed in 2008–2010 and released to the public in 2010. *Healthy People 2020* envisions "a society in which all people live long, healthy lives" and sets the following broad national health objectives:[16]

■ Eliminate preventable disease, disability, injury, and premature death. This objective involves activities such as taking more concrete steps to prevent diseases and injuries among individuals and groups, promoting healthy lifestyle choices, improving the nation's preparedness for emergencies, and strengthening the public health infrastructure.

■ Achieve health equity, eliminate disparities, and improve the health of all groups. This objective involves identifying, measuring, and addressing health differences between individuals or groups that result from a social or economic disadvantage.

■ Create social and physical environments that promote good health for all. This objective involves the use of health interventions at many different levels (such as anti-smoking campaigns by schools, workplaces, and local agencies), improving the situation of undereducated and poor Americans by providing a broader array of educational and job opportunities, and actively developing healthier living and natural environments for everyone.

■ Promote healthy development and healthy behaviors across every stage of life. This objective involves taking a cradle-to-grave approach to health promotion by encouraging disease prevention and healthy behaviors in Americans of all ages.

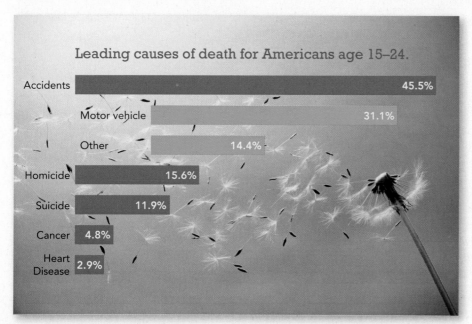

Leading causes of death for Americans age 15–24.

Accidents	45.5%
Motor vehicle	31.1%
Other	14.4%
Homicide	15.6%
Suicide	11.9%
Cancer	4.8%
Heart Disease	2.9%

figure **1.5**   **Leading causes of death for Americans age 15–24.**

Source: "Deaths: Preliminary Data for 2007," by the National Center for Health Statistics, 2009, National Vital Statistics Report 58(1).

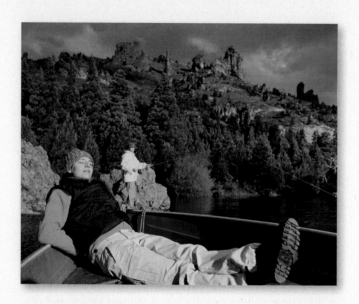

In a shift from the previous versions, *Healthy People 2020* places increased emphasis on "health determinants"—factors that affect the health of individuals, demographic groups, or entire populations. The report defines health determinants as social (including factors such as ethnicity, education level, and economic status) and environmental (including natural and human-made environments), and it emphasizes the importance of reducing the negative impact of certain health determinants on individuals and populations.

The Healthy People Initiative further identifies the nation's "leading health indicators"—a set of priority public

■ One of the goals of *Healthy People 2020* is to increase the number of rivers, lakes, and estuaries that can be used for recreational purposes.

Who's at Risk?

Variations in Leading Causes of Death Among Americans

The leading causes of death for Americans overall are heart disease, cancer, and stroke, but the top 10 causes of death vary somewhat across racial/ethnic groups. For example, HIV is the 11th leading cause of death for all groups except Blacks. Suicide is more prevalent among Whites and Asians than in other groups. Other variations can be seen in the following table. For the most part, variations in leading causes of death are a reflection of differences in social, economic, and cultural factors.

Ten Leading Causes of Death, 2006, by Race and Hispanic Origin

Rank	All	White	Black/African American	American Indian/ Alaska Native	Asian/Pacific Islander	Hispanic/Latino
1	Heart disease	Heart disease	Heart disease	Heart disease	Heart disease	Heart disease
2	Cancer	Cancer	Cancer	Cancer	Cancer	Cancer
3	Stroke	Chronic lower respiratory disease	Stroke	Unintentional injury	Stroke	Stroke
4	Chronic lower respiratory disease	Stroke	Diabetes mellitus	Diabetes mellitus	Unintentional injury	Unintentional injury
5	Unintentional injury	Unintentional injury	Unintentional injury	Stroke	Diabetes mellitus	Diabetes mellitus
6	Diabetes mellitus	Diabetes mellitus	Chronic lower respiratory disease	Chronic lower respiratory disease	Influenza/ pneumonia	Chronic lower respiratory disease
7	Influenza/ pneumonia	Influenza/ pneumonia	Homicide	Chronic liver disease/cirrhosis	Chronic lower respiratory disease	Influenza/ pneumonia
8	Suicide	Suicide	Influenza/ pneumonia	Influenza/ pneumonia	Suicide	Chronic liver disease/cirrhosis
9	Chronic liver disease/cirrhosis	Chronic liver disease/cirrhosis	HIV	Suicide	Chronic liver disease/cirrhosis	Homicide
10	Homicide	Homicide	Chronic liver disease/cirrhosis	Homicide	Homicide	Suicide

Source: Health, United States, 2009, *by National Center for Health Statistics, 2010, Hyattsville, MD: National Center for Health Statistics.*

health issues that can be targeted and measured. In *Healthy People 2020*, the initiative reported the leading health indicators as follows:

- Physical activity
- Overweight and obesity
- Tobacco use
- Substance abuse
- Responsible sexual behavior
- Mental health
- Injury and violence
- Environmental quality
- Immunization
- Access to health care

The indicators are intended to motivate individuals and communities to action by helping to determine where action is necessary.

Individual Choice Versus Societal Responsibility The ecological model of health shows us that individual lifestyle choices are embedded in layers of social/environmental determinants. When we consider these interrelationships, some interesting questions arise. If behavior choices like smoking, inactivity, and poor diet contribute to the incidence of heart disease, cancer, diabetes, and other chronic conditions, and if it is in the interest of society at large to reduce the incidence of these diseases, what are the rights and responsibilities of individuals? If you have a fundamental right to freely choose how you live, do you have a responsibility to make wise choices? If you make poor choices, are your resulting health conditions your own responsibility? Should you be held responsible for the costs to society, medical or otherwise?

Conversely, what are the responsibilities of society to protect you and others from poor choices? When should society take action to prevent you from participating in risky behaviors? When are restrictions on your rights justified for the benefit of your community?

Your life is influenced daily by policies related to these questions. Consider, for example, seat belt and helmet laws, speed limits, taxes on tobacco and alcohol, gun control laws, liquor licenses, urban development requirements for parks and green space, and health insurance premiums geared to health habits like smoking. Each of these regulations, policies, and rules is designed either to nudge individuals into making what society considers to be better choices or to reduce the societal costs of their "poor" choices. When you are analyzing a proposed restriction or regulation, consider these questions: How great a risk does a certain behavior pose for an individual and for the community? How strongly do individuals oppose restrictions on their ability to participate in the behavior? How much evidence is there that imposing a restriction will impact the behavior?

Access to Health Care A specific challenge facing our society is the crisis in health care related to costs. In 2008, an estimated 47 million Americans (20 percent of the population under age 65) were without health insurance.[17] Another 25 million Americans were underinsured, meaning that they had insurance but their policies did not cover all their expenses and/or the amount they had to pay exceeded their ability to pay.[18] Most Americans are insured through an employer, with public programs covering some people with low incomes (Medicaid) and those over the age of 65 (Medicare).

Reasons people give for being without health insurance include the high cost of coverage, loss of a job or change in employment, having an employer who does not provide coverage, and refusal of coverage by insurance companies.[19] Without insurance, people are less likely to receive health care in a timely fashion; they do not receive preventative services; and they delay seeking care until they are so sick that they have to use emergency services.[20] For these reasons, as many as 45,000 Americans die each year because they lack health insurance.[21] Even with health insurance, the costs related to care can be significant. Nearly 62 percent of all bankruptcies filed in 2007 were linked to medical expenses,

If you have a fundamental right to freely choose how you live, do you have a responsibility to make wise choices?
If not, should you be held responsible for the costs to society?

and nearly 80 percent of those filing for bankruptcy had health insurance.[22]

The health care industry already accounts for one-fifth of the U.S. economy, and the amount spent on health care is increasing faster than the rate of inflation,[23] a course considered unsustainable. The personal and societal impact of the current health care crisis is enormous, both in terms of cost and in terms of health implications. The issue is relevant even to those with adequate coverage, because costs for the uninsured are shifted to those who can pay, primarily through taxes.

Currently, health care in the United States is rationed based on ability to pay, with the uninsured and underinsured receiving poorer or less timely care than those with adequate insurance. As a society we have to ask, Do we believe health care should be accessible to all, regardless of ability to pay? If so, how will we design a system that allows equitable access and yet keeps health care affordable?

LOOKING AHEAD

Clearly we have many challenges on both the personal and the community/societal level. Throughout this book, we will ask you to consider your personal health and health choices within the context of your environment. As you read each chapter, reflect on your current level of health in that

area. Is there a behavior you would like to change? First, assess your readiness to change; then develop a behavior change plan based on the guidelines in this chapter and throughout the rest of the book.

At the same time, think about the influences that shape your decisions. What factors impact your options, whether restricting your choices or supporting them? Consider your family and friends, your classmates and peers, your school and instructors, the community you live in, government policies, and the prevailing socioeconomic and political climate. What do you have to take into account to be successful at behavior change? To help you think more deeply about these issues, we have provided a Personal Health Portfolio section at the end of the book. It includes assessments and critical thinking activities for every chapter.

Even if you decide not to make a personal change right now, perhaps you can share health information with a family member or encourage a friend to change a worrisome habit. Maybe you can do something to make a difference in your community, such as participating in a community garden or a recycling drive. Or maybe you will become involved in the health care debate or in activities aimed at improving quality of life for underserved segments of the population. The ecological model of health is not just about how your environment influences you—it's also about how your efforts shape your environment.

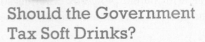

You Make the Call

Should the Government Tax Soft Drinks?

"Lifestyle taxes" are taxes imposed on products that are deemed unhealthy, such as alcohol and tobacco. Such taxes have two functions—they raise revenue for governments and they are believed to discourage people from buying the unhealthy products, thus contributing to lower health care costs and a healthier nation overall. Recently, the U.S. Senate and several states have been considering taxes on soda and other beverages sweetened with sugar, high fructose corn syrup, and other caloric sweeteners. The purpose would be to combat obesity in Americans by reducing intake of these beverages and to raise money to help pay soaring health care costs.

The current "obesity epidemic" is a major health concern in the United States and, to an increasing extent, throughout the developed world. More than two-thirds of American adults and one-fifth of American children are overweight or obese. The prevalence of obesity in the United States increased by 37 percent between 1998 and 2006 and continues to rise. Excess

weight is a risk factor for numerous diseases and conditions, including Type-2 diabetes, heart disease, stroke, some cancers, sleep apnea, and many others. Medical costs associated with obesity are estimated to exceed $147 billion annually—more than 9 percent of U.S. health care costs—half of which are paid by the government through Medicaid and Medicare. The medical costs for an obese person are 42 percent higher than they are for a person of normal weight.

Although many factors are involved in weight gain, sugar-sweetened beverages are believed to play a major role. Some scientific studies have found that sugar in liquid form does little to produce feelings of satiety (fullness), so that people consume the calories in sweetened beverages and still eat the same amount of solid food. Between 1997 and 2002, consumption of soft drinks doubled across all age groups in the United States, paralleling the rise in obesity. American adults and children consume an average of 175 calories per day from sugar-sweetened drinks.

Proponents of a tax on sugar-sweetened beverages argue that it would reduce consumption of soft drinks, just as increases in taxes on tobacco have been shown to reduce the purchase of tobacco products.

A reduction of 175 calories per day per person would slow the obesity epidemic, resulting in a healthier population that would require less medical care and thus pose less of a burden on the health care system. The American Medical Association and the Center for Science in the Public Interest have both come out in favor of a soda tax. At the same time, revenue from the taxes could be used to help finance health promotion programs. A national tax of 1 cent per ounce of beverage would generate an estimated $14.9 billion in the first year alone, and state taxes could raise additional revenue.

Opponents of such a tax argue, first, that it would be regressive—that is, it would disproportionately impact people with lower incomes, who tend to consume more soft drinks. Proponents counter that poorer people have the highest rates of obesity-related illness and would benefit the most from improving their diets. They would also benefit if revenues from the taxes were put back into their community in the form of measures that promote childhood nutrition or address obesity. Opponents also argue that obesity has many causes and should be addressed through a wide range of actions. It makes no sense to single out the soft drink industry and not tax other products that also promote obesity (e.g., television and video games). At the same time, not everyone who drinks soda becomes obese, making taxation an inefficient way to address this problem. If weight reduction is the goal, there are more direct ways to address it than a poorly targeted tax. In addition, the American Beverage Association has partnered with Coca-Cola, Pepsi-Cola, and the Corn Refiners Association to oppose the tax, claiming that reduced consumption would hurt business and lead to a loss of jobs in the beverage manufacturing sector.

Finally, some opponents argue that the government is engaging in "social engineering" when it attempts to encourage or discourage certain behaviors through tax policy. These critics believe that the tax system should be used to raise revenue for necessary programs in a straightforward way, not to control individual behavior or achieve broader social goals. They point out that every party and organization has an agenda it would like the tax system to discourage or promote, ranging from gun control to gay marriage. They believe the solution is not an across-the-board tax on risky health choices but a health care system in which individuals who require more health care as a result of their behaviors bear the cost of their choices themselves.

In sum, proponents support a tax on sugary drinks as a way to curb obesity and raise much-needed revenue. Opponents argue that among other things such a tax is a misguided attempt to control people's lifestyle choices. What do you think?

PROS

- A tax on sugar-sweetened beverages would reduce calorie consumption, especially among people with lower incomes, leading to a decrease in obesity and obesity-related health problems. People could be expected to switch to healthier beverages like juice and water.

- Taxpayers and governments have the right to recoup some of the costs they bear when people without health insurance incur medical expenses, and lifestyle taxes are one way to do so.

- Tax revenue could be used to implement health promotion activities as well as to finance reform of the health care system.

- Lifestyle taxes have long been a common and accepted way of discouraging unwanted behaviors.

CONS

- The tax would unfairly impact people with lower incomes as well as people who are not obese. If the purpose is to reduce obesity, there are more efficient ways to target the problem.

- Reduced consumption of beverages would negatively impact an important industry and lead to job loss and unemployment.

- Policy makers are inappropriately trying to implement social change through the tax system. Individuals should have the freedom to make their own choices and should also bear responsibility for the consequences.

Sources: "The Public Health and Economic Benefits of Taxing Sugar-Sweetened Beverages," by K.D. Brownell, R. Farley, W.C. Willett, et al., 2009, The New England Journal of Medicine, 361(16):1599–1605; "New York State Tax on Soda Cheered by CSPI," Center for Science in the Public Interest, 2010, retrieved March 13, 2010, from http://www.cspinet.org/new/201001191.html; "Reduction in Consumption of Sugar-Sweetened Beverages Is Associated With Weight Loss: The PREMIER Trial," by L. Chen, L.J. Appel, C. Loria, et al., 2009, American Journal of Clinical Nutrition 89(5): 1299–1306; "Recommended Community Strategies and Measurements to Combat Obesity in the United States," by L.K. Khan, K. Sobush, D. Keener, et al., 2009, Morbidity and Mortality Weekly Report 58(RR-7), July 24.

IN REVIEW

How are health and wellness defined?

Health is defined by the World Health Organization as a state of complete physical, mental, social, and spiritual well-being, not just the absence of disease. *Wellness* is defined as the process of adopting patterns of behavior that lead to better health and greater life satisfaction, encompassing several dimensions: physical, emotional, intellectual, spiritual, interpersonal or social, environmental, and, in some models, occupational. Very often, people want to have good health as a means to achieving wellness, an optimum quality of life.

What factors influence a person's health?

Individual health-related behavior choices play a key role in health, but economic, social, cultural, and physical conditions—referred to as the social determinants of health—are also important, along with the person's individual genetic makeup. Community health and public health actions are needed to ensure the personal health of individuals.

What is health-related behavior change?

The process of changing a health behavior (for example, quitting smoking, changing your diet) has been conceptualized in the Stages of Change Model as unfolding over several "stages of change," from precontemplation to maintenance of new behavior.

What health-related trends are occurring in our society?

As the United States becomes more multiethnic and multicultural, concepts of health and wellness from other cultures are being integrated into Western health care. At the same time, advances in medicine and health care have not reached many minority groups in the United States. Eliminating health disparities among different segments of the population is one of the broad goals of the national health initiative *Healthy People 2020*.

What health challenges do we face?

Health challenges for individuals include learning to be more informed consumers of health information and making lifestyle decisions that enhance rather than endanger their health. Health challenges for society include finding a balance between the freedom of individuals to make their own choices and the responsibility of society to protect individuals from poor choices and to offer increasing access to affordable health care.

Web Resources

Centers for Disease Control and Prevention: The CDC provides a national focus for disease prevention and control as well as for health promotion and education. Its Web site features health and safety topics and offers authoritative information for use in making health decisions.
www.cdc.gov

National Health Information Center: A health information referral service, NHIC is designed to connect consumers and professionals who have health questions with the organizations best suited to answer them. Its database includes 1,400 organizations and government offices offering health information.
www.health.gov/nhic

National Institutes of Health: This Web site provides health information through its A–Z index, health hotlines, and databases. MEDLINEplus, a database associated with the National Library of Medicine, is a resource for finding and evaluating health information on the Web.
www.nih.gov

U.S. Department of Health and Human Services: This site offers a wide range of health information on topics such as diseases and conditions, safety and wellness, drug and food information, and disasters and emergencies. Its news section includes daily updates on statements and reports by the DHHS.
www.os.dhhs.gov

U.S. Food and Drug Administration: The FDA site provides information on the many products this government agency regulates, such as food, drugs, medical devices, biologics, and cosmetics. Its news section highlights hot topics in health.
www.fda.gov

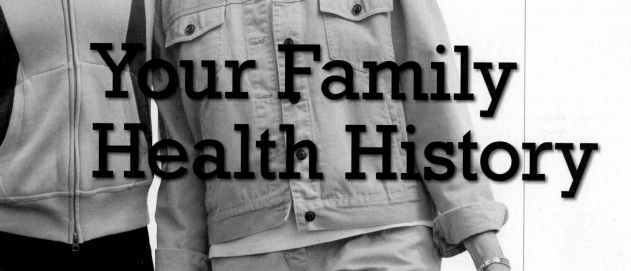

Your Family Health History

2

Ever Wonder...?

if alcoholism can run in families?

if heart disease could be genetic?

how much your parents' health predicts your own?

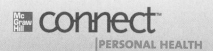

connect™ | PERSONAL HEALTH

http://www.mcgrawhillconnect.com/personalhealth

It is perhaps the biggest inheritance you will ever receive. It gives you the potential to be tall or short; apple- shaped or pear-shaped; brown-eyed or blue-eyed; blonde, brunette, or bald. This inheritance may give you the athletic potential to climb to the top of the Olympic podium, grace you with a talent for languages, or require you to use a wheelchair for mobility each day. It gives you a unique bundle of strengths, vulnerabilities, and physical characteristics. It is your genetic makeup.

People have long been curious about what contribution their genetic inheritance makes to their overall makeup as individual human beings and what contribution their upbringing makes—the classic "nature versus nurture" debate. Are people the way they are as a result of their genetic endowment or because of experiences they have had? The answer isn't black and white. Who we are as individuals is the result of a complex, ongoing interaction among

- Our genetic inheritance
- Our lifestyle choices
- Environmental factors of many kinds

This last category includes everything from our prenatal environment, to our family and community, to our ethnic or cultural group, to our society and the world at large.

What we can say definitively about genetic inheritance is that it plays a key role in establishing some of the outside parameters of what you can be and do in your life. You can think of genetic inheritance as your blueprint, or starting point. The blueprint is filled in and actualized over the course of your entire life.

Genetic inheritance is also the starting point for understanding your personal health. It is important for two reasons:

- If you know what special health risks you may have, such as a predisposition for heart disease, a particular type of cancer, or even alcoholism, you have the opportunity to make more informed lifestyle choices.

- If you know of any genetic disorders you may be at risk for and you plan to have children, you have more options for addressing the risks for future generations, especially as advancing technology improves our ability to prevent and treat genetic disorders.

This chapter will help you understand your genetic inheritance and use that knowledge to enhance your health.

Your Family Health History

You do not have to be a scientist to realize that traits can be passed from one generation to the next. As with the color of your skin, hair, and eyes, some health traits are passed from one generation to the next. Your grandmother's history of colon cancer may mean you have inherited an increased risk for colon cancer from her side of the family. Your uncle's heart attack at age 40 may mean you have received an increased risk of heart disease from his side of the family. How can you take this information and organize it in a useful way?

- While these Asian American students share similar physical characteristics, each has a unique genetic endowment that carries both limits and opportunities.

CREATING A FAMILY HEALTH TREE

A **family health tree**, also called a genogram or genetic pedigree, is a visual representation of your family's genetic history. Creating a health tree can help you see your family's patterns of health and illness and pinpoint any areas of special concern or risk for you.

family health tree
Diagram illustrating the patterns of health and illness within a family; also called a genogram or genetic pedigree.

To construct your family health tree, you need to assemble information concerning as many family members as you can. (A sample tree is shown in Figure 2.1.) The more detailed and extensive the tree, the easier it will be for you to see patterns. Basic information for each family member should include date of birth, major diseases, and age and cause of death for any deceased relatives. You might include additional data, such as the age of a family member when his or her disease was diagnosed, disabilities, major operations, allergies, reproductive problems, mental health disorders, or behavioral problems. In addition, you can think about lifestyle habits, community factors, and even public policies and the roles each may play. For example, consider the family described in Figure 2.1. Perhaps the grandfather's obesity played a role in his heart attack at age 50. Perhaps the uncle

would have survived the motor vehicle injury if seat belt laws had been in place in 1964. Your tree should include parents, siblings, grandparents, cousins, aunts, and uncles. The Personal Health Portfolio activity for this chapter at the end of this book provides detailed instructions on how to put together your own family health tree.

Gathering family health information to construct a tree may not be an easy process. Only one-third of Americans report that they have tried to gather and write down this information. In recognition of the importance of the task, the U.S. surgeon general has launched a national public health campaign called the U.S. Surgeon General's Family History Initiative. As part of the initiative, Thanksgiving Day has been declared National Family History Day. When families gather, they are encouraged to discuss and record health problems that seem to run in the family.[1] This may be easier for some people than for others. In some cultures, families do not like to discuss the dead. In other cultures, some diseases may be considered taboo, such as cancer, depression, or HIV. Such cultural views may influence the information you are able to collect. In addition, if you were adopted, you may not have the same access to your biological family's health history. Several organizations can aid in the search for such information; see the Web Resources at the end of this chapter for a start.

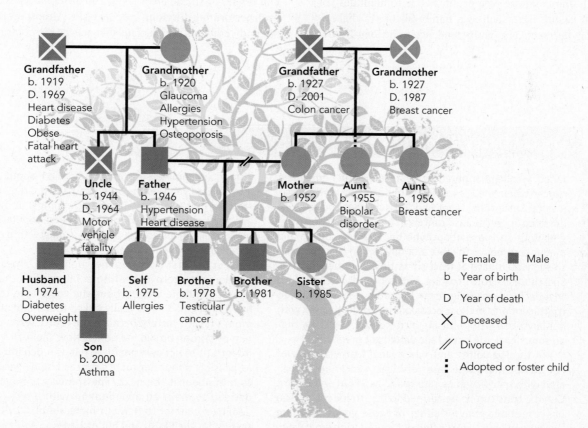

figure **2.1**   **A family health tree.**

WHAT CAN YOU LEARN FROM YOUR HEALTH TREE?

Certain patterns of illness or disease suggest that the illness is more likely to be genetically linked, as in the following instances:

- An early onset of disease is more likely to have a genetic component.

- The appearance of a disease in multiple individuals on the same side of the family is more likely to have a genetic correlation.

- A family member with multiple cancers represents a greater likelihood of a genetic association.

- The presence of disease in family members who have good health habits is more suggestive of a genetic cause than is disease in family members with poor health habits.

If you discover a pattern of illness or disease in your health tree, you may want to consult with your physician or a genetic counselor about its meaning and implications (see the box "Janet: A Family History of Breast Cancer"). You may want to implement lifestyle changes, have particular screening tests, or watch for early warning signs. Again, a pattern of illness does not automatically mean that you will be affected. The main use of a health tree is to highlight your personal health risks (such as a family history of diabetes) and strengths (such as a family tendency to be long-lived).

hot tip

The next time you're e-mailing your parents, ask them what diseases their parents and extended family have had. Save their response and take it to your next doctor's appointment.

You and Your Genes: The Basics of Heredity

In the 1850s, two defining events (and people) shaped the path of modern genetics. Charles Darwin, after years of studying plants and animals around the world, noticed that how something looks or acts changes randomly. He called this *random variation in traits*. He observed that certain traits are favored in particular environments and can be passed to future generations in a process he labeled *descent with modification*. During the same period but unknown to Darwin, Gregor Mendel proposed that traits are passed from parents to offspring as discrete units. He determined the patterns of inheritance by breeding generations of garden peas. Neither Darwin nor Mendel understood how the units were passed to future generations, but we now know that the units of heredity are **genes**. So what are genes and how do they work? Let's review some basic science.

gene
Sequence of DNA that encodes a protein or other functional product; the unit of heredity.

DNA AND GENES

Our bodies are made up of about 260 different types of cells, each performing different, specific tasks. Almost every cell in the body contains one nucleus that acts as the control center

---

Janet: A Family History of Breast Cancer

Janet, a college sophomore, lost her mother to breast cancer when she was 10 years old and her mother was just 34. Since then, Janet had felt sure that she too was destined to get breast cancer. In high school she struggled with decisions about whether to go to college and pursue a career or to start a family as early as she could so she would have at least some time with her children. She chose to go to college, but her ambivalence about that decision was reflected in her often risky approach to contraception. On those occasions when she had sex with her boyfriend without using birth control, she knew that on some level, she hoped she would get pregnant.

A turning point came when Janet learned in one of her classes that some cases of breast cancer are associated with specific genes, referred to as BRCA1 and BRCA2. Genetic tests can be performed to determine if a person has a mutated copy of either of these genes. Learning this empowered Janet to find out more. Using her college library and online sources, she learned about options available to high-risk people like herself. They included starting mammograms (breast screenings) at an earlier age than recommended for the general population, taking certain medications, and even mastectomy (breast removal) to prevent cancer.

For the first time since her mom died, Janet felt she had some control over her future. She couldn't change her genes, but there were actions she could take to reduce her risk. She had never really talked to her dad about her mom's health history because she didn't want to upset him by stirring up sad memories. Now she realized it was important to her own health to get as much information as possible about her mom's cancer. She decided to talk to him about it the next time she was home. She also decided to make an appointment with a genetic counselor to find out more about testing for the BRCA1 and BRCA2 genes.

connect ACTIVITY

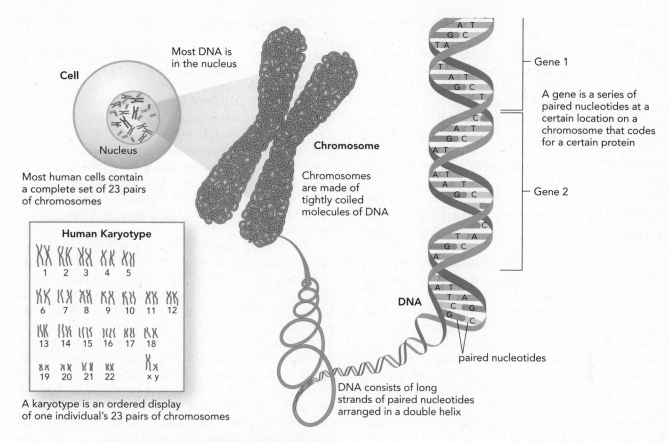

figure **2.2** **Chromosomes, genes, and DNA.**

(only red blood cells have no nucleus). Within the nucleus is an entire set of genetic instructions stored in the form of tightly coiled, threadlike molecules called **deoxyribonucleic acid**, or **DNA**. If we were to uncoil the DNA (and magnify it thousands of times), we would find it consists of two long strands arranged in a double helix—a kind of spiraling ladder (Figure 2.2). DNA has four building blocks, or bases, called adenine (A), guanine (G), cytosine (C), and thymine (T). The two strands of DNA are held together with bonds between the building blocks; an A on one strand always connects to a T on the opposite strand, and a G on one strand connects to a C on the opposite strand. The consistent pairing is important—each strand is an image of the other (Figure 2.2).

The complete set of DNA is called a person's **genome**. Within the nucleus, DNA is divided into 23 pairs of **chromosomes** (one set of each pair comes from each parent). One pair of chromosomes—the sex chromosomes—is slightly different and is labeled with an X or a Y rather than a number. Females have two X chromosomes; males have an X and a Y chromosome.

deoxyribonucleic acid (DNA)
Nucleic acid molecule that contains the encoded, heritable instructions for all of a cell's activities; DNA is the genetic material passed from one generation to the next.

genome
The total set of an organism's DNA.

chromosome
Gene-carrying structure found in the nucleus of a cell, composed of tightly wound molecules of DNA.

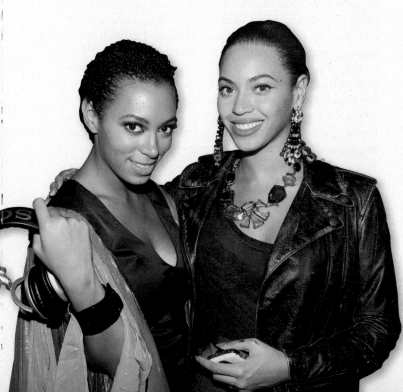

■ Family resemblance—like that between siblings Beyoncé and Solange Knowles—is just the most obvious indicator of all that family members share genetically.

DNA is the body's instruction book. The four bases are like a four-letter alphabet. Just as the letters in our 26-letter alphabet can be arranged to make thousands of words with different meanings, a series of thousands or millions of A-T-G-C combinations can be arranged to form a distinct message; this message is a gene. Each chromosome contains hundreds or thousands of genes located at precise points along the chromosome. Genes serve as a template and are transcribed into *RNA*, a temporary message that can travel out of the nucleus and is further translated into protein. Proteins, structures composed of amino acids arranged in a specific order, direct the activities of cells and functions of the body.

differentiation
The process by which an unspecialized cell divides and gives rise to a specialized cell.

stem cell
An undifferentiated cell that is capable of giving rise to different types of specialized cells.

mutation
Alteration in the DNA sequence of a gene.

Although our cells contain the same full set of genes, most of the cells in our body become specialized—that is, they take on characteristic shapes or functions, such as skin, bone, nerve, or muscle. Genes turn on or off to regulate this activity in a process called **differentiation**. Once a cell is differentiated, it can no longer become other cell types (it is as if certain "chapters" of the DNA instruction book are locked shut). Unspecialized cells, called **stem cells**, are present in an embryo (embryonic stem cells) and are retained within tissues (adult stem cells).

Scientists expected humans to have some 100,000 genes, given our complexity as an organism. However, they were surprised to discover that a human may have only 20,000 to 25,000 genes—the same number as a mouse.[3] Genes range in size from 2,000 to 2 million base-pairs. Another surprising finding was that only an approximate 2 percent of human DNA is used in protein-coding genes. The rest of the DNA used to be called "junk DNA." However, ongoing work of a related consortium suggests the story is more complicated. Genes may actually overlap one another and interact with genes on other chromosomes. The areas of DNA between genes, so-called junk DNA, are constantly being transcribed into RNA and contain signals and messages that are not well understood.[4]

The scientific implications of the HGP are vast, as are the potential applications in medicine and pharmaceuticals. There are also ethical, legal, and social implications of possessing such detailed genetic information about human beings. The HGP allows us to revisit age-old questions and assumptions, and it raises many new questions. For example, the HGP has allowed us to examine the relationship between race and genetics. Human genetic diversity occurs on a continuum with no clearly defined breaks between so-called racial groups. Thus the HGP has helped confirm that race has more to do with social and cultural interactions than a clear biological basis. Race categories are far too simple to describe the true genetic diversity of people.

Health disparities between racial groups have little to do with genetic differences *and more to do with culture, diet, socioeconomic status, health care access, education, and environment.*

THE HUMAN GENOME PROJECT

By the early 20th century, scientists had discovered chromosomes and genes and determined that DNA was the genetic material. In 1953 James Watson and Francis Crick discovered the shape and structure of DNA. By the 1980s DNA technology and knowledge had reached such an advanced state that scientists began to think about the possibility of sequencing and mapping the location of all genes on the 23 chromosomes in the human genome. *Genetic sequencing* is the process of determining the order of the DNA bases (A-T-G-C) in human DNA. *Genetic mapping* is the process of determining the position of genes in relation to one another and their location on the chromosomes.

In 1990 the Human Genome Project (HGP) was launched, organized as an international, collaborative research consortium of 20 groups in six countries: China, France, Germany, Great Britain, Japan, and the United States. In 2003 the consortium announced that the sequencing of the human genome was complete. The project determined that the human genome contains approximately 3.2 billion bases and identified the sequence of 99 percent of the bases.[2]

As discussed in Chapter 1, health disparities between racial groups have little to do with genetic differences and more to do with culture, diet, socioeconomic status, health care access, education, and environment. However, population genetics (the study of the genetic makeup of large groups of people) does show us that some traits occur more frequently in populations from similar geographical areas of the world. Thus, until we can more clearly identify ancestral origin, race may sometimes still serve as an imperfect surrogate. Other implications of genetic research are discussed in greater detail later in this chapter.

THE ROLE OF MUTATIONS

When you were conceived, you inherited one set of chromosomes from each of your parents and thus have two copies of each gene (excluding genes on the sex chromosome). The position of each gene is in a corresponding location on the same chromosome of every human. However, your two copies may be slightly different because every so often, changes occur in a gene; such a change is called a **mutation**. The change may involve a letter being left out (for example, a series A-T-G becomes A-G), an incorrect letter being inserted (for example, a series A-T-G becomes A-A-G), or an entire series of letters being left out, duplicated, or reversed. The location of the mutation determines the effect. If we go back to the analogy of the alphabet, consider what happens to the following sentence when a single letter change is made:

"When my brother came home, he lied."

If we change one letter to a "d," it can turn the sentence into nonsense:

"When my drother came home, he lied."

Or it can change the meaning entirely:

"When my brother came home, he died."

Something similar happens with a mutation in a gene. Many mutations are neither harmful nor beneficial (such as changes that lead to blue eyes or brown eyes). Other mutations may be harmful and cause disease. For example, in sickle cell disease (discussed later in the chapter), an adenine (A) is replaced by a thymine (T) in the gene for hemoglobin (a protein that carries oxygen in red blood cells). This single change at a crucial spot changes the gene's instructions and causes it to produce an altered form of hemoglobin that makes red blood cells stiff and misshapen.

While some mutations are harmful, other mutations can be beneficial or have no effect. The important thing about mutations is that they allow for human diversity. Alternative forms of the same gene are called **alleles**. You share 99.9 percent of the same DNA with your classmates. Slight differences in the remaining 0.1 percent account for all the genetic variation you see in appearance, functioning, and health.[3]

Most characteristics (like height or skin color) are determined by the interaction of multiple genes at multiple sites on different chromosomes. However, some traits are determined by a single gene. To understand the relationship between genes and appearance, let's consider a single-gene trait. An individual inherits two alleles for each gene (one copy from mom, one copy from dad). The two alleles can be the same version of the gene or they may be different versions. If they are different, one version may be dominant over the other. This version is then said to be the *dominant allele*, since it will be expressed and will determine appearance. The other version is said to be a *recessive allele*—it is hidden by the dominant allele and is not expressed. A recessive allele is expressed only if both copies of the gene are the recessive version.

As an example, let's consider earlobe appearance. A single gene appears to determine whether earlobes are attached or detached. We all have two copies of the "earlobe" gene. Let's call the two gene versions the "detached allele" and the "attached allele." The detached allele is dominant, meaning a single copy will make the earlobes appear detached (remember, if a dominant allele is present, it determines appearance). The attached allele is recessive, meaning two copies are required for the earlobes to appear attached. Think about your parents and siblings; can you figure out which alleles you have?

This is an example of the simplest relationship between alleles. There are other possible relationships. Some alleles have incomplete dominance or codominance, meaning that both alleles affect appearance in varying degrees. Many traits have more than two alleles. Most traits involve the interaction of multiple genes, each with multiple alleles.

allele
Alternate form of a gene.

single-gene disorder
Disease caused by a mutation within one gene.

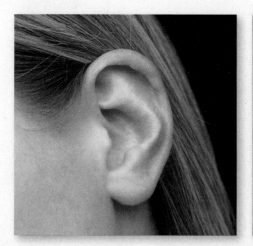 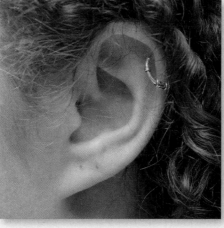

■ Earlobe appearance is an example of a trait determined by a single gene, with detached earlobes (left) dominant and attached earlobes (right) recessive. Most physical traits and conditions are determined by multiple genes interacting with each other and with environmental factors.

Genetic Inheritance

How does genetic inheritance play out in a person's life? In this section we consider some of the ways individuals are shaped by their genes—whether in terms of health conditions and disorders or simply in terms of who they are as individuals.

When genetic mutations occur, they can cause genetic disorders, as in the case of sickle cell disease. Genetic disorders are passed through families following certain rules or probabilities, so certain patterns in a family health tree can signal inherited disorders.

multifactorial disorder
Disease caused by the interaction of genetic and environmental factors.

chromosomal disorder
A disorder that is the result of altera-tion in an entire chromosome.

autosomal chromosome
Any of the chromo-somes (22 in humans) that do not contain genes that determine sex.

sex-linked chromosome
Chromosome that includes genes that determine sex.

carrier
A person who has one copy of an autosomal recessive mutation; this person shows no signs of the disease but may pass the disease on to his or her offspring.

A mutation in just one gene that causes a disease or disorder is called a **single-gene disorder**. Most disorders are caused by interactions among one or more genes and the environment; these are called **multifactorial disor-ders**. Many personal characteristics, predispositions, and behaviors are also the results of interactions among genes and multiple environmental factors. A third type of genetic disorder occurs as a result of alterations in entire chromo-somes; these are called **chromosomal disorders**.

SINGLE-GENE DISORDERS

As with the innocuous characteristic of earlobe appearance, some diseases are caused by the alteration of a single gene. Although each disease is rare, there are more than 6,000 single-gene diseases, and so, as a group, they affect a lot of people. They follow distinct patterns in family health trees depend-ing on whether they are dominant or recessive disorders and whether they are on the **autosomal chromosomes** (chromosomes 1–22) or the **sex-linked chromosome** (chromosome X or Y).

In an *autosomal dominant disor-der*, the gene is on one of the autosomal chromosomes and the disease allele is dominant, so only one copy of the disease allele is required for the disorder to be present. In a family health tree, males and females are affected equally, and the disease does not skip generations. People with an autosomal dominant disorder have a 50 per-cent chance of passing the condition on to their children. Hundreds of known autosomal dominant conditions exist (see the box "Sudden Death in Young Athletes").

In an *autosomal recessive disorder*, the gene is again on one of the autosomal chromosomes but the disease-causing allele is recessive, so two copies are required for a disease to be present. In a family health tree, again both males and females are affected equally, but the disease may skip generations. For a person to show signs of the disease, he or she must inherit two copies of the disease-causing allele. A person with one healthy allele and one abnormal allele will not have the disorder. This person is said to be a **carrier**, because he or she carries the abnormal gene but does not show signs of the disease. Each carrier has a 50 percent chance of passing the recessive allele on to his or her children. If two carriers have children, each child has a 25 percent chance of not receiving the disease-causing allele, a 50 percent chance of being a carrier, and a 25 percent chance of having the disease.

Sex-linked disorders follow slightly different patterns of inheritance. Most sex-linked disorders are caused by genes on the X chromosome. The Y chromosome is small and contains few genes and no known diseases. Therefore, sex-linked diseases are sometimes called *X-linked diseases*. Most are recessive. A female would need two copies of an abnormal allele for the disease to be expressed (females have two X chromosomes). If she has only one copy, she is

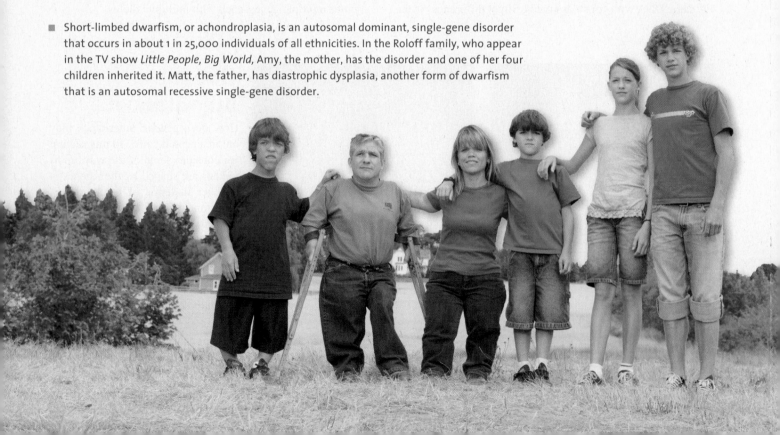

■ Short-limbed dwarfism, or achondroplasia, is an autosomal dominant, single-gene disorder that occurs in about 1 in 25,000 individuals of all ethnicities. In the Roloff family, who appear in the TV show *Little People, Big World*, Amy, the mother, has the disorder and one of her four children inherited it. Matt, the father, has diastrophic dysplasia, another form of dwarfism that is an autosomal recessive single-gene disorder.

Sudden Death in Young Athletes

The sudden death of a high school or college athlete receives extensive media attention. Collapse and death on the playing field is catastrophic and hard to understand. Exercise and athletics are supposed to be healthy, not life-threatening.

The most common cause of these deaths is a heart condition called *hypertrophic cardiomyopathy*—a thickening of the heart muscle that increases the risk for fatal arrhythmias (abnormal heartbeats). This rare condition is inherited, often in an autosomal dominant pattern, and has been linked to mutations in 1 of 12 genes.

Each summer or early fall, thousands of athletes across the country schedule their sports physicals so that they can be screened for this condition. Hypertrophic cardiomyopathy often appears during adolescence or early adulthood. Athletes are asked if they experience symptoms such as breathlessness during exercise, chest pain, fainting spells, or rapid heart rate, and the physician or health care provider listens for a certain type of heart murmur. The physician or health care provider also asks the most important screening question: Is there a family history of hypertrophic cardiomyopathy or the sudden death from an unexplained cause in an athlete's family member?

If an abnormality is suspected, it should be evaluated fully prior to the athlete's starting training or competition, as the risk of sudden death is greatest during or immediately after exercise. If an abnormality is confirmed, the athlete may be fitted with a device that can reduce the risk of death if an arrhythmia occurs. The athlete will also need to consider modifying the type of sports in which he or she participates.

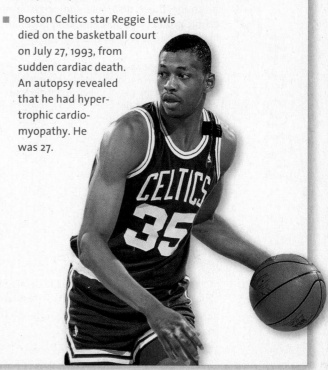

■ Boston Celtics star Reggie Lewis died on the basketball court on July 27, 1993, from sudden cardiac death. An autopsy revealed that he had hypertrophic cardiomyopathy. He was 27.

Sources: "Recommendations and Considerations Related to Preparticipation Screening for Cardiovascular Abnormalities in Competitive Athletes: 2007 Update. A Scientific Statement from the American Heart Association Council on Nutrition, Physical Activity, and Metabolism," by B.J. Maron, P.D. Thompson, M.J. Ackerman, et al., 2007, Circulation, 115, pp. 1643–1655.

---

a carrier. A male requires one copy of an abnormal allele to have the disease (males have one X and one Y chromosome). Thus X-linked diseases usually affect males.

Let's consider three single-gene disorders that occur with an increased frequency in certain populations. Because of the way different human groups have moved around the planet over the course of human evolution, often remaining isolated from other groups for hundreds of generations, some genetic patterns occur more frequently in particular groups or populations than in others (see the box "Ancestral Origin and Genetic Disorders"). Individuals from the same populations are more likely to have the same gene variants (alleles) than are individuals from other populations. If, when you consider your family tree, you find that your relatives come from particular geographical regions in the world, you may have an increased risk for certain gene disorders.

Sickle Cell Disease   If you have descended from people who lived in Africa, South or Central America (especially Panama), the Caribbean islands, Mediterranean countries (such as Turkey, Greece, and Italy), India, or Saudi Arabia, you may have an increased risk of carrying the gene for sickle cell disease. Sickle cell disease is caused by a mutation in a gene that codes for a component of hemoglobin, the protein in red blood cells that carries oxygen (see the box "Living With Sickle Cell Disease"). Because it is an autosomal recessive disorder, two copies of the gene are needed for a person to have the disease. About 1 in 400 African

Carrying a single copy of the sickle cell gene appears to offer an advantage *in areas where malaria has historically been a common cause of death.*

Who's at Risk?

Ancestral Origin and Genetic Disorders

Some genetic variants or alleles are more likely to occur in people who trace their ancestry to a particular geographical region. Although these disorders can occur in any ethnic group or population, they occur with increased frequency in these groups.

Population group	Genetic disorder
African, African American, South or Central American, Caribbean Islander, Mediterranean, Indian, and Saudi Arabian	Sickle cell disease
Ashkenazi Jews (from eastern and central Europe), French Canadian, Louisiana Cajun, Pennsylvania Dutch, Irish American	Tay-Sachs disease
Chinese and Southeast Asian	Beta thalassemia (a form of anemia)
Ashkenazi Jews (from eastern and central Europe)	Breast cancer gene (BRCA)
Southeast Asian, African, African American, Native American	Lactose deficiency
Southeast Asian	Acetaldehyde dehydrogenase deficiency (causes facial flushing when alcohol is consumed)
Scandinavian	Alpha-antitrypsin deficiency (a deficiency of an enzyme in the liver)
European Caucasians	Cystic fibrosis
Irish, northern European, Turkish	Phenylketonuria (PKU)

Americans has sickle cell disease. About 1 in 12 African Americans is a carrier, meaning he or she has a single copy of the mutated gene and has a 50 percent chance of passing a copy on to his or her children.

You may wonder why certain populations have such a high incidence of the gene for sickle cell disease. Interestingly, carrying a single copy of the gene appears to offer an advantage in areas where malaria has historically been a common cause of death. If you contracted malaria and had one copy of the gene, you had a greater chance of surviving the illness.[5] This is an example of how the environment can shape our genetics!

Tay-Sachs Disease   If you have descended from people of Ashkenazi (eastern European) Jewish, French Canadian, Pennsylvania Dutch, Louisiana Cajun, or Irish American ancestry, you may have an increased risk for carrying a gene for Tay-Sachs disease, a fatal degenerative brain disorder. Like sickle cell disease, it is an autosomal recessive disease. Children born with Tay-Sachs disease seldom live more than a few years. The aforementioned populations who are at higher risk have between a 1 in 27 and 1 in 30 chance of carrying a single copy of the mutation. The widespread use of genetic testing has made it rare for infants in the United States, Canada, and Israel to be born with Tay-Sachs disease.[6,7]

Cystic Fibrosis   If you have descended from people of white European ancestry, you may have an increased risk for cystic fibrosis. In cystic fibrosis a mutated gene codes for a defective protein that causes the body to produce thick, sticky mucus that clogs the lungs, obstructs the pancreas, and interferes with digestion. The majority of people are diagnosed before the age of 3. In the past, individuals with cystic fibrosis seldom survived childhood due to infections but with advances in treatment, more are living to adulthood and even into their 50s and 60s.

Cystic fibrosis is another autosomal recessive disorder. Although cystic fibrosis occurs more frequently among Caucasians (1 out of every 3,200 live births), it can—like sickle cell disease, Tay-Sachs disease, and any other genetic disease—occur in people of any ancestry. For example, cystic fibrosis does occur among African Americans (1 out of every 15,000 live births) and among Asians (1 in 31,000 live births).[7,8]

MULTIFACTORIAL DISORDERS

Although single-gene conditions can be easier to see in a family health tree, many diseases and traits can result from interactions between many genes and the external environment. These *multifactorial disorders* include heart disease, cancer, diabetes, obesity, schizophrenia, and a broad range of other disorders. Because so many diseases with a genetic component are multifactorial, paying attention to the lifestyle and environmental factors that contribute to them is crucial. Figure 2.3 shows the relative contribution of genetic and environmental factors to some common diseases and incidents. Notice that there is no clear distinguishing line between environment and genetics because the precise roles of each are not always clear. For instance, a poisoning may seem to have purely environmental causes, but some children may be genetically more predisposed to take risks and thus more prone to eat or drink unknown substances.

When a single gene causes a disease, the disease can be found by genetic testing or by noticing its pattern of occurrence

Challenges & Choices

Living With Sickle Cell Disease

Nearly 70,000 Americans are living with sickle cell disease. Most cases are diagnosed at birth through newborn screening. The diagnosis is important, because good health care helps people with the disorder live longer, more productive lives.

In sickle cell disease, a mutated gene causes red blood cells to become sickle-shaped (C-shaped) rather than round. The misshapen cells clump together and don't move easily through blood vessels. Clumps of cells can block blood flow to various parts of the body, causing pain, infections, and damage to organs, including the eyes, lungs, kidneys, and liver. A painful episode of blockage is called a sickle cell crisis.

Sickle cells also have a shorter lifespan than normal red blood cells (about 16 days compared to up to 120 days). This can lead to anemia, which can cause the person to feel tired, short of breath, and weak. The person may require blood transfusions if the anemia is severe.

Each person with sickle cell disease will have a different experience. Some have a very mild disease with rare crises, while others have frequent, severe crises requiring hospitalization. Regular medical care is important to reduce pain, treat infections, provide vaccinations (for example, pneumonia and meningitis vaccines to reduce the risk of infections), and monitor for complications.

Individuals with sickle cell disease can make certain lifestyle choices that reduce the risk of problems:

- Eat a healthy diet and take a folic acid supplement to help make red blood cells
- Drink plenty of water throughout the day to stay hydrated
- Sleep regular hours and avoid stress
- Avoid extremes of hot and cold weather and high altitude
- Exercise regularly but avoid extreme exercise
- Report any signs of infection (such as a fever) immediately to your physician
- Get regular health checkups and keep vaccinations up-to-date

Sources: "What Is Sickle Cell Anemia?" National Heart, Lung, and Blood Institute, U.S. Department of Health and Human Services, National Institutes of Health, retrieved October 1, 2009, from www.nhlbi.nih.gov/health/dci/Diseases/Sca/SCA_WhatIs.html; "Sickle-Cell Anaemia," World Health Organization, 2006, retrieved October 1, 2009, from http://www.who.int/gb/ebwha/pdf_files/WHA59/A59_9-en.pdf.

in a family health tree. Multifactorial diseases are more difficult to decipher. To determine the relative contribution of genetic and environmental factors of a particular disease, researchers look at how often it occurs among family members of a person with that disease (by examining the family health tree) compared with how often it occurs in the general population. If a disease has a genetic link, it usually occurs more frequently among first-degree relatives (mother, father, brother, or sister) of a person with the illness than it does in the general population. These studies are called family or familial studies. Because family members often share environmental conditions as well as genes, familial studies don't necessarily provide clear-cut evidence that disorders are genetic.

More definitive findings come from twin studies. Because identical twins have the same set of genes, an illness with a significant genetic contribution should occur more frequently among them than among fraternal twins (who are only as closely genetically related as any siblings). With advancing genetic technology, the specific genes that play a role in multifactorial diseases are being identified.

Heart Disease   Many environmental factors increase the risk for heart disease, including smoking tobacco, having a sedentary lifestyle, and being overweight. In addition, multiple studies have shown that you have two to three times the risk of heart disease if you have a first-degree relative with

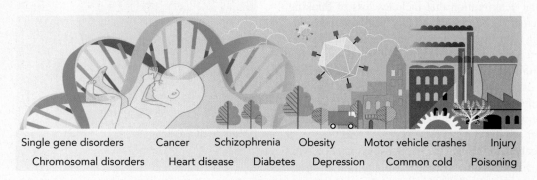

| Single gene disorders | Cancer | Schizophrenia | Obesity | Motor vehicle crashes | Injury |
| Chromosomal disorders | Heart disease | Diabetes | Depression | Common cold | Poisoning |

figure **2.3**   **Relative contribution of environment and genetics.**

heart disease. Genetics appears to play an even stronger role in heart disease when heart disease occurs at an early age (prior to age 50) than at older ages. For most forms of heart disease, there are probably several genes involved, with each contributing only 5 or 10 percent toward the disease. Genetic mutations may lead to unhealthy cholesterol levels, high blood pressure, or structural abnormalities of the heart. Researchers have begun to identify some of the specific genes involved, and it may be possible in the near future for individuals to receive genetic screening for these genes.[9,10]

Schizophrenia, Depression, and Bipolar Disorder   Many mental disorders are believed to have a genetic component. A family link has long been suspected for schizophrenia, a mental disorder characterized by delusions (distortions in thought, not being able to determine what is real), hallucinations, disorganized speech, emotional withdrawal, and bizarre behavior. Most people who develop schizophrenia show signs by their late teens to late 20s. The disorder affects about 1 percent of the population. If a person has a first-degree relative with the disorder, his or her risk is 8 to 10 percent. If a person has two parents with the disorder, his or her risk may be as high as 50 percent.[11]

An estimated 10 percent of people at some point in their lives experience major depression, which is characterized by fatigue, loss of energy, feelings of hopelessness and worthlessness, loss of interest and pleasure in daily activities, and thoughts of death or suicide. Women experience depression more often than men. The first-degree relatives of a person with depression have two to three times the risk of developing depression compared to the general population.[12]

Bipolar disorder, sometimes referred to as manic depression, is characterized by episodes of mania (euphoria, racing thoughts, excessive talkativeness, and inflated self-esteem) alternating with episodes of depression. The first-degree relatives of someone with bipolar disorder have nearly 10 times the rate of the illness experienced by the general population. Genetic research is beginning to identify some of the specific genes involved with each of these disorders. Interestingly, there appears to be a significant overlap in the genes associated with schizophrenia and bipolar disorder.[13]

Alzheimer's Disease   The most common form of dementia, Alzheimer's disease is a mental disorder marked by a gradual mental deterioration that includes loss of thinking skills and memory. The disease usually begins imperceptibly, often with a decline in alertness and interest in life, and progresses to confusion, disorientation, agitation, and a loss of contact with reality. Eventually individuals lose the ability to walk, talk, or eat. Alzheimer's disease affects less than 1 percent of the population under age 65, but risk increases progressively with age, such that it affects 24 to 33 percent of people over age 85.

A gene called APOE has the strongest association with the usual form of Alzheimer's disease. Mutations in this gene increase a person's risk of developing Alzheimer's disease two- to threefold. In a less common form called early-onset familial Alzheimer's disease, the individual exhibits symptoms of the disease before age 65. Three genes are associated with early-onset Alzheimer's; they are inherited in an autosomal dominant manner. The child of an individual with one of these genetic mutations would have a 50 percent chance of early-onset familial Alzheimer's disease.[14]

MULTIFACTORIAL INHERITANCE IN PERSONALITY AND BEHAVIOR

Genes appear to play a role in personality and everyday behavior too. Currently, researchers are studying how genetic makeup contributes to the individual differences we see among people.

Personality   Ever wonder why you like downhill bike racing while your friend is afraid to ride his bike even in designated bike lanes? Or perhaps why you like to stay home on the weekends while your friends like to go to big parties? Your personality—the sum of your mental, emotional, social, and physical characteristics—influences your behavior and responses to the environment. Among other things, personality influences what you seek out or avoid and how you communicate, react to others, express emotions, and respond to rewards. No personality type is more or less desirable than another; each contributes to the rich diversity of the human species.

Personality traits such as shyness, aggressiveness, sensation seeking, emotional reactivity, and a tendency to have an

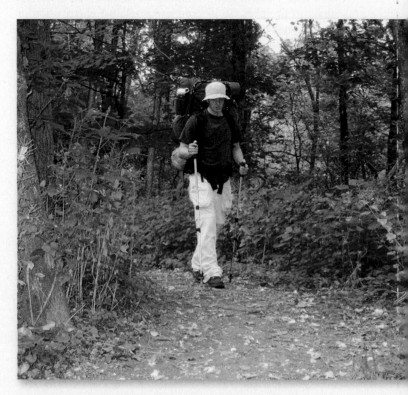

■ Personality traits that endure across a lifetime—such as shyness or introversion—may be genetically linked.

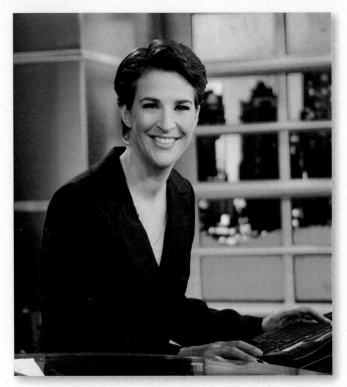

■ Sexual orientation appears to be at least partially genetic. Social and cultural factors can make it hard for people to realize they may be gay or to make their sexual orientation known to their friends and family. Television host and commentator Rachel Maddow came out as a lesbian when she was a freshman at Stanford University.

optimistic or pessimistic outlook, among others, are believed to have a genetic component. You may understand more about your own personality by exploring patterns within your family health tree.[15] Perhaps your family members tend to be novelty seekers, picking careers or hobbies that involve travel or risk taking. Or perhaps they are more reserved, choosing careers that keep them in a familiar environment. Inherited tendencies or traits are just the raw material of personality, though—environmental factors play a decisive role in shaping who we become.

Sexual Orientation   Sexual orientation appears to be another trait determined by a combination of genetic and environmental factors. Twin and family studies support a genetic component in attraction to same-sex or other-sex partners, and studies suggest genes on the X chromosome may play a role. However, to date the specific genes have not been isolated. Other biological factors appear to play a role, including birth order (with the number of older brothers increasing the likelihood of male homosexual orientation), prenatal factors, and brain development. Sexual orientation appears to exist on a continuum, ranging from heterosexuality (emotional and sexual attraction to people of the other sex), to bisexuality (attraction to people of both sexes), to homosexuality (attraction to people of the same sex). In

addition, factors influencing sexual orientation appear to be different for men and women.[16–18]

Addiction   Also known as *dependence*, addiction involves a physical or psychological need for a substance (or activity), usually with increasing amounts of the substance required to achieve the desired effect and unpleasant withdrawal symptoms occurring without it. Addiction to alcohol, tobacco, and other substances is widespread in the United States. An estimated 19.4 million adults meet the criteria for addiction to a substance such as alcohol or drugs (excluding tobacco). Addiction can also involve behaviors such as compulsive gambling, video-game playing, or binge eating. Although family and environmental factors play a role in addiction, studies suggest that genetics also plays a role. Genetics influences your likelihood of initially using a substance, your risk of continuing to use it, your risk of becoming addicted, and your risk of relapse after you quit.

Ironically, some of the best understood genes with a role in alcoholism are genes that protect against it. Several gene variations have been identified that affect the way alcohol is metabolized. These variations are found in higher frequencies among Asian and Southeast Asian populations. For people with these variations, even small amounts of alcohol cause an extremely unpleasant reaction known as flushing syndrome, which includes flushing of the skin, racing heart, nausea, and headache. These effects are a deterrent to alcohol use.

Gene variants have been identified that increase risk for both alcohol and nicotine addiction. A gene that increases risk for alcohol addiction may also play a role in nicotine or other addictions. In addition, a cluster of genes located on chromosome 15 appears to play a role in alcohol, nicotine, and cocaine addiction and increase risk for lung cancer. Such genes are often called *susceptibility genes;* they may increase an individual's risk of developing an addiction or disease, but environmental factors, including family dynamics, cultural background, availability of drugs and alcohol, socioeconomic status, and legal regulations, play a role as well. Thus, a family history of addiction increases your risk of addiction but does not inevitably lead you to addiction.[19,20] Most children of alcoholics, for example, do not become alcoholics themselves.

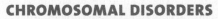

CHROMOSOMAL DISORDERS

In a chromosomal disorder, an entire chromosome may be added, lost, or altered. Many chromosomal disorders lead to fetal death or death in the first year of life. Because so much genetic information is involved, individuals with chromosomal abnormalities exhibit a broad set of symptoms, called a *syndrome*, ranging from characteristic physical traits to developmental delays to growth abnormalities. Three fairly common chromosomal disorders are Down syndrome, Turner syndrome, and Klinefelter syndrome.

In *Down syndrome*, the individual is born with an extra copy of chromosome 21. Down syndrome occurs in about 1 in every 800 live births. Risk increases with maternal age. Down syndrome is usually diagnosed during pregnancy or shortly after birth. Infants with Down syndrome have characteristic facial features and an increased risk for some heart and bowel conditions. Children with Down syndrome may take longer to learn to walk and talk and may have an increased risk for some health conditions, but the majority will live long lives, with over 80 percent reaching age 60 or older.[21]

In *Turner syndrome*, a female is born with only one copy of the X chromosome instead of the usual two. This occurs in approximately 1 of every 2,500 live births. Most females with Turner syndrome are shorter than expected (in comparison to their parents' heights) and many will not undergo puberty without taking estrogen, since their ovaries

do not function.[22] *Klinefelter syndrome* is a condition in which a male has an extra X chromosome (giving him two X chromosomes and one Y chromosome). It occurs in about 1 of every 500–1,000 live male births. Often Klinefelter syndrome is detected during the evaluation of a man for infertility. Frequently, the only signs a man may show with this disorder are lower testosterone levels and smaller testes than other men have.[23]

Diagnosing and Managing a Genetic Condition

People who have or are at risk for genetic disorders have many more options than they did in the past. The first step is genetic counseling.

GENETIC COUNSELING

The purpose of genetic counseling is to help individuals and families understand the role of genetics in a particular disorder, evaluate their risks, learn about the diagnostic tests available, and discuss treatment options. In the past, genetic counseling typically took place after a genetic disorder was diagnosed. Today, as technology improves and expands, genetic counseling is often offered before a disorder is diagnosed. (See the box "Should You See a Genetic Counselor?" for more information on this topic.)

Many people who see a genetic counselor and learn about their risks decide not to be tested, partly because of the potential consequences of such testing. In some cases, there is no treatment for a genetic disorder. In other cases, people are worried about privacy issues and how their genetic information may be used. Some of these issues are discussed later in this chapter.

GENETIC TESTING

Several different types of genetic testing are available, categorized as diagnostic tests, predictive tests, carrier tests, prenatal screening tests, and newborn screening tests.

Diagnostic Tests   If you show signs of an illness, a genetic test may help confirm or exclude the possibility of certain diseases. For example, if a 35-year-old man shows symptoms of dementia, a genetic test can be performed to confirm or exclude the presence of a gene mutation associated with early-onset familial Alzheimer's disease. In this situation, when the genetic test helps to confirm a diagnosis, it is called a diagnostic test.

Predictive Tests   If you are healthy but have a family history of a genetic disorder, a genetic test can be given to assess your risk for developing the disease in the future. Although a test may confirm the presence of a genetic mutation, it may not be able to predict when symptoms will appear or how severely affected you will be.

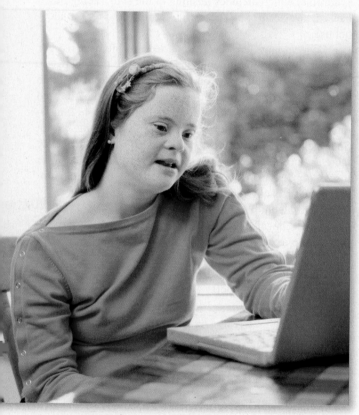

■ Down syndrome is an example of a disorder involving an entire chromosome, so many areas of functioning are affected. With improvements in treatment over the past 40 years, many individuals with Down syndrome lead satisfying and productive lives.

Should You See a Genetic Counselor?

Genetic counselors are a source of information and education about genetic disorders. They can also provide resources, reassurance, and support. A counselor can help you explore health patterns in your family and understand testing options and test results.

You may want to consider seeing a genetic counselor if

- You have a family history of a genetic condition
- Your family health tree shows a pattern suggesting a genetic condition
- You have been diagnosed with a genetic disorder
- You know or suspect you may be a carrier of a genetic disorder
- You and your partner are having trouble getting pregnant
- You or your partner have had several miscarriages
- Prenatal screening or a diagnostic test has revealed a fetal abnormality

The National Society of Genetic Counselors is a good place to start if you are trying to find a counselor. At their Web site, www.nsgc.org, you can search by zip code and the distance you are willing to travel. You can also search for the genetic specialty area you are interested in, such as infertility, cancer, or cardiac disease.

Carrier Tests   If a healthy individual has a genetic mutation for a disorder that is inherited in an autosomal recessive or X-linked recessive manner, the individual is said to be a carrier, as discussed earlier. If a genetic test is available to look for that recessive gene, it is called a carrier test. A carrier test may be offered to a healthy individual with a family member who has a certain genetic disorder or who has been identified as a carrier. Carrier tests are also offered to individuals in certain racial and ethnic groups that are known for having high carrier rates for disorders such as sickle cell disease, Tay-Sachs disease, and cystic fibrosis, as previously discussed.

Prenatal Screening Tests   As part of prepregnancy planning or during routine pregnancy care, women are assessed for their risk of genetic or chromosomal diseases. If either member of a couple has a family history of a genetic disease or belongs to a population with a high incidence of an autosomal recessive disease, the couple is counseled on the risks and benefits of genetic screening. Women are also routinely offered a blood test called a *triple screen* during the early part of pregnancy. This test cannot diagnose a genetic condition but can suggest an increased risk for a neural tube defect (problem with the spinal cord) or chromosomal abnormality. In the case of an abnormal result, the woman will be referred for an ultrasound and a test to assess fetal chromosomes (*amniocentesis or chorionic villus sampling*). As the risk for chromosomal abnormalities increases with age, pregnant women over age 35 are routinely offered testing to evaluate fetal chromosomes.

Although prenatal screening is commonplace today, the results can create a challenging situation for the prospective parents. For example, amniocentesis can tell them that their fetus has Down syndrome, but it cannot tell them how functional the child will be. Many children who have a genetic disease lead happy, productive lives with their own unique limitations and challenges. Genetic testing during pregnancy does, however, allow parents time to prepare for the upcoming birth.

Newborn Screening Tests   Newborn screening began in the 1960s with screening for phenylketonuria (PKU), an autosomal recessive disease. It became the model for newborn screening because it identified a condition at birth that could be treated when detected early. A child with PKU is unable to process an amino acid called phenylalanine, which is in many foods. If a child with PKU consumes too much phenylalanine, toxic chemicals build up that cause seizures and severe mental retardation. If the condition is detected at birth and the child is placed on a diet that restricts phenylalanine, the child can develop normally. At present, all states require newborn screening for PKU.

Newborn screening has expanded since the initial introduction of PKU screening. The American College of Medical Genetics has identified 29 core treatable conditions for which it recommends all newborns be screened, but there

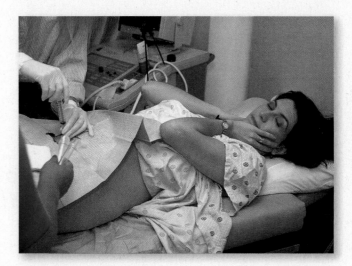

■ Amniocentesis is a prenatal screening procedure in which fluid is drawn from the amniotic sac to test for genetic disorders, birth defects, and other fetal health problems.

is no national mandate and states vary in what they offer or require. At present, the majority of babies born in the United States are screened at birth for between 29 and 54 conditions, most of which are genetic. Even though there is a parental educational component to newborn screening regulations, most parents report they are not aware of which tests their infant is receiving or of the full implications of test results.[24]

MANAGEMENT AND TREATMENT

Treatments are available for a number of genetic disorders. They include dietary modification, medications, environmental adaptations, and gene therapy.

Dietary Modification Some genetic disorders can be fully or partially treated through dietary modification, whether restriction, exclusion, or supplementation.

- *Restriction* is called for when a common food is toxic to a person with a genetic mutation, as in the case of phenylketonuria.
- *Exclusion* is required when a person has a life-threatening reaction to a particular food, as in certain food allergies. Some people are allergic to even minuscule amounts of shellfish or peanuts, and these foods have to be completely excluded from their diet.
- *Supplementation* is helpful for some genetic disorders. In cystic fibrosis, for example, the fat-soluble vitamins A, D, E, and K are poorly absorbed, so individuals with this disorder benefit from taking vitamin supplements.

Medications For some genetic disorders, drugs can decrease symptoms or prevent serious complications. For instance, people with hemophilia, who are missing a blood-clotting factor, can take a synthetic form of the factor. People at high risk of colon cancer due to hereditary colon polyps can take anti-inflammatory medicines to decrease the risk.

Environmental Adaptations Avoiding harmful environmental factors can be effective in managing many genetic and multifactorial disorders. People with albinism, for example, have an increased risk of skin cancer because they lack normal pigment in the skin, hair, and eyes; they have to avoid sun exposure more than others must. Individuals with a genetic predisposition for diabetes can lower their risk for the disorder by maintaining a healthy weight.

replace a defective gene that is responsible for a genetic disorder. The challenge is that cells are microscopic and DNA is even smaller. The miniscule section of DNA that makes up a healthy gene must be identified, collected, and then somehow inserted into the recipient's cell without destroying the cell. Once in the cell, the healthy gene must incorporate itself into the DNA of the recipient's defective cell in such a way as to function. At present, no gene therapy procedures have been approved for general use, but scientists optimistically envision a future in which single-gene and other genetic disorders can be cured by injections of healthy DNA.[25]

Implications of Genetic Research for Individuals and Society

Genetic research has conferred benefits on individuals, families, and society—but at the same time, it has raised troubling ethical issues (see "Disease Outbreaks and Genetics").

ISSUES IN GENETIC SCREENING AND TESTING

The understanding of genes and genetic disorders has far outpaced treatments and cures. Most people don't want to know they have a defective gene that might cause them harm if there is nothing they can do about it. Thus, in many instances, testing is not recommended even when a defective gene can be identified, as in the case of the gene for Alzheimer's disease. In such cases, genetic information may cause alarm and anxiety without, as yet, offering hope for a treatment or cure.

Further issues arise in the context of reproductive health and prenatal screening. Prenatal screening can identify a range of genetic conditions, but often the results can be confusing. First, the results may not be able to identify how severely a child will be affected by a condition. Second, parents may not understand the full range of diseases for which their child is being tested and they may not understand the implications of a test result. In addition, some voice concerns that identifying genetic conditions, whether life threatening or not, may put pressure on parents to terminate a pregnancy. Newborn screening also raises ethical questions. As more genes are identified that may play a role in health,

Most people don't want to know *they have a defective gene that might cause them harm if there is nothing they can do about it.*

Gene Therapy Although the treatments just described have helped people with genetic diseases to live better lives, they do not eliminate or cure the genetic disease. In 1990, the first clinical trials of gene therapy began. The goal of gene therapy is to insert a normal gene into a person's DNA to

how many and which ones should be included on newborn screens? Will newborn testing eventually expand to a state of universal DNA profiling? When should children be informed of genetic test results (for a condition that may affect them in later life)?[24,26]

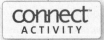

Public Health in Action

Disease Outbreaks and Genetics

- A girl in New York is admitted to the hospital with bloody diarrhea.
- An elderly man in Oregon visits his health clinic with diarrhea and dehydration.
- Three college students in Texas are evaluated at their student health center for fevers and diarrhea.

What do these people have in common? And what does it have to do with genetics?

It is possible that all of these people ate food contaminated with a disease-causing bacteria, such as *E. coli* O157:H7, *Shigella*, *Salmonella*, or *Listeria*. Each of these bacteria can cause bloody diarrhea, fever, and severe illness. In the past, when food was locally produced and eaten, it was easier to identify outbreaks of foodborne infections—everyone who was ill might have eaten at the same restaurant or church social. With current food production practices—foods being prepared and packaged in one location and then distributed widely across the United States or world—it is much more difficult. These individuals with diarrhea may have eaten the same brand of peanut butter or prepackaged salad mix. The physicians involved in their care may do a great job caring for each individual, but they would not be aware of the other cases and thus not be able to prevent more people from becoming infected.

How can we know if more cases of foodborne illness are part of a widespread outbreak? This is where genetics comes in. Bacteria have DNA and genes. As an example, let's consider *Shigella*. There are different *Shigella* strains, slightly different subtypes that arise due to genetic mutations. If each person was infected from the same source, we would expect their *Shigella* subtypes to look genetically very similar. If they were unrelated infections, the *Shigella* subtypes would be different.

In response to changing patterns of food distribution and with the increasing understanding of genetics, a program was initiated in the 1990s to aid in detecting foodborne disease outbreaks. PulseNet, a national network of laboratories and public health agencies, performs genetic testing of foodborne disease-causing bacteria. Using DNA technology, the laboratories will "fingerprint" the bacteria and send the information to a database at the Centers for Disease Control and Prevention. DNA patterns that come in from around the country are compared. If the number of submitted samples increases, and the samples have a similar DNA fingerprint, the bacteria may have come from the same source and an outbreak may be occurring. A computer alert activates health agencies so that they can evaluate cases for possible links. Ill people are interviewed to determine if they have eaten similar foods.

If a common food is identified, public health personnel can go to homes, collect samples of food, and test to see if bacteria with the same DNA profile are found. If they are, further illness can be prevented through recall of contaminated food and warnings issued to the general public not to eat that product. Inspectors can also backtrack to see where in the preparation and distribution process food was contaminated in order to prevent further disease outbreaks.

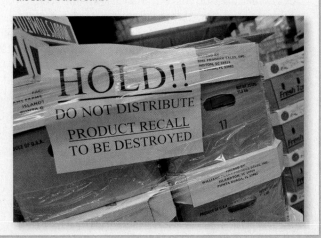

connect
ACTIVITY

ISSUES OF PRIVACY AND DISCRIMINATION

Another area of concern is the possibility of discrimination based on genetic information. Individuals who undergo genetic testing may find that they are not the only ones interested in detailed genetic information about themselves; employers and health insurance companies may also be interested in that information.

In the workplace, genetic testing has two potentially beneficial uses: It can be used to determine whether an employee is at increased risk for developing a disease if exposed to specific factors in the work environment, and it can be used to monitor a worker's genetic make-up for changes during his or her employment, thus helping to identify hazardous materials and increase worker safety. Neither

of these has been shown to be clearly useful.[27] The down side of genetic testing in the workplace is that employers may use the information to withhold promotions or refuse to hire a person—for example, someone who appears to be at risk for developing a disease or disability.

Genetic information is also of interest to insurance companies, who use information about risk for disease to help determine whom to cover and how much to charge for health insurance. There have been many cases in which people were denied health insurance because of genetic information. New health reform measures prohibiting insurers from excluding patients based on preexisting conditions may help protect individuals from losing insurance coverage.

Currently the Health Insurance Portability and Accountability Act (HIPAA), enacted in 1996, provides federal protection against genetic discrimination in health insurance. HIPAA prohibits group health plans from using past or current medical conditions, or genetic information, as a basis for denying or limiting an individual's coverage. It also states that genetic information in the absence of a current diagnosis may not be considered a preexisting condition. These protections apply only to employer-based and commercially issued group health insurance, however.

Genetic testing and genetic screening during pregnancy have paved the way for a potential new eugenics movement. When this technology is used by parents to reduce the risk of their child facing a debilitating disease, many (but not all) are comfortable. However, the technology could also be used to allow parents to select the traits they want in their child—high intelligence, athletic ability, physical appearance, and so on. Although this kind of eugenics may be different in the sense that parents are making decisions about their children's and family's future rather than having standards

> ## Eugenics was carried to an extreme by the Nazis during World War II, and it continues to occur in troubled places around the world under the guise of ethnic cleansing.

In response to gaps in HIPAA, the Genetic Information Nondiscrimination Act (GINA) was signed into law on May 21, 2008. GINA is a federal law that prohibits discrimination by health insurers and employers based on genetic information.[26]

EUGENICS

Yet another area of concern associated with genetic information is *eugenics*, the practice of selective breeding, or controlling a group's reproductive choices, in an attempt to improve the human species. A popular idea in the late 19th century, eugenics was carried to an extreme by the Nazis during World War II, and it continues to occur in troubled places around the world under the guise of ethnic cleansing.

imposed on them by a state, such practices may change how we as a society view qualities and flaws in appearance, personality, and the other varied dimensions of human difference. In some areas, the line between medical treatment and genetic enhancement may not always be clear.[24,26,28]

GENETICS, LIFESTYLE CHOICES, AND PERSONAL HEALTH

We conclude this chapter by reiterating the point we made at the outset: Genetics is simply the starting point of personal health. It determines potential but not outcome. Healthy genes do not guarantee a healthy life, nor does a genetic defect lead inevitably to a life of disability. Our genes are only one part of our overall wellness profile; other significant factors include individual lifestyle choices, socioeconomic factors, and sociocultural factors.

If you choose to explore your personal genetics, either by completing a family health tree or by having genetic tests done (for one of the reasons discussed in this chapter), keep in mind that this information is best used in helping you decide how to balance your health choices. Knowledge of your unique strengths and weaknesses, genetic and otherwise, can help you assess the risks and benefits of your actions and make the decisions that are right for you.

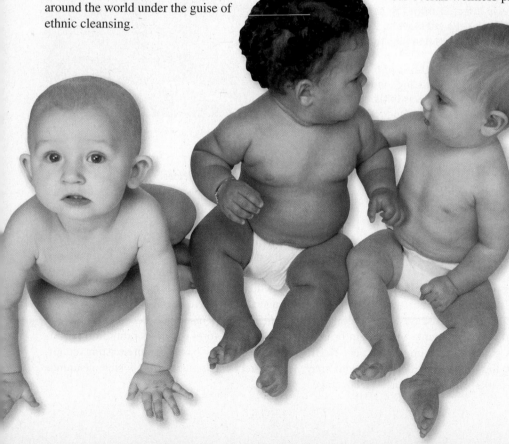

■ If parents were able to select the traits they want in their children, what would they select? How would it affect the human species as a whole?

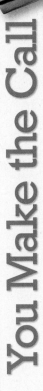

You Make the Call

Should Embryonic Stem Cell Research Be Supported?

Scientists believe that stem cells have the potential for a wide range of applications, including treatment of diabetes, many cancers, and genetic and neurological diseases like Parkinson's disease and Alzheimer's disease. However, the source of stem cells to be used in research is a subject of debate.

Stem cells, undifferentiated cells with the potential for unlimited division, can be derived from either embryonic or adult sources. Embryonic stem cells come from human embryos, usually supplied by fertility clinics. In the process of infertility treatment, fertilized eggs are allowed to develop in culture for 4–5 days to the blastocyst stage (a ball of 70–100 cells). It is common for extra blastocysts to be created and frozen until a couple decides to use them (by implantation into the uterus), donate them (for use by another infertile person), destroy them, or donate them for research purposes. If a person or couple elects to donate the embryo for research, cells from the blastocyst are allowed to grow, producing millions of embryonic stem cells—referred to as an *embryonic stem cell line*.

Adult stem cells are found in many tissues and organs in the adult body. They differ in several ways from embryonic stem cells:

- Embryonic stem cells can differentiate into all cell types in the body, but adult stem cells are generally limited to the cell types of their tissue of origin and thus are less versatile.

- Embryonic stem cells can be grown relatively easily in culture, creating millions of cells. Adult stem cells are rare, their isolation is difficult, and they are more difficult to culture in large numbers.

- Many scientists believe embryonic stem cells have greater potential than adult stem cells because of their greater versatility.

What is the controversy about? Opponents of embryonic stem cell research believe that it is unacceptable to destroy human embryos in pursuit of any goal, no matter how noble, and that adult stem cells are sufficient for use in research. President George W. Bush referred to embryonic stem cell research as "crossing a fundamental moral line" by sanctioning the destruction of human embryos that "have at least a potential for life." In 2001 the Bush administration restricted federal funding of stem cell research to adult stem cell lines and embryonic stem cell lines that existed prior to that date; however, President Barack Obama removed this restriction in 2009.

Supporters argue that while embryos represent the potential for human life, there are people already alive who are suffering from diseases and who could benefit from this research. They point out that according to most definitions, pregnancy begins when a blastocyst implants in the lining of the uterus, usually about a week after fertilization; until this point, the cluster of cells cannot really be considered potential human life. They also point out that adult stem cells do not have the vast potential of embryonic stem cells.

In addition, supporters contend that a nationally sanctioned embryonic stem cell research program keeps the United States on a par with other countries who are doing stem cell research. Allowing this research in the United States helps prevent other countries from luring away some of our most talented scientists. They argue that having a code of uniform regulations for embryonic stem cell research, as President Obama asked the National Institutes of Health to develop, will keep scientists within ethical bounds. Opponents continue to argue that embryonic stem cell research is inherently unethical. A May 2009 public opinion poll indicated that 57 percent of Americans support the use of embryonic stem cells in medical research, while 36 percent oppose it.

Embryonic stem cell research might hold out hope for millions, but opponents question the moral and ethical costs. What do you think?

PROS

- Embryonic stem cell research may eventually lead to therapies that could be used to treat diseases that afflict millions of people.

- Embryonic stem cells are derived from excess embryos created in the course of infertility treatment. Individuals must eventually decide the fate of their excess embryos, and many people are willing to donate them for research purposes.

- Adult stem cell research has resulted in therapeutic treatments. Scientists believe embryonic stem cells hold even greater promise.

CONS

- Embryonic stem cells are not needed for research; adult stem cells are sufficient.

- Embryos have a potential for life and it is unethical to destroy them.

- Scientists may purposely create new embryos solely for the purpose of stem cell research.

connect ACTIVITY

Sources: "Stem Cell Research," *Gallup, Inc., 2010, retrieved February 3, 2010, from http://www.gallup.com/poll/21676/stem-cell-research.aspx;* "Stem Cell Basics," *National Institutes of Health, 2006, retrieved February 14, 2008, from http://stemcells.nih.gov/info/basics;* "Obama Overturns Stem Cell Ban," Nature News, *March 9, 2009.*

IN REVIEW

Why is it important to know your family health history and understand your genetic inheritance?
There are two broad reasons: (1) to identify any areas where you may have an inherited predisposition for a health problem so that you have the opportunity to make informed lifestyle choices and (2) to know if your unborn children are at increased risk for any genetic disorders so that you have the opportunity to address issues associated with those disorders.

How do genes affect your health?
Although some diseases and disorders are caused by a single gene, most genetic disorders are multifactorial; that is, they are associated with interactions among several genes and interactions of genes with environmental factors, such as tobacco smoke, diet, and air pollution. Even if you have a genetic predisposition for a disease, you may never get that disease if the environmental factors are not present.

Why do some genetic disorders occur more frequently in certain ethnic or racial groups?
Because of the way different human populations have migrated around the globe over hundreds of generations, certain mutations and genetic patterns have become concentrated in certain groups. Often, a mutation that causes a disorder has persisted in the gene pool because it also provides some advantage in a particular environment.

What are the benefits and potential pitfalls of genetic research and its applications?
Some experts foresee a day when every individual will have a personalized genetic profile that will allow physicians to provide highly customized medical treatment and lifestyle recommendations, rather than broad public health recommendations. The main concern about this possibility is that genetic information may be used to discriminate against people in employment and insurance situations.

Web Resources

Access Excellence Resource Center: Associated with the U.S. Department of Health and Human Services, this national educational program provides health, biology, and life sciences information. It offers answers to questions such as the following: What are genes? What is genetic testing? How do gene mistakes occur? www.accessexcellence.org

Child Welfare Information Gateway: This is a good place to start if you are looking for information about your biological parents. www.childwelfare.gov

Gene Tests: This site offers authoritative information on genetic testing and its use in the diagnosis and management of disease and genetic counseling. Funded by the National Institutes of Health, it promotes the appropriate use of genetic services in patient care and personal decision making. www.genetests.org

Genetics Society of America: This organization includes more than 4,000 scientists and educators in the field of genetics. Through its journal *Genetics*, it publishes information on advances in genetics. www.genetics-gsa.org

Gene Watch UK: Featuring developments in genetic technologies from the perspective of public interest, environmental protection, and animal welfare, this group explores topics ranging from genetically modified crops and foods to genetic testing in humans. www.genewatch.org

National Human Genome Research Institute: The leader of the Human Genome Project for the National Institutes of Health, this institute continues to do research in genetics aimed at improving human health and fighting diseases. www.genome.gov

National Society of Genetic Counselors: This society offers FAQs about genetic counselors, such as: What is a genetic counselor? How do I find a genetic counselor near me? What can I expect on a first visit to a genetic counselor? www.nsgc.org

Mental Health and Stress

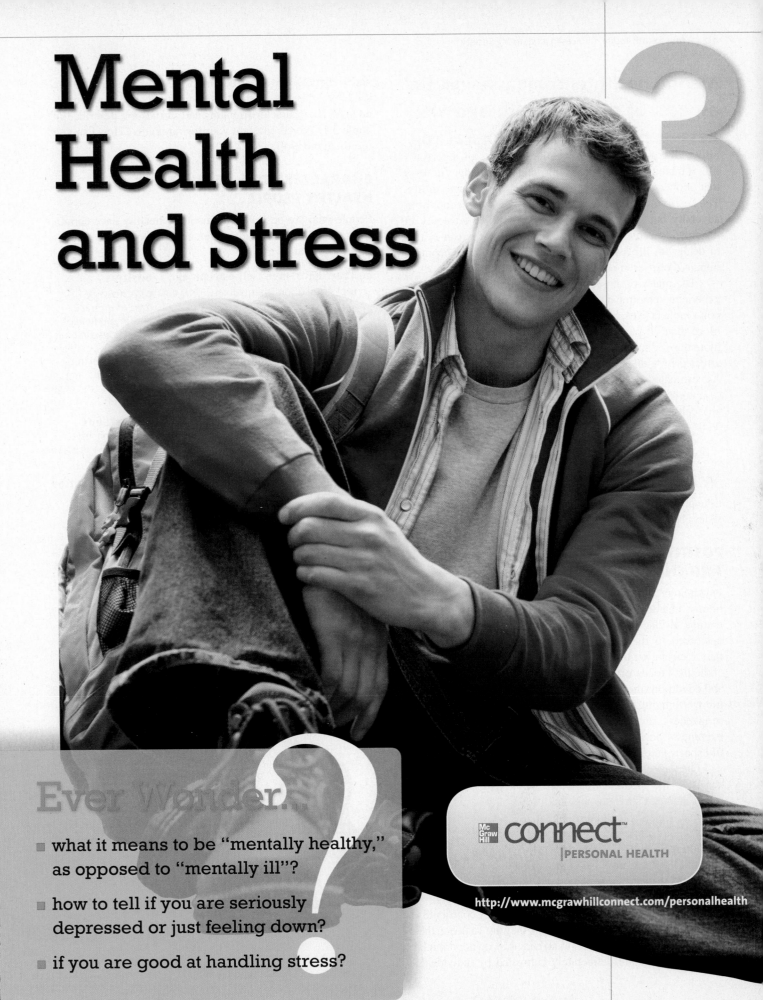

Ever Wonder...

- what it means to be "mentally healthy," as opposed to "mentally ill"?

- how to tell if you are seriously depressed or just feeling down?

- if you are good at handling stress?

Mental health encompasses several aspects of overall health and wellness—emotional, psychological, cognitive, interpersonal, and/or spiritual aspects of a person's

life. It includes the capacity to respond to challenges in ways that allow continued growth and forward movement in life. The key to mental health and happiness is not freedom from adversity but rather the ability to respond to adversity in adaptive, effective ways. A mentally healthy person is able to deal with life's inevitable challenges without becoming impaired or overwhelmed by them.

The majority of people are mentally healthy, but many experience emotional or psychological difficulties at some point in their lives, and mental disorders are fairly common. More than 26 percent of the adult American population—more than 57 million people, or one in four Americans—are affected by a diagnosable mental disorder in a given year.[1] An estimated 50 percent of Americans experience some symptoms of depression during their lifetime. Many mental health problems—as well as many general health problems—are triggered or worsened by stress.

What Is Mental Health?

Like physical health, mental health is not just the absence of illness but also the presence of many positive characteristics.

POSITIVE PSYCHOLOGY AND CHARACTER STRENGTHS

Psychologists have long been interested in such positive human characteristics as optimism, attachment, love, and emotional intelligence, but in recent years this interest has coalesced in the **positive psychology** movement. Rather than focusing on mental illness and problems, positive psychologists focus on positive emotions, character strengths, and conditions that create happiness—in short, "what makes life worth living."[2] By investigating such topics as gratitude, forgiveness, awe, inspiration, hope, curiosity, humor, and happiness, positive psychologists strive to understand the full spectrum of human experience.

One outcome of this research has been the identification of a set of character strengths and virtues that "enable human thriving" and that are endorsed by nearly all cultures across the world.[3] The six broad virtues are wisdom, courage, humanity, justice, temperance, and transcendence. Under each virtue are particular strengths that meet numerous other criteria. For example, they contribute to individual fulfillment and satisfaction, they are valued in their own right and not as a means to an end, they do not diminish others, and they are deliberately cultivated by individuals

and societies. The most commonly endorsed strengths are kindness, fairness, authenticity, gratitude, and open-mindedness. The character strengths and virtues are described in Table 3.1. Which ones are your top strengths? How can you use them more often?

CHARACTERISTICS OF MENTALLY HEALTHY PEOPLE

People who are described as mentally healthy have certain characteristics in common (often expressions of the character strengths and virtues):

- They have high **self-esteem** and feel good about themselves.
- They are realistic and accept imperfections in themselves and others.
- They are altruistic; they help others.
- They have a sense of control over their lives and feel capable of meeting challenges and solving problems.
- They demonstrate social competence in their relationships with others, and they are comfortable with other people and believe they can rely on them.
- They are not overwhelmed by fear, love, or anger; they try to control irrational thoughts and levels of stress.
- They are optimistic; they maintain a positive outlook.
- They have a capacity for intimacy; they do not fear commitment.
- They are creative and appreciate creativity in others.
- They take reasonable risks in order to grow.
- They bounce back from adversity.

positive psychology
Area of interest within the field of psychology that focuses on positive emotions, character strengths, and conditions that create happiness.

self-esteem
Sense of positive regard and valuation for oneself.

self-actualization
In Maslow's work, the state attained when a person has reached his or her full potential.

THE SELF-ACTUALIZED PERSON

Many of these healthy characteristics are found in the self-actualized person. The concept of **self-actualization** was developed by Abraham Maslow in the 1960s as a model of human personality development in his "hierarchy of needs" theory (Figure 3.1). Maslow proposed

Table 3.1   Classification of 6 Virtues and 24 Character Strengths

Virtue and Strength	Definition
1. Wisdom and knowledge	**Cognitive strengths that entail the acquisition and use of knowledge**
Creativity	Thinking of novel and productive ways to do things
Curiosity	Taking an interest in ongoing experience, openness to experience
Open-mindedness	Thinking things through and examining them from all sides
Love of learning	Mastering new skills, topics, and bodies of knowledge
Perspective	Being able to provide wise counsel to others
2. Courage	**Emotional strengths that involve the exercise of will to accomplish goals in the face of opposition, external or internal**
Authenticity	Speaking the truth and presenting oneself in a genuine way
Bravery	Not shrinking from threat, challenge, difficulty, or pain
Persistence	Finishing what one starts
Zest	Approaching life with excitement and energy
3. Humanity	**Interpersonal strengths that involve "tending and befriending" others**
Kindness	Doing favors and good deeds for others
Love	Valuing close relations with others
Social intelligence	Being aware of the motives and feelings of self and others
4. Justice	**Civic strengths that underlie healthy community life**
Fairness	Treating all people the same according to notions of fairness and justice
Leadership	Organizing group activities and seeing that they happen
Teamwork	Working well as a member of a group or team
5. Temperance	**Strengths that protect against excess**
Forgiveness	Forgiving those who have done wrong
Modesty	Letting one's accomplishments speak for themselves
Prudence	Being careful about one's choices; *not* saying or doing things that might later be regretted
Self-regulation	Regulating what one feels and does
6. Transcendence	**Strengths that forge connections to the larger universe and provide meaning**
Appreciation of beauty and excellence	Noticing and appreciating beauty, excellence, and/or skilled performance in all domains of life
Gratitude	Being aware of and thankful for the good things that happen
Hope	Expecting the best and working to achieve it
Humor	Liking to laugh and tease; bringing smiles to other people
Religiousness	Having coherent beliefs about the higher purpose and meaning of life

Source: From Character Strengths and Virtues: A Handbook and Classification, *by C. Peterson and M. Seligman, 2004, Washington, DC: American Psychological Association. Copyright © 2004 by the American Psychological Association. Reprinted with permission.*

The key to mental health and happiness is not freedom from adversity *but rather the ability to respond to adversity and manage stress in adaptive, effective ways.*

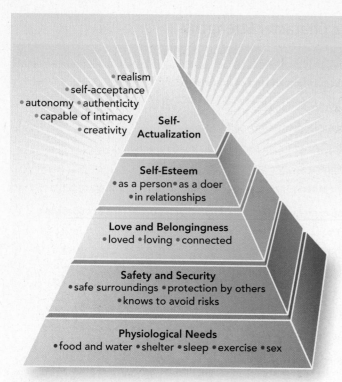

figure 3.1   Maslow's hierarchy of needs.

Source: Motivation and Personality, by Abraham H. Maslow, ed. Robert D. Frager and James Fadiman, 3rd ed., New York: Harper & Row.

that once people meet their needs for survival, safety and security, love and belonging, and achievement and self-esteem, they have opportunities for self- exploration and expression that can lead them to reach their fullest human potential. According to Maslow, a self-actualized person is realistic, self-accepting, self-motivated, creative, and capable of intimacy, among other traits. Those who reach this level achieve a state of transcendence, a sense of well-being that comes from finding purpose and meaning in life.

OPTIMISM, SELF-EFFICACY, AND RESILIENCE

A key characteristic of mentally healthy people is *optimism.* People with an "optimistic explanatory style"—the tendency to see problems as temporary and specific rather than permanent and general—seem to have better physical and mental health than more pessimistic people do.[4] Optimistic people react to failures as things they can do something about, as challenges and opportunities for learning and growth. A recent analysis of 83 studies has linked optimism to positive physical health outcomes.[5] Pessimistic people tend to attribute failure to personal defects and react with discouragement and a sense of defeat. (Of course, you also need to be realistic and recognize your own limitations; a person who disregards all the incoming information provided by successes and failures will end up only with more disappointment.)

Related to optimism is *self-efficacy,* a general sense that you have some control over what happens in your life.

Mentally healthy people have a basic belief that they can guide their own lives and take unexpected events in stride, adapt, and move on.

This ability to bounce back from adverse events is known as **resilience**, and it is another characteristic of mentally healthy individuals. People who can respond flexibly to life's challenges and redirect their energies toward positive actions tend to be more successful in life. Our lives will always have moments of adversity and vulnerability and be filled with challenging situations. Individuals who are resilient learn ways to respond to these events and situations. Resilience involves patterns of thinking, feeling, and behaving that contribute to a balanced life based on self-esteem, satisfying relationships, and a belief that life is meaningful. To discover more about your own resilience, complete the Chapter 3 Personal Health Portfolio activity at the back of the book.

Resilience research over the past two decades has suggested that most children, even those growing up in very difficult and challenging situations, not only survive but are able to build very positive lives for themselves. These children were found to be able to overcome adversity because of the protective factors or buffers that were also part of their lives.[6]

resilience
Ability to bounce back from adversity.

emotional intelligence
In Goleman's work, the kind of intelligence that includes an understanding of emotional experience, self-awareness, and sensitivity to others.

EMOTIONAL INTELLIGENCE

The concept of intelligence has been expanded by psychologist Daniel Goleman to include the idea of **emotional intelligence**. Goleman argued that such qualities as self-awareness, self-discipline, persistence, and empathy are much more important to success in life than IQ. People who are emotionally intelligent have an ability to

1. recognize, name, and understand their emotions,
2. manage their emotions and control their moods,
3. motivate themselves,
4. recognize and respond to emotions in others, and
5. be socially competent.[7]

The last ability involves skills in understanding relationships, cooperating, solving problems, resolving conflicts, being assertive at communicating, and being considerate and compassionate.[8]

Like many of the other characteristics of mentally healthy people, emotional intelligence can be learned and improved. Many groups, workshops, and self-help books assist people in learning how to control impulses, manage anger, recognize emotions in themselves and others, and respond more appropriately in social situations. However, the concept of emotional intelligence is sometimes used incorrectly to refer to a variety of qualities that have little to do with emotions or intelligence, such as motivation. When terms become part of our popular culture they often become overgeneralized and the original concept can lose meaning.[9]

People who tend to see problems as temporary and specific rather than permanent and general seem to have **better physical and mental health** *than do more pessimistic people.*

ENHANCING YOUR MENTAL HEALTH

Several other factors appear to be related to the development of mental health:

- A supportive social network
- Good communication skills
- Healthy lifestyle patterns

Social support—family ties, friendships, and involvement in social activities—is one of the primary ingredients in a mentally healthy life. These social connections can provide a sense of belonging, support in difficult times, and a positive influence when you drift toward unhealthy behaviors.

Communication skills are necessary for negotiating relationships of all kinds. The ability to be assertive—to communicate what you want clearly and appropriately without violating other people's rights—is an important part of healthy communication. Another is the ability to be an effective listener. Tips on improving your communication skills are provided in Chapter 12.

Like physical health, mental health depends on a healthy lifestyle—eating well, exercising, getting enough sleep, and so on. But it is also improved by participating in activities that challenge you mentally, emotionally, socially, and physically.

The Brain's Role in Mental Health and Illness

Human beings have always experienced mental disturbances: Descriptions of conditions called "mania," "melancholia," "hysteria," and "insanity" can be found in the literature of many ancient societies. It wasn't until the 18th and 19th centuries, however, that advances in anatomy, physiology, and medicine allowed scientists to identify the brain as the organ afflicted in cases of mental disturbance and to propose biological causes, especially damage to the brain, for mental disorders.

Since then, other explanations have been proposed, involving, for example, psychological factors, sociocultural and environmental factors, and faulty learning. Debate over the roles of these various categories of causal factors continues to this day. Although it is clear that mental disorders are best understood as the result of many factors interacting in complex ways, the central role of the brain in mental health and mental illness is beyond doubt. Mental illnesses are diseases that affect the brain.[10]

ADVANCES IN KNOWLEDGE AND UNDERSTANDING OF THE BRAIN

The human brain has been called the most complex structure in the universe.[11] This unimpressive-looking organ is the central control station for human intelligence, feeling, and creativity.

Since the 1980s, knowledge of the structure and function of the brain has increased dramatically. In fact, the 1990s were called the "decade of the brain" because of the advances made in understanding how the brain works. Most of these discoveries were made possible by advances in imaging technologies, such as computerized axial tomography (CAT scans), positron emission tomography (PET scans), magnetic resonance imaging (MRIs), and functional MRIs (fMRIs).

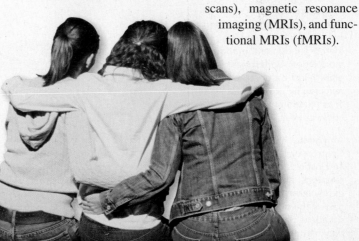

- Having a strong social support system—including friends to laugh and cry with—is an important ingredient in the maintenance of psychological health.

Research has also expanded in the physiology of the brain and the function of **neurotransmitters**. These brain chemicals are responsible for the transmission of signals from one brain cell to the next. There are dozens of neurotransmitters, but four seem to be particularly important in mental disorders: norepinephrine (active during the stress response; see later in this chapter); dopamine (implicated in schizophrenia); serotonin (implicated in mood disorders); and gamma aminobutyric acid, or GABA (implicated in anxiety).[11]

Neurotransmitter imbalances are believed to be involved in a variety of mental disorders. For example, dopamine gives us the positive feelings we experience when eating and participating in sexual activity, among other behaviors. All addictive drugs appear to trigger a dopamine release. Under consistently high levels of dopamine, a person will begin to behave erratically, with increases in sexual desire, aggressiveness, and likelihood of risk taking. Serotonin is associated with emotion and mood. Low levels of serotonin have been shown to be related to depression, problems with anger control and concentration, and a variety of other disorders. High levels of serotonin, which can be an unintended side effect of some migraine medicines and some antidepressants, can result in serotonin syndrome. Symptoms of this syndrome include nausea, vomiting, changes in blood pressure, and agitation. Many drugs have been developed to correct neurotransmitter imbalances, such as the class of antidepressants that affect levels of serotonin.

neurotransmitters
Brain chemicals that conduct signals from one brain cell to the next.

frontal cortex
The part of the brain where the executive functions of planning, organizing, and rational thinking are controlled.

THE TEENAGE BRAIN

One surprise that recent brain research produced is that the brain continues to change and grow through adolescence into the early 20s. Previously, scientists thought that brain development was completed in childhood, and in fact, 95 percent of the structure of the brain is formed by the age of 6. Scientists discovered, however, that a growth spurt occurs in the **frontal cortex**—the part of the brain where "executive functions" such as planning, organizing, and rational thinking are controlled—just before puberty. During adolescence, these new brain cells are pruned and consolidated, resulting in a more mature, adult brain by the early to mid-20s.

One implication of these findings is that the impulsivity, emotional reactivity, and risk-taking behavior that are more typical of adolescence than of adulthood may be caused in part by a still-maturing brain rather than (or in addition to) hormonal changes or other factors. Figure 3.2 shows the teenage brain and describes how its functions may differ from those of the adult brain.

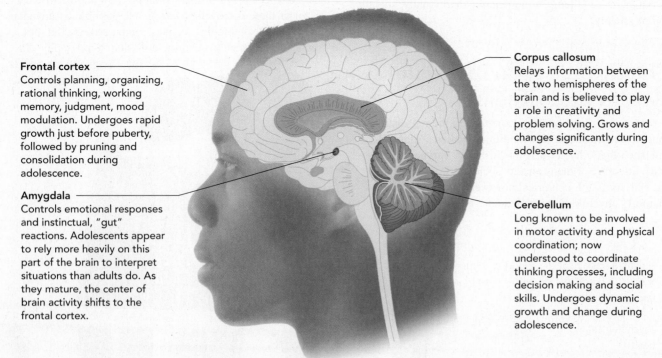

Frontal cortex
Controls planning, organizing, rational thinking, working memory, judgment, mood modulation. Undergoes rapid growth just before puberty, followed by pruning and consolidation during adolescence.

Amygdala
Controls emotional responses and instinctual, "gut" reactions. Adolescents appear to rely more heavily on this part of the brain to interpret situations than adults do. As they mature, the center of brain activity shifts to the frontal cortex.

Corpus callosum
Relays information between the two hemispheres of the brain and is believed to play a role in creativity and problem solving. Grows and changes significantly during adolescence.

Cerebellum
Long known to be involved in motor activity and physical coordination; now understood to coordinate thinking processes, including decision making and social skills. Undergoes dynamic growth and change during adolescence.

figure **3.2**   **The teenage brain.**

Sources: Adapted from "Adolescent Brains Are Works in Progress," by S. Spinks, 2005, Frontline, www.pbs.org; "Teenage Brain: A Work in Progress," 2001, National Institute of Mental Health, NIH Publication No. 01-4929, www.nimh.nih.gov.

Another implication is that because structural changes are taking place in the brain through adolescence and into early adulthood, the activities that teenagers engage in can have lifelong effects. The brain cells and connections that are used for academics, music, sports, language learning, and other productive activities—or, alternatively, for watching television and playing video games—are the ones that are more likely to be hardwired into the brain and survive.[12]

Some experts have disputed these conclusions about the teenage brain. They argue that the differences seen in brain images are not necessarily the *cause* of erratic or impulsive teen behaviors, and they point out that adolescents in other cultures are often fully ready to regulate and be responsible for their behavior. In addition, some research has indicated a relationship between impulsive, risk-taking teen behavior and exposure to movies, television, and video games. More research is needed to sort out the effects of biological versus cultural influences on teen behavior.[13]

HOW DO EVERYDAY PROBLEMS DIFFER FROM MENTAL DISORDERS?

In general, a mental disorder is diagnosed on the basis of the amount of distress and impairment a person is experiencing. According to the *Diagnostic and Statistical Manual of Mental Disorders (DSM-IV-TR)*, a **mental disorder** is a pattern of behavior in an individual that is associated with distress (pain) or disability (impairment in an important area of functioning, such as school or work) or with significantly increased risk of suffering, death, pain, disability, or loss of freedom.[11] Deciding when a psychological problem becomes a mental disorder is not easy. Nevertheless, a basic premise of the *DSM-IV-TR* is that a mental disorder is qualitatively different from a psychological problem that can be considered normal, and it can be diagnosed from a set of symptoms.

Some of the most common experiences that people struggle with in life, especially during the college years, are feeling

Worries, fears, and anxieties are common
during the college years. Most people gradually make their way, learning who they are and how they want to relate to other people.

MENTAL DISORDERS AND THE BRAIN

Although all behavior, both normal and abnormal, is mediated in some way by the brain and the nervous system, mental disorders that are caused specifically by some pathology in the brain are rare. These disorders are referred to as *cognitive disorders*; an example is Alzheimer's disease. More commonly, mental disorders are caused by complex interactions of biological factors (such as neurotransmitter levels, genetics), psychological processes, social influences, and cultural factors, especially those affecting a person during early childhood. In addition, as discussed in Chapter 2, some mental disorders, including depression, bipolar disorder, and schizophrenia, have a genetic component. Although evidence of mental disorders like depression or schizophrenia can be found in the brain, and although many disorders can be treated with drugs that act on the brain, neither of these facts means that mental disorders originate in the brain.

Mental Disorders and Treatment

Mental health is determined not by the challenges a person faces but by how the person responds to those challenges. The challenges themselves come in a range of intensities— from being turned down for a date to the death of a loved one—and people's responses also vary in how well they work in allowing the person to maintain an overall sense of balance and well-being.

sad and discouraged. These feelings can occur in response to disappointment, loss, failure, or other negative events, or they can occur for no apparent reason. Usually such experiences don't last too long; people recover and go on with their lives. If the feelings *do* go on for a long time and are painful and intense, the person may be experiencing depression.

Similarly, worries, fears, and anxieties are common during the college years. Individuals have stresses to deal with, such as grades, relationships, and learning how to live on their own without parental guidance or support. They may be feeling homesick and lonely, or they may be having problems sleeping. Most people gradually make their way, learning who they are and how they want to relate to other people. Some people, however, may develop anxiety disorders or stress-related disorders, and experience panic attacks or be overwhelmed with fears and worries.

People experience many emotional difficulties in the course of daily living that are not a cause for alarm. At the same time, it is important to be able to recognize when a person needs professional help. Far too often, people struggle with mental disorders without knowing that something is wrong or that treatments are available. They don't realize that their problems may be causing them unnecessary distress and that professional treatment can help. (See the box "Reducing the Stigma of Mental Illness.")

mental disorder According to the *DSM-IV-TR*, a pattern of behavior that is associated with distress (pain) or disability (impairment in an important area of functioning, such as school or work) or with significantly increased risk of suffering, death, pain, disability, or loss of freedom.

Public Health in Action

Reducing the Stigma of Mental Illness

In 2008 the Substance Abuse and Mental Health Services Administration (SAMHSA) of the U.S. Department of Health and Human Services launched a campaign to challenge and reduce the stigma associated with mental illness on college campuses. The effort is designed to reach 18- to 25-year-olds and to encourage them to support friends with mental health problems.

The incidence of mental health problems in this age group is the highest of any segment of the adult population, yet young adults are the least likely to get help. According to the National College Health Assessment Report, almost half of the students surveyed on U.S. college campuses said young adults felt hopeless and almost a third reported being "so depressed it was difficult to function." Suicide is the second leading cause of death for college students, according to the Centers for Disease Control and Prevention. One of the premises of the campaign is that young people will be more likely to seek mental health services if there is more social acceptance of such treatment.

The campaign, called "What a Difference a Friend Makes," emphasizes the important role of friends in recovery from mental illness. It encourages young people to offer their acceptance, companionship, and reassurance of friendship to those they know with mental illness. One of many public service announcements (PSAs) for

television and radio opens with a large group of people who state, "We're your online friends." The group slowly dwindles as it narrows down to friends from yoga class, friends you go out with on the weekends, and friends who will help you move, until there is one voice left who announces that she is the friend who will be there for you if you ever have a mental illness. The voiceover then encourages the viewer to be that friend who is there for someone with mental illness; support from a friend, the PSA says, will increase the person's chance of recovery.

The ad campaign was developed by SAMHSA and the Advertising Council and distributed, with the help of several nonprofit organizations, in the form of brochures delivered to campus bookstores, program manuals for peer educators, television and radio ads, and other outreach materials. The time for airing the ads was donated by the media. The college campaign is an extension of the National Mental Health Anti-Stigma Campaign, launched in 2006. Anti-stigma campaigns are spreading and are now under way in several states. The aim of all such programs is to counter stigma and discrimination, reduce barriers to treatment, educate people about recovery, and emphasize the importance of quality, accessible mental health services available in the community.

connect ACTIVITY

Sources: "SAMHSA and Ad Council Debut National Mental Health Anti-Stigma Campaign on College Campuses," Substance Abuse and Mental Health Services Administration, 2008, retrieved February 17, 2010, from www.samhsa.gov/newsroom/advisories/0803273627.aspx; "Friends," Substance Abuse and Mental Health Services Administration, retrieved February 17, 2010, from www.whatadifference.org.

MOOD DISORDERS

Also called depressive disorders or affective disorders, mood disorders include major depressive disorder, dysthymic disorder, and bipolar disorder (formerly called manic depression). They are among the most common mental disorders around the world.

People of all ages can get depressed, including children and adolescents, but the average age of onset for major depressive disorders is the mid-20s. In any one year, more than 20.9 million adults in the United States—about 9.5 percent of the adult population—suffer from a depressive illness. Of these individuals, a significant number will be hospitalized, and many will die from suicide.[1] Women are at significantly greater risk for depression than men, experiencing depressive episodes twice as frequently.

In many of these situations, the illness goes undiagnosed, and people struggle for long periods of time. About two-thirds of depressed individuals seek help, but many are undertreated, meaning that they don't get enough medication or they don't see a therapist on a regular basis. Many medications for depression take up to 4 weeks to begin to have an effect, and some people conclude they aren't working and stop taking them.

Major Depressive Disorder   Symptoms of **depression** include depressed mood, as indicated by feelings of sadness or emptiness or by behaviors such as crying, a loss of interest or pleasure in activities that previously provided pleasure, fatigue, feelings of worthlessness, and a reduced ability to concentrate (see the box "Symptoms of Depression"). If a person experiences one or more episodes of depression (characterized by at least five of the nine symptoms listed) lasting at least 2 weeks, he or she may be diagnosed with *major depressive disorder*.

depression
Mental state characterized by a depressed mood, loss of interest or pleasure in activities, and several other related symptoms.

Bipolar Disorder   A person with *bipolar disorder* experiences one or more manic episodes, often but not always alternating with depressive episodes. A *manic episode* is a distinct period during which the person has an abnormally elevated mood. Individuals experiencing manic episodes may be euphoric, expansive, and full of energy, or, alternatively, highly irritable. They may be grandiose, with an inflated sense of their own importance and power; they may have racing thoughts and accelerated and pressured speech. They may stay awake for days without getting tired or wake

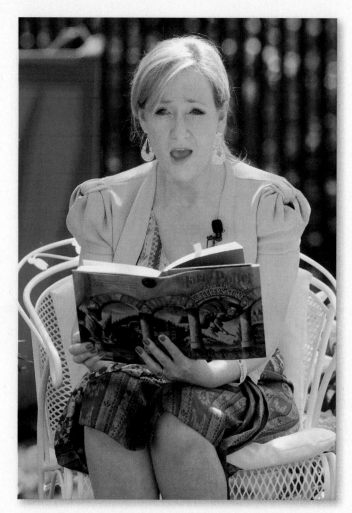

■ J. K. Rowling, author of the Harry Potter books, is one of many talented people who have spoken about their own experiences with depression. Rowling suffered a bout of depression and suicidal thoughts in her mid-twenties.

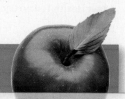

Highlight on Health

Symptoms of Depression

A person who experiences five or more of the following symptoms (including the first and second symptoms listed) for a 2-week period may be suffering from depression:

- Depressed mood, as indicated by feelings of sadness or emptiness or such behaviors as crying.
- Loss of interest or pleasure in all or most activities.
- Significant weight loss or weight gain or a change in appetite.
- Insomnia, hypersomnia, or other disturbed sleep patterns.
- Agitated or retarded (slow) body movement.
- Fatigue or loss of energy.
- Feelings of worthlessness or excessive guilt.
- Diminished ability to think, impaired concentration, or indecisiveness.
- Recurrent thoughts of death, ideas about suicide, or a suicide plan or attempt.

Source: Reprinted with permission from Diagnostic and Statistical Manual of Mental Disorders, 4th ed., Text Revision (DSM-IV-TR). *Copyright © 2000, American Psychiatric Association.*

from a few hours of sleep feeling refreshed and full of energy. People experiencing a manic episode typically are not aware they are ill.

Bipolar disorder occurs equally in men and women, with an average age at onset of about 20. Family and twin studies offer strong evidence of a genetic component in this disorder.

ANXIETY DISORDERS

Along with depression, anxiety disorders are the most common mental disorders affecting Americans. Almost 40 million Americans 18 and older—more than 18 percent of all people in this age group—have an anxiety disorder.[1]

Many of these disorders are characterized by a **panic attack**, a clear physiological and psychological experience of apprehension or intense fear in the absence of a real danger. Symptoms include heart palpitations, sweating, shortness of breath, chest pain, and a sense that one is "going crazy." There is a feeling of impending doom or danger and a strong urge to escape. Panic attacks usually occur suddenly and last for a discrete period of time, reaching a peak within 10 minutes.[14]

Panic disorder is characterized by recurrent, unexpected panic attacks along with concern about having another attack. The attacks may be triggered by a situation, or they may "come out of nowhere." Twin studies and family studies indicate a genetic contribution to this disorder. First-degree relatives of persons with panic disorder are eight times more likely to develop the disorder than the general population.[14]

A *specific phobia* is an intense fear of an activity, situation, or object, exposure to which evokes immediate anxiety. Examples of common phobias are flying, heights, specific animals or insects (dogs, spiders), and blood. Individuals with phobias realize their fear is unreasonable, but they cannot control it. Usually they try to avoid the phobic

panic attack
Clear physiological and psychological experience of apprehension or intense fear in the absence of a real danger.

panic disorder
Mental disorder characterized by recurrent, unexpected panic attacks along with concern about having another attack.

situation or object, and if they can't avoid it, they endure it with great distress. Often the phobia interferes with their lives in some way.

Agoraphobia is characterized by anxiety about being in situations where escape may be difficult or embarrassing, or where help might not be available in case of a panic attack. Such situations may include being in a crowd, on a bus, on a bridge, in an open space, or simply outside the home. Individuals with untreated agoraphobia usually structure their lives to avoid these situations; in extreme cases, they may not leave their home for years.

A *social phobia* involves an intense fear of certain kinds of social or performance situations, again leading the individual to try to avoid such situations. If the phobic situation is public speaking, individuals may be able to structure their lives so as to avoid all such situations. However, some social phobias involve simply conversing with other people. This is

addiction is continued, compulsive use of the substance or involvement in the behavior despite serious negative consequences. Individuals with a substance addiction may spend a great deal of time trying to obtain the substance, give up important parts of their lives to use it, and make repeated, unsuccessful attempts to cut down or control their use.

A person with *physiological dependence* on a substance experiences *tolerance*, reduced sensitivity to its effects such that increased doses are needed to give the same high, and *withdrawal*, uncomfortable symptoms that occur when substance use stops. Tolerance and withdrawal are indicators that the brain and body have adapted to the substance. Even without physiological dependence, the person can experience *psychological dependence*.

Typically, a person begins by using a substance to reduce pain or anxiety or to produce feelings of pleasure, excitement, confidence, or connection with others. With repeated use, users can come to depend on being in this altered state, and without the drug, they may feel worse than they did before they ever took it. Although most people don't think they will become addicted when they start, gradually the substance takes over their lives.

Addiction—*dependence on a substance or a behavior—* ## is classified as a mental disorder.

different from shyness; individuals with this disorder experience tremors, sweating, confusion, blushing, and other distressing symptoms when they are in the feared situation.

Excessive and uncontrollable worrying, usually far out of proportion to the likelihood of the feared event, is known as *generalized anxiety disorder*. Adults with this disorder worry about routine matters such as health, work, and money; children with the disorder worry about their competence in school or sports, being evaluated by others, or even natural disasters.

Obsessive-compulsive disorder is characterized by persistent, intrusive thoughts, impulses, or images that cause intense anxiety or distress. For example, the person may have repeated thoughts about contamination, persistent doubts about having done something, or a need to have things done in a particular order. To control the obsessive thoughts and images, the person develops compulsions—repetitive behaviors performed to reduce the anxiety associated with the obsession.

addiction
Dependence on a substance or a behavior.

schizophrenia
A psychotic disorder in which a person has disorganized and disordered thinking and perceptions, bizarre ideas, hallucinations (often voices), and impaired functioning.

ADDICTION

Addiction—dependence on a substance or a behavior— is classified as a mental disorder. The key characteristic of

Although addiction is usually associated with drug use, many experts now extend the concept of addiction to other areas in which behavior can become compulsive and out of control, such as gambling. Research has established that drugs cause addiction by operating on the "pleasure pathway" in the brain and changing brain chemistry (see Chapter 11 for details of this process). Some scientists speculate that compulsive behaviors may follow the same pathway in the brain, causing feelings of euphoria along with a strong desire to repeat the behavior and a craving for the behavior when it stops.

Compulsive or pathological gambling is the best known of these behavioral disorders, but people can also be addicted to Internet use, sex, shopping, eating, exercising, or other activities (Figure 3.3). The key component in these conditions is that the person feels out of control and powerless over the behavior. Both psychotherapy and self-help groups are available to assist individuals struggling with these troubling behavior patterns.

SCHIZOPHRENIA AND OTHER PSYCHOTIC DISORDERS

Psychotic disorders are characterized by delusions, hallucinations, disorganized speech or behavior, and other signs that the individual has lost touch with reality. The most common psychotic disorder is **schizophrenia**. A person with schizophrenia typically has disorganized and disordered thinking and perceptions, bizarre ideas, hallucinations (often voices),

Alcohol		AA has more than 2 million members— only a small proportion of those who are dependent on alcohol.
Drugs		More than 8 percent of the population currently use illicit drugs, with marijuana by far the most commonly used.
Tobacco		Smoking rates have declined dramatically since their peak in the 1960s, but one in five Americans still smokes.
Caffeine		The most widely used psychoactive drug in the United States, caffeine is consumed in coffee, soda, and, most recently, energy drinks with names like Red Bull and Full Throttle.
Food		Some people who are addicted to food have binge-eating disorder—a psychological disorder like anorexia or bulimia—and are likely to be overweight or obese.
Gambling		About 3–4 percent of those who gamble are believed to do so compulsively.
Shopping		A cultural emphasis on material goods, fueled by advertising, contributes to compulsive shopping.
Sex		Sex addicts are preoccupied with sexual thoughts and activities much of the time. The vast majority grew up in abusive family environments.
Internet		Internet addicts spend hours online every day instead of spending time on real-life activities and relationships.

figure **3.3** **What we're addicted to: Substances and behaviors.** The common feature in all addictions is loss of control.

and impaired functioning.[15] The symptoms are sometimes so severe that the person becomes socially, interpersonally, and occupationally dysfunctional. Age at onset is usually the early 20s for men and the late 20s for women.

Schizophrenia has a strong genetic component. First-degree relatives of individuals with schizophrenia have a risk for the disorder 10 times higher than that of the general population.[11] All of the brain scanning and visualizing technologies reveal abnormalities in the brains of people with schizophrenia. Studies indicate that these abnormalities are present before the onset of symptoms, suggesting that this illness is the result of problems in brain development, perhaps even occurring prenatally. In most cases, symptoms of the disease can be controlled with medication.

MENTAL DISORDERS AND SUICIDE

A major public health concern, particularly among young people, suicide is the second leading cause of death among college students. According to the National College Health Assessment (fall 2008), approximately 30 percent of college students have been so depressed that they could not function. About 6 percent of students seriously considered suicide, and 1 percent attempted to kill themselves in the past year.[16]

Among high school students, 14.5 percent had seriously considered attempting suicide in the past 12 months; over 18 percent of females and 10 percent of males reported having serious suicidal thoughts. Overall, during the past 12 months, 11 percent of high school students had made a plan, 6.9 percent had attempted suicide, and 2 percent of those surveyed had to receive treatment from a doctor or nurse for injuries sustained during a suicide attempt.[17]

Overall, women in U.S. society are more likely than men to attempt suicide, but men are four times more likely to succeed, probably because they choose more violent methods, usually a firearm. In the United States, firearms are used in 55–60 percent of all suicides. Women tend to use less violent methods for suicide, but in recent years they have begun to use firearms more frequently.

What Leads a Person to Suicide? Individuals contemplating suicide are most likely experiencing unbearable emotional pain, anguish, or despair. As many as 90 percent of those who commit suicide are suffering from a mental disorder, often depression. Studies indicate that the symptom linking depression and suicide is a feeling of hopelessness. Depression and alcoholism may be involved in two-thirds of all suicides. Substance abuse is another factor; the combination of drugs and depression can be lethal. People experiencing psychosis are also at risk.

Besides mental disorders and substance abuse, other major risk factors associated with suicide are a family history of suicide, serious medical problems, and access to the means, such as a gun or pills. The most significant risk factor, however, is a previous suicide attempt or a history of such attempts (see the box "Risk Factors for Suicide").

Sometimes, vulnerable individuals turn to suicide in response to a specific event, such as the loss of a relationship or job, an experience of failure, or a worry that a secret will be revealed. Other times there is no apparent precipitating event, and the suicide seems to come out of nowhere.

Highlight on Health

Risk Factors for Suicide

A number of factors place adolescents at risk for suicide. The following list highlights the leading predictors.

- Suicidal thoughts
- Psychiatric disorders
- Drug and/or alcohol abuse
- Previous suicide attempts
- Access to firearms
- Recent loss or stressful situation
- Feelings of hopelessness
- Family history of suicide

Source: Reprinted with permission from Diagnostic and Statistical Manual of Mental Disorders, *4th ed., Text Revision (DSM-IV-TR). Copyright © 2000, American Psychiatric Association.*

However, suicide is always a process, and certain behavioral signs indicate that a person may be thinking about suicide:

- Comments about death and threats to commit suicide.
- Increasing social withdrawal and isolation.
- Intensified moodiness.
- Increase in risk-taking behaviors.
- Sudden improvement in mood, accompanied by such behaviors as giving away possessions. (The person may have made the decision to commit suicide.)

How to Help   If you know someone who seems to be suicidal, it is critical to get the person help. All mentions of suicide should be taken seriously. It is a myth that asking a person if he or she is thinking about suicide will plant the seed in the person's mind. Ignoring someone's sadness and depressed mood only increases the risk. Encourage the person to talk, and ask direct questions:

- Are you thinking about killing yourself?
- Do you have a plan?
- Do you have the means?
- Have you attempted suicide in the past?

Encourage the person to get help by calling a suicide hotline or seeking counseling. Do not agree to keep the person's mental state or intentions a secret. If he or she refuses to get help or resists your advice, you may need to contact a parent or relative or, if you are a student, share your concern with a professional at the student health center. Do not leave a suicidal person alone. Call for help or take the person to an emergency room.

If you have thought about suicide yourself, we encourage you to seek counseling. Therapy can help you resolve problems, develop better coping skills, and diminish the feelings that are causing you pain. It can also help you see things in a broader perspective and understand that you will not always feel this way. Remember the saying, suicide is a permanent solution to a temporary problem.

SELF-INJURY

Self-injury, sometimes known as self-harm, self-mutilation, or self-injurious behavior, is defined as any intentional injury to one's own body. Specific behaviors include cutting, burning, scratching, branding, picking, hair pulling, and head banging. Self-injurious behaviors are sometimes mistaken for suicide attempts. Individuals who self-injure often have a history of physical and/or sexual abuse as well as coexisting problems such as substance abuse and eating disorders.

There is evidence that the incidence of self-injury is increasing, particularly among adolescents.[18] It has been estimated that approximately 17 percent of college students have engaged in at least one incident of self-injury.[16] Many of the college students reporting self-injurious behaviors had never been in therapy for any reason and only rarely disclosed their behaviors to anyone.[19] The disorder seems to be equally prevalent among men and women, and the behavior does not appear to be limited by race, ethnicity, education, sexual orientation, socioeconomic status, or religion. A variety of treatments can help people who injure themselves, including family therapy and medications.

Insurance companies often prefer to pay for medications, *which tend to produce faster, more visible, and more verifiable results, than for psychotherapy, which may last for months or years and produce results that are less objectively verifiable.*

Psychotherapy

More than 250 different models of psychotherapy exist for the treatment of mental disorders, and many different drugs can be prescribed. Most of the mild and moderate mental disorders are readily treatable with therapy and, if needed, medications.

Consumer Clipboard

Counseling Services on Campus

Counseling services on campus vary greatly. At small schools the staff may consist of just one professional, but at large universities there is typically a team of psychologists, social workers, nurse practitioners, and usually at least one psychiatrist. At many colleges the services fall somewhere in between.

If you're trying to decide whether you need professional help, ask yourself these questions:

- Am I feeling sad (homesick, lonely) a lot of the time?
- Am I having trouble studying for exams?
- Am I having more difficulty than usual with concentration?
- Do I have increased feelings of inadequacy?
- Am I feeling overwhelmed?
- Is this problem interfering with my everyday life?
- Have my friends and family asked if there's a problem?
- Have I lost interest in doing the things I usually like to do?
- Am I avoiding friends because of the problem?

Many colleges provide free psychological assessments, short-term counseling, and referrals. If you decide that you need help, consider these points:

- *Do I want to work with a professional counselor, or would another approach be better for me?* There may be support groups on campus that offer the chance to share your problems with peers. This may help put your problem in perspective, and it may be all the help you need. If you have ties to a religious organization, you may want to seek pastoral counseling in the local community.

- *Will my insurance cover mental health counseling?* Your college tuition fees or health insurance may cover some mental health services. However, if you choose to go off campus for counseling or treatment, those services may not be covered by your college benefits. If you are covered by health insurance through your parents, you will need to check with that insurance company about coverage.

- *Do I want my family to know that I'm in counseling?* Different schools have varying policies on this matter. If you're over 18, most schools will let you decide whether to tell your parents about your counseling. If you're considered to be at risk for suicide, though, most counselors will encourage you to inform your parents about the counseling.

Source: Adapted from "The Dorms May Be Great, But How's the Counseling?" by M. Duenwald, October 26, 2004, New York Times, *p. D1.*

The key feature of most forms of **psychotherapy** (or *counseling*) is the development of a positive interpersonal relationship between a person seeking help (the client or patient) and a therapist, a trained and licensed professional who can provide that help. Most therapy models agree on the central importance of this interpersonal relationship between client and therapist.

Most therapists espouse a particular theoretical orientation, but many take an eclectic approach; that is, they feel comfortable using ideas from a variety of different theories and approaches.

What should you expect if you decide to try therapy? You can expect to be treated with warmth, respect, and an open, accepting attitude. The therapist will try to provide you with a safe place to explore your feelings and thoughts. At the end of the first session, the therapist will probably propose a plan for treatment, such as a series of ten sessions or a referral to another professional (see the box "Counseling Services on Campus").

psychotherapy
Treatment for psychological problems usually based on the development of a positive interpersonal relationship between a client and a therapist.

MEDICATIONS

Until the 1950s few effective medications for the symptoms of mental illness existed. Since that time, discoveries and breakthroughs in drug research have revolutionized the treatment of mental disorders. Today the symptoms of many serious disorders can be treated successfully with drugs.

The symptoms of schizophrenia and other psychotic disorders, especially delusions and hallucinations, can be treated with *antipsychotics*. Symptoms of mood disorders can be relieved with any of several different types of *antidepressants*, most of which act on the neurotransmitters serotonin and norepinephrine. Prozac, Zoloft, and Paxil

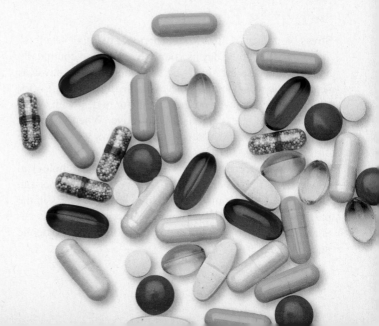

are used to treat mood disorders and are among the most frequently prescribed drugs in the United States today. The most frequently prescribed drugs overall are antidepressants. Between 2002 and 2005, prescriptions for antidepressants increased from 154 million to 170 million.[20]

Symptoms of anxiety disorders can be reduced with antianxiety drugs (or *anxiolytics*). Benzodiazepines, the most widely used antianxiety drugs, are believed to act on the neurotransmitter GABA, which has a role in the inhibition of anxiety in the brain during stressful situations. Common antianxiety medications include Valium, Xanax, and Ativan.

The use of medications has increased dramatically in recent years. The use of drugs has also increased for children and adolescents diagnosed with mental disorders, a controversial issue in our society. The controversy was highlighted in 2004 when a study showed that certain antidepressants increased the risk of suicidal thinking and behavior in adolescents.[21–24] The FDA directed manufacturers of all antidepressants to include "black box" warnings to physicians and parents on their labels.

More recent studies indicate that antidepressants also significantly increase the risk of suicidal thoughts and behaviors in young adults aged 18–24, usually during the first 1–2 months of treatment. The FDA has proposed that warnings on antidepressants be updated to include young adults.[25]

The increase in the use of drug treatments is due not just to improvements in the drugs themselves but also to the growing use of managed health care in the United States. Insurance companies often prefer to pay for medications, which tend to produce faster, more visible, and more verifiable results, than for psychotherapy, which may last for months or years and produce results that are less objectively verifiable. Drugs treat only the symptoms of mental disorders, and although they continue to remain the treatment of choice, research has been mixed about their overall effectiveness.[26] For understanding the root causes of problems and changing maladaptive patterns of thinking, feeling, and behaving, some form of psychotherapy is usually needed.

What Is Stress?

Stress is a fact of life; you experience varying levels of stress throughout the day as your body and mind continually adjust to the demands of living. We often think of stress as negative, as an uncomfortable or unpleasant pressure—for example, to complete a project on time or to deal with a traffic ticket—but stress can also be positive. When you get a promotion at work or when someone throws you a surprise birthday party, you also experience stress.

A survey conducted by the American Psychological Association in 2009 found that 75 percent of American adults report having moderate to high levels of stress in the past month[27] (see the box "Stress in America"). College students indicate that stress is the top impediment to academic performance.[16]

Such statistics only reinforce the need to manage the stress in our lives and to reduce its negative impact on our well-being. When excessive stress is unavoidable, having a repertoire of stress management techniques to fall back on is invaluable.

Events or agents in the environment that cause us stress are called **stressors**. They can range from being late for class to having a close friend die, from finding a parking space to winning the lottery. Your reaction to these events is called the *stress response*; this concept is discussed at length in the next section. Stressors disrupt the body's balance and require adjustments to return systems to normal. **Stress** can be defined as the general state of the body, mind, and emotions when an environmental stressor has triggered the stress response.

Because there is so much variation in individual responses to stressors, stress may be thought of as a *transaction* between an individual and a stressor in the environment, mediated by personal variables that include the person's perceptions and appraisal of the event.[28] When faced with a stressor, you evaluate it without necessarily realizing you are doing so: Is it positive or negative? How threatening is it to my well-being, my self-esteem, my identity? Can I cope with it or not? When you appraise an event as positive, you experience *eustress*, or positive stress. When you appraise it as negative, you experience *distress*.

stressors
Events or agents in the environment that cause stress.

stress
The general state of the body, mind, and emotions when an environmental stressor has triggered the stress response.

stress response or fight-or-flight response
Series of physiological changes that activate body systems, providing a burst of energy to deal with a perceived threat or danger.

THE STRESS RESPONSE

Regardless of the nature of the stressor and the individual's appraisal of it, all stressors elicit the **stress response** (also known as the **fight-or-flight response**), a series of physiological changes that occur in the body in the face of a threat. All animals, it appears—humans included—need sudden bursts of energy to fight or flee from situations they perceive as dangerous.

The stress response is carried out by the branch of the nervous system known as the *autonomic nervous system*, which controls involuntary, unconscious functions like breathing, heart rate, and digestion. The autonomic nervous system has two branches: The *sympathetic branch* is responsible for initiating the stress response, and the *parasympathetic branch* is responsible for turning off the stress response and returning the body to normal.

The stress response begins when the cerebral cortex (in the front of the brain) sends a chemical signal to the hypothalamus, which sends a signal to the pituitary gland. The pituitary gland sends adrenocorticotropic hormone (ACTH) to the adrenal glands, which release the hormones cortisol,

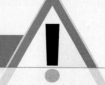

Who's at Risk?

Stress in America

All segments of the population apparently experience unhealthy levels of stress on a regular basis, but the experiences vary across gender, age, and other dimensions.

Gender
Women experience more stress than men except in the area of work.

	Women	Men
Percentage who report high levels of stress	27	19
Percentage who report money as a source of stress	75	67
Percentage who report family responsibilities as a source of stress	60	50
Percentage who report relationships as a source of stress	54	49
Percentage who report work as a source of stress	68	70
Percentage who report job stability as a source of stress	41	47

Women experience more symptoms of stress than men.

	Women	Men
Percentage who report experiencing irritability/anger as a result of stress	51	39
Percentage who report headaches as a result of stress	43	24
Percentage who report experiencing nervousness/anxiety as a result of stress	42	28

Age
Millennials are more likely to feel stress about money, GenXers are more likely to feel stress about work, Boomers are more likely to feel stress about the economy, and Matures have the lowest stress levels of any age group. *

	Millennials	GenXers	Boomers	Matures
Percentage who report money as a source of stress	81	74	71	54
Percentage who report work as a source of stress	71	75	73	31
Percentage who report the economy as a source of stress	50	66	72	57

Ethnicity
The top source of stress for Blacks and Hispanics is money; the top source of stress for Whites is work.

	Whites	Blacks	Hispanics
Percentage who report money as a source of stress	68	74	77
Percentage who report work as a source of stress	71	60	68
Percentage who report family responsibilities as a source of stress	53	64	60
Percentage who report personal safety as a source of stress	24	42	30

*Millennials: 18–30-year-olds; GenXers: 31–44-year-olds; Boomers: 45–63-year-olds; Matures: 64-year-olds and older

Source: Data from Stress in America 2009, *by American Psychological Association, 2009, Washington, DC: American Psychological Association.*

epinephrine (adrenaline), and norepinephrine (noradrenaline) into the bloodstream. Glucose and fats are released from the liver and other storage sites to provide energy.

As stress hormones surge through your body, your heart rate, breathing rate, muscle tension, metabolism, and blood pressure all increase, and other changes occur to prepare you for fight or flight (Figure 3.4). All this happens in an instant.

THE RELAXATION RESPONSE

When a stressful event is over—you decide the situation is no longer dangerous, or you complete your task—the parasympathetic branch of the autonomic nervous system takes over, turning off the stress response.[29] Heart rate, breathing, muscle tension, and blood pressure all decrease. The body returns to **homeostasis**, a state of stability and balance in which functions are maintained within a normal range. The term **relaxation response** has been used to describe this process, and we discuss it in more detail later in this chapter.

ACUTE STRESS AND CHRONIC STRESS

According to evolutionary biology, the fight-or-flight response served an important function for our ancestors. Today, most of us do not live in such dangerous environments, but this innate response to threat is still essential to our survival, warning us when it is time to fight or flee. Although the fight-or-flight response requires a great deal of energy—which is why you often feel so tired after a stressful event—your

homeostasis
State of stability and balance in which body functions are maintained within a normal range.

relaxation response
Series of physiological changes that calm body systems and return them to normal functioning.

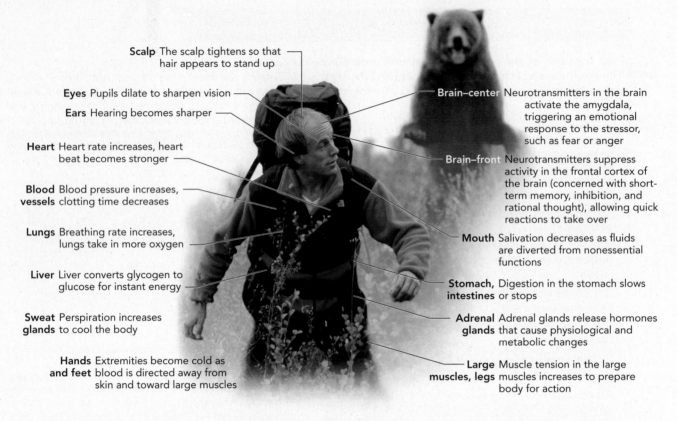

Scalp The scalp tightens so that hair appears to stand up

Eyes Pupils dilate to sharpen vision

Ears Hearing becomes sharper

Heart Heart rate increases, heart beat becomes stronger

Blood vessels Blood pressure increases, clotting time decreases

Lungs Breathing rate increases, lungs take in more oxygen

Liver Liver converts glycogen to glucose for instant energy

Sweat glands Perspiration increases to cool the body

Hands and feet Extremities become cold as blood is directed away from skin and toward large muscles

Brain–center Neurotransmitters in the brain activate the amygdala, triggering an emotional response to the stressor, such as fear or anger

Brain–front Neurotransmitters suppress activity in the frontal cortex of the brain (concerned with short-term memory, inhibition, and rational thought), allowing quick reactions to take over

Mouth Salivation decreases as fluids are diverted from nonessential functions

Stomach, intestines Digestion in the stomach slows or stops

Adrenal glands Adrenal glands release hormones that cause physiological and metabolic changes

Large muscles, legs Muscle tension in the large muscles increases to prepare body for action

figure **3.4** **The stress response: Changes in the body.**

body is equipped to deal with short-term, **acute stress** as long as it does not happen too often and as long as you can relax and recover afterward.

A problem occurs, however, when the stress response occurs repeatedly or when it persists without being turned off. In these instances, the stress response itself becomes damaging. Many people live in a state of **chronic stress,** in which stressful conditions are ongoing and the stress response continues without resolution. Chronic stress increases the likelihood that the person will become ill or, if already ill, that her or his defense system will be overwhelmed by the disease. Prolonged or severe stress has been found to weaken nearly every system in the body.

acute stress
Short-term stress, produced by the stress response.

chronic stress
Long-term, low-level stress in which the stress response continues without resolution.

General Adaptation Syndrome (GAS)
Selye's classic model used to describe the physiological changes associated with the stress response. The three phases are alarm, resistance, and exhaustion.

Stress and Your Health

Researchers have been looking at the relationship between stress and disease since the 1950s. One of the first scientists to develop a broad theory of stress and disease was Hans Selye.[30]

THE GENERAL ADAPTATION SYNDROME

Selye developed what he called the **General Adaptation Syndrome (GAS)** as a description and explanation of the physiological changes that he observed and that he believed to be predictable responses to stressors by all organisms. The process has three stages (Figure 3.5):

- *Alarm.* The body experiences the stress response. During this stage, immune system functioning is suppressed, and the person may be more susceptible to infections and illness.
- *Resistance.* The body works overtime to cope with the added stress and to stay at a peak level.
- *Exhaustion.* The body can no longer keep up with the demands of the stressor.

HEALTH EFFECTS OF STRESS

Stress plays a role in illness and disease in a variety of ways. (See the box "Symptoms of Stress.") For example, stress-triggered changes in the lungs increase the symptoms of asthma and other respiratory conditions. Stress appears to inhibit tissue repair, which increases the likelihood of bone fractures and is related to the development of osteoporosis (porous, weak bones). Stress can lead to sexual problems, including failure to ovulate and amenorrhea (absence of menstrual periods) in women and sexual dysfunction and loss of

Highlight on Health

Symptoms of Stress

Cognitive Symptoms
- Anxious thoughts
- Fearful anticipation
- Poor concentration
- Memory problems
- Continual worry
- Trouble thinking clearly
- Loss of sense of humor
- Lack of creativity

Emotional Symptoms
- Feelings of tension
- Irritability
- Restlessness
- Worries
- Inability to relax
- Depression
- Crying
- Lack of meaning in life and pursuits
- Loneliness
- Quick temper

Behavioral Symptoms
- Avoidance of tasks
- Sleep problems
- Fidgeting
- Tremors
- Grinding teeth
- Strained facial expression
- Clenched fists
- Changes in drinking, eating, or smoking behaviors
- Procrastination
- Increased drive to be with, or withdraw from, others

Physical Symptoms
- Stiff or tense muscles
- Sweating
- Tension headaches
- Feeling faint
- Feeling of choking
- Difficulty swallowing
- Stomachache, nausea, or vomiting
- Diarrhea or constipation
- Frequent or urgent urination
- Heart palpitations
- Backaches
- Fatigue

Social Symptoms
- Change in the quality of relationships

Source: Stress Management: Techniques for Preventing and Easing Stress, *by H. Benson, 2006, Cambridge, MA: Harvard Medical School Press.*

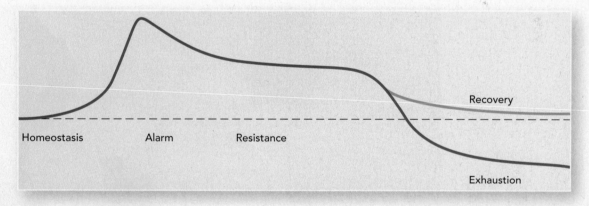

Homeostasis   Alarm   Resistance   Recovery   Exhaustion

figure 3.5   **General Adaptation Syndrome.** Selye's model describes the physiological response to stress. In the alarm stage, the body's fight-or-flight response is activated, accompanied by reduced immune system functioning. In the resistance stage, the body uses energy to adjust to the continued stress. After prolonged exposure to stress, the body may become totally depleted, leading to exhaustion, illness, and even death.

sexual desire in both men and women. Some suggest that high levels of stress can even speed up the aging process.[31]

The Immune System Since Selye's time, research has definitively shown that stress decreases immune function.

One study demonstrated a strong relationship between levels of psychological stress and the possibility of infection by a common cold virus. Other studies have found that both brief and long-term stressors have an impact on the function of the immune system.[32] Stressors as diverse as taking exams, experiencing major life events, and providing long-term care for someone with Alzheimer's disease affect the immune system. Scientists still do not fully understand why the stress response suppresses immune function or whether there is an evolutionary explanation for this suppression.

The Cardiovascular System   The stress response causes heart rate to accelerate and blood pressure to increase. When heart rate and blood pressure do not return to normal, as occurs in chronic stress, the person can experience elevated levels for long periods of time. Chronic hypertension (high blood pressure) makes blood vessels more susceptible to the development of atherosclerosis, a disease in which arteries are damaged and clogged with fatty deposits. Both hypertension and atherosclerosis increase the risk of heart attack and stroke. Overall stress levels are typically higher for individuals who have suffered heart attacks.

The Gastrointestinal System   Although not conclusive, evidence suggests that gastrointestinal problems can be stress related. More specifically, conditions such as acid reflux, indigestion, and stomach pain all seem to be more common in people who have higher levels or more frequent occurrences of stress. Irritable bowel syndrome (IBS) may be an example of individual response differences to the gastrointestinal tract by stress. When IBS patients are under stress, food seems to move more slowly through the small intestine in those individuals who are constipated; the opposite is true for those who suffer from diarrhea.

hot tip

What are the major stressors in your life right now? Brainstorm ways to get rid of them or to reduce their effects on you.

For a long time, stress was commonly believed to cause stomach ulcers. Research suggests, however, that ulcers may be caused or exacerbated by a bacterial infection that irritates the stomach lining. While not causing ulcers, stress may contribute to their development.

Mental Health   Both acute and chronic stress can contribute to psychological problems and the development of psychological illnesses, including anxiety disorders and depression. In *acute stress disorder*, for example, a person develops symptoms after experiencing severe trauma, such as assault, rape, domestic violence, child physical or sexual abuse, terrorist attacks, or natural disasters. Symptoms can include a feeling of numbness, a sense of being in a daze, amnesia, flashbacks, increased arousal and anxiety, and impairment in functioning.

If such symptoms appear 6 months or more after the traumatic event, the person may have *post-traumatic stress disorder (PTSD)*, a condition characterized by a sense of numbness or emotional detachment from people, repeated reliving of the event through flashbacks and/or nightmares, and avoidance of things that might be associated with the trauma (see the box "Jon: A Case of PTSD"). Years may pass after the trauma before PTSD symptoms appear.[11]

An example of a less severe stress-related disorder is *adjustment disorder*, in which a response to a stressor (such as anxiety, worry, social withdrawal) continues for a longer period than would normally be expected.

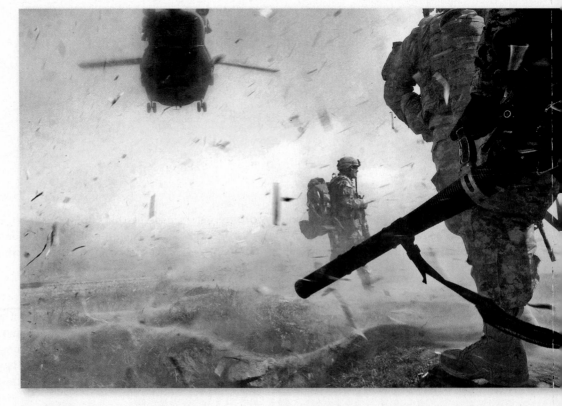

■ The stress and trauma of combat can lead to posttraumatic stress disorder in some individuals. Veterans of the conflicts in Iraq and Afghanistan have a wide range of mental health services available to them, but the stigma associated with accessing those services keeps many from getting effective treatment.

Life Stories

Jon: A Case of PTSD

Jon decided to join the army after high school. He knew he wanted to go to college, but he didn't feel like he had a good enough sense yet of what he wanted to study. Plus, his family didn't have a lot of money, and the college funding he would get from the G.I. bill would cover almost all of his education. After basic and advanced training, Jon did two tours of duty in Afghanistan, where his unit saw combat regularly.

Following his discharge from the army, Jon entered college. He was now 24, an older first-year student, who was excited about going to school to become an engineer. His life as a soldier was in the past now, as he saw it, and he was moving on to a new phase of his life. For most of his first year at school, Jon seemed to do well, but he also began to have bad dreams and intruding flashbacks of his war experiences. Anything that reminded him of his time in Afghanistan could set one off—the smell of gasoline, the slam of a door closing, or the screech of car brakes. Because he had trouble sleeping, he was consistently tired and felt on edge. He felt sad and guilty that he had survived combat while some of his friends had been

connect
ACTIVITY

wounded or killed. He didn't feel connected to anyone at school—what was the use of trying to make pointless small talk with people who had no idea about what he had been through? He even felt angry sometimes that he and his war buddies had been through so much while the younger students in his classes had such easy lives. As his sleep troubles, flashbacks, and social isolation worsened, Jon found it difficult to concentrate in class and complete his assignments. He tried to forget his problems by getting drunk, but that just made everything worse.

Jon didn't know what to do. Drop out of school? Reenlist in the army? Talk to someone? It was his nature to keep things inside and get through hardships on his own, but as he saw his life slipping out of control he decided to go for some counseling and get the help he needed before he destroyed himself or hurt others. Jon began to take part in individual and group therapy offered by the Department of Veterans Affairs; he found group therapy especially helpful because it made him feel less isolated and alone. With the help of counselors, his family, and his fellow veterans, he began the process of recovery.

Low-level, unresolved chronic stress can also be a factor in psychological problems. Stress can diminish wellness and reduce the ability to function at the highest level even without an identifiable disorder. Symptoms such as irritability, impatience, difficulty concentrating, excessive worrying, insomnia, and forgetfulness, like physical symptoms, can be addressed with stress management techniques.

Mediators of the Stress Response

Different people respond differently to stressors. Among the factors that may play a role in these differences are past experiences and overall level of wellness. Also critical are personality traits, habitual ways of thinking, and inborn or acquired attitudes toward the demands of life.

PERSONALITY FACTORS

In the 1970s two cardiologists, Meyer Friedman and Ray Rosenman, described and named the **Type A behavior pattern**.[33] Type A individuals tend to be impulsive, need to get things done quickly, and live their lives on a time schedule. They are hard driving, achievement oriented, and highly competitive. Some estimates are that more than 40 percent of the population of the United States and possibly half of all men might be Type As.

Individuals who fit this description are prime candidates for stress-related illnesses. The relationship between Type A personality traits and heart disease has been known for some time. More recently, there have been indications that a Type A personality can mean increased risk for a number of other diseases, including peptic ulcers, asthma, headaches, and thyroid problems.

However, not all the characteristics of this personality seem to be harmful. Many Type As are achievement oriented and successful and yet remain healthy. According to recent research, a key culprit is **hostility**, defined as an ongoing accumulation of irritation and anger. Hostile individuals are generally cynical toward others, frequently express anger, and display aggressive behaviors.[34] Research has indicated that hostility, by itself, is related to coronary heart disease, and it may also contribute to premature death.[35]

Friedman and Rosenman also described a constellation of personality traits they labeled Type B. In contrast to the Type A personality, the Type B personality is less driven and more relaxed. Type Bs are more easygoing and less readily frustrated. All other things being equal, Type Bs are less susceptible to coronary heart disease.

Other experts have expanded on Friedman and Rosenman's research and have found two additional personality types. Type C personalities are introverted, detail-oriented

Type A behavior pattern
Set of personality traits originally thought to be associated with risk for heart disease. Type A individuals are hard driving, competitive, achievement oriented, and quick to anger; further research has identified hostility as the key risk factor in the pattern.

hostility
Ongoing accumulation of irritation and anger.

people who may have trouble communicating and appear to be very cautious and reserved. Type D individuals appear to hold in negative emotions and are not very expressive. They experience negative emotions like anger, anxiety, and sadness while fearing negative judgments from others. Type Ds are also at risk for negative health outcomes, including arterial disease, heart failure, and poor health ratings.[36]

COGNITIVE FACTORS

Until you decide that an event is actually a threat and/or beyond your ability to cope, it remains merely a potential stressor. Experts suggest that people create their own distress with their habitual thinking patterns—illogical thinking, unrealistic expectations, and negative beliefs.[28] For example, a person may think she has to get straight As in order to be a worthy human being. If she gets a B, she will experience much more stress than if she had more realistic expectations about herself and was more self-forgiving. Her ideas can transform a relatively neutral event into a stressor.

Other common illogical ideas and unrealistic expectations are "life should be fair," "friends should be there when you need them," "everyone I care about has to love and approve of me," and "everything has to go my way." When everyday experiences don't live up to these ideas, people who

■ Many performers lack the resources needed to handle the stress of celebrity and constant media attention. In a February 2010 interview, actress Lindsay Lohan admitted that she had used alcohol and drugs to mask her problems. Five months later, she was sentenced to 90 days in jail for failing to attend court-ordered alcohol education classes.

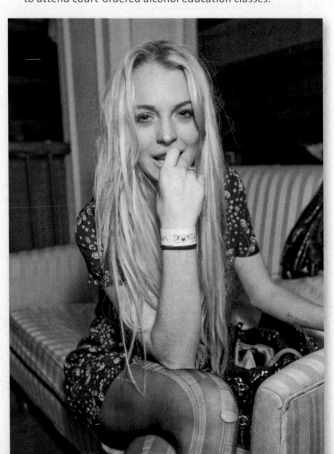

hold them end up feeling angry, frustrated, disappointed, or demoralized. (For more on cognitive distortions, see the box "Challenge Your Thinking.") With a more realistic attitude, they can take things in stride and reduce the frequency and intensity of the stress response. This doesn't mean they should have unrealistically low expectations. When expectations are too low, people may experience underachievement, depression, resignation, and lowered self-esteem. The goal is a realistic balance.

RESILIENCE AND HARDINESS

Just as resilience is a factor in mental health, it is also a factor in the ability to handle stress. Stress-resistant people also seem to focus on immediate issues and explain their struggle in positive and helpful ways. For example, a poor grade on one exam might motivate the stress-resilient person to study harder, using the grade as motivation. A person who is not so resilient may react to a poor grade by feeling like a failure and giving up.

Another line of research has developed the concept of **hardiness**, an effective style of coping with stress. Researchers have studied people who were exposed to a great deal of stress but never seemed to become ill as a result.[37,38] The researchers suggest that positive ways of coping with stress may buffer the body from its effects. They call this style *hardiness* and have suggested that people high in hardiness are more resistant to illness.

These researchers found that hardy people (1) perceive the demands of living as a challenge rather than a threat, (2) are committed to meaningful activities, and (3) have a sense of control over their lives.

Having a sense of control may be especially critical in avoiding illness and responding to stressful situations. In sum, these researchers found that people who demonstrate an ability to see life as a challenge, who are committed to what they do, and who believe they are in control tend to do better.

hardiness
Effective style of coping with stress, characterized by a tendency to view life events as challenges rather than threats, a commitment to meaningful activities, and a sense of being in control.

Daily hassles such as arguments, car problems, and money worries can lead to a **state of chronic, low-level stress,** *especially if they pile up and you don't have a period of recovery.*

Challenges & Choices

Challenge Your Thinking

Distorted thinking can increase your stress levels unnecessarily. Learning to recognize your negative thinking patterns, challenging them, and replacing them with healthier, more balanced ways of thinking can be an effective stress-buster. If you notice a distorted thought, try to examine it logically. For example, is it really likely that not getting one job offer means you'll never get a job you want? Or that not having a date this weekend means you'll never find the right romantic partner? It takes vigilance and practice to take the power out of habitual thinking patterns, but the effort is worth it. Your stress levels will go down and your sense of well-being will go up!

Common Patterns of Distorted Thinking

- Focusing on the negative; filtering out the positive.
- Magnifying the bad things; minimizing the good things.

- Catastrophizing—expecting the worst.
- Overgeneralizing—creating expectations based on one incident.
- Blaming others for everything; blaming yourself for everything.
- Personalizing—thinking everything going on around you is about you.
- Mind reading—assuming you know what others are thinking and feeling without checking it out with them.
- Being perfectionistic—thinking you have to be perfect and it's not okay to make a mistake.
- Thinking in black and white—thinking if it's not one way, it's the other, when really there are always shades of gray; seeing only options 1 and 10 and missing all the options in between.

Sources of Stress

Contemporary life presents us with nearly limitless sources of stress, ranging from major life events to our interpersonal relationships to some of our own feelings. In this section we describe some of these stressors, along with a variety of tips for handling them.

LIFE EVENTS

Can stressful life events make people more vulnerable to illness? Thomas Holmes and Richard Rahe, medical researchers at the University of Washington, observed that individuals frequently experienced major life events before the onset of an illness. They proposed that life events—major changes and transitions that force the individual to adjust and adapt—may precipitate illness, especially if several such events occur at the same time.[39] Holmes and Rahe developed a scale of stressful life events and compared it to the onset of illnesses. From this work they developed the Holmes-Rahe Social Readjustment Scale, a list of life events that require the individual to adjust and adapt to change. The higher a person's score on the scale, the more likely that person is to experience symptoms of illness.

The most stressful event on this scale is the death of a spouse, followed by such events as divorce, separation, a personal injury, and being fired from a job. Less stressful events on the scale include moving, going on vacation, experiencing a change in sleeping habits, and dealing with a minor violation of the law.

DAILY HASSLES

Surprisingly, everyday hassles can also cause health problems. In fact, daily hassles are related to subsequent illness and disease to a greater degree than are major life events.[40] Daily hassles include arguments, car problems, deadlines, traffic jams, long lines, money worries, and so on. All of these events can lead to a state of chronic, low-level stress, especially if they pile up and you don't have a period of recovery.

College Stress   College students experience a great deal of life change, and some studies even suggest that the college years may be the most stressful time in people's lives.[41,42] In

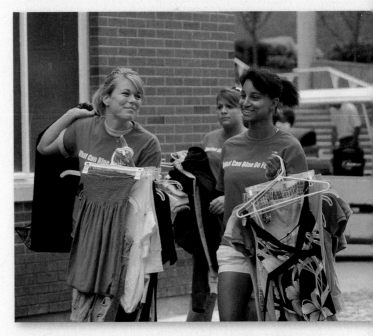

- Starting college is a major life transition with unique stressors. Individuals with the qualities of resilience and hardiness are able to take the challenges in stride and respond with energy and excitement.

one survey of college students, stress was identified as the top health concern, with 27 percent of respondents reporting that stress affected their academic performance.[16] Considering the health effects of stress, it should not be surprising that colds, mononucleosis, and sexually transmitted diseases are familiar on college campuses.

Besides the effect of this major life transition, common sources of stress for college students include academic work, exams and grades, sleep deprivation, worries about money, relationship concerns, and uncertainty about their futures. The pressure of college may be growing even more intense, particularly for young women. In one survey, 30 percent of first-year students described themselves as frequently feeling overwhelmed. Women were nearly twice as likely to feel this way as men.[43]

Rising tuition costs also appear to affect stress levels of many students. A record number of students say they have to work to afford college, and again, women in greater numbers describe themselves as feeling the pressure to work. Concern about the economy and being successful also has an impact on students.

College officials indicate that although more young people are going to college, they might also be less prepared to deal with college stressors and expectations. Almost all college students describe themselves as being depressed during their college experience, although the depression is often moderate and of a short duration. These episodes are often related to specific stressors, such as difficulties in a relationship, poor grades, and general adjustment concerns. When the intensity of the situation increases or the student is unable to find support, symptoms such as changes in appetite or increases in risk-taking behaviors, self-injurious behaviors, and smoking may appear.

Many college students adopt habits to deal with stress that are ineffective, counterproductive, and ultimately unhealthy:

- *Use of tobacco*. The chemicals in tobacco can make a smoker feel both more relaxed and more alert. However, nicotine is highly addictive, and smoking causes a host of health problems. Tobacco use is the leading preventable cause of death in the United States.

- *Use and abuse of alcohol*. Moderate use of alcohol can lower inhibitions and create a sense of social ease and relaxation, but drinking provides only temporary relief without addressing the sources of stress. Heavy drinking and binge drinking carry risks of their own, including the risk of addiction. All too often, what began as a solution becomes a new problem.

- *Use and abuse of other drugs*. Like alcohol, illicit drugs alter mood and mind without solving problems, and they often cause additional problems. For example, stimulants like

hot tip

Practice polite ways to decline invitations when you're feeling overwhelmed or aren't really interested in the event.

methamphetamine and cocaine increase mental alertness and energy, but they can induce the stress response and disrupt sleep. Opiates like oxycodone (OxyContin) and hydrocodone (Vicodin) can relieve pain and anxiety, but tolerance develops quickly, making dependence likely. Marijuana can cause panic attacks, and even caffeine raises blood pressure and levels of stress hormones.

- *Use of food to manage feelings*. Many people overeat or eat unhealthy foods when they feel stressed. According to one survey, the top "comfort foods" are candy, ice cream, chips, cookies and cakes, fast food, and pizza, in that order.[27] Other people eat less or skip meals in response to stress. For most of us, eating is a pleasurable, relaxing experience, but using food to manage feelings and stress can lead to disordered eating patterns as well as overweight and obesity.

Other approaches to stress management popular with college students are listening to music, socializing with friends, going to movies, and reading. Though not unhealthy, these sedentary activities need to be balanced with more active stress management techniques, such as walking or exercising.

Colleges usually offer resources to help students deal with stress, and at some major universities 40 percent of all undergraduates visit the counseling center. However, a sign that not enough students are getting the help they need is the fact that suicide is the second leading cause of death on college campuses. More effort must be made to reach and educate students about stress reduction and stress management techniques, including time management, relaxation techniques, exercise, and good nutrition.

Job Pressure   More than two in three Americans say that work is a significant source of stress, and stress has been found to impact productivity.[27] Half of all employees stated that they lost productivity at work due to stress, and a large portion of young people (60 percent) report being less productive because of work stress.[27] Satisfaction with one's employer remains low, and about one in three workers reports an intention to seek employment elsewhere.[27]

Job pressure contributes to many stress-related illnesses, including cardiovascular disease, and may be related to the incidence of back pain, fatigue, muscular pain, and headaches. The costs are high in terms of dollars and worker performance, seen in accidents, absenteeism, turnover, reduced levels of productivity, and insurance costs.

Over the past century many jobs have become physically easier, but expectations have grown that people will work more. Managers and professionals seem to work the longest days and are subject to associated stresses.[44] They bring work home and thus never really leave the job. Almost 35 percent of American workers do not take all their allotted vacation time each year, and almost 25 percent check their

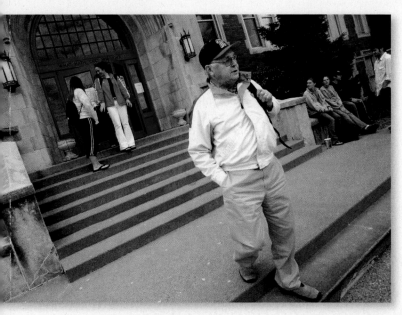

■ Returning or reentry college students experience their own stressors, including worries that they may not measure up, concerns about fitting in, and the need to balance school, work, and family obligations.

e-mail or voicemail while on vacation.[45] Many people who want to be successful become *workaholics*, never taking a break from work and setting themselves up for burnout.

burnout
Adverse work-related stress reaction with physical, psychological, and behavioral components.

Burnout is an adverse, work-related stress reaction with physical, psychological, and behavioral components.[46] The symptoms of burnout include increasing discouragement and pessimism about work; a decline in motivation and job performance; irritability, anger, and apathy on the job; and physical complaints.[47]

Money and Financial Worries   Over 70 percent of Americans say that money is a source of stress.[27] Financial worries take a particular toll on young people, with 80 percent of 18–30-year-olds, more than any other age group, saying that money is a source of stress.[27]

Many people experience financial stress because their income is not equal to their expenditures. Familiar sources of financial stress are fear of running short of money before the end of the month, carrying too much debt, reduced employment or unemployment, no savings to cover medical emergencies, and unexpected home or car repairs.

One of the best ways to relieve financial stress is to plan ahead. Being willing to follow a budget and make the lifestyle changes necessary to live within available funds may be the key to relief from financial stress. Simplifying your life, shedding those items and events that you can live without, can be liberating. Finding ways to ensure financial peace of mind is an excellent stress reduction technique.

FAMILY AND INTERPERSONAL STRESS

Families have to continuously adapt to a series of life changes and transitions. The birth of a baby places new demands on parents and siblings, and families must adapt as a teenager moves through adolescence to adulthood and leaves home. A family may be disrupted by death or divorce, and in fact, a growing number of children spend part of their lives in single-parent households, blended family units, or stepfamily systems.

Families may become weakened by these experiences, or they may become stronger and more resilient. Relationships of all kinds have the potential to be stressful, including intimate partnerships. Many experts agree that the key to a successful relationship is not finding the perfect partner but being able to communicate effectively with the partner you have. Whereas poor communication skills can cause interactions to escalate into arguments and fights (or deteriorate into cold silences), thoughtful communication and conflict resolution techniques can resolve issues before they become problems.

Time Pressure, Overload, and Technology   Most of us experience some degree of time pressure in our lives. Many people find that they have more and more to do, despite time-saving devices, and want to compress more activity into less time. Multitasking is common—people talk on the phone while driving, answer e-mail while eating lunch, take laptops on vacation. While many people think they are more efficient and productive when they multitask, multitasking actually causes people to become distractible and perform poorly on a variety of tasks.[48] The rush to do things quickly and simultaneously ends up increasing levels of stress.

Many people do not see their overstuffed schedules as a problem. Instead, they go to time management classes to learn how to squeeze more activities into the time they have. Although planning and good use of time are effective stress management techniques, there are limits to how much a person can do. Many times the solution is not to use time more effectively but to do less. Many "stressed-out" people are not poor stress managers; they are simply overloaded with responsibilities. Sometimes, learning to say no to others' requests is the best way to handle time management issues.

Most new technologies are designed to save time and improve life, but they can also be sources of stress. We feel pressure to learn them and master them; once they are widely accepted, we find we are expected to use them to get more done in less time.

Simplifying your life, *shedding those items and events that you can live without,* **can be liberating.**

Technology also has the effect of making us constantly available and never fully alone. Friends can reach us anytime with a text message or an e-mail, and work knows how to contact us outside of the office. With communication happening so quickly, we feel we must respond right away—even if we are doing something else or trying to relax. We may find that we have more "friends" on social networking sites than we can have meaningful contact with, but we continue to widen our social circles, simply adding stress to our lives. The idea of quality time with one's children has even been compromised. On a typical visit to a playground, you are likely to find parents checking their e-mail and reviewing their fantasy football teams on a smart phone while their children play.

of those with war zone experience in Vietnam developed PTSD.[49] Again, this is evidence of the role of mediating factors in the individual experience of stress.

Societal Issues Intolerance, prejudice, discrimination, injustice, poverty, pressure to conform to mainstream culture—all are common sources of stress for members of modern society. Exposure to racism and homophobia, for example, can cause distrust, frustration, resentment, negative emotions such as anger and fear, and a sense of helplessness and hopelessness. Experiencing racism has been associated with both physical and mental health-related symptoms, including hypertension, cardiovascular reactivity, depression, eating disorders, substance abuse, and violence.[50,51]

Exposure to racism and homophobia can cause distrust, frustration, resentment, negative emotions such as anger and fear, and a **sense of helplessness and hopelessness.**

Anger Sometimes the source of stress is within the individual. Unresolved feelings of anger can be extremely stressful. The idea that blowing off steam, or venting, is a positive way to deal with anger is generally not the case. Releasing anger in an uncontrolled way often reinforces the feeling and may cause it to escalate into rage.[28] Venting can create anger in the person on the receiving end and hurts relationships. Suppressing anger or turning it against oneself is also unhealthy, lowering self-esteem and possibly fostering depression.

If you find yourself in a situation in which you are getting angry, take a time-out, remove yourself from the situation physically, and take some deep breaths. Examine the situation and think about whether your reaction is logical or illogical and whether you could see it another way. Look for absurdity or humor in the situation. Put it in perspective. If you cannot avoid the situation or reduce your reaction, try some of the stress management strategies and relaxation techniques described later in this chapter.

Trauma The effect of traumatic experiences has received a great deal of study. The events of September 11, 2001, and military service in Iraq and Afghanistan are frequently cited as traumatic events of the highest order. Human beings are not equipped to deal effectively with events of this magnitude. They overwhelm our ability to cope and destroy any sense of control, connection, or meaning. They shake the foundations of beliefs about the safety and trustworthiness of the world.

Some people develop post-traumatic stress disorder (PTSD) in response to trauma, as described earlier in this chapter. Although the triggering event may be overwhelming, often it alone is not sufficient to explain the occurrence of PTSD. Many people who are exposed to a traumatic event never develop PTSD. For example, fewer than 40 percent

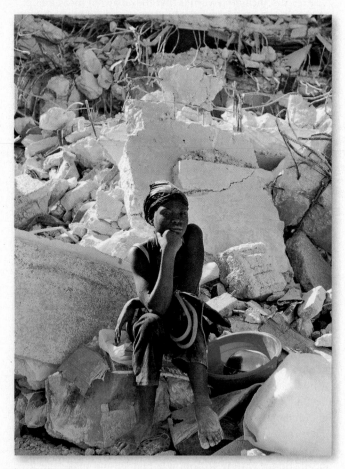

■ Natural disasters, like the 7.0 magnitude earthquake that struck Haiti in January 2010, create trauma and stress for those affected. In Haiti, the acute stress of the earthquake came on top of chronic stressors like widespread poverty, environmental degradation, and political and economic problems.

Similar effects are seen in lesbians, gay males, bisexuals, and transgender individuals when they are the targets of prejudice and homophobia.[52,53] These individuals often have higher rates of school-related problems, substance abuse, criminal activity, prostitution, running away from home, and suicide than do their nongay peers.

Managing Stress

The effects of unrelieved stress on the body and mind can range from muscle tension to a pervasive sense of hopelessness about the future, yet life without stress is unrealistic if not impossible. The solution is to find effective ways to manage stress.

CHOOSING AN APPROACH TO STRESS MANAGEMENT

There are many different ways to manage stress, but not all of them appeal to everyone. What works for someone else may not be helpful or comfortable for you. For example, some individuals feel comfortable with meditation, while others need a more active stress reduction method and might choose exercise. As you review the methods described in the following pages, consider how they might fit with your personality and lifestyle. Experiment with a few methods—and try something new—before you settle on something you think will work for you. Whatever methods you choose, we recommend practicing them on a regular basis. They will become second nature to you and part of your everyday life. They will be available during stressful moments and may even be activated naturally.

Sometimes stressful events and situations are overwhelming, and your resources and coping abilities are insufficient to support you. These times call for professional help. Don't hesitate to visit your college counseling center or avail yourself of other resources if you find that you need more support.

STRESS REDUCTION STRATEGIES

Any activity that decreases the number or lessens the effect of stressors is a stress reduction technique. Although you might not think of avoidance as an effective coping strategy, sometimes protecting yourself from unnecessary stressors makes sense. For example, try not listening to the news for a few days. You'll find that world events continue as always without your participation. If certain people in your life consistently trigger negative feelings in you, try not seeing them for a while. When you do see them, you may have

a better perspective on your interpersonal dynamics. If you have too many activities going on in your life, assert your right to say no to the next request for your time. Downscaling and simplifying your life are effective ways of alleviating stress.

Time Management   Time management is the topic of seminars and books, and some experts have devoted their entire careers to helping people learn how to manage their time. Here, we focus just on two key points: planning and prioritizing.

To improve planning, ask yourself if you are focusing on the things that are most important to you. You may be focusing on the right tasks if

- You're engaged in activities that advance your overall purpose in life
- You're doing things you have always wanted to do or that make you feel good about yourself
- You're working on tasks you don't like, but you're doing them knowing they relate to the bigger picture[54]

To make sure you focus on the things that matter to you, think about your goals in life and what you want to achieve. Are they worthy of your time? Obviously, you need time for sleeping, working, studying, and so on, but remember to allow yourself time for maintaining wellness through such activities as relaxing, playing, and spending time with family and friends. A global picture of your goals and priorities provides a framework and perspective that can give you a sense of control and reduce stress.

When you want to manage your time on the everyday level, keep a daily "to do" list and prioritize the items on it. Write the items down, because it's stressful to just keep them in your head! As you look at the list, assign each task a priority:

- Is it something you must get done today, such as turning in a paper?

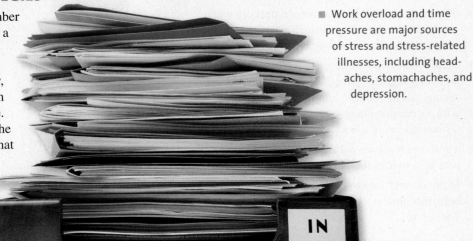

■ Work overload and time pressure are major sources of stress and stress-related illnesses, including headaches, stomachaches, and depression.

■ Is it something you would like to get done, such as catching up on the week's reading?

■ Is it something that can wait until tomorrow, such as buying a new pair of jeans?

Then organize the items into these three categories. Complete the tasks in the first category first, before moving on to tasks in the other two categories. This approach will help you be more purposeful, organized, and efficient about the use of your time, giving you more of a sense of control in your life.

In the course of evaluating your goals and prioritizing your daily tasks, you may find that you have too many commitments, an issue discussed earlier in the chapter. Trying to do more than you have time for and doing the wrong things in the time you have are stressful. Managing your time well is a key to reducing stress.

Social Support Another key to reducing stress, just as it is a key to mental health and to a meaningful spiritual life, is social support. Numerous studies show that social support decreases the stress response hormones in the body. Dr. Dean Ornish points out that people who have close relationships and a strong sense of connection and community enjoy better health and live longer than do those who live in isolation. People who suffer alone suffer a lot.[55]

Many people lack the sense of belonging and community that was provided by the extended family and closer-knit society of our grandparents' day. You may have to consciously create a social support system to overcome isolation and loneliness and buffer yourself from stress.[56,57] The benefits make the effort worthwhile. They include a shoulder to lean on and an ear to listen when you need support. Communicating about your feelings reduces stress and helps you to work through problems and feel better about yourself.

The best way to develop a support system is to give support to others, establishing relationships and building trust:

■ Cultivate a variety of types of relationships.

■ Stay in touch with your friends, especially when you know they're going through a hard time, and keep your family ties strong.

■ Find people who share your interests and pursue activities together, whether it's hiking, dancing, or seeing classic movies. You may want to join a group with a goal that interests you, such as a church group, a study group, or a book club.

■ Try to get involved with your community and participate in activities that benefit others.

■ Maintain and improve your communication skills—both listening to other people's feelings and sharing your own.

When you have a network of relationships and a community to belong to, you will be able to cope with the stress of life more effectively. And when you need support, you will have a connection that can be reciprocated comfortably.

A Healthy Lifestyle A healthy lifestyle is an essential component of any stress management program. A nutritious diet helps you care for your body and keeps you at your best. Experts recommend emphasizing whole grains, vegetables, and fruits in the diet and avoiding excessive amounts of caffeine. Getting enough sleep is also essential for wellness, as are opportunities for relaxation and fun.

Exercise is probably the most popular and most effective stress buster available. It has a positive effect on both physical and mental functioning and helps people withstand stress. Regular exercisers are also less likely to use smoking, drinking, or overeating as methods for reducing their levels of stress.[58] A growing body of evidence suggests that getting regular exercise is the best thing you can do to protect yourself from the effects of stress. While many people say they "Just don't have enough time," all you really need is a jump rope and 15–20 minutes each day.

RELAXATION TECHNIQUES

If you are in a state of chronic stress and the relaxation response does not happen naturally, it is in your best interest to learn how to induce it. Relaxation techniques seem to have an effect on a number of physiological functions, including blood pressure, heart rate, and muscle tension.[59] Here we describe just a few of the many techniques that have been developed.

Deep Breathing One relaxation tool that is simple and always available is breathing. When you feel yourself starting to experience the stress response, you can simply remember to breathe deeply. As

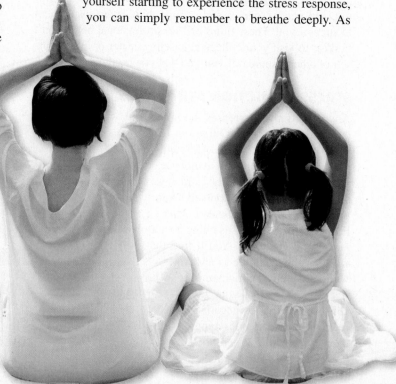

you learn to be aware of breathing patterns and practice slowing that process, your mind and body will begin to relax. Breathing exercises have been found to be effective in reducing panic attacks, muscle tension, headaches, and fatigue.

To practice deep breathing, inhale through your nose slowly and deeply through the count of 10. Don't just raise your shoulders and chest; allow your abdomen to expand as well. Exhale very slowly through your nose or through gently pursed lips and concentrate fully on your breath as you let it out. Try to repeat this exercise a number of times during the day even when you're not feeling stressed. Once it becomes routine, use it to help relax before an exam or in any stressful situation.

Progressive Relaxation Progressive muscle relaxation is based on the premise that deliberate muscle relaxation will block the muscle tension that is part of the stress response, thus reducing overall levels of stress. Progressive relaxation has provided relief when used to treat such stress-related symptoms as neck and back pain and high blood pressure.

To practice progressive muscle relaxation, find a quiet place and lie down in a comfortable position without crossing your arms or legs. Maintain a slow breathing pattern while you tense each muscle or muscle group as tightly as possible for 10 seconds before releasing it. Begin by making a fist with one hand, holding it, and then releasing it. Notice the difference between the tensed state and the relaxed state, and allow your muscles to remain relaxed. Continue with your other hand, your arms, shoulders, neck, and so on, moving around your entire body. Don't forget your ears, forehead, mouth, and all the muscles of your face.

If you take the time to relax your body this way, the technique will provide significant relief from stress. You will also find that once your body learns the process, you will be able to relax your muscles quickly on command during moments of stress.

Visualization Also called *guided imagery*, visualization is the mental creation of visual images and scenes. Because our thoughts have such a powerful influence on our reactions, simply imagining a relaxing scene can bring about the relaxation response.[48] Visualization can be used alone or in combination with other techniques such as deep breathing and meditation to help reduce stress, tension, and anxiety.

To try visualization, sit or lie in a quiet place. Imagine yourself in a soothing, peaceful scene, one that you find particularly relaxing—a quiet beach, a garden, a spot in the woods. Try to visualize all you would see there as vividly as you can,

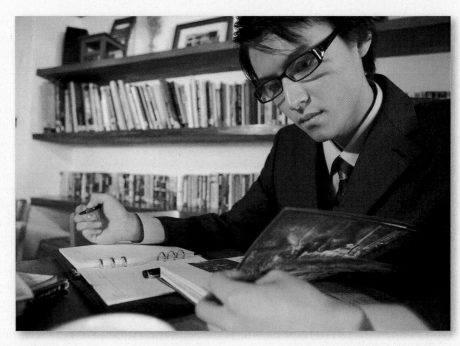

■ Time management skills are effective tools in reducing stress. Keeping a daily planner can help you stay organized and on track throughout your day.

scanning the scene. Bring in your other senses; what sounds do you hear, what scents do you smell? Is the sun warm, the breeze gentle? If you can imagine the scene fully, your body will respond as if you were really there. Commercial tapes are also available that use guided imagery to promote relaxation, but because imagery is personal and subjective, you may need to be selective in finding a tape that works for you.

Yoga The ancient practice of yoga is rooted in Hindu philosophy, with physical, mental, and spiritual components. It is a consciously performed activity involving posture, breath, and body and mind awareness. In the path and practice of yoga, the aim is to calm the mind, cleanse the body, and raise awareness. The outcomes of this practice include a release of mental and physical tension and the attainment of a relaxed state.

The most widely practiced form of yoga in the Western world is hatha yoga. The practitioner assumes a number of different postures, or poses, holding them while stretching, breathing, and balancing. They are performed slowly and gently, with focused attention. Yoga stretching improves flexibility as well as muscular strength and endurance. For yoga to be effective, the poses have to be performed correctly. If you are interested in trying yoga, we recommend that you begin by taking a class with a certified instructor. There are also commercial videos that can get you started.

T'ai Chi T'ai chi is a form of Chinese martial arts that dates back to the 14th century. Central to this method is the concept of *qi*, or life energy, and practicing t'ai chi is said to increase and promote the flow of *qi* throughout the body. T'ai chi combines 13 postures with elements of other

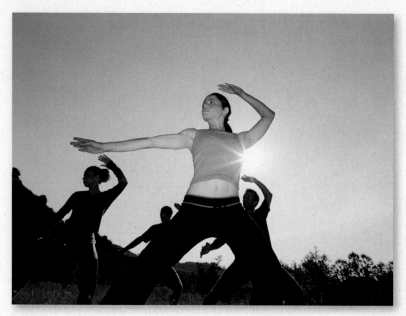

■ T'ai chi is a calming and energizing practice that can be used to elicit relaxation and manage stress.

stress-relieving techniques, such as exercise, meditation, and deep breathing. Research has shown that t'ai chi is beneficial in combating stress, although exactly how it works is unclear. You can take t'ai chi classes in a group setting, although these are not as widely available as yoga classes. Using instructional videos to learn t'ai chi is another option.

Biofeedback   Biofeedback is a kind of relaxation training that involves the use of special equipment to provide feedback on the body's physiological functions. You receive information about your heart rate, breathing, skin temperature, and other autonomic nervous system activities and thus become more aware of exactly what is happening in your body during both the relaxation response and the stress response. Once you have this heightened awareness, you can use relaxation techniques at the first sign of the stress response in daily life. Biofeedback can be used to reduce tension headaches,

affirmations
Positive thoughts that you can write down or say to yourself to balance negative thoughts.

chronic muscle pain, hypertension, and anxiety.[60] If you are interested in trying biofeedback, check with your school to see if the special equipment and training are available.

Affirmations   The literature is clear that when people have an optimistic attitude and a positive view of themselves, they are less likely to suffer the negative effects of stress. **Affirmations** are positive thoughts that you can write down or say to yourself to balance the negative thoughts you may have internalized over the course of your life. Repeatedly reciting such negative, distorted thoughts can increase stress levels. Although they may seem silly to some people, affirmations can help you shift from a negative view of yourself to a more positive one. The more often you repeat an affirmation, the more likely you are to believe it.

To create affirmations for yourself, think about areas of your life in which you would like to see improvements, such as health, self-esteem, or happiness, and then imagine what that change would look like. Here are some examples:

■ I make healthy choices for myself.

■ I am the right weight for me.

■ The more grateful I am, the more reasons I find to be grateful.

■ I love and accept myself.

■ I attract only healthy relationships.

■ I have abundant energy, vitality, and well-being.

■ I can open my heart and let wonderful things flow into my life.

We have provided a sampling of stress reducing techniques; there are many others. Many people develop their own relaxation strategies, such as listening to soothing music, going for walks in a beautiful setting, or enjoying the company of a pet. Whatever your preferences, learn to incorporate peaceful moments into your day, every day. You will experience improved quality of life today and a better chance of avoiding stress-related illness in the future.

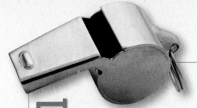

You Make the Call

Should Teachers and Administrators Be Responsible for Recognizing Mental Health Problems in Students?

On Friday, November 1, 1991, a physics student in a PhD program at the University of Iowa shot and killed three faculty members, one administrator, and a fellow physics student and permanently paralyzed a student employee. The student, Gang Lu, then killed himself. Lu was upset that he had not won a dissertation prize. In news reports following the murders, Lu was described as being extremely bright and capable but having a very bad temper and psychological problems.

On Tuesday, April 20, 1999, two students at Columbine High School in Littleton, Colorado, carried out a shooting rampage, which killed 12 students and a teacher and wounded 24 others, before committing suicide. Three years earlier, one of the students, Eric Harris, had begun a blog that included instructions on how to make bombs and expressed threats of violence against other students and teachers. The county sheriff's office was notified of the site, but no action was taken. In 1998 Harris and his friend Dylan Klebold were caught with stolen computer equipment and sentenced to juvenile diversion. They attended anger management classes, and Harris started seeing a psychiatrist. He was prescribed antidepressants and was taking them at the time of the shootings.

On April 16, 2007, Seung-Hui Cho killed 33 people and wounded 25 before killing himself at Virginia Tech University in Blacksburg, Virginia. Cho had been accused of stalking two female students in 2005 and was declared mentally ill by a Virginia special justice. An English professor had found Cho's writing so disturbing that she asked to have him removed from her creative writing class to protect the other students. During Cho's time at Virginia Tech, at least one professor had recommended that he seek counseling.

On February 14, 2008, Steven Kazmierczak, a graduate of Northern Illinois University, killed 5 students and injured 16 others when he entered a lecture hall and opened fire. Kazmierczak was seeing a psychiatrist and reportedly taking Xanax (for anxiety), Ambien (for insomnia), and Prozac (for depression). He had discontinued the Prozac about 3 weeks before the shooting, and his subsequent behavior was described as erratic.

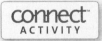

Four separate incidents, with one striking thing in common—people in authority, including mental health professionals, were aware of how troubled these individuals were. Although treatment was recommended, mandated, or even in progress, tragedies still occurred.

Some observers believe that faculty and administrators should have recognized the students' mental health problems and done more to prevent the shootings. They believe people in authority should be proactive about intervening when they see red flags suggesting a person is mentally disturbed. They argue that such individuals should be required to participate in mental health treatment or be expelled from school. They also argue that counselors in college counseling centers should breach confidentiality if they believe a client poses a threat to other students. (State laws vary regarding the circumstances that justify or require breaking client-therapist confidentiality.)

Opponents respond that such a hypervigilant attitude would have a chilling effect on free speech and could result in civil rights violations for some eccentric but harmless individuals. They point out that mass killings, though tragic and catastrophic, are very rare and proposed measures are an overreaction. They also argue that it's unrealistic and unfair to place the responsibility for recognizing mental illness on untrained persons. What do you think?

PROS

- The safety of students and staff should be the highest priority of any college administration. Schools should be safe havens.

- Those who have the most contact with troubled individuals—faculty and other students—are most likely to be able to recognize a dangerous individual. The more people who report such an individual, the more likely that person is to get help.

- Even if some innocent or harmless people are embarrassed or feel harassed, it's worth it to prevent mass killings.

CONS

- Free speech and protection of civil rights should be the highest priority of college administrations. Encouraging students and faculty to identify persons they view as a threat could create a climate of suspicion, reminiscent of a witch hunt.

- Students and professors are not qualified to make mental health assessments; most of their referrals are likely to be inappropriate.

- Harmless individuals who are identified as threats or who are forced to get an assessment will be needlessly harassed, stigmatized, and traumatized.

- If client-therapist confidentiality can be breached, individuals who need treatment and could benefit from it —for example, by talking about their anger instead of acting on it—would be less likely to seek help.

IN REVIEW

What is mental health?

Mental health is usually conceptualized as the presence of many positive qualities, such as optimism, a sense of self-efficacy, and resilience (the ability to bounce back from adversity). Some specific approaches include positive psychology's focus on "character strengths and virtues," Maslow's self-actualization model, and Goleman's concept of emotional intelligence.

How is mental illness treated?

The two broad approaches to treatment are medications and psychotherapy. Both are effective.

What is stress?

Stress is defined as a general state of the body, mind, and emotions when an environmental stressor has triggered the stress response. It can be thought of as a transaction between an individual and a stressor, mediated by personal variables that include the person's perceptions and appraisal of the event. The stress response, also known as the fight-or-flight response, is the set of physiological changes that occurs in the body in the face of a threat.

What are the main approaches to managing stress?

Stress can be managed by using stress reduction strategies such as time management and eliciting social support; by maintaining a healthy lifestyle that includes a balanced diet, exercise, and adequate sleep and that excludes self-medicating with alcohol, drugs, and tobacco; and by practicing relaxation techniques. These techniques include deep breathing, progressive relaxation, visualization, yoga, t'ai chi, biofeedback, and affirmations.

Web Resources

American Institute of Stress: This organization is a clearinghouse for information on all stress-related topics. Its monthly newsletter, *Health and Stress*, presents the latest advances in stress research and related health issues.
www.stress.org

American Psychiatric Association (APA): This organization offers a helpful fact sheet series and a Let's Talk Facts pamphlet series, both designed to dispel myths about mental illness. The Web site also includes information about mental health treatment and related insurance issues.
www.psych.org

American Psychological Association (Help Center): This organization offers information on many topics, such as work/school issues, family and relationships, stress, and health and emotional wellness.
http://helping.apa.org

Harvard Mind-Body Medical Institute: Highlighting the work of Herbert Benson, M.D., author of *The Relaxation Response,* this organization presents information on mind-body basics and wellness. It offers ways to deal with stress in everyday life.
www.mbmi.org

National Alliance for the Mentally Ill (NAMI): NAMI is a nonprofit organization for people affected by severe mental illness. Its Web site focuses on informing yourself about mental health issues, finding support, and taking action.
www.nami.org

National Institute of Mental Health (NIMH): This division of the National Institutes of Health focuses on dispensing health information to the public and sponsoring research on mental health and illness. Its authoritative information ranges from breaking news to explanations of common mental disorders.
www.nimh.nih.gov

National Mental Health Association (NMHA): This organization's resource center offers brochures on mental health and referrals to treatment centers, support groups, and other national organizations. Answers to frequently asked questions about mental health are especially helpful.
www.nmha.org

Spirituality

4

Ever Wonder...

- if you can be spiritual without belonging to an organized religion?

- what your personal values are?

- how to deal with the loss of a loved one?

Someone once said that the longest journey is the journey inward. The spiritual journey is deeply personal and individual. It may begin as a yearning for connection with what is universal and timeless or a belief in a power in the universe that is greater than oneself. It often involves a search for meaning and purpose or a desire for a more intense participation in life. Many people now believe that spiritual health enhances their psychological and physical well-being, and they pursue spiritual wellness as one of the important dimensions of total wellness.

It seems that all people in all times have experienced spiritual aspirations. Worldwide, there are more than 20 major religions and thousands of other forms of spiritual expression. In the spirit of modern genetics, some scientists have been searching for a biological basis for human spirituality—a gene or genes that would account for our spiritual experiences and yearnings—and one researcher, Dean Hamer of the National Cancer Institute, believes he

guided by my values, or am I drifting without a moral compass? What gives my life meaning? Searching for answers to these questions is part of life's spiritual journey.

Connection to Self and Others   Being connected to yourself involves knowing who you are, developing self-awareness, and building self-esteem. Growth in these areas is an incremental process in which you develop a reservoir of inner strengths through such practices as becoming more compassionate or learning to be a better listener.

Spirituality also includes being responsible for yourself and taking charge of your life. Your spiritual health affects your capacity for love, compassion, joy, forgiveness, altruism, and fulfillment. It can be an antidote to stress, cynicism, anger, fear, anxiety, self-absorption, and pessimism.

Connection with significant others through positive relationships is also essential to spiritual health and growth.

> **spirituality**
> The experience of connection to self, others, and the community at large, providing a sense of purpose and meaning.

Your spiritual health affects your **capacity for love, compassion, forgiveness, and fulfillment.** *It can be an antidote to stress, cynicism, fear, self-absorption, and pessimism.*

has found such a gene.[1] No matter what the role of biology, however, spiritual experience and expression are clearly the product of complex interactions between individuals and their cultures.

What Is Spirituality?

Because spirituality may involve different paths for different people, it has been defined in many ways. In health promotion literature, **spirituality** is commonly defined as a person's connection to self, significant others, and the community at large. Many experts also agree that spirituality involves a personal belief system or value system that gives meaning and purpose to life.[2] For some individuals this personal value system may include a belief in and reverence for a higher power, which may be expressed through an organized religion. For example, according to recent surveys, more than 8 in 10 Americans identify with a religion and believe in God or a universal spirit or higher power.[3] For others the spiritual dimension is nonreligious and centers on a personal value system that may be reflected in activities such as volunteer work. In either case, spirituality provides a feeling of participation in something greater than oneself and a sense of unity with nature and the universe.

SPIRITUALITY IN EVERYDAY LIFE

All of us have questions about our existence: Am I connected to something, or am I alone, isolated, and cut off? Is my life

■ Participating in activities that reinforce feelings of connectedness with others is a way of enhancing spirituality in everyday life.

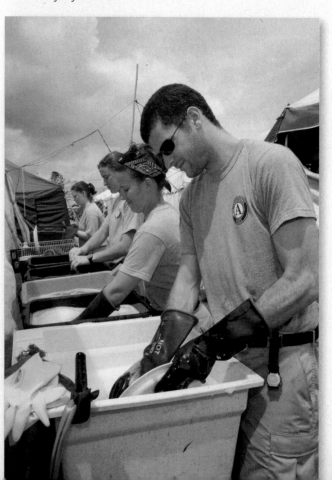

Healthy relationships involve a balance between closeness and separateness and are characterized by mutual support, respect, good communication, and caring actions. Having strong personal relationships improves health and self-esteem and gives greater meaning to life.[4,5]

Connection with the community includes enjoying constructive relationships at school, in the workplace, or in the neighborhood. Several studies have demonstrated links between social connectedness and positive outcomes for individual health and well-being.[5-7]. Evidence shows that social participation and engagement are related to the maintenance of cognitive function in older adulthood and to lowered mortality rates. In general, the size of a person's social network and his or her sense of connectedness are inversely related to risk-related behaviors such as alcohol and tobacco consumption, physical inactivity, and behaviors leading to obesity.[5,6,8]

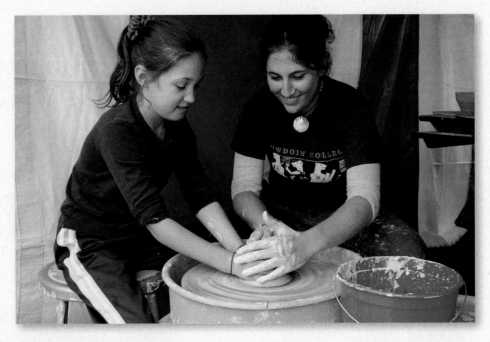

■ Engagement in meaningful activities—such as sharing one's expertise and passion with a younger person—is a major source of happiness and satisfaction for most people.

A Personal Value System   Another aspect of spirituality involves developing a personal **value system**, a set of guidelines for how you want to live your life. *Values*, the criteria for judging what is good and bad, underlie moral principles and behavior. Your value system shapes who you are as a person, how you make decisions, and what goals you set for yourself. When you develop a way of life that makes sense and enables you to navigate the world effectively, the many choices you face each day become much less complex and easier to handle. Your value system becomes your map, providing a structure for decision making that allows flexibility and the possibility of change.

value system
Set of criteria for judging what is good and bad that underlies moral decisions and behavior.

Meaning and Purpose in Life   Why am I here? This question has been asked by people all over the world, in all eras, and at all stages of life. For young people, the answer may involve developing relationships and connections. For adults, the answer may be caring for others. For older adults, it may be working for a healthier planet. Positive psychology contributes the idea that meaning in life comes from using one's personal strengths to serve some larger end.

HAPPINESS AND LIFE SATISFACTION

The study of happiness is part of the positive psychology movement, with its focus on what makes life worth living (see Chapter 3). Surveys indicate that happiness is typical rather than unusual—9 out of 10 Americans report being very happy or pretty happy.[9] According to one poll, wealth, education, IQ, and youth have little impact on happiness; instead, the top source of happiness is connections with family and friends (Figure 4.1).[10] Other sources of happiness include contributing to the lives of others, having a sense of control over one's life, and having a religious or spiritual life.

In their research, positive psychologists have found that happiness involves three components: positive emotion and pleasure (savoring sensory experiences); engagement (depth of involvement with family, work, romance, and hobbies); and meaning (using personal strengths to serve some larger end).[8] The happiest people are those who orient their lives toward all three, but the latter two—engagement and meaning—are much more important in giving people satisfaction and happiness.

Happiness research has found that people can increase their level of happiness by practicing certain "happiness exercises":[11]

■ *Three Good Things in Life.* Write down three things that went well each day and their causes every night for a week.

■ *Using Signature Strengths in a New Way.* Using the classification of character strengths and virtues (see Table 3.1), take inventory of your character strengths and identify your top five strengths, your "signature strengths." Use one of these top strengths in a new and different way every day for a week.

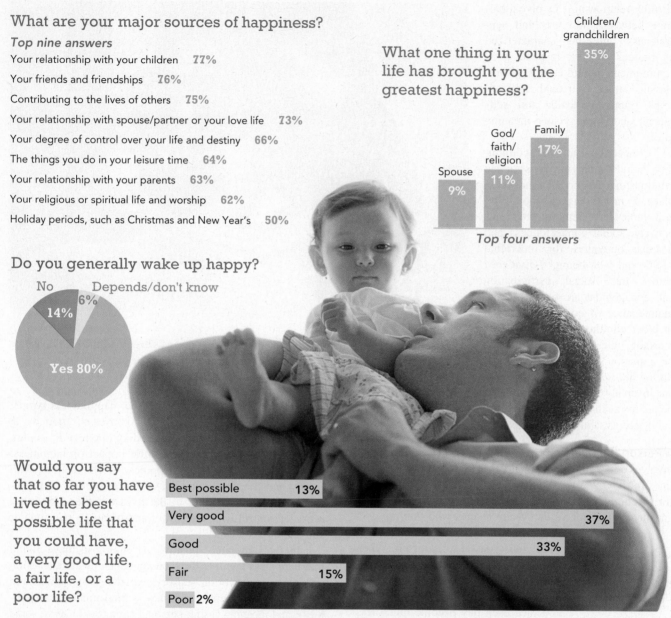

What are your major sources of happiness?

Top nine answers

Your relationship with your children **77%**

Your friends and friendships **76%**

Contributing to the lives of others **75%**

Your relationship with spouse/partner or your love life **73%**

Your degree of control over your life and destiny **66%**

The things you do in your leisure time **64%**

Your relationship with your parents **63%**

Your religious or spiritual life and worship **62%**

Holiday periods, such as Christmas and New Year's **50%**

What one thing in your life has brought you the greatest happiness?

Spouse 9% | God/faith/religion 11% | Family 17% | Children/grandchildren 35%

Top four answers

Do you generally wake up happy?

No 14% | Depends/don't know 6% | Yes 80%

Would you say that so far you have lived the best possible life that you could have, a very good life, a fair life, or a poor life?

Best possible **13%**

Very good **37%**

Good **33%**

Fair **15%**

Poor **2%**

figure **4.1** **Sources of happiness and other happiness facts reported by Americans.**

Source: Adapted from "The New Science of Happiness," by C. Wallis, January 17, 2005, Time.

■ *Gratitude Visit.* Write a letter of gratitude and then deliver it in person to someone who has been especially kind to you but whom you have never thanked properly.

Research found that two of these exercises—Three Good Things and Using Signature Strengths in a New Way—increased happiness and decreased depressive symptoms for 6 months. The Gratitude Visit caused large positive changes for 1 month.

Related research has identified other ways to increase happiness and life satisfaction, including performing acts of kindness, savoring life's joys, and learning to forgive (see the box "Steps to a More Satisfying Life"). Positive psychologists say that happiness exercises give meaning to life by helping people feel more connected to others. Almost everyone feels happier when they are with other people, even those who think they want to be alone.

The down side is that people may have a happiness "set point," determined largely by genetics. That is, no matter what happens in life, people may have a tendency to return to their norm. The notion that people can increase their happiness reinforces Western cultural biases about how individual initiative and a positive attitude can solve complex problems.[7] In addition, because happiness research focuses

Steps to a More Satisfying Life

Want to be happier? Here are some practical suggestions, based on research findings by psychologist Sonia Lyubomirsky and other positive psychologists:

1. *Count your blessings.* Keep a gratitude journal in which you write down three to five things for which you are grateful once a week.

2. *Practice acts of kindness.* Being kind to others has many positive effects, including a greater sense of connection with the people around you.

3. *Savor life's joys.* Pay attention to moments of pleasure and wonder; keep a store of such memories so that you can call on them in less happy times.

4. *Thank a mentor.* Express your appreciation to those who have been kind to you.

5. *Learn to forgive.* Write a letter of forgiveness to anyone who has hurt or wronged you. Letting go of anger and resentment allows you to move on.

6. *Invest time and energy in friends and family.* Strong personal relationships are the biggest factor in life satisfaction.

7. *Take care of your body.* Practicing good self-care—getting enough sleep, exercising, smiling and laughing—makes your daily life more satisfying.

8. *Develop strategies for coping with stress and hardship.* For some people, religious faith offers help. For others, secular beliefs—even "this too shall pass"—serve as coping tools.

Sources: *"Positive Psychology Progress: Validation of Interventions,"* by M. Seligman, T. Steen, N. Park, and C. Peterson, 2005, American Psychologist, 60(5), pp. 410–421; *"The New Science of Happiness,"* by C. Wallis, January 17, 2005, Time.

on internal processes, little or no attention is paid to the very real sources of unhappiness in people's lives that are connected to their social and economic circumstances.

Health Benefits of Spirituality

According to a *Newsweek* poll, 73 percent of Americans believe that prayer holds the power to heal,[12] and according to a 2004 study, one-third of Americans use prayer, in addition to conventional medical treatments, for health concerns.[13]

The connection between spirituality and health is gaining serious attention from the medical and scientific communities.[14,15] Hundreds of studies have been conducted on spirituality and health, and more than half the nation's medical schools now offer courses on spirituality and medicine, whereas only three did 20 years ago. The National Institutes of Health have spent millions of dollars on "mind-body" medicine.[16] The pursuit is not without its skeptics, however, and the connection between spirituality and health remains an area of controversy and debate.

PHYSICAL BENEFITS

Can prayer cure cancer or slow its progression? Can it lower blood pressure? Does spirituality speed healing after accidents or help people recover from surgery? Do religious people live longer?

There are no definitive answers to these questions, but a majority of 350 studies of physical health and 850 studies of mental health suggest a direct relationship between religious involvement and spirituality, on the one hand, and better health outcomes, on the other.[17] Research has found that religious involvement and spirituality are associated with lower blood pressure, decreased risk of substance abuse, less cardiovascular disease, less depression, less anxiety, enhanced immune function, and longer life.[18] Meditation and prayer in combination with traditional medical treatments are reported to relieve medical problems such as chronic pain, depression, anxiety, insomnia, and premenstrual syndrome.[19] There are enough positive results to spur further inquiry.

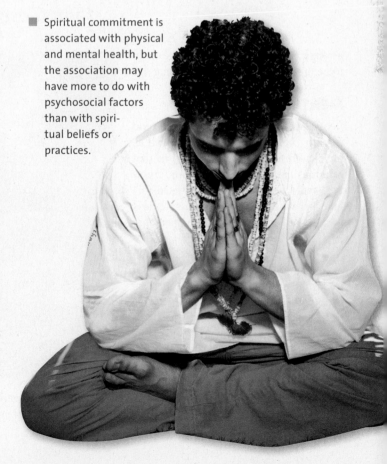

■ Spiritual commitment is associated with physical and mental health, but the association may have more to do with psychosocial factors than with spiritual beliefs or practices.

One of the most consistent research findings is that spiritually connected persons stay healthier and live longer than those who are not connected.[18,20] One study found that people who attend church regularly live an average of seven years longer than their non-churchgoing counterparts.[21] An important reason for this outcome is that people who are religious or spiritually connected generally have healthier lifestyles. They smoke less, drink less alcohol, have better diets, exercise more, and are more likely to wear seat belts and to avoid drugs and unsafe sex. However, these factors don't seem to account for all of the health-related benefits of religious and spiritual commitment. Studies find that the positive differences in death rates persist even after controlling for factors such as age, health, habits, demographics, and other health-related variables.[18]

Another explanation for better health among people who are spiritually involved is that they react more effectively to health crises. People who are religious or spiritual seem to be more willing than those who are not spiritually connected to alter their health habits, to be proactive in seeking medical treatment, and to accept the support of others. People who have strong ties to a religious group or another community segment may receive help and encouragement from that community in times of crisis.[22] Friends may transport them to the doctor and to church, shop for them, prepare meals,

such as meditation, yoga, and hypnotherapy, reduce the secretion of stress hormones and their harmful side effects.

Depression may also be mediated by spiritual involvement. Some studies indicate that people who are religiously involved suffer less depression and recover faster when they are depressed.[28,29] Religious people are also less likely to consider suicide.[12]

Studies have shown that spiritual connectedness appears to be associated with high levels of *health-related quality of life*, the physical, psychological, social, and spiritual aspects of a person's daily experience. Spiritual connectedness is especially important when a person is coping with serious health issues such as cancer, HIV infection, heart disease, limb amputation, or spinal cord injury.[18] This positive relationship persists even as physical health declines with serious illness.[30]

A DIFFERENT VIEW

Although the majority of studies indicate that spiritual connectedness has health benefits, many studies have found no relationship between health and spirituality. Some researchers have even suggested that spirituality can have negative outcomes for physical and mental health. For example, several studies indicate that when people experience a spiritual conflict in association with a health crisis, there is a

One of the most consistent research findings is that
spiritually connected persons stay healthier and live longer
than those who are not connected.

arrange child care, and encourage them to get appropriate medical treatment.

MENTAL BENEFITS

People who are spiritually involved tend to enjoy better mental health as well as physical health. One reason may be that religious people tend to be more forgiving, and recent research has linked forgiveness with lower blood pressure, less back pain, and overall better personal health.[23]

In addition, spiritual practices such as meditation, prayer, and worship seem to promote positive emotions such as hope, love, contentment, and forgiveness, which can result in lower levels of anxiety. This in turn may help to minimize the stress response, which suppresses immune functioning.[24–26] Many people may even turn to religion in times of stress.[27] Studies have also shown that prayer and certain relaxation techniques,

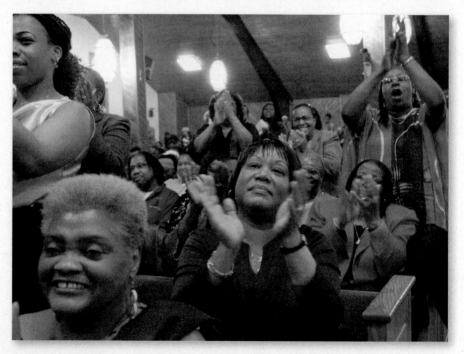

■ People who have strong ties to a religious or community group are more likely to have a network of people who can support and help them in time of need.

Who's at Risk?

Spirituality and Health

Do people with spiritual or religious beliefs and practices have better health outcomes than people without such beliefs and practices? Many research studies have been conducted to investigate various aspects of this question, with contradictory and inconsistent results. The findings of a few of them are described here:

- A combination of frequent religious attendance, prayer, Bible study, and strong beliefs predicted a faster recovery from depression.[a]

- HIV-positive patients who underwent spiritual transformation (the development of spirituality or an increase in the level of spirituality) had a higher survival rate than those who did not undergo spiritual transformation.[b]

- Attendance and public participation in religion did not affect hypertension rates among adults; however, prayer was associated with an increased likelihood of hypertension, and forgiveness was associated with a lower risk of hypertension.[c]

- Cardiac patients who received intercessory prayer (prayer by strangers) fared no better than patients who did not receive such prayer.[d]

- Religious struggles and negative religious coping (for example, "questioning God's love") were correlated with higher risk of death in hospitalized older adults.[e]

- Among older adults (66–95 years old), men received more mental health benefits from religion than did women, and women with high, moderate, and low levels of organizational involvement in religion received similar levels of benefits regardless of their level of involvement.[f]

- Neither self-reported spirituality, frequency of church attendance, nor frequency of prayer was associated with recovery from heart attack.[g]

- An increase in religiosity/spirituality after a diagnosis of HIV infection was correlated with slower disease progression after 4 years.[h]

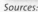

Sources:
[a] *"Religion and Remission of Depression in Medical Inpatients with Heart Failure/Pulmonary Disease," by H.G. Koenig, 2007,* Journal of Nervous and Mental Disease, *195, pp. 389–395.*
[b] *"Spiritual Transformation, Psychological Well-Being, Health, and Survival in People With HIV," by G. Ironson and H. Kremer, 2009,* International Journal of Psychiatry in Medicine, *39(3), pp. 263–281.*
[c] *"An Examination of the Relationship Between Multiple Dimensions of Religiosity, Blood Pressure and Hypertension," by A.C. Buck et al. 2008,* Social Science and Medicine, *68(2), pp. 314–422.*
[d] *"Music, Imagery, Touch, and Prayer as Adjuncts to Interventional Cardiac Care," by M.W. Krucoff et al., 2005,* Lancet, *366, pp. 211–217.*
[e] *"Religious Struggles as a Predictor of Mortality Among Medically Ill Elderly Patients," by K.I. Pargament et al., 2001,* Archives of Internal Medicine, *161, pp. 1881–1885.*
[f] *"Religion and Mental Health Among Older Adults: Do the Effects of Religious Involvement Vary by Gender?" by M.J. McFarland, 2009,* Journal of Gerontology: Social Sciences, *10, p. 1093.*
[g] *"Spirituality, Religion, and Clinical Outcomes in Patients Recovering From an Acute Myocardial Infarction," by J.A. Blumenthal et al., 2007,* Psychosomatic Medicine, *69, pp. 501–508.*
[h] *"An Increase in Religiousness/Spirituality Occurs After HIV Diagnosis and Predicts Slower Disease Progression Over 4 Years in People With HIV," by G. Ironson, R. Stuetzie, and M.A. Fletcher, 2006,* Journal of General Internal Medicine, *21, pp. S62–S68.*

negative impact on their health status.[18,31–34] And one study concluded that people who knew they were receiving intercessory prayer (prayer by strangers) may have experienced increased anxiety and more complications than those who were unsure they were being prayed for.[35] It seems that the connection between spirituality and health can have both positive and negative implications and needs more study (see the box "Spirituality and Health").

Enhancing Your Spirituality: Looking Inward

How do you build a spiritual life? Greater connectedness and meaning can be found through a variety of practices, especially if they are done on a regular basis.

MEDITATION

Human beings are engaged in a constant inner monologue, reviewing the past, commenting on the present, and speculating about the future. This inner chatter can keep us from being fully present in our lives. **Meditation** is a way to slow your racing thoughts and quiet your mind by focusing on a word, an object (such as a candle flame), or a process (such as breathing). With practice, meditation can help you become calmer as you go about your daily routines. There are many ways to meditate, but all involve introspection and attention to your inner life.

If you are interested in trying meditation as a way to build a spiritual life, follow the guidelines in the box

meditation
Technique for quieting the mind by focusing on a word, an object (such as a candle flame), or a process (such as breathing).

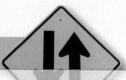

Challenges & Choices

Learning to Meditate

Meditation is an ancient technique with modern adaptations. Various forms of meditation have been developed, but their common goals are to calm the mind, raise awareness, and increase attention to what is happening in the present moment. Here are some guidelines for a type of meditation in which you focus on your breathing:

- Sit in a comfortable place—on a pillow on the floor or in a chair, for example—in a quiet room where you won't be disturbed. Close your eyes.

- Breathe deeply. Feel the breath as it enters your nostrils and fills your chest and abdomen; then release it.

- Focus your attention on your breathing and awareness of the moment. Try to be silent and still.

- Remain passive and relaxed as your thoughts come and go, noticing them without judging them. At

first, your mind will fill with memories, worries, and random thoughts. Let go of the thoughts and feelings and return to the awareness of breath. Eventually, you will be able to concentrate for longer periods of time, and these periods of concentration may be accompanied by feelings of great tranquility.

Meditate for brief periods of time each day. Start out with 5 minutes and gradually build up to 15 minutes or more. Make a commitment to continue meditating for 3 months; you will not experience any changes or benefits unless you practice. Experiment until you find a place, time, and approach that work for you. If you would like more information about techniques, contact a meditation center, consult a teacher or book, search online, talk with more experienced meditators, or listen to a tape.

"Learning to Meditate." Although meditation may not appeal to everyone, the practice can offer many benefits. It is widely used in stress management and stress reduction programs. Proponents claim that meditation provides deep relaxation, promotes health, increases creativity and intelligence, and brings inner happiness and fulfillment.

Mindfulness is both a form of meditation and the practice of living fully in the moment. By learning to be conscious of your thoughts as they pass by—observing them, not judging them—you develop your ability to control and stop habitual, impulsive, or undesirable reactions. You become more capable of responding in a "thoughtful" and "mindful" way rather than becoming overwhelmed with negative emotions or self-criticism.[36] As you learn to focus on the present moment, you can be more in touch with your life as it is happening.

- Meditation is a calming and centering spiritual practice.

When people learn to live fully in the moment, they sometimes experience a phenomenon known as **flow**, a feeling of being completely absorbed in an activity and a moment. In this state, people forget themselves, lose track of time, and feel as if they have become one with what they are doing. Writers describe times when words seem to come through them; athletes refer to being "in the zone." Flow has been described as one of the most enjoyable and valuable experiences a person can have.[37] When you learn to be mindful and live in the moment, you are more likely to experience flow in your daily activities.

mindfulness
Awareness and acceptance of living fully in the moment.

flow
Pleasurable experience of complete absorption and engagement in an activity.

Mindfulness is celebrated by the noted Vietnamese monk Thich Nhat Hanh in these words:

Our true home is in the present moment.
To live in the present moment is a miracle.
The miracle is not to walk on water.
The miracle is to walk on the green Earth in the present moment,
To appreciate the peace and beauty that are available now.[38]

JOURNALING

Another approach to building a spiritual life is *journaling*. As you record your feelings, thoughts, breakthroughs, and desires in a private journal, you will begin to understand yourself more clearly.

Psychologist James Pennebaker has found that writing about emotional upheavals can improve physical and mental health. He suggests writing about any of the following:

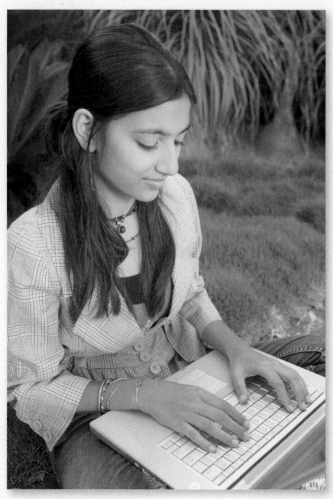

■ Journaling offers a way to explore your feeelings, deepen your self-understanding, and discover what is important to you.

■ Something that you are thinking or worrying about too much.

■ Something that you are dreaming about.

■ Something that you feel is affecting your life in an unhealthy way.

■ Something that you have been avoiding for days, weeks, or years.[39]

The more honest you are, the better. Don't censor yourself as you write; just let your thoughts flow. Try to move beyond the superficial telling to asking yourself, Why am I feeling this way?

Journaling is an effective way to learn about who you are and where you have been. Listening to your inner dialogue may offer you a sense of peace and a positive outlook on your experiences. In some cases, journaling can be painful, stirring up emotions that may be difficult to handle on your own. If you find yourself feeling overwhelmed, consider contacting a professional for counseling.[40]

RETREAT

A *retreat* is a period of seclusion, solitude, or group withdrawal for prayer, meditation, or study. Retreats are intended to reenergize your life and restore your zest for living. A spiritual retreat might offer a balance of activities that encourage growth, foster learning, and restore energy, so that when you return to your normal surroundings, you may live life to the fullest in a purposeful way.

Many kinds of facilities offer retreats, workshops, and programs for spiritual growth, but you can use your home for a retreat as well. Set aside a weekend and plan to give up all social events, phone calls, errands, television, newspapers, Internet, and all nonessential housework. Then prepare for exploration. You might meditate, journal, draw, write poetry, take walks to enjoy the beauty of nature, listen to music, read—whatever you want to do that you find deepening and centering. At their best, retreats stimulate the mind, enhance self-awareness, and refresh the spirit. They provide food for the body, mind, and spirit.

THE ARTS

Scholar Joseph Campbell once asserted, "The goal of life is rapture. Art is the way we experience it. Art is the transforming experience." Experiencing the arts—whether sculpture, painting, music, poetry, literature, theater, storytelling, dance, or some other form—is another way to build a spiritual life. Experiencing great art can inspire you, through felt experience, to think about the purpose of life and the nature of reality.[41] By engaging your heart, mind, and spirit, art can give you fresh insights, challenge preconceptions, and trigger inner growth.

When you enjoy and appreciate the arts, you embrace diverse cultures past and present and frequently discover in them the universal themes of human existence— love, loss, birth, death, isolation, community, continuity, change. When you express yourself creatively, you may be able to experience a spiritual connection between your inner core and the natural world beyond yourself. Both experiences—art appreciation and artistic expression—can be transforming. If the visual or performing arts are not part of your life right now, try to schedule time to visit a museum or attend a concert. Make notes or sketches in a journal reflecting on your experiences. Doing so may stimulate new spiritual connections in your life.

hot tip

To gain some perspective on values and meaning in life, go to YouTube and watch Randy Pausch's inspiring "Last Lecture," delivered after the popular professor had been given a prognosis of 3–6 months left to live.

LIVING YOUR VALUES

Building a spiritual life also means bringing your deepest beliefs and intentions into the world—that is, living your values. A 2010 report conducted by the Pew Research Center found that students of the Millennial generation (ages 18–29) have values similar to those of older generations. Although Millennials set themselves apart by their racial diversity, immersion in technology, and love of self-expression and social media, like older generations, they rate being a good parent as one of the most important things in life (see Figure 4.2).[42] And although this generation has grown up in an age where almost anyone can become a YouTube star, gain a large following writing a blog, or exchange tweets with minor celebrities, 86 percent say that becoming famous is not important to them.[42]

Can you articulate what is most important to you in life? Are you living and acting in accordance with it? (See the box

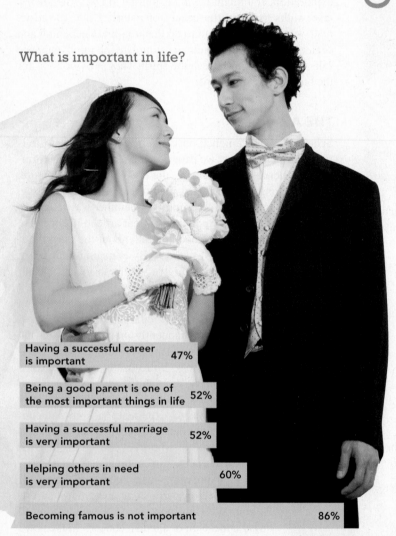

What is important in life?

Having a successful career is important — 47%

Being a good parent is one of the most important things in life — 52%

Having a successful marriage is very important — 52%

Helping others in need is very important — 60%

Becoming famous is not important — 86%

figure 4.2   **The Millennial generation and their values.**

Source: "Millennials: A Portrait of Generation Next." *Pew Research Center,* accessed February 24, 2010, from http://pewsocialtrends.org/assets/pdf/ millennials-confident-connected-open-to-change.pdf.

Challenges & Choices

Understanding Your Personal Values

Many people are unaware of their core values and the guiding principles by which they live their lives. We seldom think through our values until we are faced with a difficult choice, and even then we may make a choice without being aware of our values. For inspiration we can look to people who stood up for their values despite enormous pressure to conform and foreseeable negative consequences. A prime example is Rosa Parks, who sparked the civil rights movement when she refused to sit in the back of the bus.

How would you articulate your own core values? Consider the following list of major life values and check off the ones that are important to you:

☐ achievement   ☐ honesty
☐ autonomy   ☐ integrity
☐ compassion   ☐ learning
☐ connectedness   ☐ love
☐ creativity   ☐ personal growth
☐ education   ☐ prestige
☐ family   ☐ relationships
☐ financial well-being ☐ service
☐ freedom   ☐ social justice
☐ health   ☐ spirituality
☐ home   ☐ status

Which of these (or others) are most important and meaningful to you? Write your top three here:

_____

_____

_____

What guiding principles can you derive from them? How can you embody them in your life?

"Understanding Your Personal Values.") Try writing a "purpose statement" that will remind you of who you truly are and why you believe you are here on earth. Then ask yourself, Do I stay "on purpose" in my daily interactions and activities? Commit your purpose statement to memory, and read or recite it daily. It may be "to live and learn" or "to know my higher being and teach and express love."

Adopting a new habit, such as putting your best intentions into practice, takes time and work. Experts say that you have to continue to take action for 60 to 90 days to make a behavior change stick. As Aristotle understood almost 2,500 years ago, "We are what we repeatedly do. Excellence is not an act, then, but a habit."

Enhancing Your Spirituality: Looking Outward

Many believe that people can develop their spirituality by participating in their communities in a positive way. Unpaid work directly promotes community well-being through the services provided, whether that means caring for an elderly relative or working on a community project. It also has indirect benefits by building the social networks that contribute to optimal well-being.

SERVICE LEARNING

One way that people can connect classroom activities to community service and community building is through **service learning**. The purpose of integrating community service with academic study is to enrich learning, teach civic responsibility, and strengthen communities. Students are encouraged to take a positive role in their community, such as by tutoring, caring for the environment, or conducting oral histories with senior citizens. All of these activities are meant to teach people how to extend themselves beyond their enclosed world, taking a risk to get involved in the lives

service learning
Form of education that combines academic study with community service.

■ Volunteers benefit others and themselves when they serve their communities. President Obama has emphasized the importance of volunteering by participating in several community service projects since his inauguration, and his administration has created a Web site, www.serve.gov, to put people in touch with volunteer opportunities in their communities.

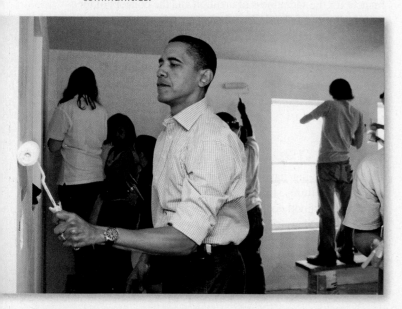

of others. In this way they learn about caring and taking care of—two particularly important concepts for personal growth.

VOLUNTEERING

Volunteering is another way to be connected with other people. Volunteers may experience a "helper's high," similar to a "runner's high."[43] Research shows that people who give time, money, and support to others are likely to be more satisfied with their lives and less depressed.[44]

Not all kinds of volunteering have the same effect, however. One-on-one contact and direct involvement significantly influence the effect of volunteering on the volunteer. Working closely with strangers appears to increase the potential health benefits of the experience. Liking the volunteer work, performing it consistently, and having unselfish motives further increase the feelings of helper's high and the health benefits associated with it.[45,46] Simply donating money or doing volunteer work in isolation does not seem to have the same positive effect.

Just as the high of helping may create enjoyable immediate benefits, the calm of helping may result in significant long-term health benefits. For example, volunteering may reduce the negative health effects of living with high levels of stress for long periods of time. Those who have experienced a helper's high have noted specific improvements in their physical well-being. These improvements included a reduction in arthritis pain, lupus symptoms, asthma attacks, migraine headaches, colds, and episodes of the flu. Volunteering may even result in longer life for the volunteer.[47,48]

SOCIAL ACTIVISM AND THE GLOBAL COMMUNITY

Some people connect with their communities—local, national, and global—through social activism. A social cause, such as overcoming poverty or fighting illiteracy, can unite people from diverse backgrounds for a common good. Many people find it meaningful to participate in global citizenship by joining organizations such as those described in the box "Global Activism."

If you are interested in social activism, look for ways to participate through your school, your religious community, or groups you locate on the Internet. When you volunteer for such an organization, you commit yourself to building a foundation for a better world, making a contribution through service to others, and creating opportunities for mutual understanding.

How is spirituality related to community involvement? Some claim that when we attend to our inner life, we nurture our compassionate responses to human need and develop a passion for social justice. Others believe that contributing to community welfare and striving for justice are the ways to a rich inner life.

Some people turn away from social activism because they think it's "just politics." We hear news stories that use

Highlight on Health

Global Activism

Many organizations help individuals put their values into practice in the world. Here are a few:

- The Peace Corps was inspired by President John F. Kennedy's call to college students to give two years of their lives to help people in developing nations. Today, it is still sending people to developing nations like Ecuador, Ghana, and Ukraine with the goal of promoting world peace and friendship. Its volunteers do everything from helping teachers develop their teaching methodologies, to raising awareness about health issues like HIV/AIDS, to teaching environmental conservation strategies, to teaching computer skills.

- Habitat for Humanity is widely known for its work providing housing for needy people in the United States, but it also works on its goal of eliminating poverty and homelessness on a global level. So far, the organization has built more than 350,000 houses in more than 90 countries.

- Greenpeace focuses on the most crucial worldwide threats to the planet's biodiversity and environment. Greenpeace has been campaigning against environmental degradation since 1971, bearing witness in a nonviolent manner.

- The Earth Charter Initiative is an international organization dedicated to building a sustainable world based on respect for nature, universal human rights, economic justice, and peace. A basic premise of the Earth Charter is that these attributes must be cultivated at the local community level before they can emerge at the national and global levels.

---

catchphrases associating traditional values with the religious right and social justice with the liberal left. Any action can be cloaked in the guise of religiosity, and distinguishing politics with a religious flavor from the practice of authentic spiritual values can be difficult. The former is designed to manipulate people's feelings for political gain; the latter has no hidden agenda or ulterior motive.

The question for the individual is, How can I best put my passion into action while respecting the beliefs of others? Some social activists have transcended their religious and social conditioning and become universal spiritual beings, ready to serve all. Both Mahatma Gandhi and the Reverend Martin Luther King, Jr., developed an integrated worldview and worked to create global community.

NATURE AND THE ENVIRONMENT

The impulse that propels people to the mountains or seashore for their holidays is the same impulse that drives pilgrims to sites of religious importance—the need to reconnect with the natural world. Many cultures in history, including many Native American cultures, did and do have a strong spiritual connection to nature or "Mother Earth." These cultures promote reverence for the universe, which results in a strong spiritual connection to nature.

Some people combine ecological, ethical, and spiritual interests and beliefs into what has been called *eco-spirituality*. They may participate in retreats or periods of reflection to deepen their connections to the earth. They may advocate respect for the sacredness of creation and the concept of tending (caring for, nurturing, and participating in nature). Daily activities that incorporate environmental values might include recycling, composting, and walking or riding a bike instead of driving. As with volunteerism and social activism, when you are environmentally active, the benefits flow back to you, sustaining your spirituality and adding meaning to life.

Death and Dying

Death and dying have great spiritual significance for people of all cultures. In one study, 89 percent of Americans described a "good death" as one that included making peace with God.[49] Many also included prayer and discussing the meaning of death in their description of a good death.

When someone you love dies, the experience is extremely personal, yet it is one that you also share with others. Life and death are part of the cycle of existence and the natural order of things. Many report that because of their personal faith, they do not fear death, since they know that their lives have had meaning within the context of a larger plan.

STAGES OF DYING AND DEATH

In 1969 Elisabeth Kübler-Ross published *On Death and Dying*, one of the first books to propose a set of stages that people go through when they believe they are in the process of dying.[50] The five stages are (1) denial and isolation, (2) anger, (3) bargaining, (4) depression, and (5) acceptance. Over time, further study has shown that these stages are not linear—individuals may experience them in a different order or may return to stages they have already gone through—nor are they necessarily universal—individuals may not experience some stages at all.

Many believe that life is full of transitions, with death being the last. A shared sense of mortality can be the basis for feeling connected with other human beings. Recently, health care professionals have begun to describe ways to *live* with an illness rather than simply looking at the diagnosis as the point at which one begins to prepare for death. As medical care has improved, many individuals diagnosed with cancer or HIV infection have recovered or lived with the disease for many years. The critical thing to remember is that one need not go on a "death watch" after a diagnosis; usually, there is time to repair relationships, to build memories, and to review one's life. The dying person may find comfort and strength in talking through the process with family and friends or with a spiritual advisor.

Research has found that terminally ill persons derive strength and hope from spiritual and religious beliefs. In fact, terminally ill adults report significantly greater religious involvement and depth of spiritual perspective than do healthy adults. Studies suggest that, unrelated to belief in an afterlife, religiously involved people at the end of life are more accepting of death than those who are less religiously involved. In addition, religious involvement and spirituality are associated with less death anxiety.[18]

HEALTHY GRIEVING

Grief is a natural reaction to loss. Besides the loss of loved ones to death, we grieve many kinds of losses throughout our lives: divorce, relocation, traumatic experiences, loss of health and mobility, and even expected life transitions such as having the last child leave home. Grief is often expressed by feelings of sadness, loneliness, anger, and guilt. These feelings are part of the process of healing, since we do not begin to feel better until we have acknowledged and felt sorrow over our loss.

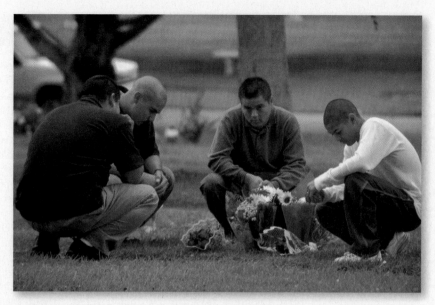

■ Spiritual beliefs and rituals can help people deal with grief and pain when a loved one dies.

Physical symptoms of grief may include crying and sighing, aches and pains, sleep disturbances, headaches, lethargy, reduced appetite, and stomach upset. The intense emotions you feel at the time of a loss can have a negative impact on immune system functioning, reducing your ability to fight off illness. Studies have shown that surviving spouses may have increased risk for heart disease, cancer, depression, alcoholism, and suicide.[51,52] Ten to 15 percent of bereaved people struggle for several years or longer with grief reactions that interfere with their ability to function.[53] Everyone has higher risk for disease after the loss of a loved one, but those who are more resilient may cope with the loss better. Resilient people seem to be more likely to find comfort in talking and thinking about the deceased and are flexible enough to either suppress or express emotions about a death.[53]

Bereavement after the loss of a loved one typically involves four phases:

■ *Numbness and shock.* This phase occurs immediately after the loss and lasts for a brief period. The numbness protects you from acute pain.

■ *Separation.* As the shock wears off, you start to feel the pain of loss, and you experience acute yearning and longing to be reunited with your loved one.

■ *Disorganization.* You are preoccupied and distracted; you have trouble concentrating and thinking clearly. You may feel lethargic and indifferent. This phase can last much longer than you anticipate.

■ *Reorganization.* You begin to adjust to the loss. Your life will never be the same without your loved one, but your feelings have less intensity and you can reinvest in life.

If you experience the death of a loved one, it is important to take care of yourself while you are grieving. There

Public Health in Action

End-of-Life Decision Making

Many physicians believe it is important to discuss end-of-life decisions with their patients—to talk about whether a patient wants anything and everything done to prolong life or whether, in certain circumstances, the patient would prefer comfort over invasive treatments. Research has found that when physicians have end-of-life discussions with their patients, the quality of care increases while costs decrease. Overall, it appears that palliative or hospice care leads to more comfortable deaths, while aggressive care does not necessarily prolong life. There will always be isolated "miracle" situations where life is prolonged due to an aggressive intervention, but overall the data indicate that the quality of life and life itself are not prolonged through extreme measures.

However, like any health care service or treatment, having an end-of-life discussion with a physician costs money. In 2003, Congress passed a law that covered these discussions for terminally ill people with Medicare, the national insurance plan for people 65 and older. This meant that terminally ill patients would not have to pay out of pocket to have end-of-life discussions with their doctors and that doctors would be fairly compensated for their time spent on these discussions, thus increasing the likelihood that these conversations would occur.

In 2009, a congressional committee in the House of Representatives proposed that as part of health care reform Medicare's coverage of end-of-life discussions be expanded to include such discussions for older people who were not terminally ill. Every five years, Medicare would pay for a doctor to discuss with the patient issues like setting up a living will, designating a health care proxy, or obtaining hospice care. The goal of the legislation, as with the 2003 bill, was to improve the quality of life for older Americans and decrease rapidly rising health care costs. However, some opponents of the bill termed these optional conversations "death panels" that would force people to die early and against their will. Because of this widespread misunderstanding, the proposal was ultimately stripped from the final House bill.

Even though coverage for end-of-life discussions has not yet been expanded to senior citizens who are not terminally ill, those who have been diagnosed with a terminal illness can still have their end-of-life conversations with their doctors covered by Medicare. And under a 1991 act passed during George H.W. Bush's Administration, hospitals are required to ask all adult patients whether they have an advanced directive and to inform them of their right to refuse treatment.

Although discussions about end-of-life care are never easy, having them improves the quality of life for a patient and provides peace of mind for the patient's family. When not being mislabeled as "death panels," government advocacy and support for end-of-life advance decision making appears to make good sense.

connect ACTIVITY

Sources: "Oh, Those Death Panels," by A. Sullivan, 2009, Time, accessed February 24, 2010, from www.time.com; "Health Care Costs in the Last Week of Life: Associations with End-of-Life Conversations," by B. Zhang et al., 2009, Archives of Internal Medicine 169(5), pp. 480–488.

is no right or wrong way to grieve and no specific timetable. Friends who suggest that it's time to move on need to understand that you are on your own journey and cannot be rushed. You need to give yourself permission to feel the loss and take time to heal. Some people seem to cope better if they talk about the death rather than internalizing their feelings. During the grieving process it is vital that you eat a balanced diet, exercise regularly, drink plenty of fluids, and get enough rest. Keeping a journal and talking about the person who has died can also be part of the healing process. Finally, you should not hesitate to ask friends for support, since having a nurturing social network is particularly helpful in coping with loss.

If intense grief persists for more than a year, or if you find yourself losing or gaining weight or not sleeping, consult a health professional to get a treatment referral. Treatment options might include support groups, family therapy, individual counseling, or a psychiatric evaluation.

RITUALS AROUND DEATH

Beliefs about death and rituals for marking the loss of loved ones vary across cultures. In some cultures, mourners have wakes and parties that last for days; in others, they sing and play music; in still others, they cover mirrors so they cannot see what they look like during times of grief.

Many rituals that surround death and dying are actually for the living, to help people cope with the loss of a loved one. Rituals help mourners move through the emotional work of grieving. When a person has been important to us, we never forget that person or lose the relationship. Instead, we find ways of "emotionally relocating" the deceased person in our lives, keeping our bonds with them while moving on. Cultural rituals can facilitate this process.

END-OF-LIFE DECISIONS

Many people dread a situation in which they or those they trust will have no say in decisions about their end-of-life treatment[50] (see the box "End-of-Life Decision Making"). To avoid this situation, they can make known their preferences through the use of formal legal documents that grant a **durable power of attorney for health care (DPOAHC)**

durable power of attorney for health care (DPOAHC) Formal legal power to make health care decisions for someone who is no longer able to do so for himself or herself.

Consumer Clipboard

How to Create an Advanced Directive

No matter how healthy you feel, it is wise to create an official document that outlines your wishes in the case that you are unable to make medical decisions for yourself—an advanced directive. Even if you have no current health problems, a sudden injury (e.g., from a motor vehicle accident) could leave you unable to communicate your wishes with regard to your medical treatment.

The main types of advanced directives are a living will and a durable power of attorney for health care, though they are sometimes referred to by different names in various states. It's a smart idea to have both. These need not be complicated documents, and you do not need a lawyer to have them created, though you should check your state's laws and guidelines before creating one. There are software packages you can buy to create these documents, but your state should have forms that you can download and fill out yourself.

Living Will

■ This document outlines the kind of care you do or do not want to receive in the event you are unable to voice your preferences yourself.

■ It does not allow someone else to make decisions for you.

■ A living will is only for health care. It is not the same thing as a conventional will.

■ When writing a living will, consider the kinds of treatments that are commonly administered to very ill patients and in what circumstances you do or do not

wish to receive them. For example, if you fall into a permanent coma, do you want to continue to be kept alive with a feeding tube?

■ Some treatments to consider: life-prolonging medical care (dialysis, blood transfusions, medical tests, use of a respirator, CPR), food and water (and whether you want these continued if you are in a vegetative state), and palliative care.

Durable Power of Attorney for Health Care

■ This document designates someone to be your health care proxy. This person will be able to make medical decisions for you in the event you are unable to make them yourself.

■ You can give the person as much or as little decision-making power as you would like.

■ In general, your health care proxy will be able to take the following actions unless you specifically prohibit them: allow or refuse treatment, hire or fire medical personnel, access your medical records, choose medical personnel and facilities, and visit you.

■ You should discuss with your health care proxy your treatment wishes (see suggested topics in the "End-of-Life Decisions" section).

After you create your advanced directive, have the document notarized and distribute copies to your doctor and family members.

Sources: Adapted from "The Living Will and Power of Attorney for Health Care: An Overview," by Shae Irving, Nolo Press, retrieved March 3, 2010, from www.nolo.com/legal-encyclopedia/article-29595.html; "End-of-Life Decisions: Advance Directives," National Hospice and Palliative Care Organization, retrieved March 3, 2010, from www.caringinfo.org/UserFiles/File/PDFs/AdvanceDirectives/ENGLISH_Advance_Dir.pdf.

---

living will
Formal legal document that outlines the medical treatment a person does or doesn't want to receive when he or she is no longer able to make such decisions.

hospice
Program that provides care for the terminally ill and their loved ones.

to someone they trust or through a **living will**, in which they outline what types of medical treatment they do or don't want to receive (see the box "How to Create an Advanced Directive"). These directives may cover any issue the patient considers important.

A common concern is whether life-sustaining treatment should be withdrawn when there is no hope of recovery. These decisions should be made in supportive consultation with family members, close friends, a spiritual advisor, and health care professionals. Such decisions must take into account the patient's values, the most common ones being family and interpersonal relationships, spiritual beliefs or religion, and independence.[54]

When terminally ill patients do decide to have treatment withdrawn, they often turn to **hospice**. Hospice is not a place

but a concept of care. The goal is to improve the quality of life in a patient's last days by providing *palliative care*—pain management, comfort, and attention to the person's physical, spiritual, emotional, and social needs. Hospice programs also provide support for family members, including help with caring for their loved one.

Beyond medical decisions, there are also practical concerns to take care of at the end of life. Organ donation is one consideration, especially since there are more people who need organ donations than there are organ donors. Over 100 people die every week in the United States from the lack of available organs for transplant.[55] Organ donors need not be in perfect health at the time of death, and all costs associated with organ donation are paid by the recipient, not the donor. Anyone over the age of 18 can become an organ donor by indicating so on his or her driver's license, but this decision should also be discussed with family members as they may be asked to sign a consent form before the donation can be carried out. People also need to let their loved ones know whether they want to be buried or cremated, what kind of funeral or memorial service they prefer, and who will administer their financial and legal affairs.

There are also profound emotional issues to work through, including the grief of both the dying person and the loved ones who will be left behind.

LIFE AFTER DEATH

Belief in an afterlife is a tenet of most faith traditions. Although some investigators say no proof of life after death exists, other researchers argue that there is empirical evidence from individuals who have been resuscitated following a near-death experience.[56,57] It would be comforting to know that there is some afterlife and that we will be reunited with our loved ones in another state of existence. However, such comforts cannot be provided by science; they remain in the realm of faith and belief.

You Make the Call

Do You Have the Right to Choose?

Ethical questions about the right to die have become more prominent since the 1975 case of Karen Ann Quinlan. She was brought to the hospital in a coma and subsequently declared to be in a persistent vegetative state. After many years of court battles, her parents were finally granted their request to have her life support discontinued. Since then, similar cases have been fought in the public spotlight, including the case of Terri Schiavo, who was taken off life support in 2005 after 2 years in a persistent vegetative state.

It is now generally acknowledged that patients have the right to refuse life-sustaining treatment, and all states authorize written advance directives by means of which individuals can state their wishes. More controversial than withdrawing treatment is the practice of actively hastening a person's death, referred to as *active euthanasia* or *physician-assisted suicide*. In this case, a physician helps a terminally ill patient administer a lethal dose of drugs to himself or herself.

Oregon is currently the only state that permits physician-assisted suicide. The Oregon Death with Dignity Act requires that a patient be terminally ill with less than 6 months to live, be judged mentally competent by two physicians, and make two oral requests and one written request at least 2 weeks apart. Since its passage, more than 200 people have taken advantage of the provisions of the bill. The legality of the act was upheld by the U.S. Supreme Court in 2006.

Proponents of physician-assisted suicide, sometimes referred to as the right to die, believe that individuals have the right to choose how they will die, just as they have the right to choose how they will live. The rights of patients to refuse life support and to sign do-not-resuscitate orders are currently protected, and they are not so different from the right to actively choose how and when to die, according to this view.

Opponents of the right to die argue that human life is unconditionally valuable and that allowing physician-assisted suicide opens the door to abuse. They believe that if more attention were paid to palliative care at the end of life, people would not need to request physician-assisted suicide.

Do terminally ill people have the right to end their lives on their own terms, or is assisted suicide a violation of our cultural values? You make the call.

PROS

- Although life should be protected, people should be allowed to die with dignity when they are terminally ill or in unbearable pain. It is the humane thing to do.

- Loss of autonomy and control are among the most feared aspects of dying. Allowing people the right to die lets them maintain their sense of personal identity until the end of their lives.

- Medical and financial resources are used, keeping people alive who are ready to die. These resources could be freed up for other uses if terminally ill patients were allowed to choose to die.

CONS

- Life is unconditionally valuable, and commitment to life is a value of virtually all societies. Physician-assisted suicide undermines this value, legitimizes suicide, and gives "permission" to more people to commit suicide.

- The vow to "do no harm" is part of the physician's oath. Any compromise in this commitment would undermine the public's faith in the medical profession.

- The practice opens the door to abuse. Some people may feel pressured to end their lives to relieve financial or emotional strains on their families, and in some cases, family members may apply such pressure.

- If attention is paid to pain management and palliative care, people can live out their days and die a natural death. Pain should be managed and depression treated so that people don't feel the need to end their lives.

connect
ACTIVITY

IN REVIEW

How is spirituality defined?

Spirituality is often defined as a person's connection to self, others, and the community at large. It usually involves a personal belief system or a value system that gives meaning and purpose to life. It provides a feeling of participation in something greater than oneself and a sense of unity with nature and the universe.

How does a person build a spiritual life?

Anyone can develop a regular spiritual practice. Examples include meditation, mindfulness, journaling, retreat, experiencing the arts, and developing a daily routine that embodies one's values. Some people develop their spirituality through community involvement, such as volunteering or social activism, and others find their spiritual connection in nature.

What health benefits are associated with spirituality?

Spiritually connected people tend to enjoy better mental and physical health than those who do not describe themselves as spiritually connected, although the reasons for these differences are a matter of debate. Spiritual connectedness appears to be related to higher levels of health-related quality of life—the physical, psychological, social, and spiritual aspects of a person's daily experiences.

What kinds of experiences are associated with death and dying?

Death is a natural part of the cycle of existence, but most people experience anxiety when facing the prospect of their own death or the death of a loved one. People with spiritual beliefs tend to derive strength and hope from their beliefs and may be more accepting of death. Hospice care can make the end of life a more comfortable and peaceful experience.

Web Resources

A Campaign for Forgiveness Research: This organization is dedicated to promoting forgiveness around the world as a way of improving the human condition. The site features myths and truths about forgiveness and offers ways to make forgiveness a part of your life.
www.forgiving.org

American Meditation Institute for Yoga Science and Philosophy: As an introduction, this Web site describes a systematic procedure for meditation. For those interested in learning meditation, the organization advocates finding a qualified teacher for personal instruction.
www.americanmeditation.org

Hospice Foundation of America: Focusing on hospice as a concept of care, this site describes the growth of the hospice movement and explains its goals. Hospice is presented as a unique source of comfort for patients and families facing death.
www.hospicefoundation.org

Organ Donation: This official U.S. government Web site for organ donation and transplantation describes the myths and facts associated with organ donation. It features a donor card that you can sign and carry.
www.organdonor.gov

5 Sleep

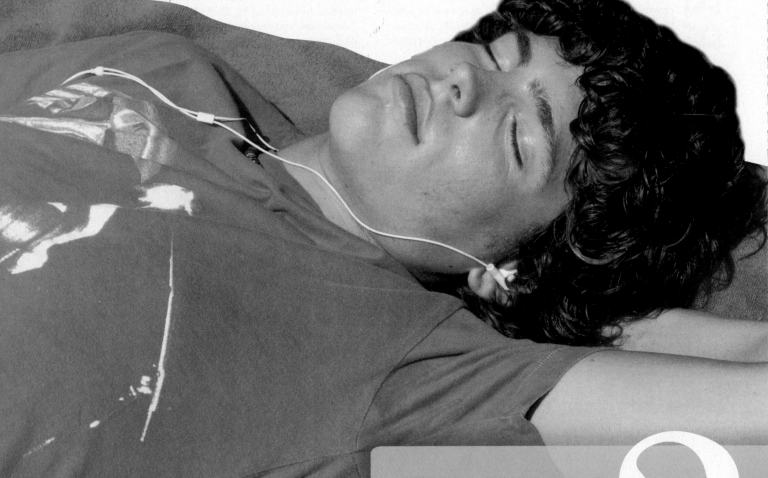

Ever Wonder...

- if pulling an all-nighter is worth it?
- why it sometimes takes so long to fall asleep?
- if it's okay to exercise right before sleep?

McGraw Hill **connect** |PERSONAL HEALTH

http://www.mcgrawhillconnect.com/personalhealth

College students often have a reputation for missing early-morning classes or falling asleep in class. It doesn't necessarily mean that they've been out partying. Most young adults have a **circadian rhythm**—an internal daily cycle of waking and sleeping—that tells them to fall asleep later in the evening and to wake up later in the morning than older adults. These circadian rhythms, accompanied by a demanding college environment, make college students vulnerable to chronic sleep deprivation. Most adults need about 8 hours of sleep each night, but the typical college student sleeps only 6 to 7 hours a night on weekdays.[1] Lack of sufficient sleep impairs academic performance. According to a survey by the American College Health Association, 23 percent of college men and 25 percent of college women rated sleep difficulties as the third major impediment (after stress and illness) to academic performance.[2]

Unfortunately, sleeping in on the weekends does not fully recapture lost sleep. Colleges and universities are exploring ways to help their sleep-deprived students. Duke University, for example, has eliminated classes that start before 8:30 a.m. Other colleges and universities are including programs on sleep and health as part of summer orientation for freshmen.

According to the 2009 Sleep in America Poll[3] conducted by the National Sleep Foundation (NSF), many Americans are not sleeping enough to sustain optimum health. Of the poll's respondents—adults aged 18 to 54—72 percent reported sleeping less than 8 hours on weekdays, and 20 percent said they slept less than 6 hours. On average, the respondents reported sleeping about 6.7 hours on weekdays and 7.1 hours on weekends.[3] Many people are unaware of the vital role that adequate sleep plays in good health.

circadian rhythm
Daily 24-hour cycle of physiological and behavioral functioning.

sleep
Period of rest and recovery from the demands of wakefulness; a state of unconsciousness or partial consciousness from which a person can be roused by stimulation.

sleep deprivation
Lack of sufficient time asleep, a condition that impairs physical, emotional, and cognitive functioning.

Sleep and Your Health

Sleep is commonly understood as a period of rest and recovery from the demands of wakefulness. It can also be described as a state of unconsciousness or partial consciousness from which a person can be roused by stimulation (as distinguished from a coma, for example). We spend about one-third of our lives sleeping, a fact that in itself indicates how important sleep is.

HEALTH EFFECTS OF SLEEP

Sleep is strongly associated with overall health and quality of life. During the deepest stages of sleep, restoration and growth take place. Growth hormone stimulates the growth and repair of the body's tissues and helps to prevent certain types of cancer. Natural immune system moderators increase during deep sleep to promote resistance to viral infections. When sleep time is deficient, a breakdown in the body's health-promoting processes can occur.

Sleep deprivation and sleep disorders are often associated with serious physical and mental health conditions, including these:

- Cardiovascular diseases (congestive heart failure, hypertension, heart attacks, strokes)
- Metabolic disorders (diabetes mellitus)
- Endocrine disorders (osteoporosis)
- Immunological disorders (influenza)
- Respiratory disorders (asthma, bronchitis)
- Mental health disorders (depression, suicide)
- Overweight and obesity (the mechanism for this connection is still unknown)

Sleeping less than 7 hours—sometimes called *short sleep*—increases the risk for negative health outcomes in both men and women. (Sleeping 10 hours or more—*long sleep*—has not been found to have negative health outcomes.) Studies strongly support the conclusion that sufficient quantity and quality of sleep are as vital to a healthy lifestyle as are good nutrition and exercise.[4–7]

SLEEP DEPRIVATION

Sleep deprivation refers to sleep of shorter duration than the average basal need of 7 to 8 hours. Most of us know what it feels like when we don't get enough

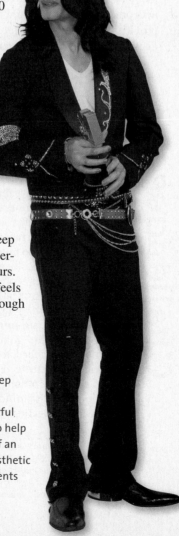

- Michael Jackson's chronic sleep problems led the pop star to become dependent on powerful anesthetics, which he used to help himself fall asleep. He died of an overdose of propofol, an anesthetic normally used to sedate patients for surgery.

sleep—we feel drowsy, our eyes burn, we find it hard to pay attention. The effects of sleep deprivation can be much more serious than this, however. Studies have shown that individuals with severe sleep deprivation (staying awake for 19 to 24 hours, for example) score worse on performance tests and alertness scales than do people with a blood alcohol concentration (BAC) of 0.1 percent—legally too drunk to drive.

Sleep deprivation has effects in all domains of functioning. Heightened irritability, lowered anger threshold, frustration, nervousness, and difficulty handling stress are some of the emotional effects. Reduced motivation may affect school and job performance, and lack of interest in socializing with others may cause relationships to suffer. Performance of daily activities is affected, as is the brain's ability to learn new material. Reaction time, coordination, and judgment are all impaired. Individuals who are sleep deprived may experience microsleeps—brief episodes of sleep lasting a few seconds at a time—which increase their risk of being involved in accidents.[6,8–10]

The impact of sleep deprivation on memory is well documented. Sleep scientists believe sleep is the time when the hippocampus and neocortex (two brain memory systems) communicate with each other. Initial memories are formed in the hippocampus. To be retained, the formed memory must be transmitted from the hippocampus to the neocortex, where it is stored as a long-term memory. Sleep provides the optimal time for this transmission. Some sleep experts believe that for every two hours a person stays

Individuals with severe sleep deprivation score worse on performance tests and alertness scales than people who are **legally too drunk to drive.**

awake, his or her brain will need an hour of sleep to support communication between the hippocampus and neocortex.[11]

Sleeping less than you need causes a **sleep debt**.[12] Your sleep debt accumulates over time, so that sleeping 1 hour less than you need every night for a week, for example, feels to your body like staying up all night. College students are especially vulnerable to building up a sleep debt, such as by pulling an all-nighter to prepare for an exam. (See the box "Study and Stimulants: Taking a Risk.") Many college students and others who build up a sleep debt during the week—night-shift workers, for example—try to cancel the debt by sleeping more on the weekends. This "solution," however, can actually worsen sleep deprivation during the week by disrupting sleep structure.[5,13,14] Getting

sleep debt
The difference between the amount of sleep attained and the amount needed to maintain alert wakefulness during the daytime, when the amount attained is less than the amount needed.

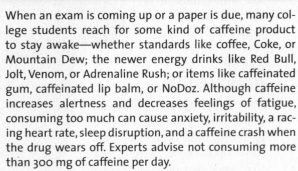

Challenges & Choices

Study and Stimulants: Taking a Risk

When an exam is coming up or a paper is due, many college students reach for some kind of caffeine product to stay awake—whether standards like coffee, Coke, or Mountain Dew; the newer energy drinks like Red Bull, Jolt, Venom, or Adrenaline Rush; or items like caffeinated gum, caffeinated lip balm, or NoDoz. Although caffeine increases alertness and decreases feelings of fatigue, consuming too much can cause anxiety, irritability, a racing heart rate, sleep disruption, and a caffeine crash when the drug wears off. Experts advise not consuming more than 300 mg of caffeine per day.

A growing number of students, between 4 and 35 percent, are turning to a different source when they want to keep going without sleep—stimulant medications prescribed for conditions such as attention deficit/hyperactivity disorder (ADHD), chronic fatigue, and depression. Among the more commonly abused of these drugs are Ritalin, Adderall, and Provigil. These medications work by affecting the levels of different neurotransmitters

in the brain, including dopamine, serotonin, and norepinephrine. They can cause irregular heartbeat, high blood pressure, high body temperature, seizures, heart attacks, and strokes. They can also be psychologically and physically addictive, and their long-term effects are not known.

Some college administrators are concerned that students may fake symptoms of ADHD to obtain prescription stimulants for their own use, to share with friends, or to sell, even though selling the drugs is a felony. On some campuses, physicians won't prescribe them or will only prescribe a supply for 15 or 30 days at a time. Many students resist the message that stimulant drugs can be dangerous. They view the illegal use of such drugs as morally acceptable since they are primarily used for academic performance rather than social recreation. They say the drugs help them focus better, give them an extra edge, and help them meet the time demands of active social lives and academic schedules. Health experts warn that the risks aren't worth it.

Sources: Data from "Illicit Use of Prescription ADHD Medications on a College Campus: A Multimethodological Approach," by A.D. DeSantis, E.M. Webb, and S.M. Noar, 2008, Journal of American College Health, 57(3), pp. 315–323; "Prevalence and Motives for Illicit Use of Prescription Stimulants in an Undergraduate Sample," by C.J. Teter, S.E, McCabe, J.A. Cranford, et. al. 2005, Journal of American College Health, 53, pp. 253–262; "Performance and Alertness of Caffeine, Dextroamphetamine, and Modafinil During Sleep Deprivation," by N.J. Wesenton, D. William, S. Kilgore, and T.J. Balkin, 2005, Journal of Sleep Research, 14(3), p. 225.

the same sufficient amount of sleep each night strengthens sleep structure.

How can you tell if you are getting enough sleep? A prime symptom of sleep deprivation is daytime drowsiness. If you feel alert during the day, you are probably getting enough sleep. If you are sleepy in sedentary situations such as reading, sitting in class, or watching television, you may be sleep deprived. Another measure of sleep deprivation is how long it takes you to fall asleep at night. A well-rested person will need 15 to 20 minutes to fall asleep.[5] If you fall asleep the instant your head hits the pillow, there is a good chance that you are sleep deprived.

What Makes You Sleep?

Over the course of the day, your body undergoes rhythmic changes that help you move from waking to sleep and back to waking. These *circadian rhythms* are maintained primarily by two tiny structures in the brain, the *suprachiasmic nuclei* (SCN), located directly behind the optic nerve in the hypothalamus (Figure 5.1). This internal "biological clock" controls body temperature and levels of alertness and activity. These controls are active in the daytime, increasing wakefulness, and inactive at night, allowing the body to relax and sleep. They are also less active in the early afternoon. In addition, the SCN control the release of certain hormones. They signal the pineal gland to release **melatonin**, a hormone that increases relaxation and sleepiness, and they signal the pituitary gland to release growth hormone during sleep, to help repair damaged body tissues.

Also important in maintaining circadian rhythms are external, environmental cues, especially light. Neurons in the SCN monitor the amount of light entering the eyes, so that as daylight increases, the SCN slow down the secretion of melatonin and begin to be more active.[12] This process keeps your sleep/wake cycles generally synchronized with the changing lengths of day and night. The process is sensitive to artificial light as well as natural light, and even relatively dim lights in the evening (for example, from a lamp or a computer screen) may delay when your biological clock induces sleepiness.

melatonin
A hormone that increases relaxation and sleepiness, released by the pineal gland during sleep.

The biological clock operates even without the cues of daylight or darkness, though not in perfect synchrony with a 24-hour day. Without the stimulation of light and dark, human beings would have a daily cycle several minutes longer than 24 hours. Every morning your body resets your biological clock to adjust to the next 24-hour period.[5] Your body easily tolerates a 1-hour adjustment. However, when bedtimes and awakening times differ greatly from their established norms, the adjustment is more difficult. Working night shifts and flying across several time zones, for example, can wreak havoc with your biological clock.[12,15]

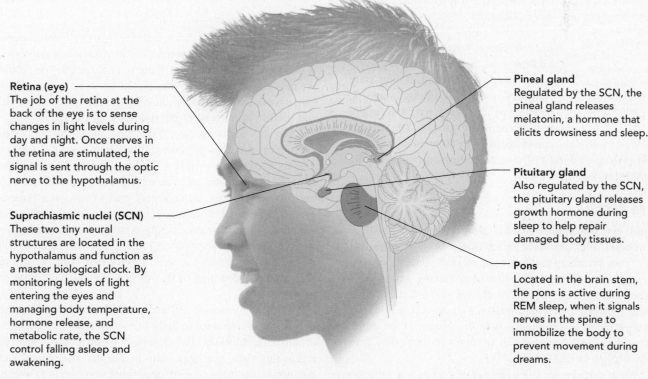

Retina (eye)
The job of the retina at the back of the eye is to sense changes in light levels during day and night. Once nerves in the retina are stimulated, the signal is sent through the optic nerve to the hypothalamus.

Suprachiasmic nuclei (SCN)
These two tiny neural structures are located in the hypothalamus and function as a master biological clock. By monitoring levels of light entering the eyes and managing body temperature, hormone release, and metabolic rate, the SCN control falling asleep and awakening.

Pineal gland
Regulated by the SCN, the pineal gland releases melatonin, a hormone that elicits drowsiness and sleep.

Pituitary gland
Also regulated by the SCN, the pituitary gland releases growth hormone during sleep to help repair damaged body tissues.

Pons
Located in the brain stem, the pons is active during REM sleep, when it signals nerves in the spine to immobilize the body to prevent movement during dreams.

figure **5.1** Brain structures involved in sleep and waking.

The Structure of Sleep

Studies have revealed that sleep consists of distinct stages in which muscle relaxation and nervous system arousal vary, as do types of brain waves and levels of neural activity. The brain cycles into two main states of sleep: non–rapid eye movement sleep, divided into four stages, and rapid eye movement sleep.

NREM SLEEP

You spend about 75 percent of your sleep time in **non–rapid eye movement (NREM) sleep**, a time of reduced brain activity with four stages.

Stage 1 of NREM sleep is a transitional, light sleep—a relaxed or half-awake state. Your heart rate slows and your breathing becomes shallow and rhythmic. This stage may last from 10 seconds to 10 minutes and is sometimes accompanied by visual imagery. People awakened in stage 1 often deny that they were asleep.[12,16]

In stage 2, your brain's activity slows further, and you stop moving. This lack of movement decreases muscle tension and brain stem stimulation so that sleep is induced. Stage 2 lasts about 10 to 20 minutes and represents the beginning of actual sleep. You are no longer consciously aware of your external environment. People awakened in stage 2 readily admit that they were asleep.[12,16]

During stages 3 and 4 your blood pressure drops, your heart rate and respiration slow, and the blood supply to your brain is minimized. If you were suddenly awakened during stage 4, referred to as *deep sleep*, you would feel momentarily groggy. You usually spend about 20 to 40 minutes at a time in deep sleep, and most of your deep sleep takes place in the first third of the night.[12,16]

REM SLEEP

Rapid eye movement (REM) sleep begins about 70 to 90 minutes after you have fallen asleep. As you enter this stage, your breathing and heart rate increase, and brain wave activity becomes more like that of a waking state. REM sleep is characterized by noticeable eye movements, usually lasting between 1 and 10 minutes. During this period you are most likely to experience your first dream of the night. Although dreams may occur in all stages of sleep, they generally happen in REM sleep.[5,12]

When you dream, there are periods when you have no muscle tone and your body cannot move, except for your eyes,

non–rapid eye movement (NREM) sleep
Type of sleep characterized by slower brain waves than are seen during wakefulness as well as other physiological markers; divided into four stages of increasingly deep sleep.

rapid eye movement (REM) sleep
Type of sleep characterized by brain waves and other physiological signs characteristic of a waking state but also characterized by reduced muscle tone, or sleep paralysis; most dreaming occurs during REM sleep.

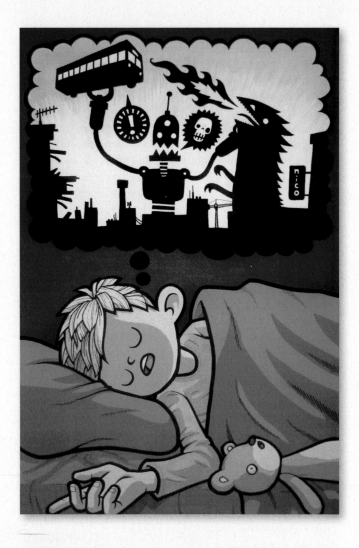

diaphragm, nasal membranes, and erectile tissue (such as penis or clitoris).[5] This state is referred to as *REM sleep paralysis*. If you were not immobilized, there is a danger that you would act on—or act out—your dreams. REM sleep is sometimes called *paradoxical sleep*, because the sleeper appears peaceful and still but is in a state of physiological arousal.

Dreams and dreaming have long intrigued people in every part of the world. Probably the best-known theory of dreams in Western culture is that of Sigmund Freud, who believed that the purpose of dreaming was the gratification of unconscious desires. By dreaming about them in disguised, symbolic form while we are sleeping, we fulfill wishes we would find unacceptable during waking life. At the opposite pole is a theory proposed in the 1970s that dreams are the product of random neural activity that goes on during REM sleep. According to this theory, dreams have little or no meaning.[5]

Still, many people believe that dreams do have some meaning and relevance to daily life, often reflecting changes or shifts in emotions. By examining your dreams, according to this view, you may gain insight into the mental and emotional processes you are applying to problems or events in your life.

Besides giving us time to dream, REM sleep also appears to give the brain the opportunity to "file" important ideas and thoughts in long-term storage, that is, in memory. This reorganization and consolidation may account for the fact that we are able to solve problems in our dreams. Scientists further believe that creative and novel ideas are more likely to flourish during REM sleep, because we have easier access to memories and emotions. Because ideas are filed in long-term storage during REM sleep, memory may be impaired if sleep time is insufficient. As a result of such memory impairment, the ability to learn new skills is also impaired. Performance in learning a new skill does not improve until an individual has had 6 hours of sleep; performance improves even more after 8 hours of sleep.[5,17,18]

The importance of REM sleep to the brain is demonstrated by what is called the **REM rebound effect**. If you get inadequate sleep for several nights, you will have longer and more frequent periods of REM sleep when you have a night in which you can sleep longer.[18]

REM rebound effect
Increase in the length and frequency of REM sleep episodes that are experienced when a person sleeps for a longer time after a period of sleep deprivation.

NREM stage 2 and REM sleep (Figure 5.2). After each successive cycle, the time spent in REM sleep doubles, lasting from 10 to 60 minutes at a time.[5,12]

The sleep cycle pattern changes across the lifespan, with children and young adolescents experiencing large quantities of NREM stages 3 and 4 sleep (deep sleep). Sleep needs are constant across adulthood, but as people get older, high-quality sleep may become more elusive, and older adults may experience less deep sleep and REM sleep and more NREM stage 1 sleep and wakefulness.[5] The production of melatonin and growth hormone declines with age, and the body temperature cycle may become irregular. All of these changes decrease total nighttime sleep.[19]

Medical conditions also affect sleep in older adults. Sleep is disrupted by such conditions as arthritis, heartburn, osteoporosis, Parkinson's disease, heart and lung diseases, dementia, incontinence, and cancer, as well as by some of the drugs used to treat these conditions. Additionally, sleep disorders are more common in middle and later life (see the next section).

However, many healthy older individuals have few or no sleep problems.[20] Some experts believe sleep problems are caused more by lifestyle choices—changes in diet, lack

If you were not immobilized during REM sleep paralysis, there is a danger you would act on—or act out—*your dreams.*

SLEEP CYCLES

After your first REM period, you cycle back and forth between REM and NREM sleep stages. These cycles repeat themselves about every 90 to 110 minutes until you wake up. Typically, you experience four or five sleep cycles each night. After the second cycle, however, you spend little or no time in NREM stages 3 and 4 and most of your time in

of exercise, decreased mental stimulation, daytime naps, and going to bed too early—than by biological changes. Older adults who maintain healthy lifestyle practices may still be able to get a good night's sleep.

There are also some gender differences in sleep cycles. Some of these differences begin as early as 6 months of age. Although the structure of sleep is essentially the same for

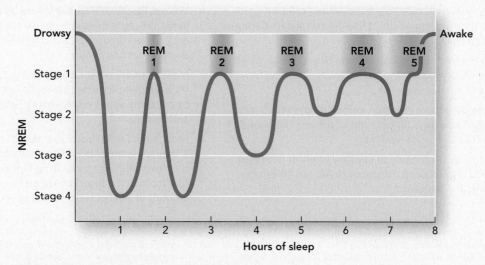

figure **5.2** **One night's sleep cycles.**

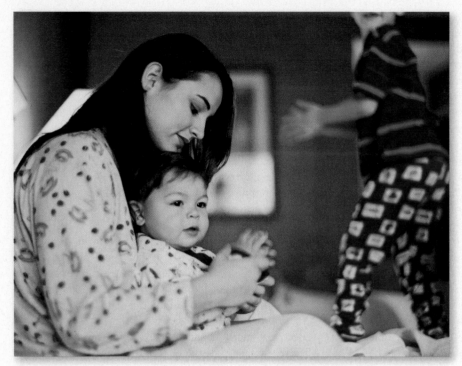

■ Women are more likely than men to get insufficient sleep. New mothers are particularly at risk for sleep deprivation.

men and women, women tend to have more slow-wave sleep (NREM stages 3 and 4) than men do and to experience more insomnia. Men have more REM periods. Men and women also tend to have some differences in habits and behaviors related to sleep. For example, women tend to get less sleep than they need in order to feel alert during the week, and men tend to get more sleep than they need. A majority of women (60 percent) say they do not get enough sleep most nights of the week.[21] However, men and women get about the same amount of sleep on the weekends.[21]

Sleep Disorders

The National Institutes of Health estimate that at least 40 million Americans suffer from long-term sleep disorders each year; another 20 million experience occasional sleep problems (see the box "Sleep Problems"). Because many sleep disorders are undiagnosed or not reported to physicians, many people who are chronically exhausted may not know why. Sleep disorders can be divided into dyssomnias and parasomnias.

DYSSOMNIAS

Sleep disorders associated with difficulty in falling asleep or staying asleep or with excessive sleepiness—the timing, quality, and quantity of sleep—are labeled **dyssomnias**.

Insomnia   In a poll conducted by the National Sleep Foundation (NSF), 30 to 40 percent of adults reported experiencing one or more

dyssomnias
Sleep disorders in which the timing, quality, and/or quantity of sleep is disturbed.

Who's at Risk?

Sleep Problems

- Sleepwalking is more common among children aged 4–12 than among adults. It usually disappears during adolescence.

- Men are more likely than women to experience sleep apnea. Being obese and having a large neck circumference also increase risk.

- Insomnia is more common among women than men. Women also have higher rates of depression, a condition that can cause insomnia.

- Whites are more likely to say they rarely or never get a good night's sleep compared to African Americans, Asians, and Hispanics.

- Whites, Blacks, and Hispanics are all about twice as likely as Asians to have a sleep disorder. Sleep apnea occurs more frequently among Blacks than within any other ethnic group

- More than other ethnic groups, Hispanics report that their sleep is disturbed at least a few nights a week by concerns about employment, relationships, money, and health.

- Older adults are at particular risk for sleep disruption if they consume alcohol. The ability to metabolize alcohol slows after age 50, causing higher levels of alcohol to remain in the blood and brain than when the same amount of alcohol is consumed at younger ages.

Sources: From "Sleepwalking," MedlinePlus, 2009, retrieved from http://www.nlm.nih.gov/medlineplus/ency/article/000808.htm; "Sleep Apnea Facts," American Association for Respiratory Care, retrieved from http://www.yourlunghealth.org/lung_disease/sleep_apnea/facts/; "Insomnia," The National Women's Health Information Center, 2010, retrieved from http://www.womenshealth.gov/faq/insomnia.cfm#c; "Drug and Alcohol Related Sleep Problems," WebMD, 2008, retrieved from http://www.webmd.com/sleep-disorders/drug-alcohol-related; "Sleep in America, 2010," The National Sleep Foundation, 2010, Washington DC: National Sleep Foundation.

Public Health in Action

Sleeping Smart

The National Sleep Foundation (NSF) has partnered with the pharmaceutical company Sanofi-Aventis U.S. to launch the Sleeping Smart campaign. Sleeping Smart targets Americans with sleep problems and aims to educate them about the importance of good sleep behaviors and the negative consequences of insomnia. It also seeks to motivate them to talk to their doctor about their sleep problems and help them understand how to safely and appropriately use sleep medications. The 2009 Sleep in America Poll was conducted as part of the campaign to raise awareness about the prevalence of sleep problems. According to the poll, 64 percent of Americans reported experiencing a sleep problem at least a few times a week, and 41 percent reported sleep problems every night of the week. However, half of those who reported sleep problems had not talked with their doctor about them. Insomnia was the primary sleep problem reported.

connect ACTIVITY

To kick off the campaign, the NSF released America's Sleep Report Card, based on the results from its 2009 sleep poll. Key findings included:

1. More than one-third of Americans are at increased risk for insomnia.
2. Although most survey respondents could identify health and performance consequences of insomnia, most did not have a clear understanding of insomnia itself.

3. Two-thirds of respondents at increased risk for insomnia did not consider themselves to have insomnia.
4. Many respondents who were at increased risk for insomnia engaged in stimulating activities an hour before getting into bed at least a few nights a week: 90 percent watched TV; 33 percent used the computer or Internet; and 43 percent did household chores.
5. Respondents at increased risk for insomnia reported this condition impacted their personal lives: 73 percent said it affected their mood; 63 percent said it affected their attention/concentration; 42 percent said it affected their family relationships; and 36 percent said it affected their job performance.

Insomnia can be a serious health condition. To help combat this problem, the Sleeping Smart campaign Web site includes a "study hall" and "faculty lounge." The study hall informs people of the many treatment options available for insomnia, which include behavioral or cognitive therapy, relaxation training, and medication. The faculty lounge features video clips of sleep professionals discussing when and how to talk to your doctor about a sleep problem and why it is important to seek treatment for insomnia. You can access this campaign at www.sleepfoundation.org.

Source: From "National Sleep Foundation: Sleeping Smart," retrieved March 7, 2010, from www.sleepfoundation.org/sleep-facts-information/sleeping-smart.

symptoms of **insomnia**—defined as difficulty falling or staying asleep—at least a few nights a week (see the box "Sleeping Smart").[2] Clinical symptoms of insomnia include (1) taking longer than 30 minutes to fall asleep, (2) experiencing five or more awakenings per night, (3) sleeping less than a total of 6½ hours as a result of these awakenings, and/or (4) experiencing less than 15 minutes of deep/slow-wave sleep.[22]

According to the NSF, insomnia can be caused by stress, anxiety, medical problems, poor sleep environment, noisy or restless partners, and schedule changes (due to travel across time zones or shift work, for example).[23] For adult women, more than half of whom report symptoms of insomnia during any given month, additional causes may include depression, headaches, effects of pregnancy, premenstrual syndrome, menopausal hot flashes, and overactive bladder. Often the person with insomnia has become distressed by his or her inability to fall asleep, which increases arousal and makes it even harder to fall asleep. In time, the bedroom, bedtime, or sleep itself becomes associated with frustration instead of relaxation, and a vicious cycle sets in.

Chronic insomnia is difficult to treat, but individuals may be able to break the cycle and experience relief through such approaches as improving their sleep habits and sleeping environment and using relaxation techniques such as deep

breathing and massage. See the section "Getting a Good Night's Sleep" later in this chapter for more strategies and tips on dealing with insomnia.

Sleep Apnea   Also known as breathing-related sleep disorder, **sleep apnea** is a condition characterized by periods of nonbreathing during sleep. Some health experts estimate that almost 40 percent of the U.S. population have some form of sleep apnea and that half of those afflicted may have a severe condition. Some 80 to 90 percent of these cases are undiagnosed. The condition occurs in all ethnic, age, and socioeconomic groups, although men are more at risk for developing sleep apnea than women are.[3,24–26]

Scientists have distinguished two main types of sleep apnea, central sleep apnea and obstructive sleep apnea. In *central sleep apnea*, a rare condition, the brain fails to regulate the diaphragm and other breathing mechanisms correctly. In *obstructive sleep apnea*, by far the more common type, the upper airway is obstructed during sleep.[3] Individuals with obstructive sleep

insomnia
Sleep disorder characterized by difficulty falling or staying asleep.

sleep apnea
Sleep disorder characterized by periods of nonbreathing during sleep; also known as breathing-related sleep disorder.

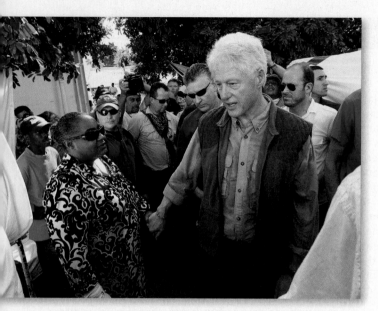

In 2010 former president Bill Clinton was briefly hospitalized for a blocked artery. After he was released, Clinton reflected that his hectic schedule over the past month, during which he got little sleep, had probably contributed to his heart problems.

apnea are frequently overweight and have an excess of bulky soft tissue in the neck and throat. When the muscles relax during sleep, the tissue can block the airway (Figure 5.3).

In obstructive sleep apnea, the individual stops breathing many times during sleep, often for as long as 60 to 90 seconds. The person's breathing pattern is usually characterized by periods of loud snoring (when the airway is partially blocked), alternating with periods of silence (when the airway is completely blocked), punctuated by sudden loud snores or jerking body movements as the person awakens for a few seconds and gasps for air. The individual is usually not

blood vessel abnormalities may occur. If sufficient oxygen is not delivered to the brain, death may occur during sleep.[25–28]

In children, sleep apnea is usually associated with enlarged tonsils. In adults, obstructive sleep apnea occurs most often in overweight, middle-aged men, although it becomes almost equally common in women after menopause. It is associated with larger neck circumferences (greater than 17 inches in men and 16 inches in women). People with the disorder often smoke, use alcohol, and/or sleep on their backs. There is sometimes a family history of sleep apnea, suggesting a genetic link.

narcolepsy
Sleep disorder characterized by frequent, irresistible "sleep attacks."

If sleep apnea is not severe, it can be addressed with a variety of behavioral strategies. They include losing weight, forgoing alcoholic nightcaps or sedatives, avoiding allergens, not smoking, using a nasal decongestant spray, using a firm pillow and mattress, and not sleeping on the back. In addition, adjustable mouthpieces are available that extend the lower jaw, adding room to the airway. They are expensive, however, and may not be covered by health insurance.[5]

In cases of severe sleep apnea, one treatment option is a continuous positive airway pressure (CPAP) machine. Through a comfortable mask, a CPAP machine gently blows slightly pressurized air into the patient's nose. Other treatment options include surgery to cut away excess tissue at the back of the throat and a new technique called *samnoplasty* that involves shrinking tissue in the back of the throat with radio-frequency energy.[29]

Narcolepsy   The neurological disorder **narcolepsy** is characterized by frequent, irresistible "sleep attacks," in which the individual unintentionally falls asleep in inappropriate situations, such as while driving a car. A person with narcolepsy experiences excessive daytime sleepiness, falls asleep

> *In obstructive sleep apnea, the individual*
> ## stops breathing many times during sleep,
> *often for as long as 60 to 90 seconds.*

aware of this pattern of snoring and gasping, although bed partners and other members of the household often are. The chief complaint of those with obstructive sleep apnea is daytime sleepiness, not nighttime awakening. Other symptoms include difficulty concentrating, depression, irritability, sexual dysfunction, and learning and memory difficulties.

Obstructive sleep apnea is a potentially dangerous condition; occasionally, it is even fatal. It is frequently seen in association with high blood pressure, and it can increase the risk of heart disease and stroke. Oxygen saturation of the blood decreases and levels of carbon dioxide rise when a person stops breathing, increasing the likelihood that heart and

for 10 to 20 minutes, and awakes feeling refreshed. Within 2 to 3 hours, however, the person once again feels sleepy.

Narcolepsy affects about 3 to 6 people in 10,000. Nearly 80 percent of cases of narcolepsy are not diagnosed. A person who has a relative with narcolepsy has a 3 percent chance of developing this disorder—a risk 60 times greater than that of someone with no family history of narcolepsy. If a person has one parent with narcolepsy, the odds are 1 in 20 that the person will have the disorder. Narcolepsy occurs as early as age 3 but usually does not begin until puberty, which suggests that maturation of the brain may play an important role in onset.[5,30]

(a)

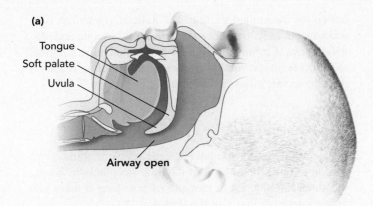

Tongue
Soft palate
Uvula

Airway open

(b)

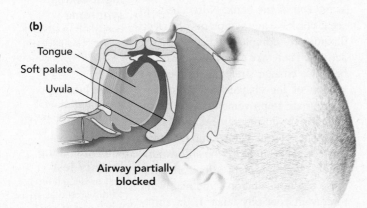

Tongue
Soft palate
Uvula

Airway partially blocked

(c)

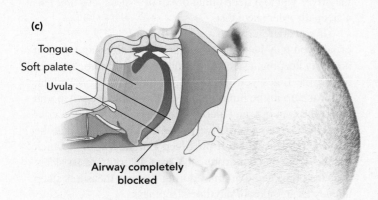

Tongue
Soft palate
Uvula

Airway completely blocked

figure 5.3 **Obstructive sleep apnea.** (a) Normally, the airway is open during sleep. (b) When the muscles of the soft palate, tongue, and uvula relax, they narrow the airway and cause snoring. (c) If these structures collapse on the back wall of the airway, they close the airway, preventing breathing. The efforts of the diaphragm and chest cause the blocked airway to become even more tightly sealed. For breathing to resume, the sleeper must rouse enough to cause tension in the tongue, which opens the airway.

There is no cure for narcolepsy, but symptoms may be reduced by taking a 10- to 20-minute nap every 2 hours throughout the day, avoiding alcohol and sleeping pills, and getting sufficient sleep on a regular basis.[30] Stimulant medications such as amphetamines have been used to treat pervasive daytime sleepiness.

Restless Legs Syndrome As the name suggests, **restless legs syndrome (RLS)** is a sleep disorder characterized by disagreeable sensations in the limbs, usually the legs. These uncomfortable and sometimes painful feelings, such as creeping, tingling, or burning, create an almost irresistible urge to move the legs. Discomfort is relieved by vigorously stretching and crossing the legs and, sometimes, walking about for a short time. The symptoms and the individual's responses to them can delay and disturb sleep, leading to daytime sleepiness. Sleep experts estimate that about 10 percent of the population have this syndrome.[30,31] Taking iron and vitamin E supplements may help reduce RLS symptoms. Avoiding late-night alcohol and engaging in moderate exercise are also encouraged.[31]

PARASOMNIAS

Whereas dyssomnias involve the timing, quality, or quantity of sleep, **parasomnias** involve physiological functioning or behavior during sleep. Body systems become activated as if the person were awake, usually during specific stages of sleep.

Sleepwalking Disorder People with **sleepwalking disorder** rise out of an apparently deep sleep and act as if they are awake. They do not respond to other people while in this state, or, if they do, it is with reduced alertness. Sleepwalking affects between 1 and 15 percent of the general population.[32] Sleepwalking takes place during the first third of the night's sleep. Episodes typically last less than 10 minutes.[5] If sleepwalkers are awakened, they are often confused for several minutes; if they are not awakened, they may return to bed and have little or no memory of the episode the next day.

Although there may be a genetic link to sleepwalking, most sufferers do not have a family history of this disorder. Episodes may be brought on by excessive sleep deprivation, fatigue, stress, illness, excessive alcohol consumption, and the use of sedatives.[5,32]

Nocturnal Eating Disorder A person with **nocturnal eating disorder** rises from bed during the night and eats and drinks while asleep. About three quarters of people with this disorder are female. The person may consume bizarre

restless legs syndrome (RLS)
Sleep disorder characterized by disagreeable sensations in the limbs, usually the legs.

parasomnias
Sleep disorders in which physiological functioning or behavior during sleep is disturbed.

sleepwalking disorder
Sleep disorder in which a person rises out of an apparently deep sleep and acts as if awake.

nocturnal eating disorder
Sleep disorder in which a person rises from bed during the night and eats and drinks while asleep.

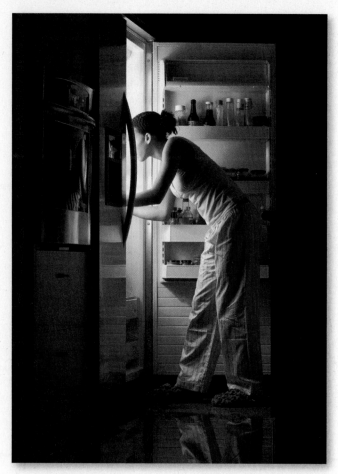

■ Night-time eating can be associated with a sleep disorder. People with nocturnal eating disorder binge eat without waking up; people with night eating syndrome consume a large portion of their daily calories during the night.

concoctions but has no memory of these experiences in the morning. Fifty percent of people suffering from this disorder binge eat without awakening. Although they may binge up to six times a night, they do not experience indigestion or feelings of fullness after the binge.[5,7]

Distinct from nocturnal eating disorder is a newly identified sleep disorder, **night eating syndrome**, in which affected persons binge eat late at night, have difficulty falling asleep, repeatedly awaken during the night and eat again, and then eat very little the next day. Some people with night eating syndrome consume more than 50 percent of their daily calories at night. Sleep experts estimate that the syndrome's frequency is about 1.5 percent in the general population and up to 10 percent among obese people seeking treatment for their weight. Treatments include medications and behavior management techniques.[5,7]

Sexsomnia Sexsomnia involves masturbating, fondling another person, or actual intercourse with a nonconsenting person while asleep. Most people who experience sexsomnia have no memory of the event. An intriguing legal question is whether a person committing a sexual assault while asleep has committed a crime. The judicial system has been inconsistent in its decisions concerning sexsomnia and sexual assaults. Curbing alcohol use and maintaining a regular sleep cycle are prevention factors. This condition is one of the remote side effects of the sleep drug Ambien.[12]

Evaluating Your Sleep

How can you tell if you have a sleep problem? First, get a sense of your general level of daytime sleepiness by taking the **sleep latency** test (a measure of how long it takes you to fall asleep) in Part 1 of the Personal Health Portfolio activity for Chapter 5 at the end of the book. Next, check to see if you have any symptoms of a sleep disorder by completing Part 2 of the activity. Then take a look at the various behavior change strategies in the next section of the chapter and make any appropriate improvements. Of course, the most basic recommendation is to make sure you are getting enough hours of sleep every night. If you still experience a sleep problem after following these recommendations, you may want to consult your physician. If the problem is serious enough, your physician may refer you to a sleep clinic or lab or a sleep disorder specialist.

If you are referred to a sleep clinic or lab, you may be asked to monitor your sleeping habits at home by keeping a sleep diary for a week or more. You will record the times you go to bed, awaken during the night, and wake up in the morning, as well as what and when you eat in the evening, any alcohol, tobacco, or drugs you consume, and so on. Alternatively, you may be evaluated at the lab. You may take a **Multiple Sleep Latency Test**, in which you lie down in a dark room and are told not to resist sleep. This test, repeated five times during the day, measures sleep latency as an index of daytime sleepiness.

night eating syndrome Condition in which a person eats excessively during the night while awake.

sleep latency Amount of time it takes a person to fall asleep.

Multiple Sleep Latency Test Test of sleep latency, administered as an index of daytime sleepiness and usually given five times in a sleep clinic.

Getting a Good Night's Sleep

What is the best way to ensure healthy sleep patterns over the course of the lifespan? In this section we provide several strategies and tips that will help you get a good night's sleep.

ESTABLISHING GOOD SLEEP HABITS

Several habits and behaviors concerning when and where you sleep and what you do before you sleep can help you sleep better and solve sleep problems (see the box "Cole: A Case of Insomnia").

Maintain a Regular Sleep Schedule Try to get about 8 hours of sleep every night, 7 days a week. With a regular

Life Stories

Cole: A Case of Insomnia

connect ACTIVITY

Cole is a 19-year-old sophomore majoring in psychology. During his freshman year, he had grant money to cover his tuition, but this year he is on his own. So when school started 3 months ago, he got a job working the evening shift at an upscale restaurant. On paper, it seemed like a logical setup: work till 11 p.m., study till 1 a.m., and wake up at 8 a.m. for a 9 o'clock class. But a month into the school year, Cole began having trouble falling and staying asleep. Sometimes he'd lie in bed for hours, staring at the ceiling, trying to think himself to sleep. Eventually he decided to just spend time on the computer playing games and messaging his friends on Facebook until he finally felt sleepy, usually between 3 and 4 a.m. He only averaged about 5 hours of sleep on weekdays, but he was grateful for the weekends, when he could sleep in and try to catch up on sleep.

At first, Cole felt okay during the day with the help of some caffeine. He stopped by Starbucks on the way to class in the morning to pick up a Venti coffee. Whenever he started feeling tired during the day or during his study time at night, he'd grab a Red Bull or a RockStar or take a caffeine pill like Vivarin. But eventually the caffeine stopped having any effect. Midterms were coming up in a few weeks and Cole felt stressed. He was in a fog during the day and couldn't fall asleep at night. He bought some Adderall from a classmate to help him stay awake and focus on studying. He also tried Tylenol PM for a few days to help him sleep, but it didn't work. The breaking point came when Cole could not fall asleep for two days straight and felt like he was going a little crazy. He knew his strategies were not working, so he made an appointment at the student health clinic to get help.

sleep schedule, you fall asleep faster and awaken more easily, because you are psychologically and physiologically conditioned for sleep and waking. Most students have an irregular sleep schedule.[2,5] As noted earlier, such a schedule throws off your internal biological clock and disrupts the structure of sleep.

Create a Sleep-Friendly Environment Your bedroom should be a comfortable, secure, quiet, cool, and dark place for inducing sleep. Your mattress should be hard enough to allow you to get into a comfortable sleep position. If it is too hard, however, it may not provide an adequate cushion to prevent painful pressure on your body.[5]

Noise can reduce restful sleep. Research on people who live near airports has found that excessive noise may jog individuals out of deep sleep and into a lighter sleep. Street noises have a similar effect.[33] Noise levels above 40 decibels (about as loud as birds singing) can disturb sleep. College residence halls and apartment complexes often have noise levels that exceed 40 decibels. Earplugs and earphones can reduce noise levels by as much as 90 percent.

If it isn't possible to eliminate noise, try creating *white noise*, a monotonous and unchanging sound such as that of an air conditioner or a fan. Noise generators that create soothing sounds such as falling rain, wind, and surf have been proven effective in protecting sleep.[7,34] If you can't find an inexpensive noise generator, start with a fan.[34]

Temperature is important too. You sleep best when the temperature is within your specific comfort zone. A temperature below or above that zone often causes fragmented sleep or wakefulness. The ideal is usually 62° F to 65° F. Generally, temperatures above 75° F and below 54° F cause people to awaken.[5]

Finally, don't expect to get a good night's sleep if you cannot lie down. Research has shown that people sleeping in an upright position have poorer quality sleep than those sleeping in a horizontal position. The amount of slow-wave sleep a person experiences in a sitting position is almost zero. If you fall asleep while standing up, your body begins to sway so that you quickly awaken. Perhaps the brain operates in a similar fashion when you are sleeping in a seated position. With your body mainly upright, your brain may interpret this position as not sufficiently safe to allow deep sleep.[5]

Avoid Caffeine, Nicotine, and Alcohol Caffeine, a stimulant, disrupts sleep, whether it comes in coffee, tea, chocolate, or soda. Caffeine enters your bloodstream quickly, reaches a peak in about 30 to 60 minutes, and it may take up

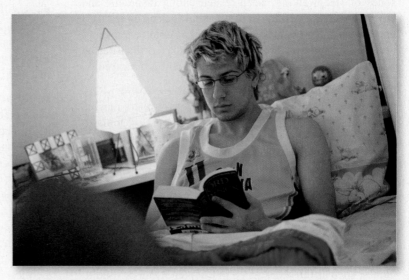

■ One key to getting a good night's sleep is creating a pleasant environment and establishing a relaxing bedtime routine.

to 4 to 6 hours for half of caffeine intake to clear the blood system of a young adult. A single cup of coffee may double the amount of time it takes an average adult to fall asleep. It may also reduce the amount of slow-wave or deep sleep by half and quadruple the number of nighttime awakenings.[12] Avoiding caffeine intake 6 to 8 hours before going to bed may improve sleep quality.

Like caffeine, nicotine is a stimulant that can disrupt sleep. People who smoke a pack of cigarettes a day have been shown to have sleep problems. Brain wave pattern analysis indicates that they do not sleep as deeply as nonsmokers. Smoking also affects the respiratory system by causing congestion in the nose and swelling of the mucous membranes lining the throat and upper airway passages. These physiological factors increase the likelihood of snoring and aggravate the symptoms of sleep apnea. They also decrease oxygen uptake, which leads to more frequent awakenings.[5,34–37]

Alcohol induces sleepiness and reduces the amount of time it takes to fall asleep, but it causes poorer sleep and restlessness later in the night. Even if consumed 6 hours before bedtime, alcohol can increase wakefulness in the second half of the night, probably through its effect on serotonin and norepinephrine, neurotransmitters that regulate sleep. Because alcohol is a depressant, it prevents REM sleep from occurring until most of the alcohol has been absorbed. After absorption, vivid dreams are more likely. Sleep experts call this an *alcohol rebound effect*, in which the body seems to be trying to recover REM sleep that was lost earlier.

Additionally, alcohol can aggravate sleep disorders such as obstructive sleep apnea and trigger episodes of sleepwalking, sleep-related eating disorders, and other disorders. The impact of alcohol on sleep apnea is of particular concern; it can even be deadly. Alcohol consumption makes throat muscles even more relaxed than during normal sleep; it also interferes with the ability to awaken.[36]

Get Regular Exercise but Not Close to Bedtime
Regular exercise during the day or early evening hours may be beneficial for sleep. Exercising within 3 hours of going to bed, however, is not recommended, because exercise stimulates the release of adrenaline and elevates core body temperature. It takes 5 to 6 hours for body temperature to drop enough after vigorous exercise for drowsiness to occur and deeper sleep to take place.[5,34]

Manage Stress and Establish Relaxing Bedtime Rituals
Stress increases physiological arousal and can adversely affect sleep patterns. Stress management and reduction techniques, such as those described in Chapter 3, can be used to help induce sleepiness. For example, keep a worry book by your bedside and record bothersome thoughts and problems

in it that keep you awake at night. Once you've written them down, tell yourself you'll work on them during daylight hours, and then let go of them. Use your notes to focus energy and attention on these problems over the course of the next few days.

It can also be helpful to develop a bedtime ritual, such as reading, listening to soothing music, or taking a warm (but not too hot) bath; your mind and body will come to associate bedtime with relaxation and peacefulness. Avoid stressful or stimulating activities before bedtime, such as working or paying bills, and dim the lights to let your internal clock know that drowsiness is appropriate. Experiment until you find a method of calming down and relaxing at bedtime that works for you.

If you do have a hard time falling asleep, don't stay in bed longer than 30 minutes. Get up, leave the room, and listen to soothing music or read until you feel sleepy.

Avoid Eating Too Close to Bedtime
Try not to eat heavy meals within 3 hours of bedtime, particularly meals with high fat content. When you are lying down, the force of gravity cannot assist the movement of food from the stomach into the small intestine to complete digestion, and you may experience acid indigestion, or heartburn.

Also avoid caffeinated beverages, citrus fruits and juices, and tomato-based products such as pasta sauce, because these foods can temporarily weaken the esophageal sphincter. When weakened, this sphincter allows stomach contents to move back into the esophagus, a condition known as *acid reflux*. If you have acid reflux, try raising the head of your bed 6 to 8 inches, which will allow gravity to help empty stomach contents into the small intestine. Tilting the bed is more effective than elevating the upper body with pillows. For those who are overweight, moderate weight loss may reduce discomfort, because excessive stomach fat can cause abdominal pressure that contributes to heartburn.[5,7]

Be Smart About Napping
The typical North American adult takes one or two naps a week, and about a third of adults nap more than four times a week. About a fourth never take a nap. If you are a napper, sleep experts recommend naps of only 15 to 45 minutes, which can be refreshing and restorative. If you nap longer than 45 minutes, your body can enter stage 4 deep sleep. It is more difficult to awaken from this stage, and you are likely to feel groggy.[5,7]

If you know you will be going to bed later than usual, you may want to take a "preventive nap" of 2 to 3 hours. Research suggests that people who take preventive naps increase their alertness by about 30 percent over that of people who do not nap. Napping 15 minutes every 4 hours until you attain 2 hours of preventive napping is also recommended. This

Critters in Your Bed and Bedroom

Dust mites are extremely common bedroom pests. A typical used mattress may have as many as 100,000 to 10 million microscopic dust mites inside, and 10 percent of the weight of a 2-year-old pillow may be made up of dust mites and their droppings. If not controlled, dust mites can spread throughout the house. To control dust mites, follow these precautions:

- Replace pillows frequently.
- Use synthetic rather than down pillows.
- Vacuum your mattress thoroughly, or cover it with a plastic case that can be wiped with a damp cloth.
- Wash your bed linens weekly in hot water (at least 130° F).
- Vacuum the bedroom carpet frequently.
- Choose hardwood floors over carpet.

Bed bugs are another bedroom pest. For unknown reasons, many cities have recently experienced an upsurge in bed bug infestations. Bed bugs are small, brownish, flattened insects that feed on the blood of animals. Adults are about $1/4$ inch long. They are active primarily at night and during the day prefer to hide in the tiny crevices provided by the mattress, box spring, bed frame, or headboard. Their bites, usually on the arms or legs, cause welts and itching that are often mistaken for mosquito bites. Professional pest control may be needed to control a bed bug problem.

Another bedroom pest is the brown recluse spider, found primarily in the central midwestern states southward to the Gulf of Mexico. This spider is about $3/8$ inch long and is sometimes referred to as a fiddleback or violin spider because of the faint violin-shaped marking on its back. The brown recluse is not an aggressive spider; people are usually bitten when they accidentally crush, handle, or disturb it, as can happen if it has crawled into bedding. Most bites leave only a small reddish mark, but in some cases the bite can cause a deep, painful wound that can blister, enlarge, and cause a general systemic reaction that includes agitation, itching, fever, chills, nausea, vomiting, or shock. Children, older adults, and people with immune suppression disorders are more vulnerable to systemic reactions.

To prevent bites by the brown recluse or any other spider, follow these precautions:

- Inspect bedding and towels before use.
- Move your bed away from the wall.
- Shake out clothing and shoes before getting dressed.
- Dust and vacuum regularly.
- Eliminate clutter in closets.
- Seal and caulk crevices where spiders can enter your home.
- Wear gloves when handling cardboard boxes, firewood, or rocks.

Many commercial pesticide products are effective for spider control, but if the problem is widespread, you may need to use a pest management company.

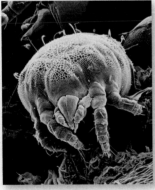 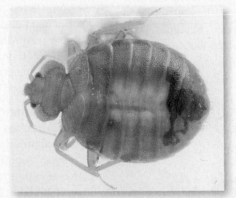 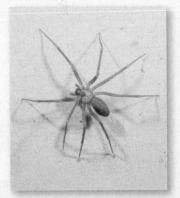

Dust mites (left) are microscopic. Bed bugs (center) are about $1/4$ inch in length. The brown recluse spider (right) has a body about $3/8$ inch in length.

short nap strategy has been effectively used by physicians and law enforcement officers, who must perform in emergency situations for long hours.[38]

Get Rid of Dust Mites and Other Bedroom Pests Dust mites are microscopic insects that feed on dead skin cells. They live primarily in pillows and mattresses. Dust mite droppings become airborne and are inhaled while people are sleeping, causing allergic reactions and asthma in sensitive individuals. If you experience itchy or watery eyes, sneezing, wheezing, congestion, or difficulty breathing in your bedroom, the culprit may be dust mites. For guidelines on preventing and controlling dust mites, and for information on other bedroom pests, see the box "Critters in Your Bed and Bedroom."

Consider Your Bed Partner Snoring is a major disrupter of partners' sleep, and body movement during sleep can also be a problem for partners. Avoiding alcohol before bedtime, using nasal sprays, sleeping on your side, and using a humidifier may help reduce snoring.

Men tend to thrash around in bed more than women do, and older couples tend to move in less compatible ways than do younger couples. A mattress with low motion transfer may help prevent sleep disruption caused by a partner's movement. Sleep can also be disrupted if a partner has a different sleep schedule or has a sleep disorder. If your partner's sleep habits create a problem for you, encourage your partner to improve his or her sleep habits or to see a sleep disorder specialist. As a last resort, you or your partner may have to sleep in a different bed or room.

USING SLEEP AIDS

Because sleep is so influential in your daily functioning, and because sleep problems are so common, it should not be surprising that many people resort to sleep aids of one kind or another to help them get a good night's sleep. About 15 percent of adults use a prescription sleep medication and/or an over-the-counter sleep aid to help them sleep a few nights a week.[34]

Prescription Medications Safe and effective sleep medications are those that can be taken at higher doses, are not addictive, do not produce serious side effects, and wear off quickly so that you are not drowsy the next day. Sleep experts disagree about whether today's sleep medications meet these criteria.[5] No sleep medication should be used for longer than two weeks without physician consultation.

The most frequently prescribed, longer acting sleep medications are the benzodiazepines Restoril, Dalmon, and Doral. These drugs induce sleep but suppress both deep sleep and REM sleep. Their effects can last from 3 to 24 hours, and daytime side effects include decreased memory and intellectual functioning. People quickly build tolerance to long-lasting benzodiazepines, which are addictive and lose their effectiveness after 30 nights of consecutive use. There are some shorter acting benzodiazepines on the market that do not suppress deep sleep and REM sleep.[34]

A new category of sleep medications is the imidazopyridines. The National Sleep Foundation considers these drugs the best prescription sleeping aids.[34] One drug in this category, zolpidem, sold under the trade name Ambien, has become the best-selling prescription sleep aid in the United States, but it has been associated with some disturbing side effects (see the box "Sleep Aids and Bizarre Behaviors").

Over-the-Counter Medications Nonprescription, or over-the-counter, medications can be useful for treating transient or short-term insomnia, such as may occur under conditions of great stress or trauma. They should be discontinued once the cause of the problem has been eliminated, ideally within 2 weeks. The recommended maximum use is 4 weeks.

Many over-the-counter sleep products contain antihistamine, a type of drug developed to treat allergies. The effects of antihistamines are general throughout the body; besides drowsiness, they cause dehydration, agitation, and constipation. Additionally, you can quickly develop tolerance to antihistamines, and when you stop taking them, you may experience **rebound insomnia**—insomnia that is worse than what you experienced before you started taking the medication.[34] Rebound insomnia can be avoided by gradually reducing the dose. Over-the-counter products like Tylenol PM that contain acetaminophen should also be used with caution. Large doses of acetaminophen are toxic to the liver and can cause severe liver damage.

rebound insomnia Insomnia that occurs after a person stops taking sleep medication and that is worse than it was before the medication was started.

Complementary and Alternative Products and Approaches Complementary and alternative products and approaches to sleep problems include herbal products, dietary supplements, and aromatherapy. The herbal product most commonly used for insomnia is valerian, which has a tranquilizing or sedative effect. Hops is another product currently receiving attention as a possible sleep aid. Both are widely available in health food stores. Herbal products can interact with other medications and drugs, including caffeine and alcohol; it is strongly recommended that you consult with your physician before trying any herbal remedies.[39]

Melatonin is a dietary supplement that has been marketed as a sleep aid, but health experts are divided on its effectiveness. As noted earlier in this chapter, melatonin is a hormone naturally secreted by the pineal gland in response to darkness. It lowers body temperature and causes drowsiness. Most experts agree that the 3-milligram dose of synthetically

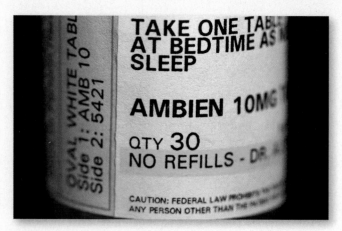

■ Ambien belongs to a class of drugs considered the best prescription sleep aids, but use of this medication is associated with unusual side effects, including eating, driving, and having sex while asleep.

Consumer Clipboard

Sleep Aids and Bizarre Behaviors

Sleep medications commonly have such side effects as next-day drowsiness, dizziness, headaches, confusion, agitation, and even hallucinations. More bizarre reactions are said by drug manufacturers to be "remote," defined as fewer than 1 episode per 1,000 users. But in recent years, there have been reports of people eating, cooking, and driving in their sleep after taking Ambien, a sleep aid.

A study by the Minnesota Regional Sleep Center found that thousands of Ambien users have experienced sleep-eating and sleep-driving behaviors. Sexsomnia—engaging in sexual behavior while asleep—is also associated with Ambien. Scientists believe that sleep-aid medications may suppress the brain's arousal system and cause these and other bizarre behaviors.

Another condition associated with sleep medications is "traveler's amnesia." Sleep aids typically cause temporary amnesia, lasting for a few hours after the drug is taken. Temporary memory loss is usually not a problem,

because the user is asleep. But when a sleep medication is taken by someone who is traveling, the person may have to wake up before the drug has worn off. Many people in this situation have found they have amnesia for the hours when the drug was still active.

The side effects of sleep medications can vary, depending on the person's general health, drug tolerance, and other medications. Most of these sleep medications, however, have not been tested for long-term use, and the U.S. Food and Drug Administration has requested that manufacturers use stronger language on their labels warning of potential risks. Some physicians question the value of these drugs, since users fall asleep faster than nonusers by only about 15 to 20 minutes.

If you use sleep aids, consult with your physician or pharmacist about proper dosage and possible side effects. Sleep medications should not be crushed or chewed, and alcohol should not be used in combination with sleep aids.

Sources: A Good Night's Sleep, by L.J. Epstein, 2007, New York: McGraw-Hill; "Ambien Linked to 'Sleep Eating,'" by D. DeNoon, retrieved from www.webmd.com/content/Article/120/113595.htm?pagenumber=3.

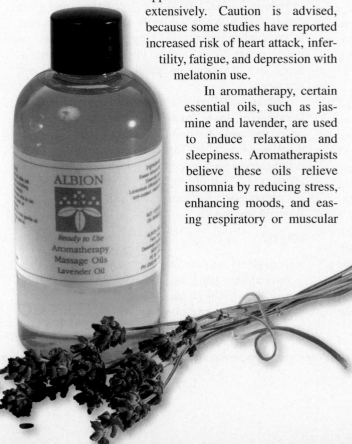

produced melatonin available in health food stores is too high and that a dose of 0.1 milligram is as effective as a higher dose.[34,39] Potential side effects, interactions with drugs, and long-term health effects of melatonin supplements have not been studied extensively. Caution is advised, because some studies have reported increased risk of heart attack, infertility, fatigue, and depression with melatonin use.

In aromatherapy, certain essential oils, such as jasmine and lavender, are used to induce relaxation and sleepiness. Aromatherapists believe these oils relieve insomnia by reducing stress, enhancing moods, and easing respiratory or muscular

problems, but no strong scientific evidence supports these claims.[39] Aromatherapy oils may be applied to the skin by full body massage, or a drop may be placed on the wrist or at the base of the throat so the scent is inhaled during sleep. Scented sprays can be used on bed linens, but aromatherapy candles should not be used when you are sleeping. Aromatherapy products are generally available in health food stores. If you are interested in trying this approach, however, it is recommended that you consult a trained aromatherapist before making any purchases.

* * *

As noted, it is not surprising that people go to great lengths to get enough high-quality sleep. Nothing is as refreshing and restorative as a good night's sleep, giving us a fresh perspective and renewed energy for facing the demands of the day. Shakespeare called sleep the "balm of hurt minds, chief nourisher in life's feast." Sleep, he wrote, "knits up the ravell'd sleeve of care." Conversely, almost nothing is as distressing as being unable to avail ourselves of the respite provided by sleep. Chronic sleep deprivation can interfere with physical, emotional, and cognitive functioning and leave us fatigued, depressed, and more susceptible to illness and disease. As with so many other facets of lifestyle, good sleep habits and practices, established early in life, can help you maintain wellness in both younger and older adulthood.

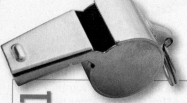

You Make the Call

Should Drowsy Drivers Be Criminally Liable for Crashes They Cause?

Maggie McDonnell, a 20-year-old college student from Washington Township, New Jersey, was killed in July 1997 when the car she was driving was hit head-on by a van that had crossed three lanes of traffic. The driver of the van told police he had not slept in 30 hours and had smoked crack cocaine a few hours before the crash. He was charged with vehicular homicide.

At the time, conviction for vehicular homicide under New Jersey law required driver recklessness. A person who drove while knowingly fatigued and caused a fatal crash could be charged only with careless driving. The jury was not allowed to consider driver fatigue as a factor in this case. The first trial ended in a deadlock on the charge of vehicular homicide, and the second trial ended in acquittal. The driver was fined $200 and received two points on his driving record.

In 2003, New Jersey passed the first statute to specifically cite driver fatigue as a factor that could be considered under the charge of vehicular homicide. New Jersey's Drowsy Driving Act, called Maggie's Law, explicitly allows a jury to find a driver reckless if he or she was awake for 24 hours prior to causing a fatal crash. Maggie's Law prevents the defense from using an inadequate law as a tool to defend the guilty. A motorist violating the law can be charged with vehicular homicide, punishable by up to 10 years in prison and a fine of $150,000.

Since Maggie's death, the number of criminal prosecutions and civil suits involving driver-fatigue crashes has increased. A Virginia man who killed two people when he fell asleep at the wheel received a 5-year jail sentence. This sentence exceeded state sentencing guidelines. McDonald's Corporation paid $400,000 to the family of a victim killed by a teenage McDonald's employee in Oregon who had only 7 hours of sleep in the previous 48 hours due to his work and school schedule. The accident occurred when the employee was driving home from work. The Los Angeles City Council approved a $16 million settlement to the family of a woman permanently disabled by a city maintenance truck when the driver fell asleep at the wheel.

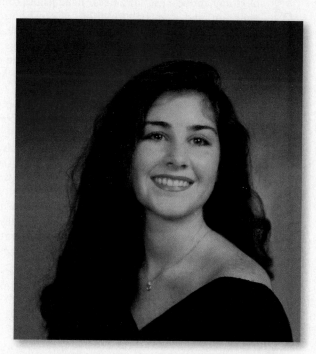

In 2002, a bill named Maggie's Law: National Drowsy Driving Act of 2002 was introduced in the U.S. House of Representatives. Although it never became law, the bill would have encouraged states and communities to develop traffic safety programs to reduce crashes related to driver fatigue and sleep deprivation, to create a driver's education curriculum, to standardize reporting of fatigue-related crashes on police report forms, and to implement countermeasures such as continuous shoulder rumble strips and rest areas.

Many states besides New Jersey have passed laws making driver drowsiness a form of recklessness under the vehicular homicide charge. Proponents of these measures claim that stringent laws with severe consequences are needed to get sleep-deprived drivers off the roads, but opponents argue that the measures are unnecessary, ineffective, and difficult to enforce. What do you think?

PROS

- Almost 55 percent of adults who drive say they have driven their vehicles while feeling drowsy, and 28 percent of adults report falling asleep while driving. An estimated 60 million Americans

connect ACTIVITY

are operating vehicles each day without adequate sleep. These people need to be held responsible for the outcomes of their choices.

- Driving fatigue has been underestimated as a factor in driving performance. The National Highway Traffic Safety Administration conservatively estimates that 100,000 police-reported crashes are the direct result of driver fatigue each year, resulting in 1,550 deaths and 71,000 injuries.

- Investigation of driver fatigue can be improved with new technology. States may mandate that cars come equipped with eyelid-measuring devices. Post-crash investigators could use this information to determine if a driver involved in a crash was significantly impaired by drowsiness.

CONS

- Most police officers are not trained to properly investigate driver drowsiness accidents. This lack of training makes it difficult to collect sufficient evidence for prosecution and wastes taxpayers' money on cases that can't be won.

- The point of New Jersey's Drowsy Driving Act was to make driver drowsiness akin to driving while intoxicated. Research suggests similarities between these two conditions, but it is much more difficult for a police officer to detect driver fatigue than to detect intoxication. A driver involved in a crash or pulled over for erratic driving may experience an adrenaline rush that masks fatigue symptoms.

- It is easy for people to lie about how many hours they have been awake in order to avoid prosecution.

- Under this law, people with diagnosed sleep disorders that can cause daytime drowsiness, such as sleep apnea or narcolepsy, could be punished for having conditions they can't help and could be held liable for outcomes for which they are not really responsible.

Sources: "Testimony of the Impact of Driver Fatigue. Report Before the Subcommittee on Highways and Transit, Committee on Transportation and Infrastructure," June 27, 2002, retrieved from www.drowsydriving.org; "A Place to Crash: The Dangers of Driving While Drowsy," by A. Dalton, retrieved June 1, 2008, from www.legalaffairs.org/printerfriendly.msp?id=843; "Sleep in America" Poll, National Sleep Foundation, 2009, Washington DC: National Sleep Foundation.

IN REVIEW

How does sleep impact your health?
Quantity and quality of sleep are strongly associated with overall health and quality of life. Adequate sleep gives the body time for repair, recovery, and renewal. Sleep deprivation is associated with a wide range of health problems, ranging from cardiovascular disease to depression to overweight and obesity.

What makes you sleep?
Sleep is induced by the activity of a specific set of structures in the brain, in combination with environmental cues such as darkness. Humans have a circadian rhythm slightly longer than 24 hours; every morning the body resets this biological clock to adjust to the next 24-hour cycle.

What is the structure of sleep?
Every night, people cycle through several stages of sleep, characterized by different brain waves, different states of muscle relaxation, and different nervous system activity.

NREM sleep includes stages of deep sleep, whereas REM sleep includes dreaming and brain activity related to the consolidation of learning and memory.

What are sleep disorders?
Problems associated with falling or staying asleep are classified as dyssomnias; they include insomnia, sleep apnea, narcolepsy, and restless legs syndrome. Problems associated with behavior during sleep are classified as parasomnias; examples are sleepwalking, nocturnal eating disorder, and a disorder sometimes associated with sleep medications, sexsomnia.

How can you enhance the quality of your sleep?
The key to a good night's sleep is establishing good sleep habits, such as maintaining a regular sleep schedule, creating a sleep-friendly environment, and avoiding stimulants late in the day. Sleep aids, whether prescription, over the counter, or herbal, can help with situational sleep problems but shouldn't be used over the long term.

Web Resources

American Academy of Sleep Medicine: This professional organization focuses on the advancement of sleep medicine and sleep research. Its Web site offers links to several sleep journals and other sleep organizations.
www.aasmnet.org

American Sleep Apnea Association: This organization focuses on increased understanding of sleep apnea disorders. It is dedicated to reducing injury, disability, and death from sleep apnea and to enhancing the well-being of those affected by this common disorder.
www.sleepapnea.org/asaa.html

National Sleep Foundation: From the basics of getting a good night's sleep to understanding sleep problems and disorders, this site offers helpful information. It features interactive sleep quizzes, brochures, and a variety of tools for better sleep.
www.sleepfoundation.org

SleepNet: If you want to locate a sleep lab, take a sleep test, understand sleep terms, and learn about sleep disorders, this site is the place to visit. It highlights various sleep problems, offering clear explanations, and features related readings.
www.sleepnet.com

Sleep Research Society: This organization is dedicated to scientific investigation of all aspects of sleep and sleep disorders. It promotes the exchange of knowledge pertaining to sleep.
www.sleepresearchsociety.org

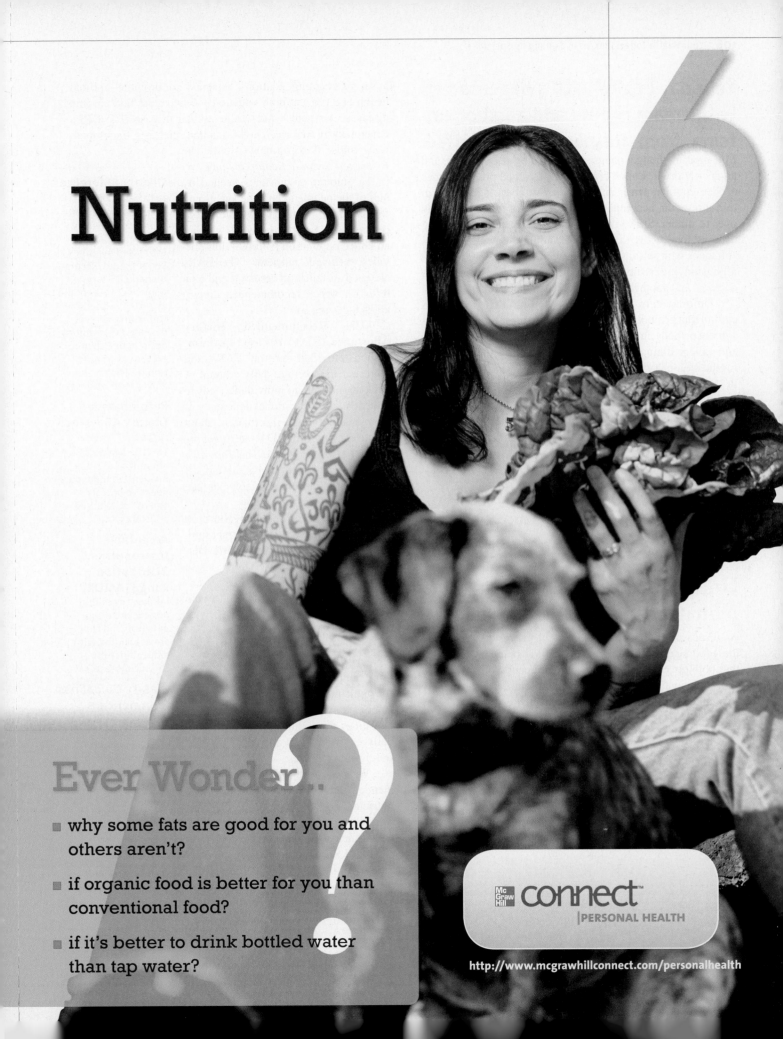

Nutrition

6

Ever Wonder...

- why some fats are good for you and others aren't?
- if organic food is better for you than conventional food?
- if it's better to drink bottled water than tap water?

McGraw Hill **connect** |PERSONAL HEALTH

http://www.mcgrawhillconnect.com/personalhealth

Your day begins with a bagel spread with cream cheese and a jolt of caffeine from freshly brewed coffee. Mid-morning hunger pangs are relieved by an energy bar and an energy drink. Lunch at the local fast-food place includes a cheeseburger, fries, and a soda. Another energy bar in mid-afternoon, accompanied by a bottle of water, tides you over to dinner. Still, you're so hungry when you get to the campus food court that you overindulge, downing several soft tacos with salsa, shredded lettuce, and sour cream. Late-night studying is supported by the consumption of popcorn, cookies, and another energy bar. Welcome to college dining!

Unfortunately, healthy dining can be a challenge in a culture that promotes the consumption of fast foods and convenience foods in shopping malls, sports arenas, airports, and college dining halls. Many people have acquired a taste for the high-calorie, full-fat, heavily salted foods so plentiful in our environment. It *is* possible to choose a healthy diet, however, and this chapter will help you see how.

Many people have acquired a taste for the high-calorie, full-fat, heavily salted foods *so plentiful in our environment.* However, it is possible *to choose a healthy diet.*

Understanding Nutritional Guidelines

As discussed in Chapter 1, society has a vested interest in the good health of its citizens. A natural outcome of this is that both governmental and nongovernmental organizations support scientific research in nutrition and have developed several different kinds of guides to healthy eating.

In 1997 the National Academies' Food and Nutrition Board introduced the **Dietary Reference Intakes (DRIs)**, a set of recommendations designed to promote optimal health and prevent both nutritional deficiencies and chronic diseases like cancer and cardiovascular disease. The DRIs, developed by American and Canadian scientists, encompass four kinds of recommendations. The *Estimated Average Requirement (EAR)* is the amount of nutrients needed by half of the people in any one age group, for example, teenage boys. Nutritionists use the EARs to assess whether an entire population's normal diet provides sufficient nutrients. The EARs are used in nutrition research and as a basis on which recommended dietary allowances are set.

The **Recommended Dietary Allowance (RDA)** is based on information provided by the EARs and represent the average daily amount of any one nutrient an individual needs to protect against nutritional deficiency. If there is not enough information about a nutrient to set an RDA, an *Adequate Intake (AI)* is provided. The *Tolerable Upper Intake Level (UL)* is the highest amount of a nutrient a person can take in without risking toxicity.

In 2002 the Food and Nutrition Board introduced another measure, the **Acceptable Macronutrient Distribution Range (AMDR)**. These ranges represent intake levels of essential nutrients that provide adequate nutrition and that are associated with reduced risk of chronic disease. If your intake exceeds the AMDR, you increase your risk of chronic disease. For example, the AMDR for dietary fat for adult men is 20–35 percent of the calories consumed in a day. A man who consumes more than 35 percent of his daily calories as fat increases his risk for chronic diseases.

Whereas the DRIs are recommended intake levels for individual nutrients, the *Dietary Guidelines for Americans*, published by the U.S. Department of Agriculture (USDA) and the U.S. Department of Health and Human Services, provide scientifically based diet and exercise recommendations designed to promote health and reduce the risk of chronic

Dietary Reference Intakes (DRIs)
An umbrella term for four sets of dietary recommendations: Estimated Average Requirement, Recommended Dietary Allowances, Adequate Intake, and Tolerable Upper Intake Level; designed to promote optimal health and prevent both nutritional deficiencies and chronic diseases.

Recommended Dietary Allowance (RDA)
The average daily amount of any one nutrient an individual needs to protect against nutritional deficiency.

Acceptable Macronutrient Distribution Range (AMDR)
Intake ranges that provide adequate nutrition and that are associated with reduced risk of chronic disease.

Dietary Guidelines for Americans
Set of scientifically based recommendations designed to promote health and reduce the risk for many chronic diseases through diet and physical activity.

■ College life often offers limited opportunities for healthy eating. Students may have to go out of their way to make sure they get healthy foods like fresh fruit.

MyPyramid
Graphic nutritional tool developed to accompany the 2005 *Dietary Guidelines for Americans*.

Daily Values
Set of dietary standards used on food labels to indicate how a particular food contributes to the recommended daily intake of major nutrients in a 2,000-calorie diet.

essential nutrients
Chemical substances used by the body to build, maintain, and repair tissues and regulate body functions. They cannot be manufactured by the body and must be obtained from foods or supplements.

kilocalorie
Amount of energy needed to raise the temperature of 1 kilogram of water by 1 degree centigrade; commonly shortened to *calorie*.

disease. The *Dietary Guidelines*, first published in 1980 and revised every 5 years, is the cornerstone of U.S. nutrition policy. The most recent version was published in 2010.

To translate DRIs and the *Dietary Guidelines* into healthy food choices, the USDA also publishes **MyPyramid**, a graphic nutritional tool that can be customized depending on your calorie needs. Also developed by the USDA, the **Daily Values** are used on food labels and indicate how a particular food contributes to the recommended daily intake of major nutrients in a 2,000-calorie diet.

Before we explore how you can use these tools to choose a healthy diet, we take a look at the major nutrients that make up our diet. For each nutrient, we include general recommendations for intake based on either the DRIs or the AMDRs.

Types of Nutrients

As you engage in daily activities, your body is powered by energy produced from the food you eat. Your body needs the **essential nutrients**—water, carbohydrates, proteins, fats, vitamins, and minerals—contained in these foods, but not only to provide fuel. They are also needed to build, maintain, and repair tissues; regulate body functions; and support the communication among cells that allows you to be a living, sensing human being.

These nutrients are referred to as "essential" because your body cannot manufacture them; they must come from food or from nutritional supplements. People who fail to consume adequate amounts of an essential nutrient are likely to develop a nutritional deficiency disease, such as scurvy from lack of vitamin C or beri-beri from lack of vitamin B$_1$. Nutritional deficiency diseases are seldom seen in developed countries because most people consume an adequate diet.

We need large quantities of *macronutrients*—water, carbohydrates, protein, and fat—for energy and important functions like building new cells and

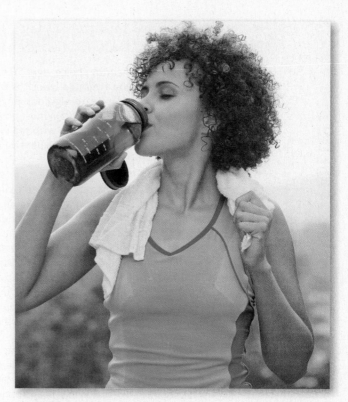

■ Water is an essential nutrient. In most communities in the United States, the quality and safety of tap water are equal or superior to the quality and safety of bottled water.

facilitating chemical reactions. We need only small amounts of *micronutrients*—vitamins and minerals—for regulating body functions.

When food is *metabolized*—chemically transformed into energy and wastes—it fuels our bodies. The energy provided by food is measured in kilocalories, commonly shortened to *calories*. One **kilocalorie** is the amount of energy needed to raise the temperature of 1 kilogram of water by 1 degree centigrade. The more energy we expend, the more kilocalories we need to consume. We get the most energy from fats—9 calories per gram of fat. Carbohydrates and protein provide 4 calories per gram. In other words, fats provide more calories than do carbohydrates or proteins, a factor to consider when planning a balanced diet that does not lead to weight gain.

WATER—THE UNAPPRECIATED NUTRIENT

You can live without the other nutrients for weeks, but you can survive without water for only a few days. We need water to digest, absorb, and transport nutrients. Water helps regulate body temperature, carries waste products out of the body, and lubricates our moving parts.[1]

The right *fluid balance*—the right amount of fluid inside and outside each cell—is maintained through the action of

Consumer Clipboard

Bottled Water: Healthy or Hype?

Drinking bottled water is a healthy choice, right? Yes and no. Drinking water keeps you hydrated, which is especially important during moderate to vigorous physical activity and when the weather is hot. But in most parts of the country you can fill a reusable bottle with tap water and get water of the same quality as the expensive kind you purchase—if not better.

Many people assume bottled water is purer and safer than tap water, but for the most part the water supply in the United States is well regulated and very safe. The Environmental Protection Agency (EPA) sets standards for water quality and inspects water supplies for bacteria and toxic chemicals. (Some bottled water is drawn from municipal water supplies, including Coca-Cola's Dasani and Pepsi's Aquafina, despite ads and labels showing pristine springs and snowy mountain peaks.) You can check the quality of your community's water supply at the National Tap Water Quality Database (www.ewg.org/tapwater/yourwater).

In contrast, bottled water is regulated by the FDA only if it is shipped across state lines. About 70 percent is bottled and sold within the same state, so it is exempt from FDA inspection. Bottled water has been found to contain contaminants, and health experts warn that it lacks fluoride, which is added to most water supplies and prevents tooth decay.

What about water that's been enhanced with vitamins, minerals, and other nutrients? Although they offer a colorful and flavorful alternative to plain water, they add little nutritional value to the typical American diet, since the average American adult consumes 100 percent of the DRI for most vitamins. They do pack a wallop when it comes to added sugars, however. A 20-ounce bottle of Vitaminwater, for example, has 32.5 grams of sugar (two heaping tablespoons) and 125 calories, about the same as a soft drink. In 2007 the company that produces Vitaminwater, Glaceau, was bought by Coca-Cola.

Aside from their effect on health, bottled waters have a huge impact on the environment. About 1.5 million tons of plastic are used in the manufacture of water bottles for global consumption every year, creating 1.5 million tons of plastic garbage. Although plastic bottles can be recycled, 80 percent of them are thrown out and end up in landfills or in the world's oceans. According to Food and Water Watch, about 47 million gallons of oil are used to produce the bottles, in addition to the gasoline expended in transporting the bottles to market. Some bottled water producers pump water from springs, depleting underground aquifers and disrupting ecosystems.

Consuming bottled water is hard on your wallet as well. Tap water is estimated to cost about $0.0015 per gallon, compared to $1.25 per gallon for bottled water, a thousandfold cost difference. Americans spent more than $7 billion for bottled water in 2002, and sales are increasing at a phenomenal rate. No wonder food industry giants Coca-Cola, Pepsi, and Nestle are staking their claim in the bottled water business and multinational corporations are purchasing groundwater rights around the world.

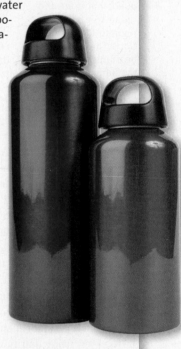

The Sierra Club urges consumers to use containers they can fill with tap water when away from home. If there is a problem with water quality or taste, they suggest buying a water filter for your tap water, still a much less expensive option than bottled water. They also urge people to advocate for good public management of municipal water systems and to monitor unusual land purchases near natural springs. The Sierra Club points out that safe and affordable water is a natural resource that many feel is a basic human right—not a commodity.

Sources: "5 Reasons to Not Drink Bottled Water," Light Footstep, 2007, retrieved April 4, 2008, from http://lightfootstep.com; "Corporate Water Privatization: Bottled Water Campaign," Sierra Club, 2004, retrieved April 4, 2008, from www.sierraclub.org/committees/cac/water/bottled_water; "Is Vitaminwater Good for You?" Scienceline, 2007, retrieved April 4, 2008, from http://scienceline.org/2007/12/03/ask-intagaliata-vitaminwater.

substances called **electrolytes**, mineral components that carry electrical charges and conduct nerve impulses. Electrolytes include sodium, potassium, and chloride. Water, in combination with a balanced diet, replaces electrolytes lost daily through sweat.[2]

Your water needs vary according to the foods you eat, the temperature and humidity in your environment, your activity level, and other factors (see the box "Bottled Water: Healthy or Hype?").

electrolytes
Mineral components that carry electrical charges and conduct nerve impulses.

Adults generally need 1 to 1.5 milliliters of water for each calorie spent in the day. If you expend 2,000 calories a day, you require 2 to 3 liters—8 to 12 cups—of fluids.[3] Heavy sweating increases your need for fluids. You obtain fluids not only from the water you drink but also from the water in foods, particularly fruits such as oranges and apples. Caffeinated beverages and alcohol are not good sources of your daily fluid intake because of their dehydrating effects, although some recent research suggests that the water in such beverages may offset these effects to some extent.[3]

CARBOHYDRATES—YOUR BODY'S FUEL

Carbohydrates are the body's main source of energy.[3] They fuel most of the body's cells during daily activities; they are used by muscle cells during high-intensity exercise; and they are the only source of energy for brain cells, red blood cells, and some other types of cells. Athletes in particular need to consume a high-carbohydrate diet to fuel their high-energy activities.

Carbohydrates are the foods we think of as sugars and starches. They come almost exclusively from plants (the exception is lactose, the sugar in milk). Most of the carbohydrates and other nutrients we need come from grains, seeds, fruits, and vegetables.[2]

Simple Carbohydrates   Carbohydrates are divided into simple carbohydrates and complex carbohydrates. **Simple carbohydrates** are easily digestible carbohydrates composed of one or two units of sugar. Six simple carbohydrates (sugars) are important in nutrition: glucose, fructose, galactose, lactose, maltose, and sucrose. Glucose is the main source of energy for the brain and nervous system. Sugars are absorbed into the bloodstream and travel to body cells, where they can be used for energy. Glucose also travels to the liver and muscles, where it can be stored as **glycogen** (a complex carbohydrate) for future energy needs.

When you eat food containing large amounts of simple carbohydrates, sugar enters your bloodstream quickly, giving you a burst of energy, or a "sugar high." It is also absorbed into your cells quickly, leaving you feeling depleted and craving more sugar. Foods containing added sugar, such as candy bars and sodas, have an even more dramatic effect.

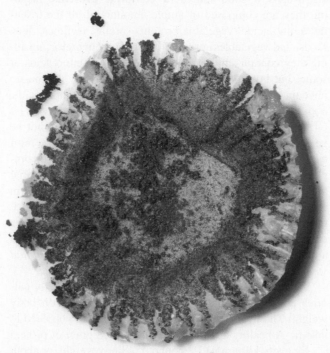

■ Foods high in sugar may give you a brief energy boost, but they will ultimately leave you feeling less energetic.

Consumption of sugar has been linked to the epidemic of overweight and obesity in the United States and to the parallel increase in the incidence of diabetes, a disorder in which body cells cannot use the sugar circulating in the blood.

Complex Carbohydrates   The type of carbohydrates called **complex carbohydrates** is composed of multiple sugar units and includes starches and dietary fiber. **Starches** occur in grains, vegetables, and some fruits. Most starchy foods also contain ample portions of vitamins, minerals, proteins, and water. Starches must be broken down into single sugars in the digestive system before they can be absorbed into the bloodstream to be used for energy or stored for future use.

The complex carbohydrates found in whole grains are often refined or processed to make them easier to digest and more appealing to the consumer, but the refining process removes many of the vitamins, minerals, and other nutritious components found in the whole food. Refined carbohydrates include such foods as white rice, white bread and other products made from white flour, pasta, and sweet desserts. Like sugar, refined carbohydrates can enter the bloodstream quickly and just as quickly leave you feeling hungry again. Whole grains (such as whole wheat, brown rice, oatmeal, and corn) are preferred because they provide more nutrients, slow the digestive process, and make you feel full longer. The consumption of whole grains is associated with lowered risk of diabetes, obesity, heart disease, and some forms of cancer.[4–6]

The RDA for carbohydrates is 130 grams for males and females aged 1 to 70 years. The AMDR for carbohydrates is 45–65 percent of daily energy intake, which amounts to 225 to 325 grams in a 2,000-calorie diet (even though only about 130 grams per day are enough to meet the body's needs). In the typical American diet, carbohydrates do contribute about half of all calories, but most of them are in the form of simple sugars or highly refined grains. Instead, carbohydrates should come from a diverse spectrum of whole grains and other starches, vegetables, and fruits.[7]

The Food and Nutrition Board recommends that no more than 25 percent of calories come from added sugars, and many health professionals recommend only 10 percent.[5] According to the American Heart Association, most American women should consume no more than 100 calories per day of sugar (about 6 teaspoons) and men no more than 150 calories per day (9 teaspoons). To cut back on sugar, check for food label ingredients like sugar, corn syrup, fructose, dextrose, molasses, or evaporated cane juice. You may

simple carbohydrates
Easily digestible carbohydrates composed of one or two units of sugar.

glycogen
The complex carbohydrate form in which glucose is stored in the liver and muscles.

complex carbohydrates
Carbohydrates that are composed of multiple sugar units and that must be broken down further before they can be used by the body.

starches
Complex carbohydrates found in many plant foods.

dietary fiber
A complex carbohydrate found in plants that cannot be broken down in the digestive tract.

functional fiber
Natural or synthetic fiber that has been added to food.

total fiber
Combined amount of dietary fiber and functional fiber in a food.

protein
Essential nutrient made up of amino acids, needed to build and maintain muscles, bones, and other body tissues.

essential amino acids
Amino acids that the body cannot produce on its own.

complete proteins
Proteins composed of ample amounts of all the essential amino acids.

incomplete proteins
Proteins that contain small amounts of essential amino acids or some, but not all, of the essential amino acids.

be surprised at the relatively high sugar content of many foods. For example, two servings of spaghetti sauce contain almost five-and-a-half teaspoons of sugars.[4]

Fiber   Dietary fiber, a complex carbohydrate found in plants, cannot be broken down in the digestive tract. A diet rich in dietary fiber makes stools soft and bulky. They pass through the intestines rapidly and are expelled easily, helping to prevent hemorrhoids and constipation.[8,9] Some foods contain **functional fiber**, natural or synthetic fiber that has been added to increase the healthful effects of the food. **Total fiber** refers to the combined amount of dietary fiber and functional fiber in a food.

Dietary fiber that dissolves in water, referred to as *soluble fiber*, is known to lower blood cholesterol levels and can slow the process of digestion so that blood sugar levels remain more even. Dietary fiber that does not dissolve in water, called *insoluble fiber*, passes through the digestive tract essentially unchanged. Because it absorbs water, insoluble fiber helps you feel full after eating and stimulates your intestinal wall to contract and relax, serving as a natural laxative.

The RDAs for fiber are 25 grams for women aged 19 to 50 and 38 grams for men aged 14 to 50 (or 14 grams of fiber for every 1,000 calories consumed). For people over 50, the RDA is 21 grams for women and 30 grams for men.[1] The typical American diet provides only about 14 or 15 grams of fiber a day. If you want to increase the fiber in your diet, it is important to do so gradually. A sudden increase in daily fiber may cause bloating, gas, abdominal cramping, or even a bowel obstruction, particularly if you fail to drink enough liquids to easily carry the fiber through the body.[2]

Fiber is best obtained through diet. Pills and other fiber supplements do not contain the nutrients found in high-fiber foods.[2] Excessive amounts of fiber (generally 60 grams or more per day) can decrease the absorption of important vitamins and minerals such as calcium, zinc, magnesium, and iron.[2] Fruits, vegetables, dried beans, peas and other legumes, cereals, grains, nuts, and seeds are the best sources of dietary fiber.

PROTEIN—NUTRITIONAL MUSCLE

Your body uses **protein** to build and maintain muscles, bones, and other body tissues. Proteins also form enzymes that in turn facilitate chemical reactions. Proteins are constructed from 20 different amino acids. Amino acids that your body cannot produce on its own, nine in all, are called **essential amino acids**; they must be supplied by foods. Those that can be produced by your body are called nonessential amino acids.

Food sources of protein include both animals and plants. Animal proteins (meat, fish, poultry, milk, cheese, and eggs) are usually a good source of **complete proteins**, meaning they are composed of ample amounts of all the essential amino acids. Vegetable proteins (grains, legumes, nuts, seeds, and vegetables) provide **incomplete proteins**, meaning they contain small amounts of essential amino acids or some, but not all, of the essential amino acids. If you do not consume sufficient amounts of the essential amino acids, body organ functions may be compromised.

People who eat little or no animal protein may not be getting all the essential amino acids they need. One remedy is to eat plant foods with different amounts of incomplete proteins. For example, beans are low in the essential amino acid methionine but high in lysine, and rice is high in methionine and low in lysine. In combination, beans and rice form *complementary proteins*. Eating the two together at one meal or over the course of a day provides all the essential amino acids.[2] The matching of such foods is called *mutual supplementation*.

The AMDR for protein is 10–35 percent of daily calories consumed.[7] The need for protein is based on body weight: The larger your body, the more protein you need to take in. A healthy adult typically needs 0.8 gram of protein for every kilogram (2.2 pounds) of body weight, or about 0.36 gram for every pound.[10] At the upper end of the

AMDR range, the percentages provide a more than ample amount of protein in the diet.

FATS—A NECESSARY NUTRIENT

Fats are a concentrated energy source and the principal form of stored energy in the body. The fats in food provide essential fatty acids, play a role in the production of other fatty acids and vitamin D, and provide the major material for cell membranes and for the myelin sheaths that surround nerve fibers. They assist in the absorption of the fat-soluble vitamins (A, D, E, and K) and affect the texture, taste, and smell of foods. Fats provide an emergency reserve when we are sick or our food intake is diminished.

Types of Fat Fats, or lipids, are composed of fatty acids. Nutritionists divide these acids into three groups—saturated, monounsaturated, and polyunsaturated—on the basis of their chemical composition. **Saturated fats** remain stable (solid) at room temperature; **monounsaturated fats** are liquid at room temperature but solidify somewhat when refrigerated; **polyunsaturated fats** are liquid both at room temperature and in the refrigerator. Liquid fats are commonly referred to as oils.

Saturated fatty acids are found in animal sources, such as beef, pork, poultry, and whole-milk dairy products. They are also found in certain tropical oils and nuts, including coconut and palm oil and macadamia nuts. Monounsaturated and polyunsaturated fatty acids are found primarily in plant sources. Olive, safflower, peanut, and canola oils, as well as avocados and many nuts, contain mostly monounsaturated fat. Corn and soybean oils contain mostly polyunsaturated fat, as do many kinds of fish, including salmon, trout, and anchovies.

Cholesterol Saturated fats pose a risk to health because they tend to raise blood levels of **cholesterol**, a waxy substance that can clog arteries, leading to cardiovascular disease. More specifically, saturated fats raise blood levels of low-density lipoproteins (LDLs), known as "bad cholesterol," and triglycerides, another kind of blood fat. Unsaturated fats, in contrast, tend to lower blood levels of LDLs, and some unsaturated fats (monounsaturated fats) may also raise levels of high-density lipoproteins (HDLs), known as "good cholesterol."[11]

Cholesterol is needed for several important body functions, but too much of it circulating in the bloodstream can be a problem. The body produces it in the liver and also obtains it from animal food sources, such as meat, cheese, eggs, and milk. It is recommended that no more than 300 milligrams of dietary cholesterol be consumed per day. The effects of cholesterol on cardiovascular health are discussed in detail in Chapter 15.

Trans Fats Another kind of fatty acid, **trans fatty acid**, is produced through **hydrogenation**, a process whereby liquid vegetable oils are turned into more solid fats. Food manufacturers use hydrogenation to prolong a food's shelf life and change its texture. Peanut butter is frequently hydrogenated, as is margarine. With some hydrogenation, margarine becomes semisoft (tub margarine); with further hydrogenation, it becomes hard (stick margarine).[12]

Trans fatty acids (or trans fats) are believed to pose a risk to cardiovascular health similar to or even greater than that of saturated fats, because they tend to raise LDLs and lower HDLs. Foods high in trans fatty acids include baked and snack foods like crackers, cookies, chips, cakes, pies, and doughnuts, as well as deep-fried fast foods like french fries.[13] In packaged foods, the phrase "partially hydrogenated vegetable oil" in the list of ingredients indicates the presence of trans fats. In 2006

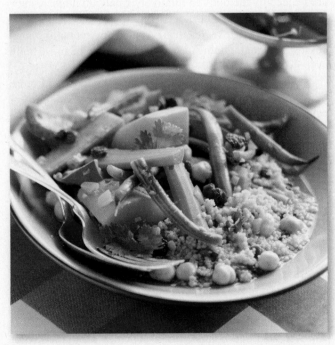

■ You can reduce your risk of chronic diseases by building your diet around colorful meals that include whole grains, legumes, two or more vegetables, and small quantities of chicken or fish.

fats
Also known as lipids, fats are an essential nutrient composed of fatty acids and used for energy and other body functions.

saturated fats
Lipids that are the predominant fat in animal products and other fats that remain solid at room temperature.

monounsaturated fats
Lipids that are liquid at room temperature and semisolid or solid when refrigerated.

polyunsaturated fats
Lipids that are liquid at room temperature and in the refrigerator.

cholesterol
A waxy substance produced by the liver and obtained from animal food sources; essential to the functioning of the body but a possible factor in cardiovascular disease if too much is circulating in the bloodstream.

trans fatty acids
Lipids that have been chemically modified through the process of hydrogenation so that they remain solid at room temperature.

hydrogenation
Process whereby liquid vegetable oils are turned into more solid fats.

the FDA began requiring that trans fat be listed on nutrition labels if a food contains more than 0.5 gram, and many food manufacturers and restaurants have stopped using trans fats in their products. Some cities, including Philadelphia and New York City, have enacted laws to ban or phase out the use of trans fats in restaurants. In 2010, California became the first state to ban the use of trans fats in restaurants.

omega-3 fatty acids
Polyunsaturated fatty acids that contain the essential nutrient alpha-linolenic acid and that has beneficial effects on cardiovascular health.

omega-6 fatty acids
Polyunsaturated fatty acids that contain linoleic acid and that have beneficial health effects.

minerals
Naturally occurring inorganic micronutrients, such as magnesium, calcium, and iron, that contribute to proper functioning of the body.

vitamins
Naturally occurring organic micronutrients that aid chemical reactions in the body and help maintain healthy body systems.

Omega-3 and Omega-6 Fatty Acids   Unlike trans fats, two kinds of polyunsaturated fatty acids—omega-3 and omega-6 fatty acids—provide health benefits. **Omega-3 fatty acids**, which contain the essential nutrient alpha-linolenic acid, help slow the clotting of blood, decrease triglyceride levels, improve arterial health, and lower blood pressure. They may also help protect against autoimmune diseases such as arthritis.[13] **Omega-6 fatty acids**, which contain the essential nutrient linoleic acid, are also important to health, but nutritionists believe that Americans consume too much omega-6 in proportion to omega-3.[14] They recommend increasing consumption of omega-3 sources—fatty fish like salmon, trout, and anchovies; vegetable oils like soybean, walnut, and flaxseed; and dark green leafy vegetables—and decreasing consumption of omega-6 sources, mainly corn, soybean, and cottonseed oils.

Although the USDA recommends two servings of fish per week, there are concerns about contamination with mercury and other industrial pollutants, which can accumulate in the tissue of certain types of fish. Mercury may cause fetal brain damage, and high levels of mercury may damage

Dietary Recommendations for Fat   How much of your daily caloric intake should come from fat? The AMDR is 20–35 percent.[7] It is recommended that Americans get about 30 percent of their calories from fats and less than one third of that (7 to 10 percent) from saturated fats. Most adults need only 15 percent of their daily calorie intake in the form of fat, whereas young children should get 30–40 percent of their calories from fat to ensure proper growth and brain development, according to the American Academy of Pediatrics. A tablespoon of vegetable oil per day is recommended for both adults and children.[13] The American Heart Association recommends limiting consumption of saturated and trans fat to no more than 10 percent of total daily calories; in a 2,000-calorie diet, that's about 22 grams.

These recommendations are designed to help improve cardiovascular health and prevent heart disease. On average, fat intake in the United States is about 34 percent of daily calorie intake.[13] You can limit your intake of saturated fat by selecting vegetable oils instead of animal fats, reducing the amount of fat you use in cooking, removing all visible fat from meat, and choosing lean cuts of meat over fatty ones and poultry or fish over beef. Limit your consumption of fast-food burgers and fries, since these foods are loaded with saturated fats.

MINERALS—A NEED FOR BALANCE

Minerals are naturally occurring inorganic substances that are needed by the body in relatively small amounts. Minerals are important in building strong bones and teeth, helping vitamins and enzymes carry out many metabolic processes, and maintaining proper functioning of most body systems.

Our bodies need 20 essential minerals. We need more than 100 milligrams daily of each of the six *macrominerals*—calcium, chloride, magnesium, phosphorus, potassium, and sodium. We need less than 100 milligrams daily of each of the *microminerals*, or *trace minerals*—chromium, cobalt, copper, fluorine, iodine, iron, manganese, molybdenum,

The food supplement industry markets vitamin and mineral supplements as a kind of insurance against nutritional deficiencies, but for most people they are unnecessary.

the hearts of adults. Polychlorinated biphenyls (PCBs) and dioxin may be associated with cancer. In 2004 the FDA and the EPA issued a joint warning stating that pregnant women, women planning to become pregnant, nursing mothers, and young children should consume no more than 12 ounces of fish and shellfish per week, should avoid certain types of fish (king mackerel, golden bass, shark, and swordfish), and should vary the kinds of fish they eat. (For more information, see the EPA fish advisory site at www.epa.gov/waterscience/fish.)

nickel, selenium, silicon, tin, vanadium, and zinc. Other minerals are present in foods and the body, but no requirement has been found for them.[15] Table 6.1 provides an overview of key vitamins and minerals.

A varied and balanced diet provides all the essential minerals your body needs, so mineral supplements are not recommended for most people.[2] (Exceptions are listed in the next section.) These insoluble elements can build up in the body and become toxic if consumed in excessive amounts.

Table 6.1   Key Vitamins and Minerals

Vitamins/Minerals	Food Sources	Adult Daily DRI*	
		Men	Women
Vitamin A	Liver, dairy products, fish, dark green vegetables, yellow and orange fruits and vegetables	900 µg	700 µg
Vitamin C	Citrus fruits, strawberries, broccoli, tomatoes, green leafy vegetables, bell peppers	90 mg	75 mg
Vitamin D	Vitamin D–fortified milk and cereals, fish, eggs	5 µg	5 µg
Vitamin E	Plant oils, seeds, avocados, green leafy vegetables	15 mg	15 mg
Vitamin K	Dark green leafy vegetables, broccoli, cheese	120 µg	90 µg
Vitamin B_1 (thiamine)	Enriched and whole-grain cereals	1.2 mg	1.1 mg
Vitamin B_2 (riboflavin)	Milk, mushrooms, spinach, liver, fortified cereals	1.3 mg	1.1 mg
Vitamin B_6	Fortified cereals, meat, poultry, fish, bananas, potatoes, nuts	1.3 mg	1.3 mg
Vitamin B_{12}	Fortified cereals, meat, poultry, fish, dairy products	2.4 µg	2.4 µg
Niacin	Meat, fish, poultry, peanuts, beans, enriched and whole-grain cereals	16 mg	14 mg
Folate	Dark green leafy vegetables, legumes, oranges, bananas, fortified cereals	400 µg	400 µg
Calcium	Dairy products, canned fish, dark green leafy vegetables	1,000 mg	1,000 mg
Iron	Meat, poultry, legumes, dark green leafy vegetables	8 mg	18 mg
Magnesium	Wheat bran, green leafy vegetables, nuts, legumes, fish	420 mg	320 mg
Potassium	Spinach, squash, bananas, milk, potatoes, oranges, legumes, tomatoes, green leafy vegetables	4,700 mg	4,700 mg
Sodium	Table salt, soy sauce, processed foods	1,500 mg	1,500 mg
Zinc	Fortified cereals, meat, poultry, dairy products, legumes, nuts, seeds	11 mg	8 mg

*For a complete listing, see the Web site of the Food and Nutrition Board (www.iom.edu/CMS/3788.aspx).

Source: "Dietary Reference Intakes," Food and Nutrition Board, Institute of Medicine of the National Academies, retrieved April 2, 2008, from www.iom.edu/CMS/3788/21370.aspx.

VITAMINS—SMALL BUT POTENT NUTRIENTS

Vitamins are organic substances needed by the body in small amounts. They serve as catalysts for releasing energy from carbohydrates, proteins, and fats; they aid chemical reactions in the body; and they help maintain components of the immune, nervous, and skeletal systems.

Our bodies need at least 11 specific vitamins: A, C, D, E, K, and the B-complex vitamins—thiamine (B_1), riboflavin (B_2), niacin, B_6, folic acid, and B_{12}. Biotin and pantothenic acid are part of the vitamin B complex and are also considered important for health. Choline, another B vitamin, is not regarded as essential.

Four of the vitamins, A, D, E, and K, are fat soluble (they dissolve in fat), and the rest are water soluble (they dissolve in water). The fat-soluble vitamins can be stored in the liver or body fat, and if you consume larger amounts than you need, you can reach toxic levels over time. Excess water-soluble vitamins are excreted in the urine and must be consumed more often than fat-soluble vitamins. Most water-soluble vitamins do not cause toxicity, but vitamins B_6 and C can build to toxic levels if taken in excess. Toxicity usually occurs only when these substances are taken as supplements.

More than half the people in the United States take vitamin and mineral supplements. The food supplement industry markets these products as a kind of insurance against nutritional deficiencies, but for most people they are unnecessary.[2] Specific groups for whom vitamin and/or mineral supplements may be recommended include

■ People with nutrient deficiencies

■ People with low energy intake (less than 1,200 calories per day)

■ Individuals who eat only foods from plant sources

- Women who bleed excessively during menstruation
- Individuals whose calcium intake is too small to preserve strength
- People in certain life stages (infants, older adults, women of childbearing age, and pregnant women)

Taking supplements to enhance your energy level or athletic performance or to make up for perceived inadequacies in your diet is not recommended.[1] Instead, try to adopt a healthy diet that provides needed nutrients from a variety of foods. Many foods provide, in one serving, the same amounts of nutrients found in a vitamin supplement pill. For a concise overview of recommended daily intakes of the macronutrients and micronutrients, see Table 6.2.

OTHER SUBSTANCES IN FOOD: PHYTOCHEMICALS

One promising area of nutrition research is **phytochemicals**, substances that are naturally produced by plants. In the human body, phytochemicals may keep body cells healthy, slow down tissue degeneration, prevent the formation of carcinogens, reduce cholesterol levels, protect the heart, maintain hormone balance, and keep bones strong.[16,17]

Antioxidants   Every time you take a breath, you inhale a potentially toxic chemical that could damage your cell DNA: oxygen.[18] If you breathed 100 percent oxygen over a period of days, you would go blind and suffer irreparable damage to your lungs. The process of oxygen metabolism in the body produces unstable molecules, called **free radicals**,

which can damage cell structures and DNA. The production of free radicals can also be increased by exposure to certain environmental elements, such as cigarette smoke and sunlight, and even by stress. Free radicals are believed to be a contributing factor in aging, cancer, heart disease, macular degeneration, and other degenerative diseases.[1]

Antioxidants are substances in foods that neutralize the effects of free radicals. Antioxidants are found primarily in fruits and vegetables, especially brightly colored ones (yellow, orange, and dark green), and in green tea. Vitamins E and C are antioxidants, as are some of the precursors to vitamins, such as beta carotene.

Most nutritionists do not recommend supplements as a source of antioxidants because of the potential toxic effects of vitamin megadoses.[16] The best source is whole foods. The top antioxidant-containing foods and beverages have been identified as blackberries, walnuts, strawberries, artichokes, cranberries, brewed coffee, raspberries, pecans, blueberries, cloves, grape juice, unsweetened baking chocolate, sour cherries, and red wine. Açai berries have been heavily marketed as a superior source of antioxidants. These berries, however, are no better than blueberries or any other berries. Also high in antioxidants are brussels sprouts, kale, cauliflower, and pomegranates.

Phytoestrogens   *Phytoestrogens* are plant hormones similar to human estrogens but less potent. Research suggests that some phytoestrogens may lower cholesterol and reduce the risk of heart disease. Other claims—that they lower the risk of osteoporosis and some types of cancer and reduce menopausal symptoms like hot flashes—have not been supported by research.

Phytoestrogens have been identified in more than 300 plants, including vegetables of the cabbage family such as brussels sprouts, broccoli, and cauliflower. Phytoestrogens are also found in plants containing lignins (a woody substance like cellulose), such as rye, wheat, sesame seed, linseed, and flaxseed, and in soybeans and soy products. Foods containing phytoestrogens are safe, but, as with all phytochemicals, research has not established the safety of phytoestrogen supplements.[1,16]

Phytonutrients   *Phytonutrients* are substances extracted from vegetables and other plant foods and used in supplements. For example, lycopene is an antioxidant found in tomatoes that may inhibit the reproduction of cancer cells in the esophagus, prostate, or stomach.[18] A group of phytochemicals known as *bioflavonoids* are believed to have a benefical effect on the cardiovascular system.[16]

To date, the FDA has not allowed foods containing phytochemicals to be labeled or marketed as agents that prevent disease. Nutritionists do not recommend taking

phytochemicals
Substances that are naturally produced by plants to protect themselves and that provide health benefits in the human body.

free radicals
Unstable molecules that are produced when oxygen is metabolized and that damage cell structures and DNA.

antioxidants
Substances in foods that neutralize the effects of free radicals.

Table 6.2   Overview of Recommended Daily Intakes

Nutrient	Recommended Daily Intake
Water	1–1.5 ml per calorie spent; 8–12 cups of fluid
Carbohydrates	AMDR: 45–65% of calories consumed
Added sugars	No more than 10–25% of calories consumed
Fiber	14 g for every 1,000 calories consumed; 21–25 g for women, 30–38 g for men
Protein	AMDR: 10–35% of calories consumed; 0.36 g per pound of body weight
Fat	AMDR: 20–35% of calories consumed
Saturated fat	Less than 10% of calories consumed
Trans fat	As little as possible
Minerals	
6 macrominerals	More than 100 mg
14 trace minerals	Less than 100 mg
Vitamins	
11 essential vitamins	Varies

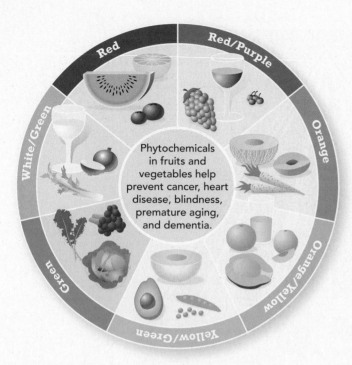

figure **6.1**   **The color wheel of foods.**
An optimal diet contains fruits and vegetables from
all seven groups.

Source: Adapted from What Color Is Your Diet? *by D. Heber, 2001, New
York: HarperCollins, p. 17. Copyright © 2001 by David Heber, M.D., Ph.D.
Reprinted by permission of HarperCollins Publishers.*

phytochemical supplements.[19,20] In 2007 the FDA announced
that manufacturers of all dietary supplements, including vitamins and herbs, must evaluate the identity, purity, strength,
and composition of their products and accurately label them
so that consumers know what they are buying. Manufacturers must comply with the new rules by 2010.[20]

National campaigns such as "Reach for It" in Canada
and "Fruits and Veggies—More Matters" in the United
States encourage consumers to select fruits and vegetables
high in phytochemicals. Because different fruits and vegetables contain different phytochemicals, a color-coded dietary
plan has been developed that helps you take full advantage
of all the beneficial phytochemicals available (Figure 6.1).

Planning a Healthy Diet

Knowing your daily nutritional requirements in grams and
percentages is not enough; you also need to know how to
translate DRIs, RDAs, and AMDRs into healthy food choices
and appealing meals. In this section we look at several tools
that have been created to help you do that.

DIETARY GUIDELINES FOR AMERICANS

The 2010 Dietary Guidelines Advisory Committee Report
notes that two-thirds of Americans are now overweight
or obese. As a result, the committee's recommendations
focused on stopping and reversing the spread of overweight
and obesity through individual, environmental, and food
supply changes. Key areas addressed by the Dietary Guidelines Advisory Committee are described in Table 6.3.

Table **6.3**   2010 *Dietary Guidelines for Americans:* Key Messages

Energy Balance and Weight Management	Increase physical activity to balance calorie intake. Limit time spent in front of the television and computer. Consume smaller portions.
Nutrient Adequacy	For most people, nutrients should come from foods, not supplements. Favor nutrient-dense foods over calorie-dense foods.
Fatty Acids and Cholesterol	Limit saturated fat to less than 7 percent of total calories and avoid consuming any amount of trans fats. Consume two servings of fish per week to obtain heart-healthy omega-3 fatty acids.
Protein	Animal sources of protein are the highest quality sources, but combinations of legumes and grains can also supply complete proteins.
Carbohydrates	Choose fiber-rich carbohydrates (including whole grains, vegetables, fruits, and cooked dry beans) over high-energy, non-nutrient dense carbohydrates (such as sugar-sweetened beverages and pastries).
Sodium and Potassium	Limit sodium consumption to 1,500 mg (less than a teaspoon) daily. Increase potassium consumption (good sources are potatoes, plain yogurt, and bananas).
Alcohol	Adults should limit alcohol consumption to an average of up to two drinks per day for men and up to one drink per day for women. Men should consume no more than four drinks on any single day; women, no more than three drinks.
Food Safety and Technology	Pay greater attention to food safety when preparing meals in the home. The health benefits of consuming cooked seafood outweigh the food safety concerns surrounding it. There are special recommendations for pregnant women and children.

Source: Report of the Dietary Guidelines Advisory Committee on the Dietary Guidelines for Americans, *U.S. Department of Agriculture and U.S. Department of Health and Human Services, 2010, retrieved from www.cnpp.usda.gov/DGAs2010=DGACReport.htm.*

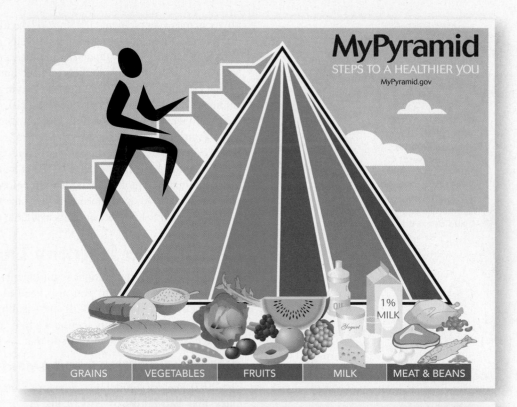

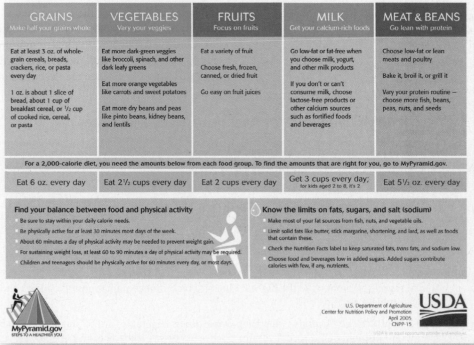

figure 6.2 **The USDA MyPyramid.** Released in 2005, this chart emphasizes whole grains, a variety of vegetables, and a balance between food and physical activity. Specific pyramids for 12 different calorie levels are available at www.MyPyramid.gov.
Source: MyPyramid, 2005, U.S. Department of Agriculture, Center for Nutrition Policy and Promotion.

The committee also outlined four main goals for Americans:

- Reduce calorie intake and increase physical activity.
- Move toward a more plant-based diet composed of nutrient-dense foods.
- Reduce intake of foods containing added sugars and solid fats and reduce overall sodium and refined grain consumption.
- Meet the 2008 Physical Activity Guidelines.

MyPyramid Like earlier food pyramid guides, MyPyramid is based on the familiar food groups (grains, vegetables, fruit, milk, meat and beans) and has some similar messages—for example, eat more of some foods than of others, eat a variety of foods, practice moderation, and so on (Figure 6.2). But MyPyramid also highlights physical activity (represented by the person climbing the steps), gradual improvement (setting small, reachable goals, as captured in the slogan "Steps to a Healthier You"), and, especially, personalization.

Go to the MyPyramid Web site (www.mypyramid.gov) and use interactive tools to assess your current diet, calculate your calorie needs, develop a customized food plan, and learn strategies for achieving a healthy weight. The Personal Health Portfolio Activity for this chapter will also help you assess your food intake. Estimate your calorie requirements based on your sex and age at three activity levels, as shown in Table 6.4. The activity levels are defined as

- *Sedentary.* Only light physical activity associated with typical day-to-day life.
- *Moderately active.* Physical activity equivalent to walking about 1.5 miles per day at 3–4 miles per hour.
- *Active.* Physical activity equivalent to walking more than 3 miles per day at 3–4 miles per hour.

The MyPyramid Plan provides specific serving recommendations (in cups, ounce-equivalents, and other specific measurements) for each of 12 different calorie levels, from 1,000 to 3,200 calories per day. Figure 6.2 shows the recommendations for a 2,000-calorie diet. The graphic also includes short statements summarizing important points from the 2005 *Dietary Guidelines*, such as "Eat more orange vegetables like carrots and sweet potatoes."

The *Dietary Guidelines* and MyPyramid differ significantly from current eating patterns in the United States. Specifically, they encourage more consumption of whole grains, vegetables, legumes, fruits, and low-fat milk products and less consumption of refined grain products, total fats, added sugars, and calories. They emphasize foods high in **nutrient density**—proportion of vitamins and minerals to total calories. Especially in a lower calorie diet, the goal is that all calories consumed provide nutrients (as opposed to "empty calories" in sodas, sweets, and alcoholic beverages). Otherwise, you reach your maximum calorie intake without having consumed the nutrients you need.

nutrient density The proportion of nutrients to total calories in a food.

If you choose nutrient-dense foods from each food group, you may have some calories left over—your discretionary calorie allowance—that can be consumed as added fats or sugars, alcohol, or other foods. At the 2,000-calorie level, your discretionary calorie allowance is 267 calories.

The DASH Eating Plan The other eating plan recommended by the *Dietary Guidelines* is the DASH Eating Plan, originally developed to reduce high blood pressure. (DASH stands for Dietary Approaches to Stop Hypertension.) The DASH plan is similar to MyPyramid, but it also has a nuts, seeds, and legumes group. For more information, visit www.nhlbi.nih.gov/health/public/heart/hbp/dash/new_dash.pdf.

Recommendations for Specific Groups The *Dietary Guidelines* also includes recommendations, where relevant, for specific population groups, including children and adolescents, older adults, pregnant and breastfeeding women, overweight adults and children, and people with chronic diseases or special medical problems. For example, women of childbearing age and women in the first trimester of pregnancy are advised to consume adequate synthetic folic acid daily in addition to eating foods rich in folate. Individuals with hypertension, African Americans, and middle-aged and older adults are advised to consume no more than 1,500 milligrams of sodium per day. Special pyramids have been developed for children (MyPyramid for Kids) and for women who are pregnant or breastfeeding (MyPyramid for Pregnancy and Breastfeeding).

Other Eating Plans and Pyramids The food pyramid concept has been extended to a variety of other food preferences and ethnic diets. The term *diet* in this context includes the

Table 6.4 Estimated Calorie Requirements at Three Levels, by Age and Gender

Gender	Age (years)	Sedentary	Moderately Active	Active
Female	14–18	1,800	2,000	2,400
	19–30	2,000	2,000–2,200	2,400
	31–50	1,800	2,000	2,200
	51+	1,600	1,800	2,000–2,200
Male	14–18	2,200	2,400–2,800	2,800–3,200
	19–30	2,400	2,600–2,800	3,000
	31–50	2,200	2,400–2,600	2,800–3,000
	51+	2,000	2,200–2,400	2,400–2,800

Source: Dietary Guidelines for Americans, U.S. Department of Agriculture and U.S. Department of Health and Human Services, 2005, retrieved from www.health.gov/dietaryguidelines.

Highlight on Health

Vegetarian Diet Planning

Vegetarian diets can be healthy if they are carefully designed to include adequate amounts of all the essential nutrients. Vegetarians need to pay careful attention to the following nutrients:

■ **Protein** Some vegetarians can get their protein from dairy products, eggs, fish, or poultry. Vegans (vegetarians who eat no animal products whatsoever) can get all the essential and nonessential amino acids by eating a variety of plant foods—whole grains, legumes, seeds and nuts, and vegetables—and consuming foods from two or more of these categories over the course of a day. Soy protein provides all the essential amino acids and can be the sole protein source in a diet.

■ **Iron** Good plant sources of iron are prune juice, dried beans and lentils, spinach, dried fruits, molasses, brewer's yeast, and enriched products, such as enriched flour. Cooking in iron cookware (cast-iron pans) also provides iron in the diet.

■ **Vitamin B_2, riboflavin** Good sources of this vitamin are dairy products, nutritional yeast, leafy green vegetables (collard greens, spinach), broccoli, mushrooms, and dried beans.

■ **Vitamin B_{12}** This vitamin is found naturally only in animal sources, so it is particularly important for vegans to make sure it is present in their diets. It can be found in some fortified (not enriched) breakfast cereals, fortified soy beverages, some brands of nutritional (brewer's) yeast, and other foods (check the labels), as well as vitamin supplements.

■ **Vitamin D** This vitamin is found in eggs, butter, and fortified dairy products. Sunlight transforms a provitamin into a substance that the body can use to make vitamin D. Vegans who don't get much sunlight may need a vitamin D supplement (but supplementation should not exceed the RDA).

■ **Calcium** Calcium is plentiful in dairy products, molasses, leafy green vegetables like kale and mustard greens, broccoli, tofu and other soy products, and some legumes. (The calcium in some foods, including spinach, chocolate, and wheat bran, is poorly used in the body.) Studies show that vegetarians absorb and retain more calcium from foods than nonvegetarians do.

■ **Zinc** Good plant sources of this essential mineral are legumes, whole grains, soy products, peas, spinach, and nuts. It is also abundant in dairy products and shellfish. Take care to select supplements containing no more than 15–18 milligrams of zinc. Supplements containing 50 milligrams or more may lower HDL ("good") cholesterol in some people.

■ **Calories** Plant foods have fewer calories than animal foods; vegetarians should make sure they are consuming enough calories to meet their bodies' energy needs.

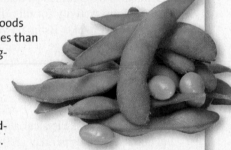

Source: Adapted from "Vegetarian Diets," American Heart Association, 2004, www.americanheart.org.

concept of cuisine, a particular style of preparing food, and *food way*, the food habits, customs, beliefs, and preferences of a certain culture.[5]

The Mediterranean pyramid was developed from the diet typical of the region in southern Europe, including Italy and Greece, where rates of cardiovascular disease and some kinds of cancer are lower than in northern Europe and North America.[1] Like MyPyramid, the Mediterranean pyramid emphasizes grains, fruits, and vegetables, but it also recommends daily servings of beans, legumes, and nuts and foods that are high in protein, fiber, and fats. In addition, it encourages the use of olive oil over other oils.

The Latin American pyramid was developed by the Latino Nutrition Coalition to combat high rates of obesity, Type-2 diabetes, and heart disease in the Latin American population. It is designed to encourage Latinos (and others who want to enjoy Latino food) to eat healthier by maintaining traditional Latin American cooking. This diet emphasizes grains (including maize and quinoa), fruits (including tropical fruits like mango and papaya), vegetables, and plant sources

of protein. You can learn more about the food plan and find meal ideas and shopping tips at www.latinonutrition.org.

The Asian food pyramid draws from the cuisines of South and East Asia. Like the Latin American pyramid, it emphasizes grains, fruits, vegetables, and plant sources of protein. At the base of the pyramid are rice and rice products, noodles, breads, millet, corn, and other minimally refined grains. Meat is at the top of the pyramid, to be consumed only monthly or, if more often, in small amounts. Dairy products that are consumed on a daily basis should also be consumed in small to moderate amounts. For more on this diet, visit www.oldwayspt.org/asian-diet-pyramid.

PLANNING A VEGETARIAN DIET

The 2005 *Dietary Guidelines for Americans* provides some direction for vegetarian choices, and several pyramids have been developed for vegetarian diets. The vegetarian pyramid has a bread, cereal, rice, and pasta group at the base and vegetable and fruit groups above that. It also has a milk, yogurt, and cheese group but allows 0–3 servings to accommodate those vegetarians who do not eat dairy products. Instead of a meat, fish, and poultry group, it has a dried beans, nuts, seeds, eggs, and meat substitutes group. This group includes soy products (for example, tofu, tempeh), legumes, and peanut butter. Vegetarians using this pyramid should also adopt the recommendations included in the *Dietary Guidelines* (such as making sure foods in the bread group are whole grain).

Vegetarian diets may offer protection against obesity, heart disease, high blood pressure, diabetes, digestive disorders, and some forms of cancer, particularly colon cancer,[21] depending on the type of vegetarian diet followed. Some research suggests that vegetarians live longer than nonvegetarians. Despite the potential benefits of vegetarian diets, however, vegetarians need to make sure that their diets provide the energy intake and food diversity needed to meet dietary guidelines.[7] (See the box "Vegetarian Diet Planning.")

DAILY VALUES AND FOOD LABELS

Daily Values are another set of standards, based on a variety of dietary guidelines and used on the food labels on packaged foods. Food labels are regulated by the FDA (labeling of meat and poultry products is regulated by the USDA).[22] The information in the Nutrition Facts panel on a food label tells you how that food fits into a 2,000-calorie-a-day diet that includes no more than 65 grams of fat (30 percent of total calories) (Figure 6.3).

The top of the label lists serving size and number of servings in the container. The second part of the label gives the total calories and the calories from fat. A quick calculation will tell you whether this food is relatively high or low in fat. Look for foods with no more than 30 percent of their calories from fat.

The next part of the label shows how much the food contributes to the Daily Values established for important nutrients, expressed as a percentage. The bottom part of the label, which is the same on all food labels, contains a footnote explaining the term "% Daily Value" and shows recommended daily intake of specified nutrients in a 2,000- and a 2,500-calorie diet.[22]

Packaged foods frequently display food descriptors and health claims, which are also regulated by the FDA to help consumers know what they are getting. For example, the term *light* can be used if the product has one-third fewer calories or half the fat of the regular product. To find out more about common nutritional claims, visit the FDA Web site.

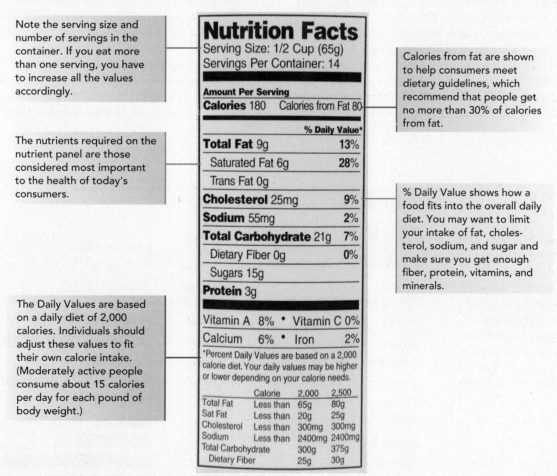

Note the serving size and number of servings in the container. If you eat more than one serving, you have to increase all the values accordingly.

The nutrients required on the nutrient panel are those considered most important to the health of today's consumers.

The Daily Values are based on a daily diet of 2,000 calories. Individuals should adjust these values to fit their own calorie intake. (Moderately active people consume about 15 calories per day for each pound of body weight.)

Calories from fat are shown to help consumers meet dietary guidelines, which recommend that people get no more than 30% of calories from fat.

% Daily Value shows how a food fits into the overall daily diet. You may want to limit your intake of fat, cholesterol, sodium, and sugar and make sure you get enough fiber, protein, vitamins, and minerals.

figure 6.3 **Nutrition Facts panel on a food label.**

Current Consumer Concerns

The food-related topics that you are likely to hear about in the media are consumer issues and concerns, such as the problems associated with soft drinks, high-sodium diets, and fast foods.

OVERCONSUMPTION OF SOFT DRINKS

Americans consume an average of 22.2 teaspoons (335 calories) of sugar each day. Sugar is believed to promote and maintain obesity, cause and aggravate diabetes, increase the risk of heart disease, and cause dental decay, gum disease, osteoporosis, and kidney stones. It should be noted, however, that scientific evidence suggests that moderate levels of sugar (no more than 10 percent of total calories) pose no health risk.[1,7,23]

Much of this sugar comes from soft drinks. These beverages represent the largest contributor of daily calories, about 7 percent of calories consumed. For teenagers, they account for 13 percent of calories consumed daily. Consumption of soft drinks doubled from the mid-1970s to the mid-1990s and increased further in the decade that followed. Soft drinks account for one in every four beverages consumed in the United States. Some experts attribute the surge in overweight and obesity among American children and adults largely to the increase in the consumption of soft drinks.

Equally important is the decreased consumption of milk, which is a major source of calcium, protein, vitamin A, and vitamin D, as well as decreased consumption of orange juice and other fruit juices.[24,25] Soft drinks contain about the same number of calories as milk and juice but none of the nutrients. Diet soft drinks don't contain sugar, but like regular soft drinks, they fill you up without providing any nutrients (Figure 6.4).

Soft drinks also contain relatively high levels of caffeine, which is mildly addictive and can lead to nervousness, irritability, insomnia, and bone demineralization. Although soft drink manufacturers claim that caffeine is added for its flavoring effects, its primary effect is to stimulate the central nervous system.[25] Nutritionists recommend limiting soft drinks in the diet and drinking water and low-fat milk instead.

HIGH-SODIUM DIETS

Another current concern is the amount of sodium consumed in our diets. Sodium is an essential nutrient, but we need only about 500 milligrams per day—about $\frac{1}{10}$ of a teaspoon. Although many foods contain sodium, we get most of our sodium—about 90 percent—from salt (which is made up of sodium and chloride). The recommended upper limit for salt is 2,400 milligrams per day, about 1 teaspoon, and the 2010 *Dietary Guidelines* recommends no more than 1,500 milligrams per day. However, most Americans consume about 4,000 milligrams per day. To promote the reduction of American salt consumption, the American Heart Association also recommended in 2010 that all Americans reduce their salt intake to less than 1,500 milligrams per day.

Salt may be a factor in causing hypertension (high blood pressure) in some "salt-sensitive" people. Even people who are not salt sensitive can benefit from reducing the salt in their diets.[1]

Many packaged foods, convenience foods, fast foods, and restaurant foods are heavily salted, primarily to enhance flavor. At one nationwide restaurant chain, for example, an order of grilled baby back ribs has between 3,300 and 5,300

figure **6.4** **Diet soda vs. fat-free milk.** Diet soda has virtually no nutritional value, but it has replaced milk in the diets of many Americans, including adolescent and young adult women, who need calcium to build bone mass. Milk is one of the best sources of calcium, protein, potassium, and many other nutrients.

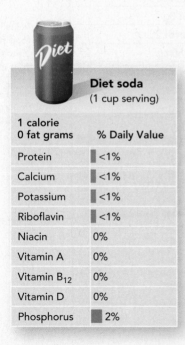

Diet soda (1 cup serving)	
1 calorie 0 fat grams	% Daily Value
Protein	<1%
Calcium	<1%
Potassium	<1%
Riboflavin	<1%
Niacin	0%
Vitamin A	0%
Vitamin B$_{12}$	0%
Vitamin D	0%
Phosphorus	2%

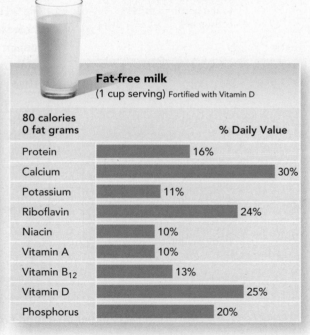

Fat-free milk (1 cup serving) Fortified with Vitamin D	
80 calories 0 fat grams	% Daily Value
Protein	16%
Calcium	30%
Potassium	11%
Riboflavin	24%
Niacin	10%
Vitamin A	10%
Vitamin B$_{12}$	13%
Vitamin D	25%
Phosphorus	20%

Many restaurant foods are heavily salted, primarily to enhance flavor. At one nationwide restaurant chain, an **order of chicken tacos has 4,400 milligrams of sodium,** *and an order of steak fajitas has more than 3,000 milligrams of sodium.*

milligrams of sodium, depending on the preparation and sauce. At the same chain, an order of chicken tacos has 4,400 milligrams of sodium, and an order of steak fajitas has more than 3,000 milligrams of sodium.[26] Canned soups, lunch meats, pickles, soy sauce, teriyaki sauce, catsup, mustard, salad dressing, and barbecue sauce are also high in sodium (see the box "Food, Diet, and Health").

food security
Having enough food at all times to support an active, healthy lifestyle.

You can reduce the amount of salt in your diet by emphasizing whole foods, like grains, vegetables, and fruits, which are naturally low in sodium. Remove the salt shaker from your table, and don't use salt in cooking. When buying packaged foods, read the labels to check for salt content, and look for descriptors such as "reduced sodium" or "low sodium." (For more guidelines on grocery shopping, see the box "Shopping Tips for College Students," on p. 122.) Highly salted food is an acquired taste; if you use less salt, you will gradually rediscover the natural taste of the food. Although scientists have found substitutes for sugar, substitutes for salt are much more elusive, since it has a distinct taste. Potassium is a salty substance that has been used as a salt substitute, but some people find it too bitter.

FOOD ALLERGIES AND FOOD INTOLERANCES

Food allergies occur when the immune system overreacts to specific proteins in food; they affect about 7 percent of children and 2 percent of adults. More than 200 food ingredients can cause an allergic reaction, but eight foods are responsible for 90 percent of food allergies—milk, eggs, peanuts, tree nuts, fish, shellfish, soy, and wheat. Allergic reactions to these foods cause 30,000 emergency room visits each year and 150 to 200 deaths.[27] The Food Allergen Labeling and Consumer Protection Act of 2004 requires that these allergens be clearly identified on all packaged foods below the list of ingredients.

Typical symptoms of allergic reactions include skin rash, nasal congestion, hives, nausea, and wheezing. Most children eventually outgrow food allergies, except for

Who's at Risk?

Food, Diet, and Health

- People with low incomes generally cannot afford healthier foods. They tend to rely more on processed foods than on fresh foods. The migration of supermarkets to the suburbs and the lack of transportation in low-income communities may contribute to malnutrition among these populations.

- About half of all African American and Latino children born in the year 2000 are expected to develop diabetes at some time in their lives. A healthy diet and a healthy body weight are essential in preventing this disease. On average, a child with diabetes at age 10 will have his or her life expectancy reduced by 17 to 26 years.

- **Food security** is defined as having enough food at all times to support an active, healthy life. It is estimated that almost 6 percent of the population do not have enough food to eat. About 40 percent of households with incomes below the poverty line experience food insecurity.

- About 20 percent of households with children report food insecurity. Children in food-insufficient households experience more headaches, stomachaches, and infections. Malnutrition impairs cognitive development in children and decreases social interaction due to low energy levels.

- Women in food-insecure households consume less than two-thirds of the DRI for calories, calcium, iron, vitamin E, magnesium, and zinc. Pregnant women experiencing food insecurity are at higher risk for providing inadequate nutrition for the fetus.

- About 33 percent of the general population are heavy consumers of sugar. Individuals who consume high levels of sugar tend to have a higher calorie intake and lower nutrient intake than those who consume low levels of sugar.

Sources: "Household Food Security in the United States, 2008," by M. Nord, M. Andrews, and S. Carlson, 2009, ERR-83, U.S. Department of Agriculture, Economic Research Service; *Perspectives in Nutrition,* by G.M. Wardlaw, J.S. Hampal, and R.A. DiSilvestro, 2006, New York: McGraw-Hill; "Neighborhood Characteristics Associated With the Location of Food Services Places," by K. Morland, S. Wing, A.D. Roux, and C. Poole, 2002, in Race, Ethnicity, and Health, ed. T.A. LaVeist, San Francisco: Jossey-Bass; *Liquid Candy,* by M.F. Jacobson, 2005, Washington, DC: Center for Science in the Public Interest.

Challenges
& Choices

Shopping Tips for College Students

- Make a shopping list before you go to the store. Better yet, make a menu for the week and buy all the things you need in one trip.

- Take a quick inventory of the food in your kitchen when making your list. You may already have many of the items you need. If you have coupons, keep them with your shopping list. They can reduce your grocery bill significantly.

- Eat something before you go to the store. Grocery stores thrive on impulse buying and are designed to take advantage of the powers of smell and sight. Almost every food looks good when you're hungry.

- Know your budgetary limits and check prices when you're shopping. Read the unit price (usually posted on the shelf below the item) and not just the package price. Unit prices will tell you cost per pound or ounce. Compare this information with similar food items, which are usually nearby on the shelf.

- Concentrate your shopping around the periphery of the store, where you'll find produce, meat, dairy products, and bakery sections. Limit your forays into the middle of the store to find beans, whole grains, cereals, pasta, and other nutrient-dense items.

- Read labels and look for foods that are minimally processed. Be sure to look at the serving size so that you'll know if the information applies to less than the whole container.

- In the produce aisle, look for brightly colored fruits and vegetables.

- In the bread aisle, look for products with the word *whole* in the first ingredient on the ingredient list (whole wheat, whole grain).

- In the snack aisle, choose pretzels, rice cakes, baked corn or potato chips, and popcorn over regular potato chips. Another healthy, inexpensive choice is peanut butter.

- Choose fresh vegetables over frozen and frozen over canned. Canned vegetables are loaded with sodium.

- Choose olive, canola, or safflower oil; if you use mayonnaise, get a light or low-fat version.

- In the dairy section, choose low-fat or fat-free milk, cottage cheese, yogurt, and cheese. Choose tub margarine over stick margarine or butter. Consider trying a soy product.

- Soup is very high in sodium. Look for low-salt versions, and try bean or lentil soup for fiber, folate, and protein.

- At the meat counter, choose lean cuts of beef and skinless poultry (or remove the skin yourself at home). Put meat in a plastic bag to catch leaks. To ensure food safety, buy meats and frozen foods last.

- Watch the scanner to make sure the register rings up the same price you saw on the shelf. If it doesn't, ask the cashier to check the price.

Sources: "Cut Three Hundred or More off Your Grocery Bill," by D.L. Montaldo, http://couponing.about.com/cs/grocerysavings/a/groceryshoptips.htm; Restaurant Confidential, by M.F. Jacobson and J.G. Hurley, 2002, New York: Workman; "Smart Food Shopping," by C. Palumbo, 2007, retrieved April 3, 2008, from www.foodfit.com/healthy/archive/healthy/About_dec01.asp.

allergies to peanuts, nuts, and seafood.[1] Generally, people suffer temporary discomfort, but approximately 30,000 people each year in the United States have an *anaphylactic shock* reaction to a food they have eaten—the throat swells enough to cut off breathing.[2] A person experiencing this type of allergic reaction needs immediate medical attention.

Most food reactions are not caused by allergies, however; most are caused by food intolerances.[3] These are less severe than allergies and can be triggered by almost any food. Lactose intolerance, a condition that results from an inability to digest the milk sugar lactose, is especially prevalent.

There is no treatment or cure for food allergies or intolerances. If you experience these reactions, the best you can do is try to avoid the offending food.[1] It can be especially hard to avoid allergenic foods when eating out, because restaurants are not required to reveal this information. Many health experts are now calling for menu labeling by restaurants, not only for health reasons but also for personal, cultural, and religious reasons. For example, McDonald's has been sued in class action suits brought by vegetarian groups and Muslim associations for flavoring french fries with small amounts of meat, milk, and wheat products without informing customers.[28]

ENERGY BARS AND ENERGY DRINKS

Energy bars are a convenient source of calories and nutrients for people with busy schedules or intense exercise regimens. Luna Bars, Power Bars, and Balance Bars are examples of these convenience foods. Most are low in saturated and trans fats and contain up to 5 grams of fiber. They are better for you than candy bars and other snack foods high in saturated fat, but they can also be high in calories and sugar. Healthier alternatives are whole foods like fruits and vegetables, with their abundant vitamins, minerals, and phytochemicals. If you do buy energy bars, check the labels for calories, total fat, saturated fat, protein, fiber, and sugar and choose the healthiest ones.[29]

Americans consume about four quarts of energy drinks each year per person. Energy drinks are marketed as a source of instant energy, improved concentration and memory, and enhanced physical performance. They have names like Red Bull, Rockstar, Full Throttle, and Monster. Energy drinks are not considered a health risk if consumed in recommended amounts, but there are no long-term studies on their side effects, if any.

Mixing hard alcohol and energy drinks has become popular with young adults. Combining a stimulant (caffeine and other herbal ingredients) with a depressant (alcohol) disguises the intoxication effects of alcohol by helping the drinker feel alert and sober. In a recent study, people who had been drinking energy drinks with liquor were three times more likely to be drunk than those who drank only alcohol and were four times more likely to say they planned to drive within the hour.[30] Multiple cocktails of energy drinks and liquor can also pose a danger to heart muscle fibers and cause extreme dehydration.

performance, but consumption should not exceed 300 milligrams per day. Caffeine levels above 400 milligrams are likely to produce negative effects, including loss of focus, racing heart rate, nausea, and anxiety. For most other additives, little or no empirical research either supports their effectiveness or details their potential dangers. The FDA does not monitor energy drinks, but it is beginning to take an interest in doing so. Sales of energy drinks have been

In a recent study, people who had been drinking energy drinks with liquor were **three times more likely to be drunk** *than those who drank only alcohol and were* **four times more likely to say they planned to drive** *within the hour.*

In addition to water, sodium, and glucose, many energy drinks contain caffeine and a variety of dietary supplements, such as ginseng, guarana, and B vitamins. Caffeine can stimulate mental activity and may increase cardiovascular

■ Energy drinks provide a brief burst of alertness, typically fueled by caffeine and usually followed by a crash. High profile celebrities like Jessica Simpson have helped popularize energy drinks like Red Bull.

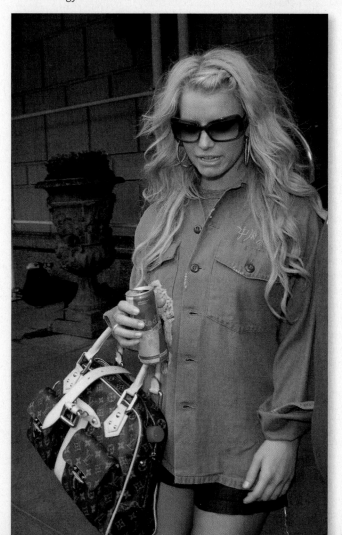

restricted in a few countries. For example, Red Bull has been banned in France, Germany, and Denmark due to health concerns.[31]

If you consume energy drinks, your maximum intake should be two 20-ounce cans a day. Consuming more than 20 ounces an hour can cause an increase in arterial pressure and in blood sugar levels. Energy drinks should not be consumed immediately after a vigorous workout or in combination with alcohol. They should not be consumed by pregnant women, children, young teens, older adults, or people with cardiovascular disease, glaucoma, or sleep disorders. The bottom line, according to many health experts, is that the risks associated with energy drinks outweigh any perceived benefits.[32]

FAST FOODS

Americans eat out more than four times a week, and every day, one in four Americans eats fast food.[33] Although plenty of people choose to eat fast food over more healthy options, people who live in *food deserts* do not have adequate access to healthy, affordable food (see the box "Food Deserts"). For these people, fast food is often the alternative. Fast-food meals tend to be high in calories, fat, sodium, and sugar and low in vitamins, minerals, and fiber. A single fast-food meal can approach or exceed the recommended limits on calories, fat, saturated fat, and sodium for a whole day's meals (Figure 6.5).

Many fast-food restaurants (and restaurants in general) are offering healthier choices these days, though, so if you know what to order, it's possible to make healthy choices:

■ Don't supersize or order extra-large servings. Standard-size orders are already very large.

■ Go easy on sauces, toppings, and condiments like sour cream, guacamole, tartar sauce, mayonnaise, and gravy.

■ Order grilled chicken or fish on a whole wheat roll, but have them hold the "special sauce."

■ Order a salad with dressing on the side or a fat-free dressing. A dinner salad without dressing may have about

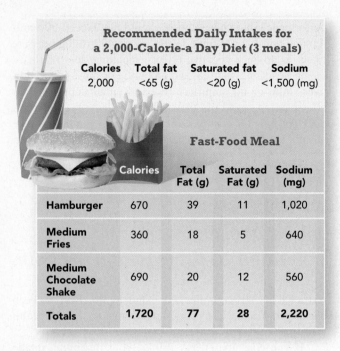

Recommended Daily Intakes for a 2,000-Calorie-a Day Diet (3 meals)			
Calories	Total fat	Saturated fat	Sodium
2,000	<65 (g)	<20 (g)	<1,500 (mg)

Fast-Food Meal				
	Calories	Total Fat (g)	Saturated Fat (g)	Sodium (mg)
Hamburger	670	39	11	1,020
Medium Fries	360	18	5	640
Medium Chocolate Shake	690	20	12	560
Totals	**1,720**	**77**	**28**	**2,220**

figure **6.5**   **A fast-food meal compared with recommended daily intakes.**

150 calories, but a Caesar salad with dressing may have almost 1,000 calories.

■ Order a baked potato with vegetables instead of butter or sour cream.

■ Instead of a soda, order orange juice, low-fat milk, or a glass of iced water.

■ Instead of pie or cake, order yogurt and fruit.

The least healthy options are fried fish or fried chicken sandwiches, chicken nuggets, croissants and pastries, onion rings, and large fries. Most fast-food restaurants will give you a nutritional brochure if you ask for it, or it may be posted; choose the healthiest options.

Food Safety and Technology

Although the FDA is charged with monitoring the safety of the U.S. food supply, consumers, too, need to learn to distinguish between safe and unsafe foods and understand key elements of food safety.

Public Health in Action

Food Deserts

The term *food desert* describes neighborhoods and communities that have limited access to affordable and nutritious food. In the United States, people who live in urban and rural low-income neighborhoods are more likely to live in food desert zones. Supermarket chains are more likely to offer healthier and affordable food choices than small grocery stores or convenience stores, but supermarkets, like any other business, do not operate stores where it is not profitable to do so.

In 2009 Congress asked a number of government agencies (the Economic Research Service of the U.S. Department of Agriculture, the Institute of Medicine, and the National Research Council) to gather more information about the health effects of living in a food desert. Previous research had focused on the factors that contribute to food deserts, but less was known about their impact on public health, particularly in relation to obesity and chronic diet-related diseases. The agencies' findings confirmed that food deserts do exist in inner city and rural low-income areas and that they are a public health concern. One study found that people living in food deserts are 32 to 55 percent less likely to have a high-quality diet. These areas also have higher rates of obesity and chronic diet-related diseases such as diabetes, heart disease, and cancer.

To date, government interventions to counter food deserts have been concentrated at the grassroots level in communities. Some states and local governments have established public transportation programs that help inner-city residents access supermarkets in the suburbs. More creative efforts have included grants and loans to build and subsidize smaller supermarkets in high-need neighborhoods. The Healthy Bodega Initiative in New York City encourages existing stores in inner-city areas to improve their offerings of healthy foods. The Food Trust in Philadelphia, which found that children there consume about 600 calories per day in mostly unhealthy snacks, works with corner stores where children shop for snacks. The organization helped corner stores set up attention-grabbing coolers with appealingly packaged fruit to increase the likelihood that children would choose fruit over processed foods for snacks.

Most recently, as part of First Lady Michelle Obama's efforts to combat childhood obesity, the Obama Administration allocated $400 million to eliminate food deserts. The money will be used for tax credits and below-market-rate loans, which are expected to help create new grocery stores and help current businesses expand their produce offerings in areas with insufficient access to healthy, affordable food.

connect ACTIVITY

Sources: "The Public Health Effects of Food Deserts: Workshop Summary," by Paula Tarnapol Whitacre, Peggy Tsai, and Janet Mulligan, Rapporteurs, National Research Council, 2009, Washington, D.C.: The National Academies Press; "Obama Administration Details Healthy Food Financing Initiative," Department of Health and Human Services, retrieved February 19, 2010, from http://www.hhs.gov/news/press/2010pres/02/20100219a.html.

Aspartame contains phenylalanine and should be avoided by people with phenylketonuria (PKU), an inherited metabolic disorder (see Chapter 2). Generally, artificial sweeteners are considered safe.[1] Still, they should be consumed only in moderation and as part of a well-balanced diet.

ORGANIC FOODS

Plant foods labeled "organic" are grown without synthetic pesticides or fertilizers,[2] and animal foods labeled organic are from animals raised on organic feed without antibiotics or growth hormone. Organic foods appeal to health- and environment-conscious consumers.[34] They tend to be more expensive than foods grown using conventional methods, however, and consumers cannot always determine exactly how some foods were grown.

The USDA regulates the use of terms related to organic foods on the labels of meat and poultry products. The label "100% organic" means that all contents are organic; "organic" means that contents are at least 95 percent organic; "made with organic ingredients" means the contents are at least 70 percent organic. Food manufacturers who comply with the USDA standards can place the seal "USDA Organic" on their labels.

Although it seems that organic foods ought to be healthier and safer than foods grown conventionally, no research has demonstrated that this is the case. Conventional food products do contain pesticide residues that can be toxic at high doses, but research has not documented ill effects from them at the levels found in foods, nor is there any evidence that people who consume organic food are healthier than those who don't.[1]

What has been documented is that organic farming is beneficial to the environment. It helps maintain biodiversity of crops; it replenishes the earth's resources; and it is less likely to degrade soil, contaminate water, or expose farm workers to toxic chemicals. As multinational food companies get into the organic food business, however, consumers

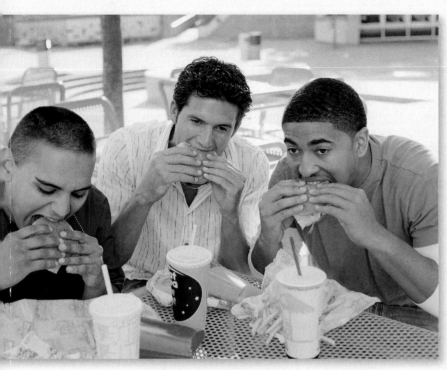

■ Fast food is readily available, inexpensive, convenient, and tasty—and sometimes the only option. Even at fast-food restaurants, though, some choices are healthier than others.

ARTIFICIAL SWEETENERS

Artificial sweeteners are just one type of food additive—substances that are added to food to maintain or improve nutrient value, aid in food preparation, and/or improve taste or appearance.[1] Currently, about 2,800 different additives are approved by the FDA, which requires that they be effective, detectable, measurable, and safe.

Artificial sweeteners enable people to enjoy a sweet taste in foods and beverages without consuming sugar. One sweetener, aspartame, has undergone rigorous study. It is marketed as Nutrasweet, Equal, and Spoonful. Many products contain it, including Diet Pepsi and Diet Coke. In the United States, the ADI (acceptable daily intake) of aspartame is 50 milligrams per kilogram of body weight; in Canada, it is 40 milligrams per kilogram.[1] This means a 150-pound person would have to consume 97 packets of Equal or 20 cans of diet soft drinks a day to exceed the ADI. The typical person consumes less than 5 milligrams of aspartame per kilogram of body weight per day.[1]

■ Organic foods aren't necessarily healthier, but organic farming is better for the environment. Many consumers are now choosing organic, locally grown produce and other foods.

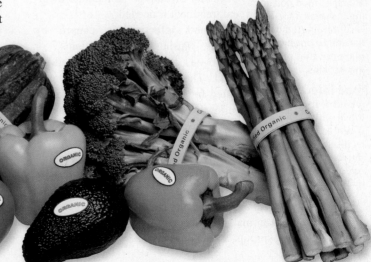

should look for foods that are not only organic but also locally grown. The average food item currently travels at least 1,500 miles to its destination, consuming massive amounts of oil for transportation. Locally grown food tastes better, keeps money in the local economy, and cuts down on the consumption of processed food. The burgeoning popularity of farmers' markets is a sign of growing interest in locally grown food.

A disadvantage of organic foods is that they may place consumers at higher risk of contracting foodborne illnesses. If you purchase organic food, buy only the amount you need immediately, store and cook the food properly, and wash organic produce thoroughly before eating it.[1,35]

Some experts recommend that consumers who want to buy organic fruits and vegetables spend their money on those that carry higher pesticide residues when grown conventionally (the "dirty dozen"): apples, bell peppers, celery, cherries, imported grapes, nectarines, peaches, pears, potatoes, red raspberries, spinach, and strawberries. Fruits and vegetables that carry little pesticide residue whether grown conventionally or organically include asparagus, avocados, bananas, broccoli, cauliflower, corn, kiwi, mangoes, onions, papaya, pineapples, and peas.[35]

FOODBORNE ILLNESSES

The Centers for Disease Control and Prevention (CDC) estimates that 76 million people get sick every year from foodborne illness, 325,000 are hospitalized, and 5,000 die.[36] Foodborne illnesses may be caused by food intoxication or by food infection; both types are commonly referred to as *food poisoning*.

Food intoxication occurs when a food is contaminated by natural toxins or by microbes that produce toxins. Botulism is an example of food intoxication. When food has been contaminated with the botulism bacterium and then improperly prepared or stored, the bacterium releases a dangerous and potentially fatal toxin. Warning signs of botulism poisoning are double vision, weak muscles, difficulty swallowing, and difficulty breathing.[1] Immediate medical treatment is needed.

Food infection is caused by disease-causing microorganisms, or pathogens, that have contaminated the food. The more commonly contaminated foods are ground beef, chicken, turkey, salami, hot dogs, ice cream, lettuce and other greens, sprouts, cantaloupe, and apple cider.

Three of the most common pathogens that cause food infection are *Escherichia coli (E. coli)*, salmonella, and campylobacter. *E. coli* occurs naturally in the intestines of humans and animals. Raw beef, raw fruits and vegetables, leafy greens, sprouts, and unpasteurized juices and cider are the foods most commonly contaminated by it. A 2007 nationwide outbreak of *E. coli* infection was traced to packaged spinach and lettuce grown in California and contaminated by domestic animals and wildlife.

One strain, *E. coli* O157:H7, is especially dangerous because it can cause *hemolytic uremic syndrome (HUS)*, which can lead to kidney failure, a potentially fatal condition. The CDC estimates that *E. coli* O157:H7 causes nearly 73,000 illnesses each year in the United States and kills 250 to 500 people.[37] Young children and older adults are particularly at risk. *E. coli* is a hearty microbe, thriving in moist environments for weeks and on kitchen countertops for days.

Salmonella enteritis can contaminate raw eggs, poultry and meat, fruits, and vegetables, and other foods. Eggs containing salmonella enteritis are the number-one cause of food poisoning outbreaks in the nation. The best way to prevent salmonella infection is to thoroughly cook eggs, chicken, and other foods to kill the bacterium. Avoid eating raw or undercooked eggs, such as in raw cake batter or cookie dough, salad dressings, and eggnog.[37] New federal safeguards are expected to reduce salmonella infections by 80,000 per year and deaths by 30 per year. The safeguards focus on mandating rodent control programs on egg-producing farms and requiring eggs to be refrigerated during storage.

Campylobacter occurs in raw or undercooked poultry, meat, and shellfish, in unpasteurized milk, and in contaminated water. Campylobacter from contaminated poultry can spread when juices from packages spill onto kitchen surfaces and other foods; it can also be spread by hand.[38] Campylobacter and salmonella together cause 80 percent of the illnesses and 75 percent of the deaths associated with meat and poultry practices.[38]

Food poisoning causes flu-like symptoms such as diarrhea, abdominal pain, vomiting, fever, and chills. More serious complications can include rheumatoid arthritis, kidney or heart disease, meningitis, HUS, and death. Some symptoms are cause for immediate medical attention:

- Bloody diarrhea or pus in the stool
- Fever that lasts more than 48 hours
- Faintness, rapid heart rate, or nausea when standing up suddenly
- Significant drop in the frequency of urination[36,39]

Although only about 20 percent of food poisoning cases occur at home, the best defense against foodborne illness is the use of safe food practices in your own kitchen (Figure 6.6).[40]

Recent foodborne-illness outbreaks, such as salmonella-tainted hot peppers from Mexico that sent over 240 people to the hospital in 2008, have prompted increased safety concerns about imported foods. Until passage of the Country-of-Origin Law (COOL) in 2009, consumers had little idea where everyday foods originated. COOL

food intoxication
A kind of food poisoning in which a food is contaminated by natural toxins or by microbes that produce toxins.

food infection
A kind of food poisoning in which a food is contaminated by disease-causing microorganisms, or pathogens.

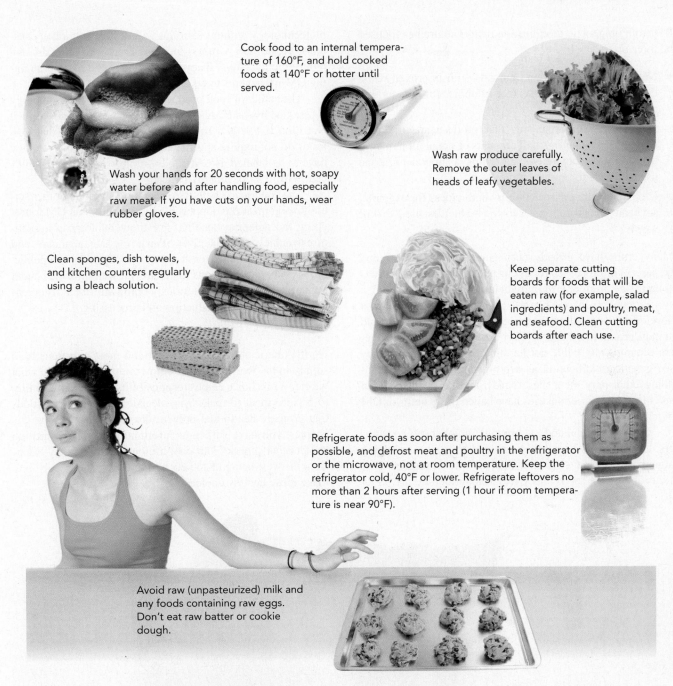

Cook food to an internal temperature of 160°F, and hold cooked foods at 140°F or hotter until served.

Wash raw produce carefully. Remove the outer leaves of heads of leafy vegetables.

Wash your hands for 20 seconds with hot, soapy water before and after handling food, especially raw meat. If you have cuts on your hands, wear rubber gloves.

Clean sponges, dish towels, and kitchen counters regularly using a bleach solution.

Keep separate cutting boards for foods that will be eaten raw (for example, salad ingredients) and poultry, meat, and seafood. Clean cutting boards after each use.

Refrigerate foods as soon after purchasing them as possible, and defrost meat and poultry in the refrigerator or the microwave, not at room temperature. Keep the refrigerator cold, 40°F or lower. Refrigerate leftovers no more than 2 hours after serving (1 hour if room temperature is near 90°F).

Avoid raw (unpasteurized) milk and any foods containing raw eggs. Don't eat raw batter or cookie dough.

figure **6.6**   **Food safety in the kitchen.**

genetically modified (GM) organisms
Organisms whose genetic makeup has been changed to produce desirable traits.

requires retailers to notify consumers of the country of origin of common unprocessed foods such as raw beef, veal, lamb, vegetables, frozen fruits, and many other foods. However, processed foods are not included under COOL; for example, raw pork chops have to be labeled, but ham and bacon do not. Butcher shops selling meat and/or seafood are also exempt.[41]

GENETICALLY MODIFIED FOODS

Farmers, scientists, and breeders have long been tinkering with the genetic makeup of plants and animals to breed organisms with desirable traits, a process known as *selective breeding*. Compared to modern techniques, however, selective breeding is slow and imprecise. Using biotechnology to produce **genetically modified (GM) organisms** is a faster and more refined process. Genetic modification involves the addition, deletion, or reorganization of an organism's genes in order to change that organism's protein production.

Research on genetic modification in agriculture has focused on three areas:

- New strains of crops and animals with improved resistance to disease and pests (for example, corn plants that resist blights)
- Strains of microorganisms that produce specific substances that occur in small amounts or not at all in nature (for example, bovine somatotropin, a growth hormone used in cattle to produce more meat)
- Crops that resist destruction by herbicides (for example, soybean plants that can survive herbicides used to kill weeds)

Many crops have already been genetically modified, and 60 percent of processed foods currently sold in supermarkets contain one or more GM ingredients.[41]

Proponents of GM crops and animals say we must develop new agricultural technologies that increase crop and animal productivity and support food growers and producers economically while not harming the environment. They see genetic modification as a promising agricultural technology that may meet these needs, and many in the food and biotechnology industries have hailed the benefits of GM organisms.[42]

On the other hand, a growing number of consumers, animal rights supporters, national consumer watchdog organizations, and environmentalists have expressed concerns about GM foods. They fear that agriculture driven by biotechnology without restraint will destroy natural ecosystems, create new viruses, increase cruelty to animals, and reduce biodiversity.[42] They have called for all foods containing GM ingredients to be labeled.

The safety of food products produced by biotechnology is assessed by the FDA's Center for Food Safety and Applied Nutrition (CFSAN). To date, the center has held that GM foods do not require any special safety testing—nor do they have to be labeled as GM foods—unless they differ significantly from foods already in use.[1,36]

The American Dietetic Association and many other scientific organizations support the FDA position on GM foods, citing the potential benefits. For biotechnology in agriculture to achieve the objectives of ensuring safe, abundant, and affordable food, however, it must be accepted by the public. Surveys suggest that consumers are not well informed about this technology but are cautiously optimistic about its potential benefits in food production and processing.[42]

* * *

North Americans enjoy the safest and most nutritious food supply in the world. We also enjoy immense choice in what we eat. With choice comes responsibility—the responsibility to be informed, to make wise decisions, to consume foods that promote health and prevent disease. After reading this chapter, you have sufficient information to make nutrition choices that support your own lifelong health and, by extension, the well-being of society at large. We encourage you to make those healthy choices!

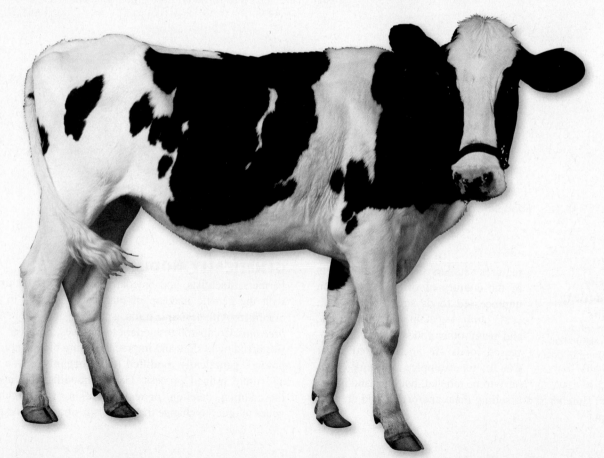

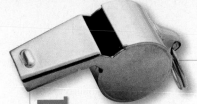

You Make the Call

Can Menu Labeling Make Us Healthier?

On March 30, 2010, President Barack Obama signed the Patient Protection and Affordable Care Act, part of which included a new requirement that all chain restaurants (restaurants with more than 20 locations, such as Denny's, Pizza Hut, and Taco Bell) provide calorie labeling on menus, menu boards, drive-through displays, and vending machines. A handful of states had previously passed their own labeling requirements, but the new law will override individual state laws. The law requires that only calories be listed, not fat grams, milligrams of sodium, or other nutritional information. The average consumer at Wendy's, for example, will now see that a Chicken BLT Salad has 790 calories and a Double Stack Cheeseburger has 360 calories. The National Restaurant Association supports the current form of the legislation but opposed previous versions that included additional labeling requirements.

The legislation is designed to address two problems: (1) that consumers don't know the calorie content of the food they eat, and (2) that they also tend to underestimate calorie content by quite a bit. One study found that people underestimate calories in food from fast-food chains by 200 to 600 calories. Most people would not guess that a small milkshake at McDonald's actually has more calories than a Big Mac.

The ultimate goals of the legislation are to help consumers make healthier choices and to reduce the rates of overweight, obesity, and chronic disease in the United States. Americans get a third of their calories from meals outside their homes. Proponents of the law say that people need accurate nutrition information to maintain a healthy weight and to decrease the risk of chronic diseases such as heart disease, stroke, cancer, and diabetes. These diseases are the leading causes of death and disability for Americans and contribute to the nation's rising health care costs. Many of these diseases are preventable through healthy lifestyle behaviors, particularly healthy diets.

connect ACTIVITY

Supporters of menu labeling argue that if people know the calorie content of restaurant foods they will make healthier dietary choices. Proponents of menu labeling also believe it will put pressure on restaurants to lower the calorie content of their meals. When laws were passed requiring that trans fats be included on food labels, many food manufacturers quickly removed trans fats from their products, fearing that consumers would stop buying them.

Opponents argue that menu labeling will not change consumer behavior or solve the nation's overweight and obesity problems. They cite a study that looked at the behavior of fast-food customers in New York after the state introduced mandatory menu labeling in 2008. It found that while close to 30 percent of those surveyed *said* the calorie labeling had changed their habits, a review of their actual receipts revealed that the labeling had not actually caused them to make healthier choices than people in New Jersey, where there was no menu labeling. Opponents of the legislation also point out that food consumption is only one factor in the development of obesity; for example, states with higher rates of obesity have lower levels of physical activity. Finally, smaller chain restaurants warn that complying with the new regulations will impose a financial burden on them, which they will be forced to pass on to consumers in the form of higher prices. The Food and Drug Administration has until March 2011 to formulate the precise details of the law, and in the meantime and thereafter opponents will probably attempt to overturn the law.

Proponents of menu labeling believe it will help people make better food choices and manage their weight more successfully. Opponents think it won't make a difference in people's health but will raise prices. What do you think?

PROS

- People want nutrition information. Without this information, it is difficult to compare food options and make informed choices. Nearly 80 percent of Americans support menu labeling. Three-quarters of adults say the nutrition labels currently on packaged food help them eat healthier foods.

- Empirical studies link eating out with obesity and higher calorie intake. Children eat almost twice as many calories at a restaurant as they do eating at home. Consumers need all the help they can get, given the popularity of eating out.

- Mandatory nutrition labeling is likely to spur restaurants to offer more healthy food choices.

CONS

- Menu labeling will not change consumer behavior. People may want to believe the information helps them make better choices, but it does not actually affect their behavior.

- Many factors other than diet, such as physical inactivity, contribute to chronic diseases. Menu labeling is likely to have marginal impact, at best, on the health of Americans.

- Adding calorie information to menus will increase costs, particularly for small restaurant chains, which will most likely pass the costs on to consumers.

Sources: "Can Menu Labeling Make Us Healthier, Cheaper, Better?" by E. Klein, 2009, Washington Post, retrieved from http://voices.washingtonpost.com/ezra-klein/2009/05/can_menu_labeling_make_us_heal.html; "Health Reform to Deliver Calorie Counts to Chain Restaurant Menus Nationwide," Center for Science in the Public Interest, 2010, retrieved from http://www.cspinet.org/new/201003211.html; "Does Menu Labeling Affect Diners?" by J. Stein, February 22, 2010, Los Angeles Times.

IN REVIEW

What are the categories of nutrients?
The macronutrients are water, carbohydrates, proteins, and fats. The micronutrients are vitamins and minerals. A balanced diet includes adequate intake of all the nutrients, primarily from nutrient-rich foods (as opposed to dietary supplements). Whole foods and especially plant foods contain additional important substances, such as antioxidants.

How do you plan a healthy diet?
The *Dietary Guidelines for Americans* translates the findings of nutritional research into daily dietary recommendations, and MyPyramid customizes these recommendations to the individual, based on activity levels and calorie needs. Many other sets of guidelines are available as well, including pyramids for vegetarians and for those who want to follow ethnic diets.

What are the main nutrition-related concerns currently affecting our society?
Americans overall do not eat a very healthy diet compared to what is recommended, and overweight and obesity are significant problems. The American diet tends to include too many calories; too much sugar, salt, and fat; and too few vegetables, fruits, and whole foods. Current concerns include the overconsumption of soft drinks, high-sodium diets, and the prevalence of fast food.

What are the main food safety–related issues?
The main safety issue is foodborne illness, typically caused by pathogens such as *E. coli* and salmonella. The American food supply is safe overall, but increasing centralization of food production and distribution creates the conditions for widespread outbreaks of foodborne illness from a single source of contamination. Other safety-related issues of interest to consumers include the use of artificial sweeteners, and genetically modified foods. Consumers are becoming increasingly interested in organic and locally grown foods.

Web Resources

American Heart Association, Face the Fats: This site provides information about dietary fats and includes an interactive feature, My Fats Translator, that guides consumers in understanding their fat intake.
www.americanheart.org/facethefats

Center for Science in the Public Interest: This advocacy organization focuses on nutrition and health, food safety, alcohol policy, and sound science.
www.cspinet.org

FDA Center for Food Safety and Applied Nutrition: This resource offers a wide range of information—from food and nutrition topics in the news to legal issues related to food safety.
http://vm.cfsan.fda.gov

Food Allergy and Anaphylaxis Network: Featuring information on common food allergens, this site offers practical approaches to living with food allergies.
www.foodallergy.org

Food Safety: This is an excellent resource for food news and safety alerts, consumer advice, and topics related to children and teens.
www.foodsafety.gov

National Institutes of Health, Office of Dietary Supplements: This government site provides reliable information on popular dietary supplements.
www.ods.od.nih.gov

Nutrition.gov: A gateway to reliable information on nutrition, from the U.S. government.
www.nutrition.gov

USDA, MyPyramid: This official site offers a wealth of information and interactive tools for using MyPyramid to improve your diet.
www.mypyramid.gov

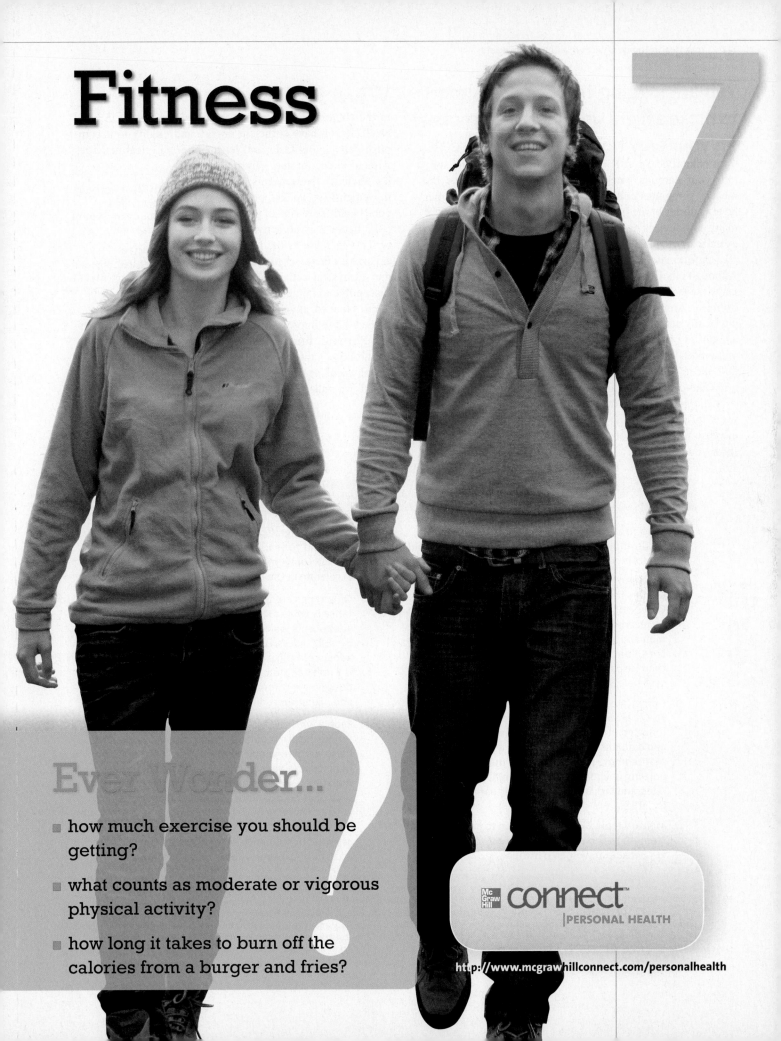

Fitness

7

Ever Wonder...

- how much exercise you should be getting?

- what counts as moderate or vigorous physical activity?

- how long it takes to burn off the calories from a burger and fries?

McGraw Hill **connect** ™
|PERSONAL HEALTH

http://www.mcgrawhillconnect.com/personalhealth

You are jogging through the airport to make a flight on another concourse on your way home for winter break.

Your Nike iPod Sport Kit shoe is blaring your favorite song into your earbuds when a voice suddenly interrupts the music: "5 minutes completed. 0.30 mile. Pace, 5 miles per hour. Calories burned, 45." The Nike iPod shoe is just one of many new devices designed to motivate the general public to exercise, particularly young adults.

Unfortunately, Americans need a lot of motivation. Although many public health campaigns are aimed at Americans' sedentary habits, the fact is that most people don't exercise. Almost 40 percent of American adults are not physically active, and only 30 percent get the recommended amount of physical activity.[1] Among adolescents, only 1 in 4 in grades 9 to 12 meet physical activity recommendations. Of college students, 32 to 47 percent are inactive.[2] (See the box "Exercise and Health.")

The good news is that there are simple and enjoyable ways to build physical activity into your lifestyle and to increase the amount of exercise you get. This chapter will show you now.

What Is Fitness?

In the context of *fitness*, you are considered to be in good health if you have sufficient energy and vitality to accomplish daily living tasks and leisure-time physical activities without undue fatigue. **Physical activity**—activity that requires any type of movement—is an important part of good health. Any kind of physical activity is better than no activity at all, and benefits increase as the level of physical activity increases, up to a point. Too much physical activity can make you susceptible to injury. **Exercise** is structured, planned physical activity, often carried out to improve fitness.

Physical fitness, in general, is the ability of the body to respond to the physical demands placed upon it. When we talk about *fitness*, we are

physical activity
Activity that requires any type of movement.

exercise
Structured, planned physical activity, often carried out to improve fitness.

physical fitness
Ability of the body to respond to the physical demands placed upon it.

Who's at Risk?

Exercise and Health

- In 2008 about 24 percent of adults reported no leisure-time physical activity. About one in four older adults is classified as sedentary.

- Less than half of all adults in the United States meet Centers for Disease Control and Prevention/American College of Sports Medicine aerobic/endurance activity recommendations for health, with 50.7 percent of men and 47.9 percent of women meeting the objectives. Caucasian adults (51.1 percent) are more likely than Hispanics (44 percent) or African Americans (41.8 percent) to meet the objectives.

- Latinos are the most physically inactive racial and ethnic group in the United States. This inactivity is reflected in their exceptionally high rates of obesity and diabetes. Many Latinos live in low-income areas that promote inactive lifestyles due to over-crowded housing environments, high neighborhood crime rates, and lack of access to public parks and recreation facilities.

- Men are more likely than women to participate in strength training, with 21.9 percent of men and 17.5 percent of women participating. Muscle strength

decreases significantly for men between the ages of 50 and 70 years and even more dramatically after age 80. For women, muscle strength losses begin to accelerate in their early 20s.

- Only 17 percent of adults walk when the trip distance is 1 mile or less. Only 31 percent of children and adolescents walk to school when the trip distance is 1 mile or less. Less than 3 percent of children and adolescents bike to school when the trip distance is 2 miles or more. Many communities are actively designing environments that will encourage walking and biking short distances.

- People with physical disabilities are at greater risk for serious health problems associated with sedentary lifestyles than people without disabilities. About 55 percent of people in this population report accumulating no leisure-time physical activity. People with physical disabilities living in neighborhoods with active living buoys (environment supports) were more likely to be involved in leisure-time physical activity. Such supports include access ramps and accessible transportation.

Sources: "1988–2008 No Leisure-Time Physical Activity Trend Chart," Centers for Disease Control, retrieved from http://www.cdc.gov/nccdphp/dnpa/physical/stats/leisure_time.htm; "Active Living in Latino Communities," by G.R. Flores, 2008, American Journal of Preventive Medicine, 34 (4), pp. 369–70; "Designed to Deter: Community Barriers to Physical Activity for People with Visual and Motor Impairments," by C.E. Kirchner, E.G. Gerber, and B.C. Smith, 2008, American Journal of Preventive Medicine, 34 (4), pp. 349–368; The Guide to Community Preventive Health Services, by S. Zara, P.A. Briss, and K.W. Harris, 2005, New York: Oxford University Press; "Physical Activity and Public Health: Updated Recommendation for Adults From the American College of Sports Medicine and the American Heart Association," by W.L. Haskell, L. I-Min, R.R. Pate, et al., 2007, Circulation, 116 (9), pp. 1081–1093.

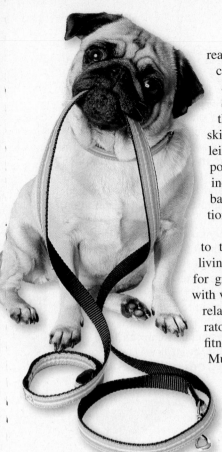

really talking about two different concepts: skill-related fitness and health-related fitness.[3]

Skill-related fitness refers to the ability to perform specific skills associated with various leisure activities or sports. Components of skill-related fitness include agility, speed, power, balance, coordination, and reaction time.

Health-related fitness refers to the ability to perform daily living activities (like shopping for groceries) and other activities with vigor.[3] Components of health-related fitness are cardiorespiratory fitness, musculoskeletal fitness, and body composition. Musculoskeletal fitness, in turn, includes muscular strength, muscular endurance, and flexibility.

BENEFITS OF PHYSICAL ACTIVITY AND EXERCISE

Why should you be physically active? Your answers to this question may include having fun, looking good, feeling good, and other excellent answers. Beyond these, however, is another reason to be physically active: People who are active are healthier than those who are not.[4] There are benefits in the domains of physical, cognitive, psychological, emotional, and spiritual health, among others. An overview of the health benefits associated with physical activity is presented in Figure 7.1.

Physical Benefits of Exercise   One benefit of physical activity is a longer lifespan: people with moderate to high levels of physical activity live longer than people who are sedentary. Physical activity and exercise are associated with improved functioning in just about every body system, from the cardiorespiratory system to the skeletal system to the immune system. A

skill-related fitness
Ability to perform specific skills associated with various sports and leisure activities.

health-related fitness
Ability to perform daily living activities with vigor.

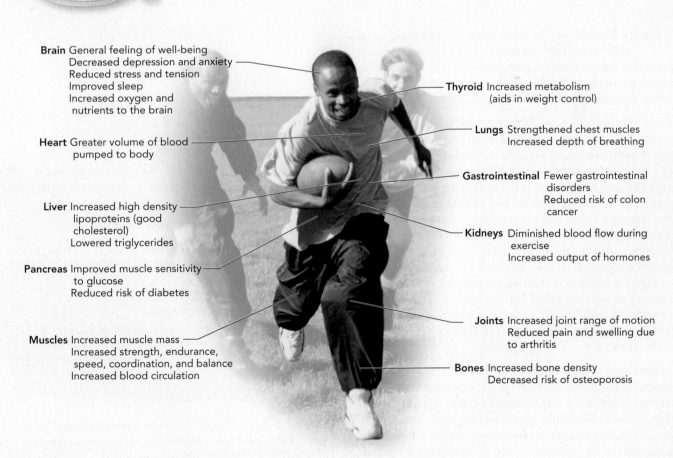

Brain General feeling of well-being
Decreased depression and anxiety
Reduced stress and tension
Improved sleep
Increased oxygen and nutrients to the brain

Heart Greater volume of blood pumped to body

Liver Increased high density lipoproteins (good cholesterol)
Lowered triglycerides

Pancreas Improved muscle sensitivity to glucose
Reduced risk of diabetes

Muscles Increased muscle mass
Increased strength, endurance, speed, coordination, and balance
Increased blood circulation

Thyroid Increased metabolism (aids in weight control)

Lungs Strengthened chest muscles
Increased depth of breathing

Gastrointestinal Fewer gastrointestinal disorders
Reduced risk of colon cancer

Kidneys Diminished blood flow during exercise
Increased output of hormones

Joints Increased joint range of motion
Reduced pain and swelling due to arthritis

Bones Increased bone density
Decreased risk of osteoporosis

figure **7.1**   **Health benefits of physical activity.**

Challenges & Choices

Exercising Your Brain

The benefits of mental activities (chess, bridge, crossword puzzles) for brain function are well established. Animal studies and some human studies are now beginning to show that physical activity is beneficial to the brain as well. Exercise stimulates the growth of new brain cells in the hippocampus (the part of the brain where learning is centered) and in the frontal cortex (the center for decision making, planning, and other executive functions). Exercise encourages brain cells to branch out, join together, and communicate with each other in new ways, and it prompts nerve cells to form denser, more interconnected webs that enable the brain to operate more quickly and efficiently.

Because the brain is not fully developed until early adulthood, exercise is vital to optimal brain development and function. In children and young adults up to about age 25, exercise facilitates the enlargement of the hippocampus and the development of the frontal lobes. Some states cite the importance of exercise for brain development in pushing for mandatory daily physical education up until ninth grade.

Exercise may also help prevent cognitive disorders like Alzheimer's disease in older adults. Some studies found that inactive individuals were twice as likely to develop Alzheimer's disease as those who participated in aerobic exercise at least 30 minutes a day three times a week. Research has particularly focused on the benefits of walking and running and has found that even non-strenuous walking can improve learning, concentration, and abstract reasoning.

A unique system of mental exercise called neurobotics has been developed by Lawrence Katz to help the brain manufacture the nutrients that strengthen, preserve, and grow new brain cells. These exercises are designed to shape daily routines in unexpected ways. An example is using your nondominant hand to control your computer mouse or to brush your teeth. The awkwardness and discomfort you feel reflect the brain's attempt to learn a new skill. Challenging your brain in such ways strengthens neural connections and even creates new ones.

Sources: "Stronger, Faster, Smarter," by M. Carmichael, March 26, 2007, Newsweek, pp. 38–55; "On Your Marks," by A. Kuchment, March 26, 2007, Newsweek, pp. 56–59; "While You Wait: The Cost of Inactivity," 2005, Nutrition Action Newsletter, 32 (10), pp. 3–6; "Exercise and the Brain," Society for Neuroscience, retrieved from www.sfn.org.

sedentary lifestyle, on the other hand, has been associated with 28 percent of deaths from the leading chronic diseases, including cancer, heart disease, osteoporosis, diabetes, high blood pressure, and obesity.[5–11] Results from just a few research studies are shown in Figure 7.2.

Cognitive Benefits of Exercise Although there is no compelling evidence that short-term exercise training significantly improves cognitive functioning,[12] some research has suggested positive effects. For example, evidence suggests that fit individuals process information more quickly than do less fit individuals of the same age. Other research has shown that aerobic fitness may prevent or slow down the loss of cognitive functions associated with advancing age.[13] However, generalizations about the influence of exercise on cognitive performance must be viewed with caution. Improvements as a result of physical activity may have more to do with overall feelings of well-being than with specific cognitive functions (see the box "Exercising Your Brain").

Psychological and Emotional Benefits of Exercise Moderate-to-intense levels of physical activity have been shown to influence mood, decrease the risk of depression and anxiety, relieve stress, and improve overall quality of life.[14] Although biological explanations have been proposed for the improved sense of well-being associated

- Each 2-hour increment in TV watching was associated with a 23% increase in obesity and a 14% increase in Type-2 diabetes.

- Inactivity over 6 months resulted in significant gains in abdominal fat.

- Active people were nearly 20% less likely to be diagnosed with depression.

- At least 1 hour of walking per week predicted lower risk of coronary heart disease in women aged 45 years or older.

- Highly active people had a 27% lower risk of stroke than low-active people.

- Midlife physical activity was associated with a decreased risk of dementia and Alzheimer's disease later in life, even in genetically susceptible individuals.

figure **7.2**   **Health risks and physical inactivity.**
Source: Studies are cited in "While You Wait," by B. Liebman, December 2005, Nutrition Action Newsletter.

with physical activity, better explanations are improved self-esteem, improved quality of sleep, more opportunities for social interaction, and more effective physiological responses to stress.

The magnitude of a person's "cardiovascular reactivity" to stress—increased heart rate, blood pressure, and so on—can be mitigated by exercise. If you are physically fit, your body is conditioned to react more calmly to stressful situa-

If you are physically fit, your body is conditioned to react more calmly *to stressful situations.*

tions. Exercise can also help you deal with stressful situations by providing a temporary distraction, increasing your feelings of control or commitment, and providing a sense of success in doing something that is important to you.[15]

Spiritual Benefits of Exercise   When you exercise, you are taking charge of your life and taking care of yourself. Exercising and being physically active give you the opportunity to connect with yourself, with other people, and with nature in deep and immediate ways. As you jog through a park, cycle on a bike path, hike in a natural area, or cross-country ski on a wilderness trail, you may find yourself feeling refreshed and reinvigorated both by a sense of physical well-being and by the natural scene around you. Thus, exercise enhances your feelings of self-esteem and mastery as well as your connection to yourself and something beyond yourself.

GUIDELINES FOR PHYSICAL ACTIVITY AND EXERCISE

Many leading health organizations publish physical activity and exercise guidelines aimed at achieving a variety of health goals. A widely accepted set of guidelines aimed at promoting and maintaining health and preventing chronic diseases and premature mortality was issued by the Department of Health and Human Services (HHS) in 2008. Its physical activity guidelines recommend that for substantial health benefits, adults should accumulate 150 minutes (2 hours and 30 minutes) of moderate-intensity exercise, or 75 minutes (1 hour and 15 minutes) of vigorous-intensity exercise a week.[16] The American College of Sports Medicine (ACSM) released its own guidelines in 2010, which are similar to those given by the HHS. The ACSM recommends that adults do moderate-intensity exercise for at least 30 minutes on 5 or more days a week (for a minimum of 150 minutes of moderate-intensity exercise a week), or vigorous-intensity for 20–25 minutes on 3 or more days a week (for a minimum of 75 minutes of moderate-intensity exercise a week).[17]

Moderate-intensity activity is defined as activity that noticeably accelerates the heart rate; an example is a brisk walk (see Table 7.1 for more examples). Vigorous-intensity activity causes rapid breathing and a substantial increase in

Table 7.1   Examples of Light-, Moderate-, and Vigorous-Intensity Activities

Light	Moderate	Vigorous
Slow walking	Walking 3.0 mph	Walking 4.5 mph
Canoeing	Cycling leisurely	Cycling moderately
Golf with cart	Golf, no cart	Jogging 7 mph
Croquet	Table tennis	Tennis singles
Fishing–sitting	Slow swimming	Moderate swimming
Billiards	Boat sailing	Volleyball
Darts	Housework/lawnwork	Basketball
Playing cards	Calisthenics	Competitive soccer
Walking the dog	Tennis doubles	Rope skipping
Grocery shopping	Yoga	Martial arts
Laundry	Playing with children	Snowboarding

heart rate, as exemplified by jogging. The recommended activity is in addition to the light activities associated with daily living.[18]

Activity should be done in bouts of 10 minutes or more and spread throughout the week. For example, a person can meet the HHS guidelines by doing 30 minutes of moderate-intensity exercise 5 days a week, or by doing 50 minutes of moderate-intensity exercise 3 days a week. Combinations of moderate-intensity activity and vigorous-intensity activity may be used to meet the recommendation. For example, you may walk briskly on a flat surface for 30 minutes 2 days a week and jog for 20 minutes 2 days a week.

These are minimum recommendations; exercise levels beyond the minimum can confer additional health benefits, such as the prevention of unwanted weight gain.[16] In general, people with disabilities should follow the same recommendations as people without disabilities. The HHS and ACSM guidelines also include recommendations for improving muscular strength and endurance; we describe these recommendations later in the chapter. The Personal Health Portfolio Activity for this chapter will help you assess your current level of physical activity.

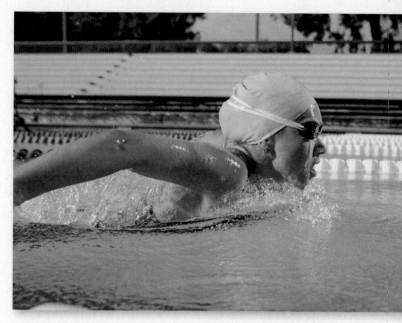

■ Swimming is an excellent way to develop cardiorespiratory fitness with a low risk of injury. Cardio training can include any form of exercise that involves continuous movement by the large muscles of the body.

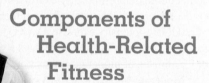

Components of Health-Related Fitness

Fitness training programs can improve each of the components of health-related fitness—cardiorespiratory fitness, musculoskeletal fitness (muscular strength, muscular endurance, and flexibility), and body composition.

The key to fitness training is the body's ability to adapt to increasing demands by becoming more fit—that is, as a general rule, the more you exercise, the fitter you become. The amount of exercise, called *overload*, is significant, however. If you exercise too little, your fitness level won't improve. If you exercise too much, you may be susceptible to injury. When you are designing an exercise program, you need to think about four different dimensions of your exercise sessions that affect overload: frequency (number of sessions per week), intensity

(level of difficulty of each exercise session), time (duration of each exercise session), and type (type of exercise in each exercise session). You can remember these dimensions with the acronym FITT.

CARDIORESPIRATORY FITNESS

Cardiorespiratory fitness is the ability of the heart and lungs to efficiently deliver oxygen and nutrients to the body's muscles and cells via the bloodstream. This should be at the center of any fitness program. It is developed by activities that use the large muscles of the body in continuous movement, such as jogging, running, cycling, swimming, cross-country skiing, and aerobic dance.

Cardiorespiratory Training Benefits of cardiorespiratory training are an increase in the oxygen-carrying capacity of the blood, improved extraction of oxygen from the bloodstream by muscle cells, an increase in the amount of blood the heart pumps with each heartbeat, and increased speed of recovery back to a resting level after exercise.

cardiorespiratory fitness
Ability of the heart and lungs to efficiently deliver oxygen and nutrients to the body's muscles and cells via the bloodstream.

Cardiorespiratory training improves muscle and liver functioning and decreases resting heart rate, resting blood pressure, and heart rate at any work level.

How do you go about developing a cardiorespiratory training program to improve your level of fitness? Start by using the FITT acronym (frequency, intensity, time, and type of activity).

Frequency In general, you must exercise at least twice a week to experience improvements in cardiorespiratory functioning. The ideal frequency for training is three times a week. Exercising five or six times a week is appropriate if weight control is a primary concern.[18]

Intensity The point at which you are stressing your cardiorespiratory system for optimal benefit but not overdoing it is called the **target heart rate (THR) zone**. The most accurate way to calculate your THR, the heart rate reserve method, is shown in the box "Calculating Your Target Heart Rate Zone Using the Heart Rate Reserve Method." The ACSM recommends that people set their THR at 55–90 percent of their MHR—that is, that they exercise at 55 percent to 90 percent of their maximum heart rate.

Another way to determine your target heart rate is using the maximum heart rate formula. The formula is 220 (MHR) minus your age times your desired intensity. For example, if you are 20 and want to work out at 60–80 percent intensity, you would subtract 20 from 220 and multiply by 0.60 and 0.80. Your target heart rate zone would be 120 to 160. The Harvard Health Studies recommend a more precise maximum heart rate formula: 208 minus (0.7 × age in years) times intensity.

target heart rate (THR) zone
Range of exercise intensity that allows you to stress your cardiorespiratory system for optimal benefit without overloading the system.

heart rate reserve (HRR)
Difference between maximum heart rate and resting heart rate.

Time Generally, exercise sessions should last from 15 to 60 minutes; 30 minutes is a good average to aim for. Duration and intensity of exercise have an inverse relation with each other, so that a shorter, higher intensity session can give your cardiorespiratory system the same workout as a longer, lower intensity session, all other things being equal.

Type of Activity There are two types of aerobic exercise: (1) exercises that require sustained intensity with little variability in heart rate response, such as running and rowing, and (2) exercises that involve "stop-and-go" activities and do not maintain continuous exercise intensity, such as basketball, soccer, and tennis. Stop-and-go activities usually have to be done for a longer period of time than do sustained-intensity activities before they confer cardiorespiratory benefits. Both types of activity can be part of a cardiorespiratory training program.

Training Progression To receive the maximum benefit from exercise, you need to adjust your level of activity by altering duration and intensity every so often. As a general rule, it takes people between the ages of 20 and 29 two weeks to adapt to a cardiorespiratory activity workload. Older people need to add 10 percent to adaptation time for each decade after age 30. A 20-year-old, for example, can expect to adjust activity workload every two weeks. A 70-year-old would adjust workload about every three weeks (40 percent longer

Highlight on Health

Calculating Your Target Heart Rate Zone Using the Heart Rate Reserve Method

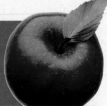

Follow these steps to calculate your target heart rate zone:

1. To determine your resting heart rate (RHR), take your pulse at the carotid (neck) or radial (wrist) artery while you are at rest. Use your middle finger or forefinger or both when taking your pulse; do not use your thumb, since it has a pulse of its own. Take your pulse for 15 seconds and multiply by 4.

2. To determine your maximum heart rate (MHR), subtract your age from 220.

3. To determine your THR objective, use the maximal **heart rate reserve (HRR)** formula, which is considered the most accurate method. Heart rate reserve is the difference between your maximum heart rate and your resting heart rate. The THR is usually 60–80 percent for young adults and 55–70 percent for older adults. Here is the HRR formula:

$$THR = X\% (MHR - RHR) + RHR$$

Example: Serena is 20 years old and just starting a cardiorespiratory training program. Her THR goal is 60–80 percent, and she has a resting heart rate of 70. For a 60 percent threshold, the THR would be calculated as follows:

$$0.6 (200 - 70) + 70$$
$$= 0.6 (130) + 70 = 78 + 70 = 148$$

For an 80 percent threshold, the THR would be calculated as follows:

$$0.8 (200 - 70) + 70$$
$$= 0.8 (130) + 70 = 104 + 70 = 174$$

Thus, Serena's THR is between 148 and 174.

is about six days). After you have obtained a satisfactory level of cardiorespiratory fitness and are no longer interested in increasing your conditioning workload, you can maintain your fitness level by continuing the same level of workout.[19]

Developing Your Own Program To develop your own regular cardiorespiratory training program, start out slowly to avoid injury and gradually build up your endurance. If you have any known medical conditions, or if you have been sedentary and are over the age of 40, see your physician for a checkup before starting. To ensure that you will stick with your program, select activities that you enjoy and that are compatible with the constraints of your schedule, budget, and lifestyle. Whether you choose running, swimming, cycling, a team sport, or another aerobic activity, try to build sessions of at least 30 minutes' duration into your schedule three times a week. If you make these sessions part of your life, they can be the foundation of a lasting fitness program.

MUSCULAR STRENGTH AND ENDURANCE

Health-related fitness also includes muscular strength and muscular endurance. Benefits of improved muscular fitness are increased lean body mass, which helps prevent obesity; increased bone mineral density, which prevents osteoporosis; improved glucose metabolism and insulin sensitivity, which prevent diabetes; and decreased anxiety and depression, which improves quality of life.[20] Muscular fitness improves posture, prevents or reduces low back pain, enables you to perform the tasks of daily living with greater ease, and helps you to look and feel better.[21, 22]

Muscular fitness has two main components: muscular strength and muscular endurance. **Muscular strength** is the capacity of a muscle to exert force against resistance. It is primarily dependent on how much muscle mass you have. Your muscular strength is measured by how much you can lift, push, or pull in a single, all-out effort. **Muscular endurance** is the capacity of a muscle to exert force repeatedly over a period of time, or to apply and sustain strength for a period lasting from a few seconds to a few minutes.

muscular strength
Capacity of a muscle to exert force against resistance.

muscular endurance
Capacity of a muscle to exert force repeatedly over a period of time.

cross training
Participation in one sport to improve performance in another, or use of several different types of training for a specific fitness goal.

Strength Training   Muscular strength and endurance are developed by strength training, also known as weight training or resistance training. This is a type of exercise in which the muscles exert force against resistance, such as free weights (dumbbells, barbells) or exercise resistance machines.

Intensity and Duration: A Strength-Endurance Continuum
The same exercises develop both strength and endurance, but their intensity and duration vary. To develop strength, you need to exercise at a higher intensity (greater resistance or more weight) for a shorter duration; to develop endurance, you need to exercise at a lower intensity for a longer duration. Duration is measured in terms of repetitions—the number of times you perform the exercise (for example, lift a barbell). If you lift a heavy weight a few times (for example, 1 to 5 repetitions), you are developing strength. If you lift a lighter weight more times (for example, 20 repetitions), you are developing endurance.

Frequency and Type of Activity   Two to three resistance training sessions a week are sufficient for building muscle

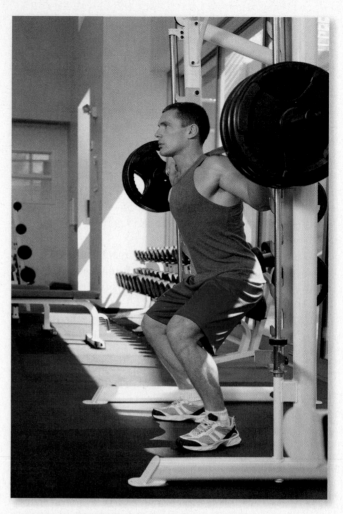

■ Muscular strength and endurance, important components of a fitness program, are developed by weight training, using either weight machines (shown here), free weights, or the weight of the body (as in calisthenics).

strength and endurance. The primary muscle groups targeted in resistance training are the deltoids (shoulders), pectorals (chest), triceps (back of upper arms), biceps (front of upper arms), quadriceps (front of thighs), hamstrings (back of thighs), gluteus maximus (buttocks), and abdomen. Other areas to exercise are the upper back, the lower back, and the calves. Whether you choose free weights or weight machines, try to exercise every muscle group during your strength training sessions.

When you participate in one activity or sport to improve your performance in another, or when you use several different types of training for a specific fitness goal, you are **cross training**. For example, you might lift weights, run, and cycle on different days of the week. Two key advantages of cross training are that you avoid the boredom of participating in the same exercise every day and you reduce the risk of overuse injuries.

Breathing and Safety   Oxygen flow is vital for preventing muscle fatigue and injury during resistance training. Inhale when your muscles are relaxed and exhale when you initiate the lifting or push-off action. Never hold your breath while performing resistance exercises.

Gender Differences in Muscle Development The amount of muscle that can be developed in the body differs by gender. Muscle mass growth is influenced by the male sex hormone testosterone, and although women do produce this hormone, they do so at levels that are only about 10 percent of the levels seen in men. Women can increase muscle mass

back injury, and sculpt the body without bulking it up. Scientific evidence in support of these claims is sparse. Exercise experts, however, argue that training programs increase muscle mass, and metabolic expenditure provides health benefits.[24]

Probably the most popular core-body training program being taught in health clubs today is Pilates (pi-**lah**-teez), an exercise system developed in the 1920s by physical trainer Joseph Pilates. The exercises, performed on special appara-

A shorter, higher intensity exercise session can give your cardiorespiratory system **the same workout** *as a longer, lower intensity session, all other things being equal.*

through strength training programs, but the increase will be less than that achieved by men.[21]

There is also a wide range of individual variability in both men and women. Regardless of gender, some people can make significantly more improvements than others can.[22] Body type (*somatotype*) plays a role in some of these differences. People with a *mesomorphic* body type (stocky, muscular) gain muscle more easily than those with an *ectomorphic* body type (tall, thin) or *endomorphic* body type (short, fat). Both men and women with mesomorphic bodies have higher levels of testosterone, and thus a greater ability to build muscle, than do those with the other two body types.

muscular power
Amount of work performed by muscles in a given period of time.

core-strength training
Strength training that conditions the body torso from the neck to the lower back.

Training for Muscular Power In addition to strength training, there are many other ways of developing the physical capabilities of the body. The amount of work that can be performed in a given period of time is known as **muscular power**. Power is determined by the amount and quality of muscle; it requires great strength and the ability to produce that strength quickly. You can train for muscular power by performing any exercise faster.

One type of exercise program developed specifically for muscular power is *plyometrics*, a program that trains muscles to reach maximum force in the shortest possible time. A muscle that is stretched before contracting will contract more forcefully and rapidly. You can experience this effect by crouching and immediately jumping. You can jump higher if you initiate the movement from a crouched position.[23]

Core-Strength Training Another type of training is **core-strength training**, also called *functional strength training*, which conditions the body torso from the neck to the lower back. The objectives of core-strength training are to lengthen the spine, develop balance, reduce the waistline, prevent

tus and a floor mat, are based on the premise that the body's "powerhouse" is in the torso, particularly the abdomen. Exercises are taught by trained instructors and are tailored to the individual.

Gaining Weight and Muscle Mass Safely When people want to gain weight it is usually to improve appearance, health, or performance. Gaining weight simply by eating more is not a productive strategy, because the weight gain will be nearly all fat. The goal is to increase muscle tissue with little or no increase in body fat stores. The healthy way to attain such a gain is through physical activity, particularly strength training, combined with a high-calorie diet. Some people, especially athletes, attempt to gain muscle tissue by using drugs, dietary supplements, or protein supplements. Most of these substances are expensive and ineffective; some are dangerous, and some are illegal.

Drugs and Dietary Supplements People who use performance-enhancing drugs and dietary supplements may enhance their athletic performance by building bigger muscles, but they also may be heading for health problems that can shorten their lives. Unfortunately, any discussion of the risks and benefits of these substances is clouded by a lack of scientific data. Scientists often don't know who is using them, what the effects of different doses are, how long

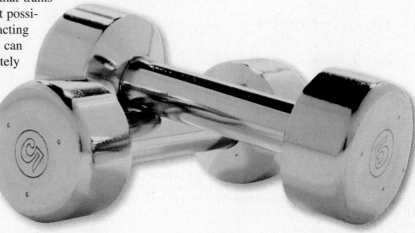

they can be taken before causing side effects, or what happens when they are taken with other drugs.[25] An overview of some of the major performance-enhancing drugs and dietary supplements, along with their possible benefits and side effects, is shown in Table 7.2.

Protein Supplements The sports and fitness industry is experiencing a boom in protein supplements.[26] The protein in these products is from natural protein sources, such as soy, eggs, milk, or chicken. Other substances, such as purified amino acids, are often added. Commercial protein supplements are expensive and do not carry all the nutrients of natural fuels. They can serve as a convenient adjunct to a balanced diet for people who are too busy to obtain enough protein in their diet, but most Americans, including athletes, get more than enough protein from their diets.

Training Programs for Weight Gain The best way to gain muscle tissue, as noted earlier, is through a weight training program combined with a high-calorie diet. Gaining a pound of muscle and fat requires consuming about 3,000 extra calories.[27] To build muscle, you need to consume 700–1,000 calories a day above energy needs or take in sufficient calories to support both the added activity energy requirements and the formation of new muscle.[26] A gain of a half pound to a pound a week is a reasonable goal. Your primary exercise activity to gain muscle should be weight training.

Developing a Strength Training Program The 2009 ACSM recommendations for strength training vary by level of experience. Novices (people who have never done resistance training or who have not done resistance training for several years) and intermediates (people who have done six months or more of resistance training) should perform 8 to 12 repetitions per set using sufficient resistance to fatigue the muscles. Novices are advised to do two to three full-body workouts a week consisting of 8 to 10 exercises that work all major muscle groups. Intermediates and more advanced people often do a split routine, where they exercise different muscle groups on different days. Intermediates can do four workouts per week on a split routine.

People who have been doing strength training for several years can also do as many as 12 repetitions per set using sufficient resistance to fatigue the muscles, or as few as 1 repetition using the maximum amount of weight they can lift. They can train four to six times a week doing a split routine. Sets and rest periods for all levels of experience will vary based on goals (strength, power, endurance), but

Table 7.2 Selected Performance-Enhancing Drugs and Dietary Supplements and Their Effects

Substance or Dietary Supplement	Effects	Side Effects
Anabolic steroid, testosterone	Promotes muscle growth by improving ability of muscle to respond to training and to recover.	Masculinization of females; feminization of males; acne; mood swings; sexual dysfunction.
Human growth hormone	Promotes muscle growth.	Widened jawline and nose, protruding eyebrows, buck teeth; increased risk of high blood pressure, congestive heart failure.
Ephedrine	Boosts energy, promotes weight loss (stimulates metabolism).	High blood pressure; irregular heartbeat; increased risk of stroke and heart attack.
Androstenedione (Andro)	Promotes muscle growth.	Decreased good cholesterol (HDL); increased levels of estrogen, promotes breast enlargement in men; increased risk of pancreatic cancer; may significantly increase testosterone levels in women (little known about Andro effects in women).
Dehydroepiandrosterone (DHEA)	May promote muscle growth.	Body hair growth; liver enlargement; aggressive behavior; long-term health effects not known.
Creatine monohydrate	May increase performance in brief high-intensity exercises; promotes increased body mass when used with resistance training.	Diarrhea; dehydration and muscle cramping; muscle tearing; long-term health effects not known.
Chromium picolinate	May build muscle tissue, facilitate burning of fat, and boost energy.	Chromium buildup with large doses and possible liver damage and other health problems; long-term health effects not known.

Sources: "The Physiological and Health Effects of Oral Creatine Supplementation," American College of Sports Medicine, 2000, Medicine and Science in Sports and Exercise, 32, pp. 706–717; "Dietary Supplements and the Promotion of Muscle With Resistance Exercise," by R.B. Kreider, 1999, Sports Medicine, 27, pp. 97–110; "How Effective Is Creatine?" by C. Nelson, 1998, Sport Medicine Digest, 73, pp. 73–81; The Ergogenic Edge: Pushing the Limits of Sports Performance, by M.H. Williams, 1998, Champaign, IL: Human Kinetics.

in general, 2 to 4 sets should be done with 1 to 2 minutes of rest between sets.[21]

Strength training can be a safe and effective form of exercise if appropriate guidelines are followed:

- Warm up by gently stretching, jogging, or lifting light weights.

- Do not hold your breath or hyperventilate. As you are lifting, breathe rhythmically.

- To protect your back, hold weights close to your body. Do not arch your back. Weight belts may prevent arching.

- When using resistance training machines, always check to make sure the pins holding weights are in place. When using free weights, make sure collars are tight.

- Lift weights with a slow, steady cadence through a full range of motion. Do not jerk the weight to complete a repetition.

- Always use a spotter when working out with free weights.

- Allow at least 48 hours between training sessions if you will be exercising the same muscle groups.

FLEXIBILITY

Another important component of musculoskeletal fitness is **flexibility**, the ability of joints to move through their full range of motion. Good flexibility helps you maintain posture and balance, makes movement easier and more fluid, and lowers your risk of injury. It is a key factor in preventing low back pain and injury.

flexibility
Ability of joints to move through their full range of motion.

Flexibility is affected by factors that you cannot change, such as genetic endowment, gender, and age, and by factors that you can change, such as physical activity patterns. A common misconception is that flexibility declines steadily once a person reaches adulthood. Flexibility does seem to be highest in the teenage years, and aging is accompanied by a shortening of tendons and an increased rigidity in muscles and joints. However,

there is also strong evidence that much of the loss of flexibility that results from aging can be reduced by stretching programs.[28]

Types of Stretching Programs Medical and fitness experts agree that stretching the muscles attached to the joints is the single most important part of an exercise program designed to promote flexibility, reduce muscle tension, and prevent injuries. However, stretching done incorrectly can cause more harm than good. Thus, understanding the right stretching techniques and progressing gradually are keys to a successful program.

In *passive stretching*, a partner applies pressure to your muscles, typically producing a stretch beyond what you can do on your own. If you can totally relax your muscle fibers, the use of pressure by another person can help prevent the problem of partial contraction of muscle fibers. Passive stretching is often used by physical therapists. There is a danger, however, of forcing a stretch beyond the point of normal relaxation of the muscles and tendons, causing tearing and injury. For this reason, passive stretching should be limited to supervised medical situations and persons who cannot move by themselves.[2]

In *static stretching*, you stretch until you feel tightness in the muscle and then hold that position for a set period of time without bouncing or forcing movement. After you have held the stretch for 30 to 60 seconds, the muscle tension will seem to decrease, and you can stretch farther without pain. Static stretching lengthens the muscle and surrounding tissue, reducing the risk of injury. Static stretching is the kind of stretching done in hatha yoga and is the type recommended for general fitness purposes.

In *ballistic stretching*, the muscle is stretched in a series of bouncing movements designed to increase the range of motion. As you bounce, receptors in the muscles, called *muscle spindles*, are stretched. Ballistic stretching is used by experienced athletes, but because it can increase vulnerability to muscle pulls and tears, it is not recommended for most people.

Proprioceptive neuromuscular facilitation (PNF) is a therapeutic exercise that causes a stretch reflex in muscles. It is used primarily in the rehabilitation of injured muscles.[29]

- Developing flexibility through stretching exercises should be part of a regular fitness program. Stretching is most beneficial and effective when the muscles are warm, as they are after a workout.

Developing Your Own Flexibility Program The ACSM recommends that stretching exercise be done for all the major joints, including the neck, shoulders, upper back and trunk, hips, knees, and ankles. Stretching should be done a minimum of 2 to 3 days a week and ideally 5 to 7 days a week. Stretch to a point of mild discomfort (not pain) and hold the stretch for 15 to 30 seconds. Do two to four repetitions of each stretch.

Stretching can be part of your warm-up for your cardio-respiratory or resistance training program as long as these stretches are gentle, slow, and steady. To prevent injury, warm up first with 5 to 10 minutes of brisk walking, marching in place, or calisthenics. This warm-up will increase your heart rate, raise your core body temperature, and lubricate your joints. You will experience the greatest improvement in flexibility, however, if you do your stretching exercises after your other exercise, when your muscles are warm and less likely to be injured by stretching.

BODY COMPOSITION

The final component of health-related fitness we consider here is **body composition**—the relative amounts of fat and fat-free mass in the body. Fat-free mass includes muscle, bone, water, body organs, and other body tissues. Body fat includes both fat that is essential for normal functioning, such as fat in the nerves, heart, and liver, and fat stored in fat cells, usually located under the skin and around organs. The recommended proportion of body fat to fat-free mass, expressed as *percent body fat*, is 21–35 percent for women and 8–24 percent for men.

---

body composition
Relative amounts of fat and fat-free mass in the body.

The relative amount of body fat has an effect on overall health and fitness. Too much body fat is associated with overweight and obesity and with a higher risk for chronic diseases like heart disease, diabetes, and many types of cancer. A greater amount of fat-free mass, on the other hand, gives the body a lean, healthy appearance. The heart and lungs function more efficiently without the burden of extra weight. Because muscle tissue uses energy at a higher metabolic rate than does fat tissue, the more muscle mass you have, the more calories you can consume without gaining weight.

We discuss body composition in more detail in Chapter 8, on body weight. Here, the basic message is that you can control body weight, trim body fat, and build muscle tissue by incorporating more physical activity into your daily life. Use the stairs rather than taking the elevator, walk or ride your bike rather than driving, and if you drive, park your car at the far end of the parking lot.

Beyond such simple steps to increase physical activity, plan to incorporate regular exercise into your life as well. According to the *2008 Physical Activity Guidelines for Americans* from the Department of Health and Human Services, maintaining weight stability requires 150 to 300 minutes of moderate- to vigorous-intensity exercise. Strength training activities are helpful in maintaining weight stability but are not as effective as aerobic exercise. Losing a substantial amount of weight or maintaining substantial weight loss requires a high amount of physical activity unless calories are reduced. People who want to lose weight or prevent weight regain may need to do more than 300 minutes a week of moderate- to vigorous-intensity exercise.[16] If you work toward these goals, you will see improvements not only in your body composition but also in many other areas of your life.

For a summary of physical activity recommendations for adults, see Table 7.3.

Table 7.3   Summary of Physical Activity Recommendations for Adults

Aerobic (Endurance) Activity	150 minutes of moderate-intensity aerobic activity per week. OR 75 minutes of vigorous-intensity aerobic activity per week. OR A combination of moderate- and vigorous-intensity physical activity that meets the recommendation.
Muscle-Strengthening Activity	8 to 10 exercises that stress the major muscle groups on 2 or more nonconsecutive days per week. Do one or more sets of 8 to 12 repetitions for each exercise using sufficient resistance to fatigue the muscles.
Flexibility	Stretching exercise for all major joints, at least 2 to 3 days per week. Stretch to the point of tension, hold for 15 to 60 seconds, and repeat 4 or more times.
Weight Management	To prevent unhealthy weight gain, 150 to 300 minutes of moderate- to vigorous-intensity physical activity per week. For substantial weight loss or to sustain weight loss, 300 minutes or more of moderate- to vigorous-intensity exercise a week.

Sources: Adapted from 2008 Physical Activity Guidelines for Americans, Department of Health and Human Services, 2009, retrieved March 28, 2010, from www.health.gov/paguidelines; "Position Stand: Progression Models in Resistance Training for Healthy Adults," American College of Sports Medicine, 2009, Medicine & Science in Sports & Exercise, 41 (3), pp. 687–708; ACSM's Guidelines for Exercise Testing and Prescription, American College of Sports Medicine, 2010, Baltimore: Lippincott Williams & Wilkins.

Improving Your Health Through Moderate Physical Activity

As noted earlier, exercise does not have to be vigorous to provide health benefits. There are many simple, easy, and enjoyable ways to use physical activity to obtain health benefits.

MAKING DAILY ACTIVITIES MORE ACTIVE

How much time do you spend in sedentary activities in your day? How can you make these minutes more active? Try getting up to change the TV channel instead of using the remote, or walk around, stretch, or do sit-ups during commercials. Ride your bike to class instead of taking the bus, take the stairs instead of the elevator at the library, or walk around while checking your cell phone messages. These kinds of unstructured physical activities can actually make a difference. In one study, researchers found that obese people sat for an average of two hours longer a day than people who were not obese, and that if the obese were to mirror the unstructured physical activities of those who were not obese, they would burn an extra 350 calories a day.[30]

You can also turn light activity into moderate activity by cranking up the intensity. For example, when you are standing in line, stretch or do isometric exercises (such as contracting and relaxing your abdominal muscles). Increase your pace while cycling, walk briskly instead of strolling, take the stairs two at a time.

Why is it important to move from light to moderate activities? Consider that an order of french fries contains about 400 calories. If you are sitting and watching television, it will take you 308 minutes, or more than 5 hours, to use up that many calories. If you are walking briskly or jogging slowly, it will take you about an hour.

WALKING FOR FITNESS

Walking is the most popular physical activity in North America,[31] and it has many health benefits. Women who do moderate or vigorous physical activity for at least 4 hours a week reduce their risk of premature death. As with other activity, increasing the pace and/or duration of walking results in greater health benefits. For tips on walking, see the box "Walking for Fitness."

Experts at the Shape Up America! program found that people could control their weight if they walked 10,000 steps each day.[32] Walking 10,000 steps (about 5 miles) expends between 300 and 400 calories, depending on body size and walking speed—well above the recommended 150 calories a day. Walking 10,000 steps a day 5 days a week expends the optimal 2,000 calories per week recommended for preventing premature death.

You can count your steps with a pedometer, a pager-sized device worn on the belt or waistband centered over the hipbone. Pedometers that convert activities into calories expended are not accurate, because they do not factor in activity intensity.

If you are interested in counting your steps, first determine how many steps you typically take each day. Record the number of steps you take every day for 7 days. Most inactive people take between 2,000 and 4,000 steps a day. Then, to set a reasonable goal, plan to increase this number by about 500 steps at a time. If you typically take 5,000 steps a day, set a goal of 5,500 steps. Once you achieve 5,500 steps, raise your goal by 500 steps, and continue until you reach 10,000 steps.[33] This is an easy and painless way to add physical activity to your day and to move from light to moderate activity levels.

TAKING THE STAIRS

Climbing stairs is an excellent activity for improving leg strength, balance, and fitness. Stair climbing is twice as taxing to your heart and lungs as brisk walking on a level surface. A Harvard Health Alumni study found that men who climb an average of eight flights of stairs a day experience 33 percent lower mortality than men who are sedentary. Always make sure the stairs are safe before taking them, though.[34]

If you have access to stair-climbing machines at your fitness center, they also provide a good workout. Dual-action climbers exercise your legs, arms, and heart. This equipment

■ Counting steps with a pedometer is one way to move toward fitness. Walking 10,000 steps a day confers health benefits and helps people control their weight.

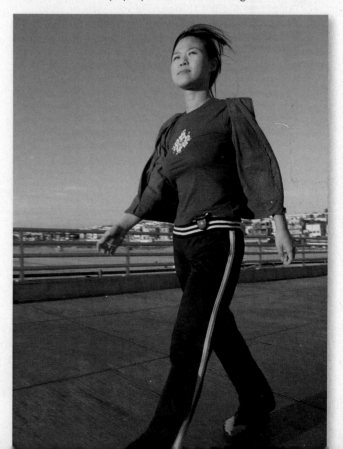

Challenges & Choices

Walking for Fitness

If you have been completely sedentary, begin a walking program with 10 minutes of walking a day. Gradually work up to 30 minutes a day, most days of the week. If you want to lose weight by walking, you will need to walk from 45 to 60 minutes a day, most days of the week. To improve your cardiovascular functioning, walk briskly (at a pace of 4–4.5 mph). In urban areas, a general rule of thumb is to count 12 average city blocks as 1 mile. If you are counting your steps, 80 steps a minute is considered a leisurely pace, 100 steps a minute is considered a brisk pace, and 120 steps a minute is considered a fast pace. The following are some guidelines for getting the most out of walking:

- Schedule your daily walk as you would an appointment. Plan it for a time of day when you're most likely to make it a permanent habit.

- Increase your walking time gradually. Don't increase duration by more than 10–20 percent a week.

- After you have walked for a couple of weeks, focus on quicker steps. As you do so, bend your arms 90 degrees at the elbow and move them when you walk. Moving your arms increases your caloric expenditure.

- Stretch at the end of your walk or after warming up. Adding 4 minutes of stretching to your daily walk can have a beneficial effect on your muscles, joints, and bones.

- Don't ignore or exercise through pain. If the pain is severe, see a physician. Pain that is not serious should be treated by rest, ice, compression, and elevation; massage may also help. Discontinue walking up or down hills if doing so causes pain.

provides a moderate- to high-intensity workout with low impact on your joints. If you don't have access to exercise machines, just take the stairs.

EXERCISE GAMING

A recent trend in the video game industry is the development of games that include physical activity. Dance Dance Revolution, introduced in 2001, spurred the development of more fitness-oriented video games.

The Nintendo Wii lets players make the moves involved in various recreational activities and sports. Some fitness clubs have incorporated Wii workout stations into circuit training programs. Users punch, run, and jump with the station's movement-sensation controller. During one 30-minute workout, the user can expend 75 to 125 calories.

Many health experts welcome this new generation of video games as a positive step by the "sedentary entertainment industry." One study found that the exercise gaming is comparable to moderate-intensity walking.[35] The games do have their downside, though. They can be expensive, they may limit social interaction, and they may send a message that being fit requires technology. Fitness video games should not be considered a substitute for active outdoor play and physical activity. They can best be viewed as part of an overall strategy to encourage children, teens, and adults to become more active.

Special Considerations in Exercise and Physical Activity

Special considerations have to be taken into account to ensure health and safety in exercise and physical activity, to accommodate the effects of certain environmental conditions, and to make exercise appropriate for particular populations.

HEALTH AND SAFETY PRECAUTIONS

Injuries and illness associated with exercise and physical activity are usually the result of either excessive exercise or improper techniques. In this section we look at several considerations related to health and safety.

Warm-Up and Cool-Down Proper warm-up before exercise helps to maximize the benefits of a workout and minimize the potential for injuries. Muscles contract more efficiently and more safely when they have been properly warmed up.

Suggested warm-up activities include light calisthenics, walking or slow jogging, and gentle stretching of the specific muscles to be used in the activity. You can also do a low-intensity version of the activity you are about to engage in, such as hitting tennis balls against a wall before a match. Your warm-up should last from 5 to 10 minutes.

A minimum of 5 to 10 minutes should also be devoted to cool-down, depending on

hot tip
Do take the stairs whenever possible, but never endanger your safety: If a stairwell is dark, if it is late at night, or if you are in a sketchy neighborhood, take a safer route to your destination.

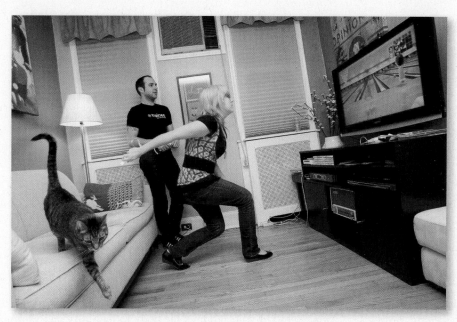

■ Exercise gaming is the latest in consumer-oriented approaches to fitness.

environmental conditions and the intensity of the exercise program. Pooling of blood in the extremities may temporarily disrupt or reduce the return of blood to the heart, momentarily depriving your heart and brain of oxygen. Fainting or even a coronary abnormality may result. If you continue the activity at a lower intensity, the blood vessels gradually return to their normal smaller diameter.

Walking, mimicking the exercise at a slower pace, and stretching while walking are all excellent cool-down activities. Never sit down, stand in a stationary position, or take a hot shower or sauna immediately after vigorous exercise.

Fatigue and Overexertion Fatigue is generally defined as an inability to continue exercising at a desired level of intensity. The cause of fatigue may be psychological—for example, depression can cause feelings of fatigue—or physiological, as when you work out too long or too hard, do an activity you're not used to, or become overheated or dehydrated. Sometimes fatigue occurs because the body cannot produce enough energy to meet the demands of the activity. In this case, consuming enough complex carbohydrates to replenish the muscle stores of glycogen may solve the problem. Athletes need to eat a high-carbohydrate diet to make sure they have enough reserve energy for their sport.[36]

Overexertion occurs when an exercise session has been too intense. Warning signs of overexertion include (1) pain or pressure in the left or midchest area, jaw, neck, left shoulder, or left arm during or just after exercise; (2) sudden nausea, dizziness, cold sweat, fainting, or pallor (pale, ashen skin); and (3) abnormal heartbeats, such as fluttering, rapid heartbeats or a rapid pulse rate immediately followed by a very slow pulse rate. These symptoms are similar to signs of a heart attack. If you experience any of these symptoms,

consult a physician before exercising again.

Soft Tissue Injury Injuries to soft tissue (muscles and joints) include tears, sprains, strains, and contusions; they usually result from a specific activity incident, such as a bicycle crash. Some injuries, known as overuse injuries, are caused by the cumulative effects of motions repeated many times. Tendinitis and bursitis are examples of overuse injuries. (For tips on preventing running-related injuries, see the box "Running Shoe Prescription.")

Soft tissue injuries should be treated according to the R-I-C-E principle: rest, ice, compression, and elevation. Immediately stop doing the activity, apply ice to the affected area to reduce swelling and pain, compress it with an elastic bandage to reduce swelling, and elevate it to reduce blood flow to the area. Do not apply heat until all swelling has disappeared. When you no longer feel pain in the area, you can gradually begin to exercise again. Don't return to your full exercise program until your injury is completely healed.

EFFECTS OF ENVIRONMENTAL CONDITIONS ON EXERCISE AND PHYSICAL ACTIVITY

Certain environmental conditions require adjustment of physical activity and exercise workload. Environmental conditions of particular concern are heat and cold, and air pollution.

Heat and Cold Heat disorders can be caused by impaired regulation of internal core temperature, loss of body fluids, and loss of electrolytes (Table 7.4).[26] Two strategies

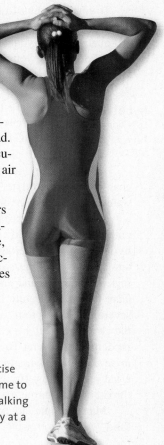

■ Cooling down after vigorous exercise gives the cardiovascular system time to return to normal. Cool down by walking or continuing your exercise activity at a much lower intensity.

Table 7.4 Heat-Related Disorders

Heat Disorder	Cause	Symptoms	Treatment
Heat cramps	Excessive loss of electrolytes in sweat; inadequate salt intake.	Muscle cramps.	Rest in cool environment; drink fluids; ingest salty food and drinks; get medical treatment if severe.
Heat exhaustion	Excessive loss of electrolytes in sweat; inadequate salt and/or fluid intake.	Fatigue; nausea; dizziness; cool, pale skin; sweating; elevated temperature.	Rest in cool environment; drink cool fluids; cool body with water; get medical treatment if severe.
Heat stroke	Excessive body temperature.	Headache; vomiting; hot, flushed skin (dry or sweaty); elevated temperature; disorientation; unconsciousness.	Cool body with ice or cold water; give cool drinks with sugar if conscious; get medical help immediately.

Source: Adapted from Nutrition for Health, Fitness and Sport, *7th ed., by M.H. Williams, 2007, New York: McGraw-Hill.*

for preventing excessive increases in body temperature are skin wetting and hyperhydration. Skin wetting involves sponging or spraying the head or body with cold water. This strategy cools the skin but has not been shown to effectively decrease core body temperature.[26]

Hyperhydration is taking in extra fluids shortly before participating in physical activity in a hot environment.[37] This practice is recommended by the ACSM and may improve cardiovascular function and temperature regulation during physical activity in conditions of excessive heat.[38]

If you are going to be exercising in very hot conditions, you can hyperhydrate by drinking a pint of water (16 ounces) when you get up in the morning, another pint 1 hour before your activity, and a final pint 15 to 30 minutes before exercising. Plan to consume from 4 to 8 ounces of fluid every 15 minutes during your exercise. After exercise, consume 24 ounces of water for every pint you lose.[26,37] The goal is to prevent excessive changes in electrolyte balance and body water loss of 2 percent or more.

hypothermia
Low body temperature, a life-threatening condition.

Exercising in excessive cold also puts a strain on the body. Symptoms of **hypothermia** (dangerously low body temperature) include shivering, feelings of euphoria, and disorientation.[39] Core body temperature influences how severe these symptoms are and whether the hypothermia is considered mild, moderate, or severe. To stay warm, dress in several thin layers of clothes and wear a hat and mittens. If cold air bothers your throat, breathe through a scarf.

Many people do not take in sufficient fluid when exercising outside during the winter. Fluid losses during the winter can be very high, since cold, dry air requires the body to humidify and warm the air, resulting in the loss of significant amounts of water. An effective strategy is to consume needed fluids 1.5 to 2 hours before exercising and to drink more fluids just before exercising.

Air Pollution If you live and exercise in a large city, air pollution can be a concern. Pollution can have an irritating effect on the airways leading to your lungs,[40] causing coughing, wheezing, and shortness of breath. To minimize the effect of air pollution, exercise early in the morning before motor vehicle pollution has its greatest impact. If possible, exercise in areas with less motor vehicle traffic, such as parks. Pay attention to smog alerts, and move your exercise indoors when air pollution is severe.

EXERCISE FOR SPECIAL POPULATIONS

In this section we look briefly at special exercise considerations for children and adolescents, people with disabilities, and older adults.

Exercise for Children and Adolescents

To obtain the direct and indirect health benefits of fitness, children should get 60 minutes or more of exercise a day. Children have smaller hearts and lungs and less blood volumes than adults, so they should not be expected to perform physically like adults.[41] Children are also more vulnerable to overheating than adults, so they need to be properly hydrated.

A serious concern is the incidence of sudden death in adolescents engaged in strenuous physical activities

Consumer Clipboard

Running Shoe Prescription

More than 30 million runners develop injuries each year; 20–30 percent of these injuries require medical care. Proper shoe selection and maintenance can reduce running-related injuries by as much as 56 percent.

Shoe Selection

- Buy shoes from a running specialty store or reputable Internet vendor to guarantee a high-quality shoe. Running magazines typically provide a list of specialty stores.

- Feet swell by the end of the day, so have your shoes fitted in the evening. Make sure there is one-half inch between your longest toe and the end of the shoe toe. Wear running socks when trying on the shoes and insert orthotics if you use these devices.

- Ask the store to allow you to run in the shoes for a short distance before buying. Select your shoes by fit, not by the size on the shoe box. Most runners use running shoes that are two sizes larger than their street shoes. Women's shoes are usually narrower than men's shoes, and the heel is slightly smaller, but about 25 percent of women runners have feet that conform more comfortably to the shape of men's shoes.

- The arch of your foot should be considered when you select exercise shoes. People with a high arch are typically under-pronators, and those with a flat or very low arch are over-pronators. Pronation is the flattening of the foot arch when stepping, which causes the foot to roll inward. Pronation is normal and necessary for loosening foot structures and enabling the foot to

adjust to surface conditions. However, excessive pronation and under-pronation can both lead to injuries. To determine your foot arch shape, place your foot in water and then step on a brown piece of paper or bag (so that your foot will leave a visible wet mark). For a high arch, the heel and ball of the foot appear like two islands with very little or no connection between them. A flat foot or very low arch is indicated by a rectangular foot shape. A shape in between these two indicates a normal arch. Athletic shoes are usually classified in three categories: stability (for normal or low arches), neutral (for high arches), and motion control (for flat arches). Buy the type appropriate for your foot.

Shoe Care

- Use your shoes only for running to preserve the motion control and cushioning of your shoes.

- Untie your shoes before taking them off. Kicking off tied shoes can damage the heel counter.

- Do not run in wet shoes; a wet midsole has 40–50 percent less shock-absorbing capability. Let wet shoes dry naturally. Excessive heat will degrade shoe components.

- Never wash your shoes in the washing machine; it destroys the shoe shape.

- Running shoes lose 30–50 percent of their shock-absorbing capability after about 250 miles of use. Unused shoes sitting on the shelf will lose a significant amount of shock-absorbing capability after 1 to 2 years.

Sources: "What Every Runner Should Know About Shoes," 2005, Physician and Sports Medicine, 33 *(1), pp. 23–24;* Running: Getting Started, *by J. Galloway, 2005, United Kingdom: Meyer & Meyer Sport.*

and competitive sports programs. About 12 young athletes die each year from heart disease while participating in vigorous sports.[42] Most of these deaths are thought to be caused by congenital heart defects, such as an abnormally enlarged heart, that go undetected until an incident occurs. (See Chapter 2 for more on sudden death in young athletes.)

New guidelines issued by the American Heart Association (AHA) urge parents, coaches, and physicians to be vigilant for symptoms that may indicate a heart defect.[42] These symptoms include fainting episodes, sudden chest pain during exercise or at rest, high blood pressure, and irregular or high heart rate at rest or during exercise. The AHA also recommends that a family history of heart disease or unexplained death be considered in evaluating whether children should be involved in vigorous physical activity.[42]

Exercise for Persons With Disabilities Physical activity and exercise are especially beneficial for persons with disabilities and chronic health problems. Immobility or inactivity may aggravate the original disability and increase the risk for secondary health problems, such as heart disease, osteoporosis, arthritis, and diabetes. The ACSM stresses the importance of physical activity for people with disabilities for two reasons: (1) to counteract the detrimental effects of bed rest and sedentary living patterns and (2) to maintain optimal functioning of body organs or systems.[43]

Not too long ago, regular physical activity was missing in the lives of many people with disabilities.[44] The reasons for this absence included lack of knowledge about the importance of physical activity, limited access to recreation sites and difficulty with transportation, a low level of interest, and the lack of exercise facilities and resources designed to accommodate people with disabilities.

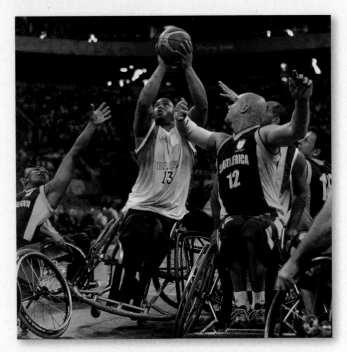

Having a disability does not mean a person can't exercise or be fit. Exercise counters the effects of immobility and inactivity, improves all body functions, and enhances self-esteem for individuals with disabilities as well as for people in the general population.

Laws have strengthened the rights of persons with disabilities and fostered their inclusion in programs and facilities providing physical activity opportunities. Increased visibility and positive images of people with disabilities engaging in physical activity, such as in the Special Olympics and wheelchair basketball, have also helped raise awareness.

recommendations for adults, the recommendations for older adults include exercises that maintain or improve balance, performed 2 days per week, for older adults at risk for falls.[16]

Physical Activity for Life

The most significant drop in physical activity occurs in the last few years of high school and the first year of college.[4] The decline accelerates again after college graduation. Certain key factors help people make physical activity a lifetime pursuit. In this section we consider two of them—commitment to change and social and community support.

MAKING A COMMITMENT TO CHANGE

Let's consider exercise in terms of the Transtheoretical Model (refer to Chapter 1 for an explanation of this stages of change model). In the precontemplation and contemplation stages, the biggest challenges for most people are barriers to exercise.[44] Common barriers to active lifestyles cited by adults are inconvenience, lack of self-motivation, lack of time, fear of injury, the perception that exercise is boring, lack of social support, and lack of confidence in one's ability to be physically active.[45] If you are in the precontemplation or contemplation stage and feel overwhelmed by these or other barriers, see the box "Strategies for Overcoming Barriers to Physical Activity."

In the preparation stage, self-assessment is critical. Ask yourself these four questions: (1) What physical activities do I enjoy? (2) What are the best days and times for me to participate in physical activities? (3) Where is the best place to pursue these activities? and (4) Do I have friends and/or family members who can join in my physical activities? In

The most significant **drop in physical activity** *occurs in the last few years of high school and the first year of college. The decline accelerates again after college graduation.*

Exercise for Older Adults The aerobic activity recommendations for older adults are the same as for adults, but the recommended intensity of aerobic activity takes into account the wide variation in aerobic fitness among older adults. Intensity of activity is gauged on a 10-point scale of perceived exertion, with sitting at 0 and all-out effort at 10. Moderate-intensity activity, which produces noticeable increases in heart rate and breathing is a 5 or 6 on this scale. Vigorous-intensity activity, which produces large increases in heart rate and breathing, is a 7 or 8.[16]

Exercises to develop muscular strength and endurance are also recommended. They should be performed on 2 or more nonconsecutive days of the week, focusing on 8 to 10 exercises for the major muscle groups and using a weight that allows 10 to 15 repetitions for each exercise. Unlike the

making specific preparations, you need to take into account your current level of fitness and your previous experiences in various physical activities. This information about yourself will help you develop an exercise program that you can commit to and maintain.

In the action stage, a key component is goal setting. Your goals should be based on the benefits of physical activity, but they should also be specific and reasonable. Achievable and sustainable goals are essential for exercise compliance. Include both short-term and long-term goals in your plan, and devise ways to measure your progress. Build in rewards along the way.

When you have been physically active almost every day for at least 6 months, you are in the maintenance stage. One key to maintaining an active lifestyle is believing that

Strategies for Overcoming Barriers to Physical Activity

Lack of time

- Identify available time slots. Monitor your daily activities for 1 week. Identify at least three 30-minute time slots you could use for physical activity.
- Add physical activity to your daily routine: Walk or ride your bike to work or shopping, organize school activities around physical activity, walk the dog, or park farther away from your destination.
- Make time for physical activity. Walk, jog, or swim during your lunch hour; take fitness breaks instead of coffee breaks.
- Select activities requiring minimal time, such as walking, jogging, or stair climbing.

Social influence

- Explain your interest in physical activity to friends and family. Ask them to support your efforts.
- Invite friends and family members to exercise with you. Plan social activities involving exercise.
- Develop new friendships with physically active people. Join a group, such as the YMCA.

Lack of energy

- Schedule physical activity for times in the day or week when you feel energetic.
- Convince yourself that physical activity will increase your energy level; then try it.

Lack of willpower

- Plan ahead. Make physical activity a regular part of your schedule and write it on your calendar.
- Invite a friend to exercise with you on a regular basis, and write the dates on both your calendars.
- Join an exercise group or class.

Fear of injury

- Learn how to warm up and cool down safely.
- Learn how to exercise appropriately considering your age, fitness level, skill level, and health status.
- Choose activities involving minimum risk.

Lack of skill

- Select activities requiring no new skills, such as walking, climbing stairs, or jogging.
- Exercise with friends who are at the same skill level as you.
- Find a friend who is willing to teach you new skills.
- Take a class to develop new skills.

Lack of resources

- Select activities that require minimal equipment, such as walking, jogging, or calisthenics.
- Identify inexpensive, convenient resources available in your community, such as park and recreation programs.

Weather conditions

- Develop a set of regular activities that are always available regardless of weather (indoor cycling, aerobic dance, indoor swimming, calisthenics, stair climbing, rope skipping, dancing).
- Think of outdoor activities that depend on weather conditions (cross-country skiing, outdoor swimming, outdoor tennis) as "bonuses"—extra activities possible when weather and circumstances permit.

Family obligations

- Trade babysitting time with a friend, neighbor, or family member who also has small children.
- Exercise with your children. Go for a walk together, play tag or other running games, get an aerobic dance or exercise tape for kids.
- Hire a babysitter and look at the cost as an investment in your physical and mental health.
- Jump rope, do calisthenics, ride a stationary bicycle, or use other home gymnasium equipment while the kids are playing or sleeping.
- Try to exercise when the kids are not around (during school hours or their nap time).
- Encourage exercise facilities to provide child care.

Source: "Physical Activity for Everyone: Making Physical Activity Part of Your Life," Centers for Disease Control and Prevention, 2005, retrieved from www.cdc.gov.

your commitment to physical activity can make a difference in your life. People who establish a personal stake in physical activity are more likely to maintain an active lifestyle. When exercise has become entrenched as a lifelong behavior—when it's as much a part of your day as eating and sleeping—you are in the termination stage.

Which stage are you in right now? If you are in an early stage, you probably do not have sufficient commitment to follow through on an exercise plan. To make any

change, you must want to change. Work on overcoming barriers and gaining more information about the health benefits of physical activity and the problems associated with a sedentary lifestyle. Knowledge is one of the best predictors of a commitment to healthy living. Being a mentor to friends and family members can also help you become or stay motivated to make exercise a lifelong habit. Remember, the more active you are, the more health benefits you will receive.

USING SOCIAL AND COMMUNITY SUPPORT

A network of friends, coworkers, and family members who understand the benefits of exercise and join you in your activities can make the difference between a sedentary and an active lifestyle. Family and friends are not enough, however; activity-friendly communities are also instrumental in promoting physical activity. Many communities have paths, trails, sidewalks, and safe streets that encourage people to become physically active.[46] There are community programs that encourage parents to walk their children to school, that promote "mall walking" (walking at shopping malls), and that sponsor biking and walking days (see the box "Creating Activity-Friendly Communities"). The health of an individual in any given neighborhood is a function of the interaction between personal competencies and environmental barriers and supports. For example, access ramps and adapted transportation are supports that can be used to overcome barriers that discourage physical activity for people with disabilities or make it difficult.[47]

What can you do to encourage community planning that promotes physical activity? You can advocate for new growth designed around public transportation hubs and for bicycle lanes incorporated into streets. As a citizen and taxpayer, you can vote on local growth measures and become active in local chapters of organizations such as New Urbanism and Smart Growth America.[48] Taking political action can work. In 2002, for example, New Jersey voters and antisprawl lobbyists were rewarded with an executive order against sprawl from their governor, which preserved open areas and focused expansion and redevelopment on existing urban and suburban areas.[49,50]

When making personal choices about where to live and work, look at a map of the immediate area and think about how communities you're considering are planned. How close are recreational areas? What types of places are within a 10-minute walking radius of home and work? Will living in this community help to make you more active and physically fit? Taking such questions into consideration will give you

Public Health in Action

Creating Activity-Friendly Communities

Physical activity levels are influenced by diverse factors that go beyond individual motivation, knowledge, and behavior. The Centers for Disease Control and Prevention (CDC) established the Task Force on Community Preventive Services to investigate how lifestyles are affected when changes are made in the physical environment, social networks, organizational norms and policies, and laws through environmental and policy initiatives. Among the task force's findings, compiled in the 2005 *Guide to Community Preventive Services*, were that community-wide campaigns to increase physical activity are effective and that creating or improving access to places for physical activity increases the percentage of people who exercise.

A related CDC program, the Active Community Environments Initiative (ACES), promotes walking, bicycling, and the development of accessible recreational and park facilities. The program draws on the expertise of several disciplines, especially public health, urban design, and transportation. The underlying idea is that activity-friendly environments play a vital role in promoting physical activity. Some ACES activities include

- Development of the Kids-Walk-to-School program.
- Promotion of National and International Walk-to-School Day.
- Partnership with the National Park Service's Rivers, Trails, and Conservation Assistance Program to facilitate the development of close-to-home parks and recreational facilities.

- Collaboration with an Atlanta-based study to assess the relationship among land use, transportation, air quality, and physical activity.
- Collaboration with the Environmental Protection Agency on a national study that surveyed attitudes of the American public toward the environment, walking, and bicycling.

In partnership with ACES, some communities have increased the safety of walking and biking by developing or improving bike lanes, and others have promoted walking by designing sidewalks and streets to ensure continuity and connectivity. Studies have found that these efforts may increase physical activity by well over 100 percent.

ACES also promotes social support in community settings. Examples include setting up buddy systems and sponsoring walking groups. Studies have found that social support in community settings can increase the time spent being physically active by 44 percent and the frequency of physical activity by 20 percent. Enhanced access to places for physical activity combined with informational outreach activities (seminars, forums, workshops, counseling, referrals to physicians for risk assessment) can be especially effective in getting people to exercise more. Studies examining this strategy found a median increase of about 48 percent in the number of people exercising three times or more a week.

connect
ACTIVITY

Sources: The Guide to Community Preventive Services, *by S. Zaza, P.A. Briss, and K.W. Harris, 2005, New York: Oxford University Press;* "Physical Activity Resources for Health Professionals: Active Environments: ACES-Active Community Environments Initiative," *Centers for Disease Control and Prevention, retrieved from www.cdc.gov/nccdphp/dnpa/physical/health/_professionals/active_environments/aces.*

■ When communities provide spaces for physical activity and improve access to those spaces, people respond by becoming more active. Thus, public policy and community planning play important roles in the physical fitness of community members.

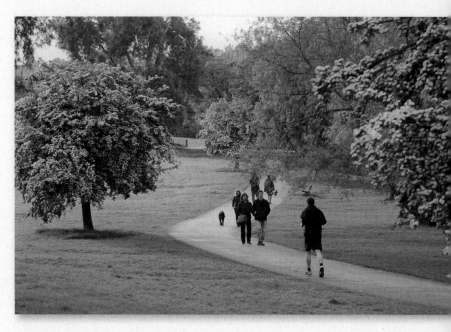

more opportunities to make physical activity and exercise a natural part of your life.

The key message of this chapter is that physical activity is a natural, enjoyable, sometimes thrilling, frequently challenging part of human life. It is a part of life that children instinctively embrace but that adults may have lost touch with living in a fast-paced, sedentary culture. We encourage you to get up, get moving, and get back in touch with the lifelong pleasures of physical activity.

You Make the Call

Should Insurers and Employers Reward Healthy Behaviors and Punish Bad Ones?

There is no doubt that healthy lifestyles make for more vital individuals and more productive workers and citizens. When people increase their physical activity, they also bring economic benefits to themselves and society. The annual cost of inactivity is estimated at $24 to $76 billion and is a contributing factor in rapidly rising health care costs. Even if you are in good physical condition, some of the money you (or your parents) pay in insurance premiums goes toward treating other people's obesity- and inactivity-related health conditions.

The benefits of physical activity are clear, but getting people to live healthier lives has been difficult. Many health insurance companies have attempted to address this problem by offering incentives to people willing to adopt healthy behaviors such as not smoking. Corporations and other institutions have undertaken similar actions by offering incentives for workers who are physically active, maintain a healthy body weight, lower their blood pressure, have healthy cholesterol levels, wear their seat belts consistently, and so on. For example,

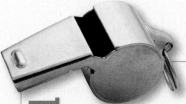

employees at the University of Louisville receive a $20 credit on their monthly insurance premiums if they adopt good eating and physical activity habits. The university reports that for every $1 it has spent on the program, it has saved $5.

Some employers have gone even further, using disincentives to encourage their employees to make healthy behavior changes. For example, employees of Whirlpool who smoke are required to pay an extra $500 a year in insurance costs. Some employers have threatened smokers with termination of employment, and others will not hire a person who smokes. In 2005, Weyco Inc., a health consulting firm, gave its employees 15 months to quit smoking and then fired all the employees who had not quit after the time had passed. At the end of the 15 months, 14 of the company's estimated 18 to 20 employees who were smokers had quit. One Cincinnati-based company fines employees an extra $15 to $75 a month in health care premiums if their body mass index is above what is considered healthy.

However, there has been a backlash against policies that either incentivize people for their good health and habits or penalize them for bad health and habits. About half of all states have passed laws prohibiting employers from firing or refusing to hire people who smoke during nonworking hours. These laws are intended to keep employers from discriminating against people who engage in a legal activity (smoking) on their own time. Some employees are reluctant to share personal data, such as their exercise, eating, and smoking habits, with their employer. Others point out that physical inactivity is only one of many factors that contribute to obesity and other health problems. Genetics play a factor, as do one's socioeconomic status and community resources. People should not be blamed for health conditions that are not entirely their fault, opponents argue.

The use of incentive programs, and especially disincentives, by employers and insurance companies to induce behavior change has been controversial. Should people who choose to take health risks be penalized for their actions? Do such practices unfairly discriminate against those with less control over their lives, such as the poor and disenfranchised? What do you think?

PROS

■ National health care costs are skyrocketing, and sedentary lifestyles are a primary cause. Encouraging people to adopt healthy behaviors will decrease health care costs.

■ The power to be more physically active is under the control of the individual.

■ Empirical evidence supports the relationship between physical inactivity and preventable diseases.

■ Insurance companies already use incentives and disincentives in their life insurance and automobile insurance plans.

CONS

■ An overemphasis on individual health is part of a victim-blaming mentality that does not take into account the impact of genetics, culture, and racial inequalities on health.

■ Use of incentives and disincentives is an invasion of privacy and a violation of personal rights.

■ Certain racial and ethnic groups, low-income people, and people with disabilities living in urban areas do not have adequate access to fitness or park and recreation facilities.

Sources: "Cost-Effectiveness of Community-Based Physical Activity Interventions," by L. Roux, M. Pratt, T.O. Teng, et al., 2008, American Journal of Preventive Medicine, 35 (6), pp. 578–588; "Michigan Health Care Company Has Strict Anti-Tobacco Policy," the Associated Press, 2005, retrieved from http://www.msnbc.msn.com/id/6870458/; "Companies Penalizing Workers with High Health Risks," the Associated Press, 2007, retrieved from http://www.usatoday.com/money/industries/health/2007-09-09-risk-penalties_N.htm.

IN REVIEW

What is fitness?
Physical fitness is generally defined as the ability of the body to respond to the demands placed upon it. Skill-related fitness is the ability to perform specific skills associated with recreational activities and sports; health-related fitness is the ability to perform daily living activities with vigor. Physical activity is activity that requires any kind of movement; exercise is structured, planned physical activity.

What are the components of health-related fitness?
The most important component is cardiorespiratory fitness; other components are musculoskeletal fitness (muscular strength, muscular endurance, and flexibility) and body composition.

What are the benefits of physical activity and exercise?
Physical activity and exercise confer benefits in every domain of wellness, ranging from improved cognitive functioning to relief from depression to better cardiovascular health. Inactivity is a leading preventable cause of premature death from such causes as cardiovascular disease and cancer. Of all the positive health-related behavior choices you can make, exercising may be the easiest, most effective, and most important.

How much should you exercise?
A widely accepted set of guidelines aimed at promoting and maintaining health and preventing chronic disease, issued jointly by the American College of Sports Medicine and the American Heart Association, calls for a minimum of 30 minutes of moderate-intensity aerobic activity 5 days a week or 20 minutes of vigorous-intensity activity 3 days a week. Activity should also be included for muscle strengthening, flexibility, and weight management.

What special exercise-related considerations and precautions are important for health and safety?
It's important to warm up and cool down before and after exercise, to avoid fatigue and overexertion, to take proper care of injuries, and to take environmental conditions into account. Everyone can benefit from exercise, as long as they follow any relevant special guidelines, such as those for older adults and people with disabilities.

Web Resources

Adult Fitness Test: The President's Council on Physical Fitness and Sports developed this adult fitness test. The test consists of three components for aerobic fitness, muscular strength, and flexibility. You can enter your test results online to see where you rank among people of the same age based on percentile.
www.adultfitnesstest.org

Aerobics and Fitness Association of America: In addition to training and certification of fitness professionals, this organization offers information on exercise, health and safety, lifestyle, and nutrition.
www.afaa.com

American College of Sports Medicine: ACSM presents various health and fitness topics, with expert commentary and tips for maintaining a lifestyle of physical fitness, through its e-newsletter and brochures.
www.acsm.org

American Council on Exercise: This site offers health and fitness information, including core stability training, healthy recipes, fitness fact sheets, and what to look for in a health club.
www.acefitness.org

Map My Run: Avid walkers, hikers, runners, and bicyclers may find this a useful site for mapping routes. Satellite images help map routes anywhere in the world. Users can save their routes, search for routes by other users, and develop a personal training log.
www.mapmyrun.com

National Center for Chronic Disease Prevention and Health Promotion: Look here for CDC recommendations on physical activity, information on measuring physical activity intensity, and strength training for older adults.
www.cdc.gov/nccdphp/dnpa

National Center on Physical Activity and Disability: This site features information on lifetime sports, competitive sports, and exercise and fitness for individuals with disabilities.
www.ncpad.org

Shape Up America! Fitness Center: This site features a variety of ways to improve your fitness and lose weight, offering assessment tools, tips on motivation, and ways to design an improvement program that matches your individual needs and goals.
www.shapeup.org/fitness.html

8

Body Weight and Body Composition

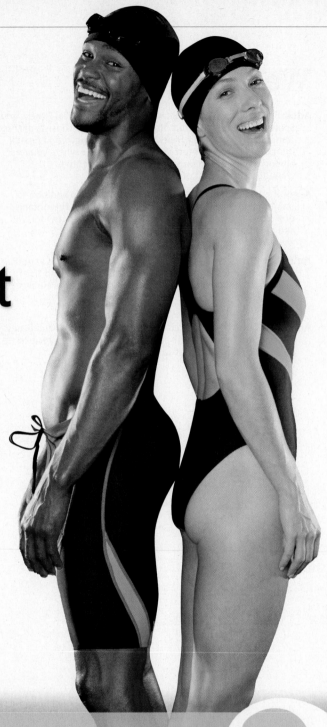

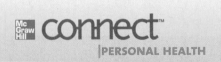 connect™

|PERSONAL HEALTH

Ever Wonder...

- what diets work?

- if being overweight can run in families?

- what normal portion sizes look like?

Overweight and obesity are increasingly worrisome problems in the United States and around the world.

Among American adults, 68 percent meet the criteria for overweight and 34 percent meet the criteria for obesity.[1] **Overweight** is defined as body weight that exceeds the recommended guidelines for good health; **obesity** is body weight that greatly exceeds the recommended guidelines.

overweight
Body weight that exceeds the recommended guidelines for good health.

obesity
Body weight that greatly exceeds the recommended guidelines for good health, as indicated by a body mass index of 30 or more.

In 1991 four states reported a prevalence rate of obesity greater than 15 percent, and no states reported prevalence greater than 20 percent. Seventeen years later, in 2008, only Colorado reported a prevalence rate less than 20 percent (see the box "Obesity Trends Among Adults in the United States").[2] If these trends continue, all Americans could be overweight within a few generations. Worldwide, an estimated 300 million people are obese; rates vary tremendously by country, ranging from less than 5 percent in parts of China, Japan, and certain African countries to more than 75 percent in urban Samoa.[3]

No sex, age, state, racial group, or educational level is spared from the problem of overweight, although the problem is worse for the young and the poor. Rates of obesity for children have steadily increased, and today an estimated 12 percent of children 2 to 5 years of age and 17 percent of children 6 to 19 years of age are obese. Among low-income children ages 2 to 4, an estimated 14.6 percent are obese.[4,5]

The trend is particularly worrisome because an elementary school child who is overweight has an 80 percent likelihood of being overweight at age 12; a person who is obese at age 18 faces odds 28 to 1 against maintaining a healthy adult weight.[5]

What Is a Healthy Body Weight?

How much should you weigh? The answer to this question depends on who is asking and why. If you are a 16-year-old varsity wrestler getting ready for your competition weigh-in, your coach and the wrestling weight classes may influence your weight goals. If you are an 18-year-old girl comparing yourself with the fashion models you see daily in magazines, your goals may be determined by a media-generated cosmetic ideal. If you are a 50-year-old woman wondering whether you should be concerned about the 25 pounds you gained last year, you may be more interested in health goals for weight and fitness.

Who's at Risk?

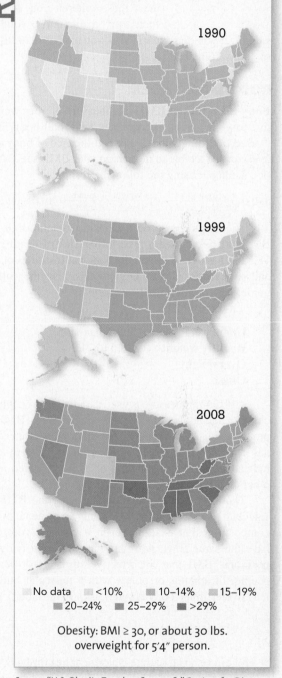

Obesity Trends Among Adults in the United States

Rates of obesity have soared since 1990 and especially since 2000. Multiple factors—some known, some still to be identified—account for this trend.

1990

1999

2008

No data   <10%   10–14%   15–19%   20–24%   25–29%   >29%

Obesity: BMI ≥ 30, or about 30 lbs. overweight for 5′4″ person.

Source: "U.S. Obesity Trends 1985–2008," Centers for Disease Control and Prevention, Behavioral Risk Factor Surveillance System, 2009, retrieved from www.cdc.gov/obesity/data/trends.html.

There is no ideal body weight for each person, but there are ranges for a healthy body weight. A healthy body weight is defined as (1) an acceptable body mass index (explained in the following sections); (2) a fat distribution that is not a risk factor for illness; and (3) the absence of any medical conditions (such as diabetes or hypertension) that would suggest a need for weight loss. If you currently meet these criteria, you will want to focus on maintaining your current weight. If you don't meet them, you may need to lose weight or gain weight.

body mass index (BMI)
Measure of body weight in relation to height.

BODY MASS INDEX

Body mass index (BMI) is a measure of your weight relative to your height; it correlates with total body fat. BMI is used to estimate the health significance of body weight. You can use a table to determine your BMI (see Table 8.1) or calculate it using the following formula:

$$BMI = \frac{\text{weight in kg}}{(\text{height in meters})^2} OR \frac{\text{weight in pounds}}{(\text{height in inches})^2} \times 703 \text{ (conversion factor)}$$

There appears to be a U-shaped relationship between BMI and risk of death. The lowest risk of death is in the 18.5 to 25 range. As such, the National Institutes of Health and the World Health Organization use the following guidelines for adult BMI categories:[2,3]

	BMI
Underweight	Less than 18.5
Healthy weight	18.5 to 24.9
Overweight	25 to 29.9
Obese	≥30

A different measure is used to define overweight in children and adolescents. For these age groups, BMI is plotted using growth charts (for either boys or girls), and a percentile ranking is determined (percentile indicates the relative position of BMI compared to other children of the same sex and age).

There are some limitations to using the BMI to calculate risk of disease. BMI is only an estimate of body composition. For example, even if you and your friend have the same BMI, you may have different body compositions. BMI may incorrectly estimate risk for some people. In athletes or others with a muscular build, BMI may overestimate body fat (and risk). In the elderly or others who have lost muscle mass, BMI may underestimate body fat (and risk).

BODY FAT PERCENTAGE

Body composition is measured in terms of percentage of body fat. There are no clear, accepted guidelines for healthy body fat ranges, although ranges of 11–20 percent have been used for men and 17–30 percent for women. Some body fat is essential to healthy function; the lower healthy range may be 5–10 percent for male athletes and 15–20 percent for female athletes. Below a certain body fat threshold, hormones cannot be produced and problems can occur, such as infertility, lack of menstruation, depression, lack of sex drive, hair loss, and loss of appetite.

At each level of BMI, there are differences in body fat percentage for certain groups. Women on average have 10–12 percent more body fat than men. African American men average slightly lower body fat percentage than White men, and Asian men average slightly higher body fat percentage than White men. As people get older, body fat percentage increases at each level of BMI.[6,7]

Because body fat percentage is considered an important component in judging the need for weight reduction, it may be measured as part of a physical examination. Several methods exist to measure body fat percentage. The most accurate methods are expensive and require special equipment. They include weighing a person underwater (immersion), or using a special type of X-ray. Two simpler but slightly less reliable methods are measuring thickness of skin and fat in several locations of the body (skinfold measurement or caliper testing) and sending a weak electrical current through parts of the body and measuring the electrical resistance of tissue to calculate body fat (bioelectroimpedence).

BODY FAT DISTRIBUTION

Not only the amount but also where you carry your body fat is important in determining your health risk. Fat carried around and above the waist is abdominal fat and is considered more "active" than fat carried on the hips and thighs. Abdominal fat (also called *central obesity*) is a disadvantage because it breaks down more easily and enters the bloodstream more readily.

A large abdominal circumference or waist circumference is associated with high cholesterol levels and higher risk for

■ BMI can be an inaccurate indicator of healthy body weight and fat percentage in athletes with a high proportion of muscle tissue. For example, basketball player LeBron James, at 6 feet, 8 inches and 250 pounds, has a BMI of 27 and would be classified as overweight.

Table 8.1 Body Mass Index (BMI)

Find your height in the left-hand column and look across the row until you find the number that is closest to your weight. The number at the top of that column identifies your BMI. The darkest shaded area represents healthy weight ranges.

BMI	18	19	20	21	22	23	24	25	26	27	28	29	30	31	32	33	34
Height																	
4'10"	86	91	96	100	105	110	115	119	124	129	134	138	143	148	153	158	162
4'11"	89	94	99	104	109	114	119	124	128	133	138	143	148	153	158	163	168
5'0"	92	97	102	107	112	118	123	128	133	138	143	148	153	158	163	168	174
5'1"	95	100	106	111	116	122	127	132	137	143	148	153	158	164	169	174	180
5'2"	98	104	109	115	120	126	131	136	142	147	153	158	164	169	175	180	186
5'3"	102	107	113	118	124	130	135	141	146	152	158	163	169	175	180	186	191
5'4"	105	110	116	122	128	134	140	145	151	157	163	169	174	180	186	192	197
5'5"	108	114	120	126	132	138	144	150	156	162	168	174	180	186	192	198	204
5'6"	112	118	124	130	136	142	148	155	161	167	173	179	186	192	198	204	210
5'7"	115	121	127	134	140	146	153	159	166	172	178	185	191	198	204	211	217
5'8"	118	125	131	138	144	151	158	164	171	177	184	190	197	203	210	216	223
5'9"	122	128	135	142	149	155	162	169	176	182	189	196	203	209	216	223	230
5'10"	126	132	139	146	153	160	167	174	181	188	195	202	209	216	222	229	236
5'11"	129	136	143	150	157	165	172	179	186	193	200	208	215	222	229	236	243
6'0"	132	140	147	154	162	169	177	184	191	199	206	213	221	228	235	242	250
6'1"	136	144	151	159	166	174	182	189	197	204	212	219	227	235	242	250	257
6'2"	141	148	155	163	171	179	186	194	202	210	218	225	233	241	249	256	264
6'3"	144	152	160	168	176	184	192	200	208	216	224	232	240	248	256	264	272
6'4"	148	156	164	172	180	189	197	205	213	221	230	239	246	254	263	271	279
6'5"	151	160	168	176	185	193	202	210	218	227	235	244	252	261	269	277	286
6'6"	155	164	172	181	190	198	207	216	224	233	241	250	259	267	276	284	293

Underweight (≤18.5)   Healthy Weight (18.5–24.9)   Overweight (25–29.9)   Obese (≥30)

Source: Adapted from "Body Mass Index Table," National Heart, Lung, and Blood Institute, retrieved from www.nhlbi .nih.gov/guidelines/obesity/bmi_tbl.htm.

heart disease, stroke, diabetes, hypertension, and some types of cancer. If your BMI is in the healthy range, a large waist circumference may signify an independent risk for disease. If your BMI is in the overweight or obese range, measuring your waist circumference can be an additional tool to determine your health risk. If your BMI is above 35, your health risk is already high.

To measure your waist circumference, use a tape measure. Measure your waist right above your hip bones, at the point where it crosses your navel. Keep the tape level. It should be snug, but not tight. A high waist circumference is[8]

Greater than 40 inches (102 cm) for men

Greater than 35 inches (88 cm) for women

Obese men tend to accumulate abdominal fat, whereas obese women tend to accumulate fat on the hips and

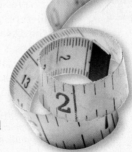

thighs. However, women have a change in body fat distribution at the onset of menopause with fat shifting to the abdomen. This shift coincides with an increased risk of heart disease for women.

HEALTH ISSUES RELATED TO OVERWEIGHT AND OBESITY

If you are overweight or obese, you are at increased risk for serious health problems. Obese people are four times more likely than people with a healthy weight to die before reaching their expected lifespan. They have an increased risk for high blood pressure, diabetes, elevated cholesterol levels, coronary heart disease, stroke, gallbladder disease, osteoarthritis (a type of arthritis caused by excessive wear and tear on the joints), sleep apnea (interrupted breathing during sleep), lung problems, and certain cancers, such as uterine, prostate, and colorectal (see the box "Diabetes and Obesity"). Women who are obese before pregnancy are at increased risk of having a baby with a birth defect.[9] Obesity is also a component of *metabolic syndrome*, a condition associated with a significantly increased risk for cardiovascular disease and the development of Type-2 diabetes (see Chapter 15). There has been some controversy over the number of annual deaths attributable to overweight and obesity; estimates range from 112,000 to 365,000.[10]

THE PROBLEM OF UNDERWEIGHT

The prevalence of obesity often obscures the problem of underweight. A sudden, unintentional weight loss without a change in diet or exercise level may signify an underlying illness and should prompt a visit to a physician. Depression, substance abuse, eating disorders, thyroid disease, infections, and cancer can all be associated with unexpected weight loss.

However, you may just have difficulty keeping on weight. In this situation, calorie intake is inadequate for energy output. To gain weight, you need to change the energy balance. Calories can be increased by eating more frequent meals (every three hours or so) and increasing servings of healthy, more energy-dense foods, such as nuts, fish, or yogurt. Adding protein powders or nutritional supplements to the diet as snacks is another option. Your pattern of physical activity can also be changed, so that aerobic exercise is reduced and weight training is increased.

What Factors Influence Your Weight?

There is no simple answer to why Americans are getting fatter. Many factors contribute to this trend, both individual and environmental. You may look to

Highlight on Health

Diabetes and Obesity

The rise in obesity in the United States has been paralleled by a rise in rates of diabetes. As overweight increasingly becomes an issue among children and adolescents, so does a disease that previously was rare in this age group.

Diabetes is a disease in which the levels of glucose circulating in the bloodstream are too high. Normally the pancreas produces the hormone insulin in response to rising glucose levels. Insulin binds to receptors in body cells, allowing glucose to enter the cells to be used for energy and keeping blood levels of glucose fairly stable. Without insulin, levels of glucose in the bloodstream rise, setting the stage for such health complications as heart disease, kidney failure, blindness, sexual dysfunction, and others.

There are two forms of diabetes. In Type-1 diabetes, little or no insulin is produced by the pancreas and has to be provided by injection or a pumping device. Type-1 diabetes is not related to obesity, and levels of this form of the disease appear to be remaining fairly stable. Type-1 diabetes is sometimes referred to as juvenile-onset diabetes, because the average age at onset is 14. In Type-2 diabetes, body cells become resistant to the effects of insulin. The pancreas produces insulin at normal or even higher than normal levels, but the body's cells do not respond, causing blood glucose levels to rise. Type-2 diabetes is sometimes called adult-onset diabetes because, previously, the average age at diagnosis was 40.

Type-2 diabetes is by far the more common form of the disease; 90–95 percent of people with diabetes have Type-2. Numerous factors contribute to its prevalence: There is a genetic component, and the disease runs in families, but there is also a lifestyle component. Obesity, high caloric intake, and low levels of exercise are important factors. In fact, the onset of Type-2 diabetes can be delayed and early Type-2 diabetes can be treated by intensive lifestyle change, including nutritional education, a low-fat, lower calorie diet with a goal of 5–7 percent weight loss, and 150 minutes of exercise per week.

The onset of Type-2 diabetes is usually gradual. Symptoms include excessive thirst, frequent urination, and fatigue. In rare cases, the first symptoms are nausea, vomiting, and confusion. If you are overweight and have a family history of diabetes, you should have your blood glucose level checked by your physician on a regular basis. Early diagnosis and lifestyle changes can prevent or delay the onset of the disease.

Source: "Diabetes Successes and Opportunities for Population-Based Prevention and Control," National Center for Chronic Disease Prevention and Health Promotion, 2009, retrieved April 1, 2010, from www.cdc.gov/nccdphp/publications/aag/pdf/diabetes.pdf.

other family members, for example, and think that it is your genes that make you overweight. Unless you are adopted, however, the people who gave you your genes also taught you how to eat, chose your neighborhood, and influenced your educational status and perhaps your occupation.

GENETIC AND HORMONAL INFLUENCES

If neither of your parents is obese, you have a 10 percent chance of becoming obese. The risk increases to 80 percent if both of your parents are obese. Adopted children also tend to be similar in weight to their biological parents, and twin studies support a genetic tendency toward obesity. These findings have led to the search for genes associated with obesity. It appears that for most people, obesity is a multifactorial disease; that is, it results from a complex interaction among multiple genes and the environment. Each gene can increase a person's susceptibility to obesity, and, together, multiple genes can further increase risk.

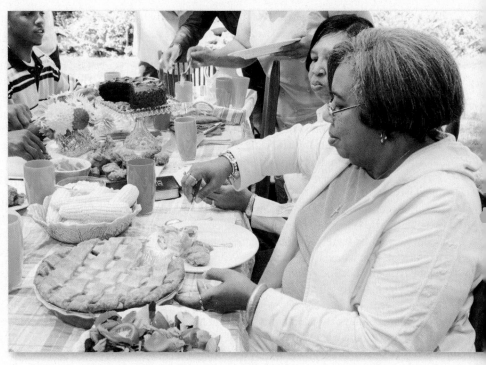

■ Genes and hormones play a role in overweight and obesity—as do family, social, cultural, and other environmental factors. These can include favorite family and ethnic foods, mealtime rules and traditions, and the kinds of restaurants and grocery stores available in the community.

Nearly two dozen hormones identified thus far play a role in appetite and energy expenditure. They act in the brain to influence when to start or finish eating; to monitor external cues for food, such as smells, sights, and texture; to monitor internal cues, such as body fat stores, glucose level, free fatty acids, and stomach fullness; and to adjust metabolic rate. It is a complex interaction that is not yet fully understood. If you are maintaining your current weight, the interaction of hormones controls your daily calorie intake to within 10 calories (a single potato chip) of balanced food intake and energy expenditure.[11]

Some medical conditions can be associated with weight gain. Thyroid disorders are a prime example. The thyroid

are slow to change, requiring generations and hundreds of years. Environmental influences, such as abundant food and a sedentary lifestyle, can produce such effects in a much shorter period.[12]

GENDER AND AGE

Most of us develop our eating patterns from our families during childhood. Poor childhood eating habits are believed to be a major cause of the recent surge in overweight and obesity. There are several crucial times in your life when you may change these patterns, a critical one being the first time you leave home for college or to live independently. Take

If neither of your parents is obese, you have a 10 percent chance of becoming obese. The **risk increases to 80 percent** *if both of your parents are obese.*

gland, located in the neck, produces a hormone that is involved in metabolism. If the gland becomes less active, metabolism slows and weight is gained. If the gland is overactive, metabolism speeds up and weight can be inappropriately lost.

Except in rare cases of a single gene mutation, genetics alone does not fully explain obesity. The rapid rise in obesity since the 1980s is too sudden to be due to genetics. Genes

advantage of this opportunity to evaluate the eating habits you learned at home and make changes if they are needed.

During puberty, boys and girls undergo significant hormonal changes that alter their respective body compositions. Female hormones begin preparing girls for childbearing with increases in body fat, especially on the hips, buttocks, and thighs. Before puberty, a girl of a healthy weight will have approximately 12 percent body fat. After puberty, the healthy range can increase to up to 25 percent body fat.

In contrast, a boy's hormones in late adolescence are geared more toward muscle development. Before puberty, a boy of healthy weight has approximately 12 percent body fat; after puberty, he levels out at approximately 15 percent body fat. In addition to experiencing the hormonal influences of puberty on body composition, the average adolescent girl is less physically active than are her male peers, an additional pressure toward increased body fat percentage. Physical activity levels for both boys and girls are declining in adolescence.[13]

Between the ages of 20 and 40, both men and women gain weight. Married men weigh more than do men who have never been married or were previously married but are currently unmarried. For women, these are the years in which pregnancy typically occurs. Weight gain is a normal part of pregnancy. The majority of women will lose most of this weight within a year of delivery. However, about 15–20 percent of women continue to maintain significant weight a year after delivery, partly as a result of changes in lifestyle associated with childrearing.[14]

As people enter their 50s, both women and men can have potentially serious problems with weight gain. Men tend to see an increase in abdominal fat. Women in their late 40s and early 50s undergo significant hormonal changes and shifts in body fat distribution.

At the age of 60 and beyond, weight tends to decline. This loss can be attributed to a number of causes, including decreased calorie needs, less muscle tissue, and less body mass. These changes give older adults thinner limbs. During these years, weight-bearing exercise, such as walking, becomes critical to maintain body mass and bone strength.

FOOD ENVIRONMENTS

The new term *obesogenic environment* has been coined to highlight the fact that our chances of becoming obese are significantly influenced by our environment.

Food Choices Your choice in foods is usually driven by three factors: taste, cost, and convenience. Your taste in food is largely developed by what you have been exposed to in the past, but you can influence it by trying new foods. Cost and convenience are also major factors. As a college student, you are probably on a limited budget and have limited time to prepare foods. This scenario will likely remain true after you leave college and enter the workforce. The ability to

---

Life Stories

Grace: Trying to Make Healthy Changes

Grace, a sociology major at a state college, is the first member of her family to attend college. Her parents and two younger siblings live in a small industrial town about 200 miles from campus. Her father has worked in an automotive parts plant for the past two decades, and her mother works part-time as the school secretary at the central high school. Both of Grace's parents are overweight, and her maternal grandmother has diabetes. Because both adults work, the family tends to eat a lot of prepared and processed foods, like macaroni and cheese, beef stroganoff, pizza, and hot dogs. When her mom cooks, she tends to make "comfort meals" like meatloaf and mashed potatoes, fried chicken with biscuits and gravy, and pot roast. No one in the family exercises.

When Grace got to college she was about 20 pounds overweight, weighing in at about 160 pounds. She had heard about the "freshman 15" and was worried she would gain more weight that year. Instead, she did so much walking around campus that she actually started to lose weight. She became friends with two women in her residence hall who were much more conscious about food choices than she was, and they often ate dinner together. Following their lead, Grace found herself frequenting the salad bar more often than the taco bar. One of them was a vegetarian, and Grace started enjoying some vegetarian dishes as well. She still ate fast food when she was rushed during exam weeks, but her weight stabilized at just about 20 pounds less than what she had weighed when she arrived on campus.

Grace spent the summer after freshman year at home, working a summer job. Her mom served the same high-fat, high-calorie meals she always had. At first, Grace talked up her new eating patterns, trying to interest her parents in a healthier diet, but her mom seemed to be hurt by Grace's suggestions, and her dad got mad that her mom was hurt. Grace even offered to do the grocery shopping one week, thinking she would get some good fruits and veggies, at least for herself, if not for the whole family. She was disappointed to see there was not much choice in produce at the local supermarket, and what was there looked wilted and unappetizing. When she brought home strawberries for dessert, her younger brother and sister ignored them and went for the ice cream.

Grace slipped back into her old eating patterns and spent more and more time watching TV with her family in the evenings. Grace had hoped to continue walking, but her neighborhood wasn't very safe for walking, and there wasn't a fitness center or gym in town. She was unhappy with herself—and could feel her clothes getting tighter—but she felt guilty trying to be different from her family, and there was a certain comfort in doing the same old things.

When the summer was over, Grace felt both sad and relieved to be leaving her family and going back to school. She would be living in a campus apartment with her two friends, and she knew it would not be such a struggle to eat well and exercise. She worried about her family and wished they had the same resources she did.

connect
ACTIVITY

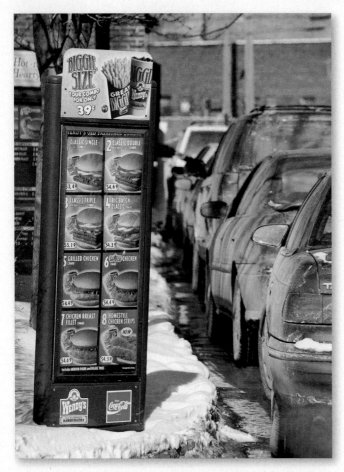

■ More and more Americans are eating out (or ordering in) on a daily basis, and many are getting their meals in the drive-through lane. This major cultural shift is one of the factors implicated in the current overweight and obesity phenomenon.

maintain a healthy diet depends on having sufficient knowledge about healthy food choices, the money to buy healthy foods, and the time to prepare a healthy meal (see the box "Grace: Trying to Make Healthy Changes").[15]

In general, unhealthy foods are more available, more convenient, more heavily advertised, and less expensive than healthy foods, especially in low-income neighborhoods. In these communities, fast-food outlets and small food markets dominate the retail food landscape, providing consumers with less healthy foods at higher prices. Obesity rates are highest among the poorest and least educated segments of the population.[16,17] In more affluent neighborhoods, where supermarkets predominate, low-fat and whole-grain foods are much more readily available, along with diverse fruit and vegetable choices. On college campuses, all-you-can-eat, buffet-style dining has been associated with increased weight gain among students.[18]

Being aware of the factors influencing your food choices can help you attain and maintain a healthy diet. A little planning ahead can go a long way toward supporting healthy food choices. If your fruits and vegetables often go bad in the fridge before you eat them, consider purchasing frozen or canned items. If you don't have healthy choices available on campus, consider packing a lunch or healthy snacks to take with you.[16,19]

EATING OUT

In the 1950s eating out was a rare event; today it has become a part of daily life. Twenty-one percent of households use some form of take-out food or food-delivery service daily.[16] The trend is likely related to the increased number of dual-career households and single-parent households and the convenience and accessibility of fast foods. The concern is that foods served in restaurants and fast-food outlets tend to be higher in fat and total calories and lower in fiber than are foods prepared at home. Increased reliance on fast foods is associated with weight gain.[19] For ideas on eating out without going overboard, see the box "Tips for Eating Out."

Challenges & Choices

Tips for Eating Out

Many people eat a healthy diet at home but have less success in restaurants, college dining halls, and food courts. Try these tips to maintain control the next time you eat out.

■ Increase the proportion of plant-based foods in your diet. Take larger servings of vegetables and fruits and smaller servings of meat, cheese, and eggs.

■ Include two vegetables in your meal or a vegetable and a salad.

■ Choose whole-wheat bread, brown rice, or whole-grain cereals. Whole-grain foods are more filling.

■ Have fresh fruit or yogurt for dessert instead of cake or ice cream.

■ Drink water instead of soda or juice.

■ Control your portion size by taking smaller servings. Don't go back for seconds.

■ Eat slowly and savor the taste of your food.

■ Stop eating when you first feel full rather than waiting until you feel stuffed.

■ Share large portions or take some home for another meal. Don't feel obligated to eat everything on your plate.

■ Don't skip meals—you'll only be inclined to eat quickly and more at the next meal.

Source: Data from "The Way We Eat Now," by C. Lambert, May–June 2004, Harvard Magazine.

Larger Portions   Serving size has increased steadily both inside and outside the home. The largest increases in serving size have occurred in fast-food restaurants and may be due to "supersized" pricing strategies.

The impact of supersizing on the caloric bottom line is dramatic. When confronted with large serving sizes in restaurants or prepackaged foods, people eat more. The larger the portion of food, the worse we become at estimating how much we are eating. (See Figure 8.1 for some visual images of portion sizes.) Paying attention to package labeling, dividing prepackaged food into smaller serving sizes, and using visual cues can help with more appropriate serving sizes.[20,21]

LIFESTYLE INFLUENCES ON WEIGHT

Before the mid-1900s, most of the population would never have considered exercise to be a necessity for health, because their daily lives involved regular physical activity.

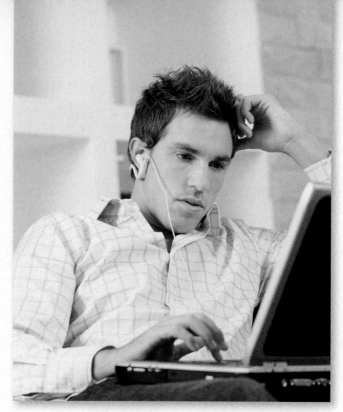

■ Most of us need to spend time in front of the computer on a daily basis, whether to study, work, or communicate with family and friends. In order to maintain a healthy body weight, we need to balance sedentary activities with physical activity.

Our current lifestyle has become so mechanized, and sedentary, however, that many of us can go through a regular day spending almost no energy on physical activity. Even the majority of college students, who often have access to recreational facilities and intramural sports, do not meet recommended physical activity levels.[16]

The automobile, television, and the computer are three technological advances that have improved our lives in many ways yet led to unhealthy habits. Surveys show that 25 percent of all trips in the United States are less than 1 mile, and yet 75 percent of these trips are taken by car.[22] Increased time spent in the car each day increases the risk of obesity.[22] Safety considerations and community structure are factors that significantly influence your method of transportation. If you live in a neighborhood or on a campus that is designed to favor walking or biking (with sidewalks, bike lanes, green space, and reliable transportation), you are more likely to incorporate regular physical activity into your life and have a lower risk of obesity than if you live in a less walkable community.[22,23]

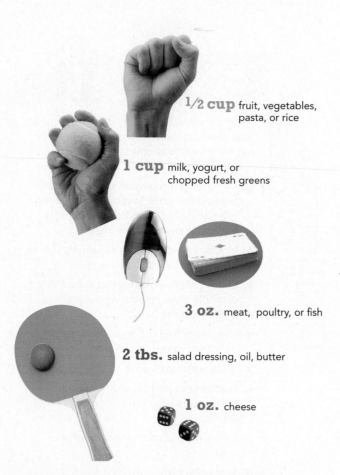

1/2 cup fruit, vegetables, pasta, or rice

1 cup milk, yogurt, or chopped fresh greens

3 oz. meat, poultry, or fish

2 tbs. salad dressing, oil, butter

1 oz. cheese

figure **8.1**   **Visual images of portion sizes.**
Half a cup of fruit, vegetables, pasta, or rice is about the size of a small fist. One cup of milk, yogurt, or chopped fresh greens is about the size of a small hand holding a tennis ball. Three ounces of meat, poultry, or fish is about the size of a computer mouse or a deck of cards. Two tablespoons of salad dressing, oil, or butter is about the size of a ping pong ball. One ounce of cheese is about the size of a pair of dice.

When **confronted with large serving sizes** *in restaurants or prepackaged foods,* **people eat more.**

Watching television continues to be the leading form of sedentary entertainment. In 2009, Americans spent an average of 4.9 hours a day watching television.[24] Studies have found an association between television watching and overweight in children, youth, and adults.[25] Computers and other technological advances have further altered the activity level of children and adults. A 2010 report by the Surgeon General found that 8- to 18-year-olds spend over 7 hours per day playing video games, going on the computer, and watching television.[26] Talking to friends, playing games, and shopping online are just a few computer activities that would previously have involved some physical activity. In addition, people who sit long hours at a computer for their work are at increased risk of gaining weight due to little energy expenditure.

Friends and social networks also appear to influence weight. If your friends gain weight, you are more likely to gain weight. The more strongly you identify a person as a friend, the more likely you are to match his or her weight gain. This effect may relate to social norms and how comfortable you are with overweight and obesity. The good news is that recruiting friends in your efforts to maintain a healthy weight or lose weight may make you more successful.[25]

DIETING AND OBESITY

Contributing to the obesity trend is the "yo-yo dieting" effect, or **weight cycling**. People frustrated with their weight often turn to fad diets in hopes of finding a solution. Fad diets do not consist of realistic food plans that can be maintained for a lifetime. People may lose weight initially, but most find it difficult to maintain the harsh restrictions, returning to their previous patterns. With rapid weight loss on a highly restrictive diet, the body can enter starvation mode, with decreased basal metabolism. When a person goes off the restrictive diet, he or she rapidly gains back the weight lost and sometimes gains even more before the body's metabolism readjusts.

THE STRESS RESPONSE

In response to stress, our bodies release several hormones, including adrenaline and cortisol. Fat cells release fatty acids and triglycerides in response to these hormones and increase the amount of circulating glucose. These responses are vital in enabling the body to handle acute stress, especially physical stress. But when stress is chronic, the constant presence of these hormones can influence fat deposits, increasing the amount of fat deposited in the abdomen. The stress response also affects eating patterns. Adrenaline is an appetite suppressant, whereas cortisol stimulates the appetite. You may find that in high-stress situations, such as the transition to college or final exams week, you eat either more than usual or less than usual. People respond differently to stress, but either pattern can affect your overall health and long-term weight.

hot tip

Keep a bag of nuts in your backpack as an emergency snack—nuts are nutritious, filling, and healthier than most of what you will find in a vending machine.

The Key to Weight Control: Energy Balance

The relationship between the calories you take in and the calories you expend is known as **energy balance**. If you take in more calories than you use through metabolism and movement (a positive energy balance), you store these extra calories in the form of body fat. If you take in fewer calories than you need (a negative energy balance), you draw on body fat stores to provide energy. Energy in must equal energy out in order to maintain your current weight. If you adjust one or the other side of the equation, you will gain or lose weight (Figure 8.2).

ESTIMATING YOUR DAILY ENERGY REQUIREMENTS

In Chapter 7 we discussed energy intake, the calories-in side of the energy equation. Here we are more interested in energy expenditure, the calories-out side. Components of energy expenditure include the thermic effect of food, adaptive thermogenesis, basal metabolic rate, and physical activity. Each of the components of energy expenditure is influenced by genetics, age, sex, body size, fat-free mass, and intensity and duration of activity.

weight cycling
Repeated cycles of weight loss and weight gain as a result of dieting; sometimes called yo-yo dieting.

energy balance
Relationship between caloric intake (in the form of food) and caloric output (in the form of metabolism and activity).

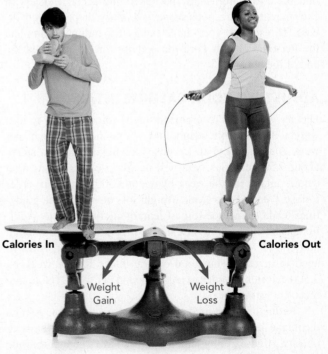

Calories In   Calories Out

Weight Gain   Weight Loss

figure **8.2** **Balancing calories in with calories out.**

The **thermic effect of food** is an estimate of the energy required to process the food you eat—chewing, digesting, metabolizing, and so on. The thermic effect of food is generally estimated at 10 percent of energy intake. If, for example, you ingested 2,500 calories of food during a day, you would burn approximately 250 calories processing what you ate. *Adaptive thermogenesis* takes into account the fact that your baseline energy expenditure varies with changes in the environment, such as in response to cold, or with physiological events, such as trauma, overeating, and changes in hormonal status.

thermic effect of food
Estimate of the energy required to process the food you eat.

basal metabolic rate (BMR)
Rate at which your body uses energy for basic life functions, such as breathing, circulation, and temperature regulation.

Basal metabolic rate (BMR) is the rate at which the body uses energy to maintain basic life functions, such as digestion, respiration, and temperature regulation. About 60–70 percent of energy consumed is used for these basic metabolic functions. BMR is affected by several factors, including age, gender, and weight.

Between 10 and 30 percent of the calories consumed each day are used for physical activity, depending on level and duration of activity. Physical activity influences the energy balance in two ways: Exercise itself burns calories, and exercise increases muscle mass, which is associated with a higher BMR.

You can estimate your daily energy expenditure by considering (1) the thermic effect of food, (2) the energy spent on basal metabolic rate, and (3) the energy spent on physical activities. The effects of adaptive thermogenesis on basal metabolic rate are usually not taken into account except in extreme situations, such as severe injury or prolonged illness. To estimate your daily energy expenditure, complete the Personal Health Portfolio activity for Chapter 8 at the end of the book.

ADJUSTING YOUR CALORIC INTAKE

Dietary guidelines recommend that if you are trying to lose weight, a reasonable weight loss of 1 pound to 2 pounds per week is a healthy goal. Because a pound of body fat stores about 3,500 calories, you will need to decrease your total calorie intake for the week by about 3,500 calories in order to lose 1 pound per week. Weight loss beyond these guidelines tends to include loss of lean tissue like muscle. Additionally, diets too low in calories may not provide enough nutrients. If you are trying to increase your weight, you will need to increase your total calorie intake for the week by 3,500 calories in order to gain 1 pound per week. (Note that these are estimates.)

Reducing your intake of fat is also important. A high fat intake leads to higher caloric intake and is linked with obesity. High-carbohydrate foods also have a greater thermic effect than do high-fat foods. Thus it takes more energy to process a high-carbohydrate diet, and less of the food's energy is available for storage as fat.

Are There Quick Fixes for Overweight and Obesity?

Time is a major issue for most Americans, and most of us would love a quick and easy way to stay at a healthy body weight. How healthy are fad diets? Are they worth the money? And do they work?

THE DIET INDUSTRY

Americans pay an estimated $58.6 billion for the diet industry's quick fixes.[27] Two prominent players in this field are fad diets and weight management organizations. Remember to be skeptical of unrealistic promises and to use your critical thinking skills when considering a diet or weight loss program. Some programs have been around for years, while others seem to come and go. For a comparison of several programs, see Table 8.2.

Fad Diets Every year, "new and improved" fad diets seduce consumers despite the fact that their safety and effectiveness are often unproven. No matter what the latest title, fad diets follow a pattern of altering the balance of carbohydrates, protein, and fat with the goal of promoting weight loss. Many will label certain foods as "good" or "bad," require the elimination of one of the five food groups, or prescribe certain "fat-burning foods." Be wary of diets with

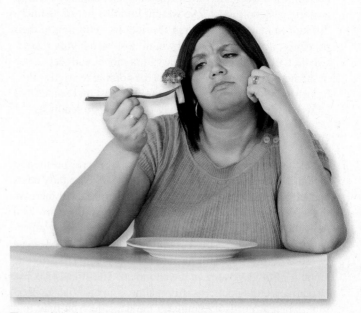

■ Any diet plan that requires you to eat only certain foods or to stop eating entire food groups is not a recipe for long-term success.

Table 8.2 A Comparison of Selected Diets and Weight Management Organizations

Diet/Organization	Theory	Pros and Cons
Volumetrics (self-help book)	Focus on low-energy-dense foods (vegetables, soup broth, nonfat milk) in place of high-energy-dense foods (chips, cookies, candy, nuts, oils) Includes physical activity	Emphasis on lifelong eating patterns Low drop-out rate* Recipes may be time-consuming to prepare
Weight Watchers (commercial organization)	Point exchange system (calorie counting equivalent) Earn or spend points with exercise and food Weekly behavioral component (group support), weigh-ins, and physical activity recommendations	Low drop-out rate* 4.6-pound weight loss at 1 year**
Jenny Craig (commercial organization)	Restrict calorie intake Prepackaged meals only Individual behavioral counseling and exercise recommendations	Expensive due to meals Minimal time for food prep Average drop-out rate* 14-pound weight loss at 1 year***
Slim-Fast (commercial products)	Meal replacement system – 1 to 2 meals a day are replaced with 400-calorie drink or bar	Convenient, minimal time involvement High drop-out rate* Reported "as effective as calorie-control diet"
Atkins (self-help book)	Low-carbohydrate diet No restriction on proteins or fats	Requires total calorie restriction for weight loss Average drop-out rate* 4.6-pound weight loss at 1 year**
Ornish (self-help book)	Low-fat diet Bans on meat, fish, oils, alcohol, sugar, white flour	Drastic diet change for most people Average drop-out rate* 3.3-pound weight loss at 1 year**
TOPS (nonprofit organization)	Group-format weekly sessions teaching skills for healthy eating and exercise Low-calorie diet emphasis Encourages exercise	Nonprofit No recent published data on weight loss or retention
Overeaters Anonymous (self-help organization)	12-step program Weekly sessions emphasizing healthy eating and physical, emotional, and spiritual recovery Assigned sponsor	May be beneficial for binge eaters or others with emotional issues attached to eating No published data on weight loss or retention

*Drop-out rate: low drop out = more than 50% continue at 1 year; average drop out = approximately 50% continue at 1 year; high drop out = less than 50% continue at 1 year.
**Independent study trials confirm weight loss amounts listed.
***Recent small randomized trial evaluating Jenny Craig versus control.

Sources: "Comparison of Atkins, Ornish, Weight Watchers and Zone Diets for Weight Loss and Heart Disease Risk Reduction: A Randomized Trial," by M.L. Daninger, J.A. Gleason, J.L. Griffith, et al., 2006, Journal of the American Medical Association, 293 (1), pp. 43–53; "Systematic Review: An Evaluation of Major Commercial Weight Loss Programs in the United States," by A.G. Tsai and T.A. Wadden, 2005, Annals of Internal Medicine, 142 (1), pp. 56–67; "Randomized Trial of a Multifaceted Commercial Weight Loss Program," by C.L. Rock, B. Pakiz, S.W. Flat, et al., 2007, Obesity, 15, pp. 939–949.

these features as no scientific data exist to support any of these claims. For some other tips, see the box "Myths and Misconceptions About Weight Gain and Weight Loss."

Most dietitians and physicians encourage people to monitor energy balance and eat a diet that emphasizes complex carbohydrates rather than trying fad diets. When evaluating a diet, consider if the food plan is something you can live with for the long haul. Remember, the factors that influence our food choices most are taste, cost, and convenience. You are unlikely to stick with a diet if it is too drastically different from your current eating patterns, if it calls for complete elimination of certain foods (especially ones you really like), if the diet requires hours of preparation, or if it requires the purchase of expensive pre-packed foods.[28]

Consumer Clipboard

Myths and Misconceptions About Weight Gain and Weight Loss

Myth Skipping meals is an effective way to lose weight.

Reality People who skip meals tend to be heavier than people who eat smaller, regular meals four to five times a day. Eating smaller meals throughout the day may help control appetite.

Myth Eating snacks late at night causes you to gain weight.

Reality How much you eat is the critical factor in determining whether you gain, lose, or maintain weight. Eating late at night in and of itself does not alter risk if total calorie intake is not increased.

Myth Certain foods, such as grapefruit and cabbage, can burn fat.

Reality No foods can burn fat. Some substances, such as caffeine, may increase metabolism in the short term.

Myth Nuts should be avoided if you are trying to lose weight as they are high in fat.

Reality Nuts are high in fat and calories, but they are also a good source of protein, fiber, and minerals. Nuts are a healthy choice if consumed in small quantities.

Myth Doing multiple sets of leg lifts every day will help "spot reduce" large thighs.

Reality Spot reducing (targeting a particular body location with exercises) does not work. Fat distribution is determined by genetics, hormones, and total body fat. Weight training may help improve muscle definition, but it won't reduce fat in a specific area unless it contributes to reduction in total body fat.

Myth You have to avoid fast foods if you want to lose weight.

Reality No food or restaurant is inherently "bad." The key is moderation. When eating at a fast-food restaurant, order grilled foods or a salad, drink water instead of soda, don't supersize your meal, and don't eat there every day.

Source: Adapted from Weight Loss and Nutrition Myths *(NIH Publication No. 04-4561), March 2004, updated August 2006, retrieved August 16, 2007, from www.win.niddk.nih.gov/publications/myths.htm#dietmyths.*

Weight Management Organizations   Weight management organizations offer group support, nutrition education, dietary advice, exercise counseling, and other services. Weight Watchers, Take Off Pounds Sensibly (TOPS), and Overeaters Anonymous are three well-known weight management organizations. TOPS and Overeaters Anonymous are free and provide group support. Weight Watchers is a commercial program. TOPS focuses on teaching. Overeaters Anonymous may be more suitable for binge eaters or others with emotional issues related to weight.[29] (See Table 8.2.)

THE MEDICAL APPROACH

Because obesity is a major risk factor for many health conditions, health centers are involved in helping people find solutions. We consider here three medical strategies used to treat obesity: very-low-calorie diets, diet drugs, and surgical procedures.

Very-Low-Calorie Diets (VLCDs)   An aggressive option for patients with high health risks because of obesity, VLCDs require a physician's supervision. These diets provide a daily intake of 800 calories or less and *must* be monitored closely.

VLCDs are used for moderately to severely obese patients (people with BMIs greater than 30) who are highly motivated but have not had success with more conservative plans. Patients with BMIs of 27 to 30 with medical conditions that could improve with rapid weight loss are also candidates. Weight loss after a 26-week program averages 20 percent of the patient's initial weight. However, maintaining weight loss is challenging.

Prescription Drugs   Because of the expense, potential for side effects, and need for medical supervision, weight loss drugs are intended for people who are at least 30 percent over their healthy body weight. There are currently only two weight-loss drugs approved by the Food and Drug Administration for long-term use in the United States. Sibutramine is an appetite suppressant. Its use results in an average weight loss of about 8 to 10 pounds when combined with lifestyle modification. Sibutramine can cause a slight increase in blood pressure and thus is not recommended for people with high blood pressure, heart disease, or a history of stroke.[30] Orlistat blocks the absorption of fat and its use results in an average weight loss of 6 pounds. Digestion of fat is reduced by approximately 30 percent, and the undigested fat passes through the body. Orlistat has some potential side effects: stomach cramps, gas, and fecal incontinence (leaking stool). In addition, the reduction in fat absorption leads to a decrease in the absorption of certain fat-soluble vitamins (Vitamins A, D, E, and K). An over-the-counter version of orlistat, called Alli, is now available. It is a reduced-strength version with the same potential side effects.[30]

Phentermine is an appetite suppressant that has been approved by the

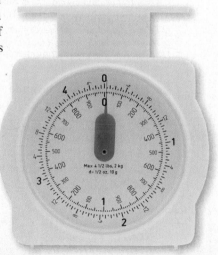

This disorder overlaps with anorexia and bulimia, and risk factors are similar. Often, a first sign of a problem is a decrease in performance, a muscle injury, or an exercise-related stress fracture. Amenorrhea is another important sign. Female athletes need to understand the importance of good eating habits and moderation in exercise and recognize the patterns and dangers of eating disorders.

ACTIVITY DISORDER

People with **activity disorder** control their bodies or alter their moods by being overly involved in exercise or addicted to exercise. People who are addicted to exercise continue to exercise strenuously even when the activity causes such problems as illness, injury, or the breakdown of relationships. At the heart of activity disorder is the use of exercise to gain a sense of control and accomplishment, to maintain self-esteem, and to soothe emotions rather than to increase fitness, relaxation, or pleasure. The disorder is not about exercise itself but about meeting psychological needs through exercise. The hallmark of activity disorder is a pattern of exercise that becomes detrimental to health rather than beneficial (see the box "Ron: A Case of Muscle Dysmorphia and Activity Disorder").

activity disorder
Excessive or addictive exercising, undertaken to address psychological needs rather than to improve fitness.

The signs and symptoms of activity disorder often resemble those of anorexia and bulimia. Physical symptoms include fatigue, reduction in performance, decreased focus, increased compulsion to exercise, decreased heart rate response to exercise, and muscle degeneration. Cycles of repetitive overuse injuries are common.

Activity disorder is more common among men than among women, a difference that may be related to childhood experiences and cultural values. Males tend to be more active than females during childhood, and our culture supports male independence and physical achievement. The association between activity and achievement may influence active people with perfectionist tendencies to become addicted to exercise.

Treatment for activity disorder is similar to that for eating disorders, although most cases of pure activity disorder can be handled in an outpatient setting. Unfortunately, activity disorder often occurs in conjunction with an eating disorder; the combination can rapidly increase the physical problems of both disorders.

Awareness and Prevention: Promoting a Healthy Body Image

Promotion of healthy eating and a healthy body image involves many components and coordinated efforts.

Life Stories

Ron: A Case of Muscle Dysmorphia and Activity Disorder

Ron had been concerned about his muscular development ever since he was a kid. At the age of 18, he still felt he wasn't big enough, even though he was bigger and stronger than the average man and quite athletic. Ron didn't socialize or go out much, mostly because he was usually at the gym working out. He avoided talking to people while he was there, because he was sure that they were all secretly laughing at how scrawny he was. Ron couldn't really enjoy a meal at a restaurant or a friend's house, either. He kept to a strict diet of high-protein foods and dietary supplements. Ron lifted weights in competition and was actually quite strong, but his muscles didn't look bulky enough to him. He thought about trying steroids to further increase his muscle size.

Not only was Ron obsessed with his muscular development; he was also using exercise to control his moods. He never really felt in control except when he was lifting weights. On a few occasions he injured himself by lifting too much weight, yet he couldn't rest long enough to heal properly. When he felt too sore to lift, he would run or do calisthenics. All the extra activity actually kept his muscles from bulking up further, but he saw the lack of new bulk as a sign that he wasn't working hard enough. Ron wasn't able to see how his pattern of exercise was hurting his health. It took the intervention of a personal trainer at the gym to help him recognize that he needed to seek psychological help.

connect
ACTIVITY

INDIVIDUAL ATTITUDES

As an individual, you can begin to challenge the way you interact with the world. Value yourself based on your goals, talents, and strengths rather than your body shape or weight. Start to look critically at the images and messages you receive from people and the media. Develop skills to handle stress in a healthy way, and avoid judging yourself or others.

COLLEGE INITIATIVES

Colleges have a role to play in ensuring that students learn how to transition successfully to new environments, new relationships, and different sociocultural pressures. These are skills that will translate well into future environments and relationships. Ideally, prevention efforts will include both individual measures and campuswide activities. Campus life typically affords many opportunities for people to recognize individuals who are at increased risk for disordered eating patterns and psychological distress. Residence advisors, professors, coaches, trainers, and other college staff can be trained to watch for signs that students are having problems with the transition to college life. Health and counseling services can be visible and accessible so that students feel comfortable accessing help early if they are feeling distressed.

PUBLIC HEALTH APPROACHES

Public health approaches focus on raising awareness about eating disorders and changing widely accepted social norms. The "Love Your Body Day" campaign is one example of a public health approach aimed at promoting healthy body images. The idea of the campaign is to encourage acceptance of physical differences, including different body shapes and sizes and the normal changes of healthy aging (see the box "Love Your Body Day").

Nationally, organizations and programs have been developed to promote healthy body image and lifestyle patterns for young people. For example, the Girl Scouts' "Free to Be Me" program emphasizes inner strength and healthy differences instead of outer appearances. It encourages girls to think about who they really are and what they like to do,

hot tip

Try going a week without making any critical comments about your body—or anyone else's.

to understand and resist peer pressure, to learn about eating disorders and substance abuse, and to celebrate their own diversity. The Boy Scouts' "Fit for Life" and "5-a-Day" badge programs, although not designed specifically to combat eating disorders, teach boys about the roles of healthy nutrition, fitness, and exercise.

Girls, Inc., is a nationwide educational and advocacy organization that encourages girls to be "strong, smart, and bold." This organization's programs focus on building girls' interest and skills in math, science, and technology; on developing media literacy, emotional literacy, strategies for self-defense, and leadership; and on helping girls participate in sports and take healthy risks in life. Dads and Daughters is an organization that recognizes the important role of parents in the lives of youth. Parents are powerful role models and can communicate a healthy body image, a healthy approach to weight management, and problem-solving skills. Parents can lead the way by emphasizing the importance of a balance between inner and outer beauty, healthy relationship patterns, and balanced achievements.

In addition to private efforts, the government sponsors a number of programs. The Office of Women's Health, operating under the U.S. Department of Health and Human Services, sponsors "Body Wise," an educational campaign aimed at increasing knowledge about eating disorders, promoting healthy eating, and reducing preoccupation with body weight and size. This office publishes information on boys and eating disorders as well.

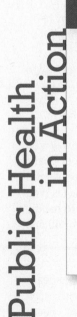

Public Health in Action

Love Your Body Day

Since 1998, on a day in October, the National Organization for Women (NOW) has sponsored Love Your Body Day. The day is promoted as a fun but serious way to help people "fight back" against Hollywood and the fashion, cosmetics, and diet industries. NOW encourages colleges and schools across the country to host events that draw attention to body image issues and that highlight the importance of diversity in body shape, size, and function.

Events have included picketing the headquarters of publications that promote offensive images of women and girls, creating T-shirts with slogans that will initiate discussions and questions (such as "This is what Barbie OUGHT to look like"), and hosting rallies and forums to discuss and highlight body image issues. Every year there is a Love Your Body poster contest; the winner receives a monetary prize, and the winning poster is distributed as the official poster for the upcoming year.

NOW provides other resources designed to help the public become active in confronting the media on the Love Your Body Web site. For example, it posts "Offensive Ads" and "Positive Ads" with explanations of why ads fall into different categories, thus enhancing media literacy skills. They also promote advocacy by asking visitors to nominate ads for posting. For further information and to find out when the next annual Love Your Body Day is scheduled, visit the Web site at www.loveyourbody.nowfoundation.org.

connect ACTIVITY

In short, to counteract unhealthy attitudes, we can begin to resist current cultural messages and become active in changing them. The media and advertising industry spend millions of dollars every year finding out what consumers want and selling products. The industry conducts research on consumer attitudes, holds focus groups, monitors sales, and pays attention to consumer reactions. By supporting healthy body images and buying products that reflect diversity, we can move our society in the direction of realistic, accepting, and healthy attitudes toward the body.

Value yourself based on your goals, talents, and strengths
rather than your body shape or weight.

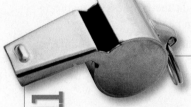

You Make the Call

Photo Enhancement in Magazines and Ads: Artful and Inspiring or Dishonest and Harmful?

- When Britney Spears shot a series of ads for Candie's in 2010, she released the untouched images from the shoot along with the retouched ads. A comparison of the two showed that her legs, arms, and waist had been thinned, cellulite removed, and skin blemishes evened out.

- The June/July 2007 issue of *Men's Fitness* magazine featured a cover photo of tennis superstar Andy Roddick that had been doctored to give him enormous biceps. Even Roddick was surprised at his appearance. One of the cover tag lines near Roddick's head was "How to Build Big Arms in 5 Easy Moves."

- A 2009 Ralph Lauren advertisement featured a photo of 23-year-old model Filippa Hamilton so heavily Photoshopped that her hips were narrower than her head. The 5′10″, 120-pound model appeared emaciated in the digitally distorted image.

Magazine cover and ad photos are routinely altered to create more perfect images of models and celebrities—at least to the eyes of the magazine editors. Photos are digitally edited to enlarge busts, reduce waists, remove cellulite, whiten teeth, lighten dark skin, darken light skin, make lines and wrinkles disappear, and change a host of other human "flaws." With the advent of digital photography and advanced software to manipulate photos, the practice is growing in sophistication and pervasiveness. Often the people portrayed in the images have little knowledge or say in the practice.

What difference does this practice make? Magazines and ads create images and ideals to which members of the general population aspire. The most famous and successful models and actors already represent a look shared by only 2 percent of the population. Research has shown that both men and women experience feelings of inadequacy, lower self-esteem,

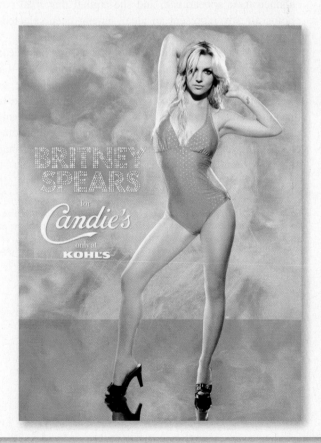

and increased dissatisfaction with their bodies after viewing fashion magazines. Further enhancements to appearance and body proportions create images that are physically unattainable and may create even more dissatisfaction among viewers. For some, comparing themselves to these images may contribute to psychological problems like depression and eating disorders.

Many people, especially adolescent girls and young women, are vulnerable to these fantasy images and have not been sufficiently trained in media literacy to recognize enhanced photos. Some critics have suggested that when images have been altered, magazines include a disclaimer to allow viewers to make informed decisions about whether to compare themselves to such impossible ideals. The suggestion has not been taken seriously by the magazine industry. When a slimmed-down version of singer Kelly Clarkson appeared on the cover of *Self* magazine, editor in chief Lucy Danziger responded to criticism by asserting that airbrushing and "post-production corrections" are well-known industry standards.

Danziger went on to say that the cover was "art, creativity, and collaboration," not journalism, and was intended to "inspire women to want to be their best." She likened photo retouching to women wearing makeup or push-up bras to enhance their appearance, and she argued that final cover photos already represent an ideal, having been selected as the best out of hundreds of shots in a photo session.

Others have pointed out that digital editing has become commonplace among the general population, with many people retouching their own photographs using home software. Some cameras even come with a "slimming" feature that automatically compresses an image vertically, shaving 5 to 15 pounds off the photo subject. With photo enhancement part of everyday life, only the very naive would take a magazine cover or ad at face value.

Some argue that digital enhancement of photos is an acceptable part of our celebrity-focused, commercial culture. Others believe photo enhancement is a damaging and unethical practice, promoting unattainable ideals for vulnerable young people, and that altered photos ought to be explicitly identified. What do you think?

PROS

- Magazines are an art form, presenting ideal images. They are not in the business of depicting reality or presenting journalistic truths. They are in the business of inspiring people to be the best they can be.

- Using Photoshop to alter an image is commonplace; everyone does it. It's not the magazine industry's job to bring everyone up to speed on current technology or well-known practices.

- Altering a photo creates the same kind of illusion that women create every day by wearing makeup or choosing a push-up bra.

CONS

- Models already represent a look shared by a fraction of the population. Further enhancement of their images results in physically unattainable ideals.

- Many people are susceptible to feelings of inadequacy and dissatisfaction with themselves when viewing photos of models and celebrities. The practice of digital enhancement preys on their vulnerabilities.

- Many people do not realize how much images have been enhanced, nor are they informed of such enhancement. They are being misled if not deceived.

connect ACTIVITY

Sources: *Photo Tampering Throughout History*, by Hany Farid, retrieved from www.cs.dartmouth.edu/farid/research/digitaltampering/; *HP Develops a Camera That Makes You Look Thinner*, retrieved from cybernetnews.com/hp-develops-a-camera-that-makes-you-look-thinner/; *Lucy's Blog—Pictures That Please Us*, by Lucy Danziger, retrieved from www.self.com/magazine/blogs/lucysblog/2009/08/pictures-that-please-us.html; *Smile and Say "No Photoshop,"* by Eric Wilson, May 27, 2009, New York Times, retrieved May 28, 2009, from www.nytimes.com/2009/05/28/fashion/28RETOUCH.html?pagewanted=1&_r=2&ref=media.

IN REVIEW

What is body image, and how is it determined?
Body image is the mental representation a person has of his or her body. It includes perceptions, attitudes, thoughts, feelings, and judgments about one's body, and it is strongly influenced by culture. Via advertising, fashion, and language, our culture sends messages about appearance, beauty, and acceptable body size and shape, especially for women but increasingly for men.

What is disordered eating, and what are eating disorders?
To meet society's standards, many people practice disordered eating behaviors like dieting or binging and purging on occasion, but some people develop full-blown eating disorders. These disorders are characterized by severe disturbances in eating behavior and by a distorted body image. They are serious, chronic illnesses and are classified as mental disorders. Related disorders are body dysmorphic disorder and activity disorder.

Why do people develop eating disorders?
Aside from social pressures and cultural messages, which affect everyone, some people may be vulnerable to eating disorders because of a genetic predisposition, family factors, or other underlying emotional problems and characteristics, such as depression, anxiety, low self-esteem, a sense of powerlessness, perfectionism, and lack of other coping skills.

What are the most common eating disorders?
Anorexia nervosa, characterized by self-starvation, is the most severe eating disorder. Bulimia nervosa, characterized by binge eating and purging, is more difficult to identify, because people with bulimia are of normal weight. Binge-eating disorder leads to obesity, but only a small percentage of obese people have this disorder. All eating disorders have serious health consequences.

How are eating disorders treated?
Because they are mental disorders, treatment usually includes psychotherapy to address psychological issues, along with weight stabilization, behavior modification, nutritional rehabilitation and education, and, in some cases, medication. For anorexia, hospitalization may be required at first to prevent starvation. Treatment usually involves the whole family, and recovery can be lifelong. Communities have a role to play in promoting healthy body images for both women and men.

Web Resources

Body Positive: This educational organization teaches critical thinking about our culture's focus on thinness. Its resources include *BodyTalk*, a video on body acceptance for teen girls and boys, and links to other organizations that offer information on body image. www.bodypositive.com

Girls, Inc.: Dedicated to inspiring all girls to be "strong, smart, and bold," Girls, Inc., offers educational programs throughout the United States, particularly to girls in high-risk, underserved areas. It teaches girls how to advocate for themselves and their communities and to promote positive change. www.girlsinc.org

National Association for Self-Esteem: The aim of this organization is to improve self-esteem among Americans. Its Web site features a self-guided tour that lets you rate your self-esteem, as well as articles, a newsletter, FAQs, and links to other resources. www.self-esteem-nase.org

National Eating Disorders Association: Promoting public understanding of eating disorders, this organization offers programs and services related to treatment and support of families affected by these disorders. www.edap.org

TeensHealth: This site offers various topics of interest to teens, including body image and self-esteem, eating disorders, cutting, and emotional changes in adolesence. www.kidshealth.org/teen

10

Alcohol and Tobacco

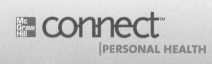

http://www.mcgrawhillconnect.com/personalhealth

Ever Wonder...

- what counts as having "too much to drink"?

- if drinking coffee or walking will help you sober up?

- if smoking occasionally is really bad for you?

Alcohol and tobacco are the most commonplace—and the most problematic—substances used in our

society. The use of both can have profound effects on the lives of individuals, families, communities, and society in general. The use of both also illustrates the tension between personal choice and the common good. For these reasons, responsible decisions about their use are particularly important.

Understanding Alcohol Use

The alcohol culture permeates the environment on many college campuses, as seen in tailgate parties, bar crawls, twenty-one-shot birthday celebrations, and an endless variety of rituals marking the end of classes, the first snowfall, or spring break. For decades, college administrators ignored or condoned this culture. But recently, chilling statistics have brought alcohol-related problems to the forefront. High-risk alcohol drinking kills 1,700 students between the ages of 18 and 24 every year and causes injury to 599,000. Sexual assaults, physical violence, vandalism, and academic casu-

for low-risk and high-risk drinking. For men, **low-risk drinking** means no more than 14 drinks per week and no more than 4 drinks on any one day. For women, it means no more than 7 drinks per week and no more than 3 drinks on any one day. Alcohol consumption above these levels is considered heavy or at-risk drinking. Another way to think about the guidelines is that *moderate drinking* is two drinks a day for men and one for women. Regardless of these specific guidelines, alcohol should not be consumed at any level in a situation that would put you or others at risk.[5] The Personal Health Portfolio Activity for Chapter 10 at the back of your book will help you determine if you are a low-risk or at-risk drinker.

"One drink" is defined by the NIAAA as 0.5 ounce (or 15 grams) of alcohol, the amount contained in about 12 ounces of beer, 5 ounces of wine, a 1.5-ounce shot of 80-proof distilled liquor, or 1.5 ounces of liquor in a mixed drink (Figure 10.1). The term *proof* refers to the alcohol

psychoactive drug
A substance that causes changes in brain chemistry and alters consciousness.

intoxication
Altered state of consciousness as a result of drinking alcohol or ingesting other substances.

low-risk drinking
Fourteen drinks a week for men and no more than 4 on one day; 7 drinks a week for women and no more than 3 on one day.

We use alcohol to feel good, to celebrate, and to toast one another and life, yet we also see the devastation that results when drinking gets out of control.

alties are additional problems associated with the campus alcohol culture.[1–4]

Ambivalence toward college drinking reflects the ambivalence of the larger culture toward alcohol. We use alcohol to feel good, to celebrate, and to toast one another and life, yet we also see the devastation that results when drinking gets out of control.

Because alcohol is a **psychoactive drug**—it causes changes in brain chemistry and alters consciousness, a state referred to as **intoxication**—it can have wide-ranging effects on all aspects of our thinking, emotions, and behavior. It is in society's interest to regulate the use of such a powerful substance, but it is up to individuals to determine what role they want alcohol to play in their lives.

WHO DRINKS? PATTERNS OF ALCOHOL USE

About 65 percent of American adults drink, at least occasionally. About 35 percent of the adult U.S. population label themselves *abstainers*. They do not drink at all, or they do so less often than once a year. Of the 65 percent who do drink, 28 percent are considered *at-risk drinkers*, and the remainder are *low-risk drinkers*.[5] The National Institute on Alcohol Abuse and Alcoholism (NIAAA) has set parameters

content of hard liquor, defined as twice the actual percentage of alcohol in the beverage; for example, 80-proof liquor is 40 percent alcohol by volume.

Drinking patterns are established by the adolescent years. Consumption of alcoholic beverages is highest between the ages of 18 and 25 for Whites and then begins a steady

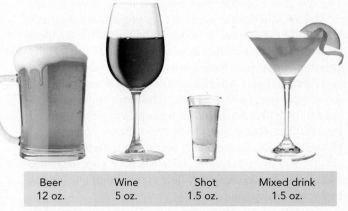

| Beer | Wine | Shot | Mixed drink |
| 12 oz. | 5 oz. | 1.5 oz. | 1.5 oz. |

figure 10.1   **What is "one drink"?** Each drink contains about 0.5 ounce of alcohol.

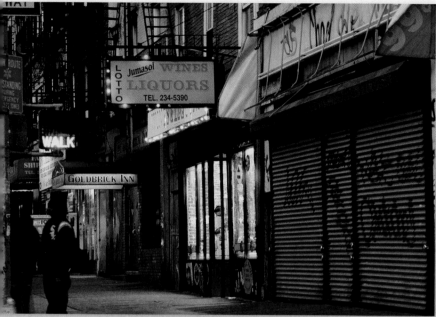

■ An oversupply of liquor stores in poor and minority neighborhoods plays a role in both the availability of alcohol and the social acceptability of alcohol use.

descent. The peak period for heavy drinking among Hispanic and African American men occurs between the ages of 26 and 30, and the decline tends to be less marked than that for White men.[6] In general, people are more likely to drink at certain stages in the lifespan, such as adolescence and early adulthood, the threshold of middle age, and following retirement.

Older adults drink significantly less than younger adults do. Women of all ages drink less than men do and start later. Alcohol consumption is higher among Whites than among African Americans across most of the lifespan.[6] Alcohol consumption is high among Hispanic/Latino men, but it is very low among Hispanic/Latina women.

Differences in alcohol consumption among ethnic groups are strongly influenced by sociocultural or environmental factors, including poverty, discrimination, feelings of powerlessness, immigration status, and degree of acculturation.[7] Economic factors, such as the heavy marketing of alcoholic beverages in minority neighborhoods, play a considerable role. For example, the number of liquor stores located in African American communities is proportionately much higher than the number in White communities.[6] Given these pressures, it is notable that alcohol consumption is generally lower among African Americans than among other groups.

Among Native Americans, alcoholism is recognized as the number one health problem.[6] The death rate from alcoholism for Native Americans is more than five times greater than that for other groups.[8] Numerous factors contribute to these disparities, most notably sociocultural factors such as poverty and discrimination. Scientists have also suggested that genetic factors may contribute to patterns of alcohol use by Native Americans.

Among Asian Americans, alcohol consumption overall is lower than among White Americans. Approximately half of all Asian Americans have a gene that impairs the metabolism of alcohol, causing a set of unpleasant reactions (facial flushing, sweating, nausea) referred to as the flushing effect.[8]

WHAT CAUSES PROBLEM DRINKING?

Why do some people develop problems with alcohol while others do not? This question has no simple answers. Instead, a complex interaction of many factors—individual, psychological, and sociocultural—is at work.

As discussed in Chapter 2, a family history of alcoholism is a risk factor for the development of alcoholism. Family dysfunction in general, even without an alcoholic parent, increases the likelihood that children will grow up to have alcohol problems. However, most children who grow up in dysfunctional family environments do not develop problems with alcohol. Sociocultural or environmental factors also play an enormous role in how alcohol is used and misused. Some cultures have higher acceptance of alcohol use, more tolerant attitudes toward drinking and drunkenness, and/or higher levels of alcohol consumption than others do. Economic factors, such as the availability and cost of alcohol, and the ease of access, also play a role, as do laws governing drinking age and the sale of alcoholic beverages.

DRINKING ON THE COLLEGE CAMPUS

Drinking rates at most colleges are very high; surveys indicate that up to 83 percent of college students drink alcoholic beverages.[9] Some students engage in binge drinking, a particularly risky way to consume alcohol.

Binge Drinking   Binge drinking is defined in this study as the consumption of five or more drinks in a row for men and four or more drinks in a row for women at least once in the previous 2-week period. In 2005, the College Alcohol Study (CAS) conducted by the National Center on Addiction and Substance Abuse at Columbia University found that about 40 percent of all college students were binge drinkers, and almost one in four were *frequent binge drinkers*, meaning they had binged three or more times in the previous 2 weeks or more than once a week on average (see the box "College Students and Binge Drinking").[10]

binge drinking
Consumption of five or more drinks in a row by a man or four or more drinks in a row by a woman.

Who's at Risk?

College Students and Binge Drinking

- Men binge drink at rates almost three times those for women. Male freshmen drink less than male upperclassmen, but female freshmen drink more than female upperclassmen.

- Binge drinking rates are similar between racial/ethnic populations. However, non-Hispanic Blacks and Hispanics reported a higher number of drinks per binge episode than Whites, and American-born Hispanics report higher binge-drinking rates than foreign-born Hispanics.

- Students at historically Black colleges and universities (HBCUs) have lower rates of binge drinking than do students at other colleges. Family expectations, peer modeling, and religion and spirituality may account for some of the difference, but the most important factor may be the stronger emphasis on community engagement and service.

- Members of fraternities have much higher rates of binge drinking than do non–fraternity members. Dormitory residents and students living off campus have about the same rates.

- Of college students who drink alcohol, about 25 percent began drinking in college, about 65 percent began drinking in high school, and about 8 percent began drinking in junior high. Students who began drinking in junior high consume more and drink more often than students who began drinking later.

- The highest prevalence of binge drinking occurs between ages 18 and 24. Binge drinking rates decrease with advancing age; only 3.7 percent of people age 65 or older binge drink.

Sources: "What We Have Learned from the Harvard School of Public Health College Alcohol Study: Focusing Attention on College Student Alcohol Consumption and the Environmental Conditions That Promote It," by H. Wechsler and T.F. Nelson, 2008, Journal of Studies of Alcohol, 69 (3), pp. 481–489; "The Hispanic Americans Baseline Alcohol Survey (HABLAS): DUI Rates, Birthplace, and Acculturation Across Hispanic National Groups," by R. Caetano, S. Ramisetty-Mikler, and L.A. Rodriguez, 2008, Journal of Studies of Alcohol, 69 (2), pp. 159–265; "Wasting the Best and the Brightest: Substance Abuse at America's Colleges and Universities," 2007, New York: National Center on Addiction and Substance Abuse at Columbia University; "A Matter of Degree: The National Effort to Reduce High-Risk Drinking Among College Students," American Medical Association, 2006, retrieved from www.ama-assn.org/ama/pub/category/3558.html.

Very often, binge drinking does not begin in college. Many students binge drink in high school and come to college expecting to continue drinking heavily.[9,10] This pattern suggests that colleges inherit the behavior of young people who binge drink. At the same time, college environments that promote drinking not only attract drinkers but also encourage drinking among people who were previously nondrinkers.

College students under the age of 21 consume 48 percent of all alcohol consumed by college students.[11] They

percent more likely to be victims of date rape, sexual battering, and unplanned sexual activity than are women who do not drink alcohol.[15] According to CAS, about one in four students reported that their drinking caused them to miss class, turn in mediocre work, fail exams, or earn failing grades.

Binge drinkers also cause problems for other students. About 9 out of 10 students reported experiencing at least one adverse consequence of another student's drinking during the school year.[16] These "secondhand effects" of binge drinking include serious arguments, physical assault, dam-

Students at historically Black colleges and universities have **lower rates of binge drinking** *than do students at other colleges.*

drink less frequently than older students do, but they are more likely to binge drink during these episodes and to drink simply to get drunk.[12] They are also more likely to be injured or encounter trouble with law enforcement than are older students who binge drink.[13]

Binge drinking can have serious physical, academic, social, and legal consequences. Individuals who have been drinking heavily are more likely to be injured, to commit a crime or fall victim to violence, and to be involved with the law. Half to two-thirds of campus homicides and serious assaults are believed to involve drinking by the offender, the victim, or both.[14] Women who binge drink are nearly 150

aged property, interrupted sleep or studying, unwanted sexual advances, sexual assault, and having to take care of a drunk student.

Binge drinkers are more likely to meet the *Diagnostic and Statistical Manual of Mental Disorders* criteria for alcohol abuse and alcohol dependence 10 years after college and are less likely to work in prestigious occupations, compared with non–binge drinkers. Alcohol-related convictions for crimes like driving under the influence, vandalism, assaults, and providing alcohol to a minor may jeopardize ambitions in many careers, including engineering, medicine, law enforcement, and teaching.

Why Do College Students Binge Drink? Students may drink to ease social inhibitions, fit in with peers, imitate role models, reduce stress, soothe negative emotions, or cope with academic pressure or for a variety of other reasons. The mistaken belief that alcohol increases sexual arousal and performance (heavy drinking actually suppresses sexual arousal) may also account for some binge drinking.[14]

Binge drinking is also promoted by easy access to alcohol and cheap prices. Thus, social norms and the campus culture contribute to patterns of drinking. Students are more likely to binge drink on campuses where heavy drinking is the norm and less likely to do so where drinking is discouraged.[17,18]

Is the Definition of Binge Drinking Realistic? Some health experts believe the CAS definition of binge drinking (five or more drinks in a row for a man, four or more for a woman) is too broad and classifies a large number of people as binge drinkers who may not have a problem. Other terms, such as *heavy drinking* or *high-risk drinking*, may be preferable to describe the drinking currently labeled *binge drinking*. The latter term could be reserved for a prolonged period of intoxication (2 days or more). This definition would direct attention to the minority of students who have real problems with alcohol consumption. The term *extreme drinking* is now being used to describe alcohol consumption that goes well beyond binge drinking, to double or triple the amounts in the CAS definition—10 to 15 drinks a day for men and 8 to 12 drinks a day for women. Many colleges and universities are now targeting such extreme drinking on campus.

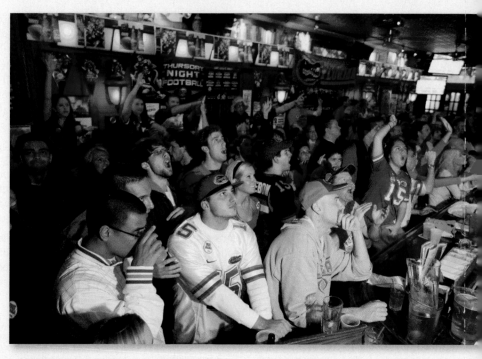

■ Alcohol consumption among college students is influenced by the social norms around drinking on their campus. In some cases, there is a gap between student-perceived levels of alcohol consumption and actual consumption by most students.

mandating treatment for substance-related offenses, educating students to resist peer pressure, helping students cope with stress and time management issues, and targeting prevention messages to high-risk times and events, such as freshman year, athletic events, and spring break.

Colleges can also implement strategies aimed more directly at changing the campus drinking culture. Some schools sponsor alcohol-free social and cultural events, while others have gone further by prohibiting alcohol at all

Colleges have focused on restricting alcohol advertising and promotion on campus, but this can be tricky because **the alcohol industry provides significant financial support** *to athletic programs at many colleges.*

Addressing the Problem The problem of excessive drinking by college students requires an integrated response at several levels. At the level of the individual student, the focus is on reducing the amount of drinking by students and identifying and helping high-risk students, such as through screenings during health care visits. Screening tools can also be used to help students compare their drinking behaviors with those of other students. Other student-level measures include enforcing college alcohol policies consistently and punishing students who violate policies or break the law,

college-sponsored events and maintaining alcohol-free residence halls and fraternity and sorority houses. Colleges have also focused on restricting alcohol advertising and promotion on campus, but this can be tricky because the alcohol industry provides significant financial support to athletic programs at many colleges.

Finally, colleges can work cooperatively with their communities to support such strategies as increased enforcement of drinking-age laws, provision of "safe rides" programs, and limits on the density of alcohol retailers near campus.

Effects of Alcohol on the Body

Within minutes of ingestion, alcohol is distributed to all the cells of the body (Figure 10.2). In the brain, alcohol alters brain chemistry and changes neurotransmitter functions. It particularly affects the cerebellum—the center for balance and motor functions—and the prefrontal cortex—the center for executive functions, such as rational thinking and problem solving.

Alcohol is a **central nervous system depressant**. While alcohol levels in the blood and brain are rising, you experience feelings of relaxation and well-being and a lowering of social inhibitions. At higher levels, and especially when blood levels are falling, you are more likely to feel depressed and withdrawn and to experience impairments in thinking, balance, and motor coordination. These effects last until all the alcohol is metabolized (broken down into energy and wastes) and excreted from the body.

central nervous system depressant
Chemical substance that slows down the activity of the brain and spinal cord.

ALCOHOL ABSORPTION

Many factors affect alcohol absorption:

- *Food in the stomach*. The type of food has not been shown to have a meaningful influence on alcohol absorption.
- *Gender*. Women absorb alcohol into the bloodstream more quickly than men do.
- *Age*. Older adults are less tolerant of alcohol.
- *Body fat*. The more body fat a person has, the less alcohol is absorbed by the body tissue and the more there is to circulate in the bloodstream and reach the brain.
- *Drug interaction*. Interactions with many prescription and over-the-counter drugs can intensify a drinker's reaction to alcohol, leading to more rapid intoxication.
- *Cigarette smoke*. Nicotine extends the time alcohol stays in the stomach, increasing time for absorption into the bloodstream.
- *Mood and physical condition*. Fear and anger tend to speed up alcohol absorption. The stomach empties more rapidly than normal, allowing the alcohol to be absorbed more easily. People who are stressed, tired, or ill may also feel the effects sooner.
- *Alcohol concentration*. The more concentrated the drink, the more quickly the alcohol is absorbed. Hard liquor is absorbed faster than are beer and wine.
- *Carbonation*. The carbon dioxide contained in champagne, cola, and ginger ale speeds the absorption of alcohol. Drinks that contain water, juice, or milk are absorbed more slowly.
- *Tolerance*. The body adapts to a given alcohol level. Each time a person drinks to the point of impairment, the body attempts to minimize impairment by adapting to that level. More alcohol is needed to overcome the body's adaptation and achieve the desired effect.

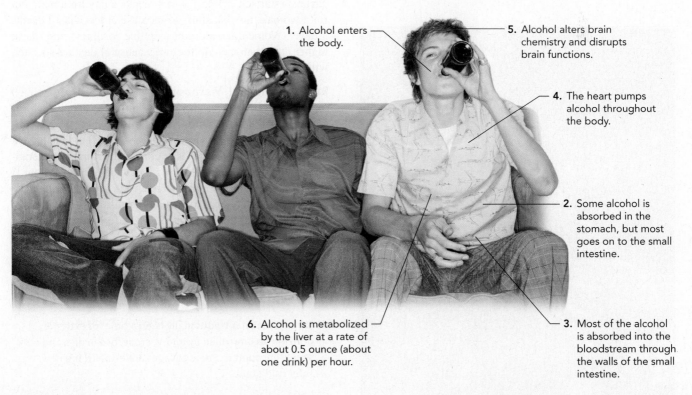

1. Alcohol enters the body.

5. Alcohol alters brain chemistry and disrupts brain functions.

4. The heart pumps alcohol throughout the body.

2. Some alcohol is absorbed in the stomach, but most goes on to the small intestine.

6. Alcohol is metabolized by the liver at a rate of about 0.5 ounce (about one drink) per hour.

3. Most of the alcohol is absorbed into the bloodstream through the walls of the small intestine.

figure **10.2** **The path of alcohol in the body.**

ALCOHOL METABOLISM

A small amount of alcohol is metabolized in the stomach, but 90 percent is metabolized in the liver. Between 2 and 10 percent is not metabolized at all; instead, it is excreted unchanged in the breath and urine and through the pores of the skin. This is why you can smell alcohol on the breath of someone who has been drinking.

In the liver, alcohol is converted to acetaldehyde, an organic chemical compound, by the enzyme *alcohol dehydrogenase (ADH)*. The ability to metabolize alcohol is dependent on the amount and kind of ADH enzymes available in the liver. If more alcohol molecules arrive in the liver cells than the enzymes can process, the extra molecules circulate through the brain, liver, and other organs until enzymes are available to degrade them.

Blood Alcohol Concentration   **Blood alcohol concentration (BAC)** is a measure of the amount of alcohol in grams in 100 milliliters of blood, expressed as a percentage. For example, for 100 milligrams of alcohol in 100 milliliters of blood, the BAC is .10 percent.

BAC provides a good estimate of the alcohol concentration in the brain, which is why it is used as a measure of intoxication by state motor vehicle laws. The alcohol concentration in the brain corresponds well with alcohol concentration in the breath, so breath samples are accurate indicators of BAC.

blood alcohol concentration (BAC)
The amount of alcohol in grams in 100 milliliters of blood, expressed as a percentage.

For this reason, breath analyzers are legal in most states for identifying and prosecuting drunk drivers.[6]

BAC is influenced by the amount of alcohol consumed and the rate at which the alcohol is metabolized by the body. Because alcohol is soluble in water and somewhat less soluble in fat, it does not distribute to all body tissues equally.[6] The more body water a person has, the more the alcohol is diluted and the lower the person's BAC will be. The more body fat a person has, the less alcohol is absorbed by body tissue and the more there is to circulate in the bloodstream and reach the brain. Thus a 150-pound person with high body fat will have a higher BAC than will a 150-pound person with more lean body tissue who drinks the same amount. Body size alone influences BAC as well; a larger, heavier person has more body surface to diffuse the alcohol (as well as a higher body water content to dilute the alcohol).

Gender Differences in Alcohol Absorption and Metabolism   Both of these factors—body size and body fat percentage—play a role in gender differences in the effects of alcohol. Women are generally more susceptible to alcohol's effects and have a higher BAC than men do after drinking the same amount. Women are generally smaller than men, and they have a higher body fat percentage.

Another factor is that women absorb more of the alcohol they drink because they metabolize alcohol less efficiently than men do.

These differences make women more vulnerable to the health consequences of alcohol, including alcohol-related liver disease, heart disease, and brain damage.[19] The risk for cirrhosis starts at 2½ drinks to 4 drinks a day for a man, but for a woman this risk starts to increase at less than 2 drinks a day.[20] Women are more susceptible to illness and die at higher rates than men do for every cause of death associated with alcohol.

Rates of Alcohol Metabolism   Alcohol is metabolized more slowly than it is absorbed. This means that the concentration of alcohol builds when additional drinks are consumed before previous drinks have been metabolized. As a rule of thumb, people who have normal liver function metabolize about 0.5 ounce of alcohol (about one drink) per hour.[19]

Because of individual differences in sensitivity to alcohol, people experience impairment at different BAC levels. The National Highway Traffic Safety Administration reports that driving function can be impaired by BAC levels as low as .02–.04 percent.[6]

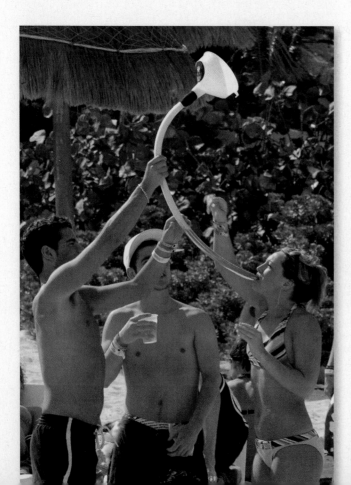

■ Spring break has traditionally been a time for extreme drinking accompanied by injury, property damage, and risky sexual encounters. Some colleges are establishing new, safer traditions.

Table 10.1 Stages of Acute Alcohol Influence/Intoxication

Blood Alcohol Concentration (grams/100 ml)	Physiological and Psychological Effects	Impaired Functions
0.01–0.05	Relaxation Sense of well being Loss of inhibition	Decreased alertness Impaired concentration Impaired judgment Impaired coordination (especially fine motor skills)
0.06–0.10	Euphoria Blunted feelings Nausea Sleepiness	Slower reflexes Impaired reasoning Impaired visual tracking Reduced depth perception
0.11–0.20	Emotional arousal Mood swings Anger or sadness Boisterousness	Slowed reaction time Staggering gait Slurred speech Impaired balance
0.21–0.30	Aggression Reduced sensations Depression Stupor	Lethargy Increased pain threshold Severe motor impairment Memory blackout
0.31–0.40	Unconsciousness Coma Death possible	Loss of bladder control Impaired temperature regulation Slowed breathing Slowed heart rate
0.41 and greater	Death	Respiratory arrest

Source: Adapted from "Information About Alcohol," Biological Sciences Curriculum Study, 2003, retrieved July 7, 2010, from http://science.education.nih.gov/supplements/nih3/alcohol/guide/info-alcohol.htm.

The behavioral effects of alcohol, based on studies of moderate drinkers, are summarized in Table 10.1. A person with a BAC of .08 percent is considered legally drunk in all states.

ACUTE ALCOHOL INTOXICATION

People who drink heavily in a relatively short time are vulnerable to **acute alcohol intoxication** (also called *acute alcohol shock* or *alcohol poisoning*), a potentially life-threatening BAC level. Acute alcohol intoxication can produce collapse of vital body functions, notably respiration and heart function, leading to coma and/or death (see the box "First Aid for Alcohol Poisoning").

Slow, steady drinking allows the vomiting reflex to be suppressed, and BAC can increase to dangerously high levels. At very high alcohol concentrations, .35 or greater, a person can become comatose, and death is possible. Some colleges have instituted "good Samaritan" rules that provide amnesty for students who seek help for themselves or others in a medical emergency in situations where drinking may have occurred in a residence hall room and/or where underage drinkers are present.

BLACKOUTS

A **blackout** is a period of time during which a drinker is conscious but has impaired memory function; later, he or she has amnesia about events that occurred during this time. The impairment is associated with changes in the hippocampus, a brain structure essential for memory and learning.[21] These changes may be temporary or permanent. Either way, a blackout is a warning sign

acute alcohol intoxication
A life-threatening blood alcohol concentration.

blackout
Period of time during which a drinker is conscious but has partial or complete amnesia for events.

First Aid for Alcohol Poisoning

People who have passed out from heavy drinking should be watched closely. All too often they are carried to bed and forgotten. For their safety, follow these measures:

- Know and recognize the symptoms of acute alcohol intoxication:
  - Lack of response when spoken to or shaken
  - Inability to wake up
  - Inability to stand up without help
  - Rapid or irregular pulse (100 beats per minute or more)
  - Rapid, irregular respiration or difficulty breathing (one breath every 3–4 seconds)
  - Cool, clammy, bluish skin
  - Bluish fingernails or lips

- Call 911. An intoxicated person who cannot be roused or wakened or has other symptoms listed above requires emergency medical treatment.

- Do not leave the person to "sleep it off." He or she may never awaken.

- Roll an unconscious drinker onto his or her side to minimize the chance of airway obstruction from vomit.

- If the person vomits, make certain his or her head is positioned lower than the rest of the body. You may need to reach into the person's mouth to clear the airway.

- Try to find out if the person has taken other drugs or medications that might interact with alcohol.

- Stay with the person until medical help arrives.

that fundamental changes have occurred in the structure of the brain.[22] Alcohol-induced blackouts are a common experience among nonalcoholics who binge drink. Some people may be genetically predisposed to experience blackouts.

HANGOVERS

Hangovers are characterized by headache, stomach upset, thirst, and fatigue. Health experts speculate that alcohol disrupts the body's water balance, causing excessive urination and thirst the next day. The stomach lining may be irritated by increased production of hydrochloric acid, resulting in nausea. Alcohol also reduces the water content of brain cells. When the brain cells rehydrate and swell the next day, nerve pain occurs. The only known remedy for a hangover is pain medication, rest, and time.

Health Risks of Alcohol Use

Alcohol is toxic and has an effect on virtually all body organs and systems as well as all aspects of a person's functioning.

MEDICAL PROBLEMS ASSOCIATED WITH ALCOHOL USE

The major organs and systems damaged by alcohol use are the cardiovascular system, the liver, the brain, the immune system, and the reproductive system (Figure 10.3). When pregnant women drink, it can cause a set of fetal birth defects known as **fetal alcohol syndrome (FAS)** (discussed in Chapter 13). Children born with FAS have permanent physical and mental impairments.

Heart Disease and Stroke   Chronic heavy drinking is a major cause of degenerative disease of the heart muscle, a condition called **cardiomyopathy**, and of heart arrhythmias (irregular heartbeat). Abnormal heart rhythm is one cause of sudden death in alcoholics, whether or not they already had heart disease. Heavy drinking also causes coronary heart disease (disease of the arteries serving the heart). In addition, long-term heavy drinking can elevate blood pressure and increase the severity of high blood pressure, which increases the risk for stroke (an interruption in the blood supply to the brain).

Liver Disease   Alcohol-related liver disease occurs in three phases. The first, called **fatty liver**, occurs when the liver is flooded with more alcohol than it can metabolize, causing it to swell with fat globules. This condition can literally develop overnight as a result of binge drinking. Fatty liver can be reversed with abstinence (usually about 30 days or so).

The second phase of liver disease is called **alcoholic hepatitis**, which includes liver inflammation and liver function impairment. This condition can occur in the absence of fatty liver, which suggests that direct toxic effects of alcohol may be the cause.[19]

The third phase of liver disease is **cirrhosis**, scarring of the liver tissue. Although other diseases can cause cirrhosis

fetal alcohol syndrome (FAS) Set of birth defects associated with use of alcohol during pregnancy.

cardiomyopathy Disease of the heart muscle.

fatty liver Condition in which the liver swells with fat globules as a result of alcohol consumption.

alcoholic hepatitis Inflammation of the liver as a result of alcohol consumption.

cirrhosis Scarring of the liver as a result of alcohol consumption.

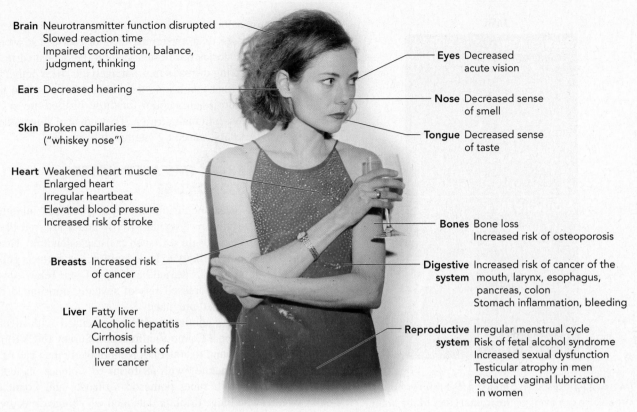

Brain Neurotransmitter function disrupted
Slowed reaction time
Impaired coordination, balance,
judgment, thinking

Ears Decreased hearing

Skin Broken capillaries
("whiskey nose")

Heart Weakened heart muscle
Enlarged heart
Irregular heartbeat
Elevated blood pressure
Increased risk of stroke

Breasts Increased risk
of cancer

Liver Fatty liver
Alcoholic hepatitis
Cirrhosis
Increased risk of
liver cancer

Eyes Decreased
acute vision

Nose Decreased sense
of smell

Tongue Decreased sense
of taste

Bones Bone loss
Increased risk of osteoporosis

Digestive Increased risk of cancer of the
system mouth, larynx, esophagus,
pancreas, colon
Stomach inflammation, bleeding

Reproductive Irregular menstrual cycle
system Risk of fetal alcohol syndrome
Increased sexual dysfunction
Testicular atrophy in men
Reduced vaginal lubrication
in women

figure **10.3** **Effects of alcohol on the body.**

(such as viral hepatitis), between 40 and 90 percent of people with cirrhosis have a history of alcohol abuse.[19] The risk rises sharply with higher levels of consumption. It usually takes at least 10 years of steady, heavy drinking for cirrhosis to develop.[19]

As cirrhosis sets in, liver cells are replaced by fibrous tissue, called collagen, which changes the structure of the liver and decreases blood flow to the organ. Liver cells die and liver function is impaired, leading to fluid accumulation in the body, jaundice (yellowing of the skin), and an opportunity for infections or cancers to establish themselves. The prognosis for people with alcoholic hepatitis or cirrhosis is poor.

Cancer Alcohol is associated with several types of cancer, particularly cancers of the head and neck (mouth, pharynx, larynx, and esophagus), cancers of the digestive tract, and breast cancer.[6] Alcohol causes inflammation of the pancreas, but the link between this inflammation and pancreatic cancer remains unproven. Substantial evidence from many countries suggests that the risk of breast cancer increases for women who consume more than three drinks per day compared with women who abstain.[6]

Brain Damage Heavy alcohol consumption causes anatomical changes in the brain and directly damages brain cells. Alcohol can cause a loss of brain tissue, inflammation of the brain, and a widening of fissures in the cortex (covering) of the brain.[21] Heavy drinking, especially binge drinking, has been shown to disrupt short-term memory and the ability to analyze complex problems.[19]

In long-term alcohol abuse, loss of brain tissue is associated with a mental disorder called alcohol-induced persisting dementia, an overall decline in intellect. Some of this loss may be reversible if the person abstains from alcohol use for a few months, but after age 40, there is little improvement even with abstinence.[21]

Because the brain continues to grow and mature until the early 20s, there is concern that heavy alcohol use during the teen years can be harmful to the developing brain. Studies have revealed that the hippocampus (a center for learning and memory) is 10 percent smaller in teenagers who drink heavily than in those who don't.[21] Research has also found differences in the prefrontal cortex, the center for executive functions (rational thinking, planning).

Body Weight and Nutrition A regular beer has about 144 calories; a glass of wine, 100–105 calories; and a shot of gin or whiskey, 96 calories.[23] Mixers add more calories, as do *alcopops* or *malternatives*—sugary, fizzy, fruit-flavored drinks popular among younger drinkers (see the box "Malternatives: 'Starter' Beverages for Young Drinkers").

MRI

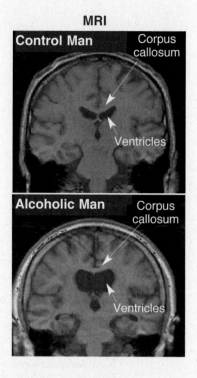

This magnetic resonance imaging (MRI) shows how chronic alcohol use can damage the frontal lobes of the brain, increase the size of the ventricles, and cause an overall reduction in brain size (shrinkage).

These calories are empty, providing almost no nutrients. It's easy to see that consuming alcohol can lead to weight gain; these calories have a tendency to be deposited in the abdomen, giving drinkers the characteristic "beer belly."

On the other hand, long-term heavy drinkers who substitute the calories in alcohol for those in food are at risk for weight loss and malnutrition. They are also vulnerable to mental disorders caused by vitamin deficiencies.

SOCIAL PROBLEMS ASSOCIATED WITH ALCOHOL USE

Alcohol reduces social inhibitions, and reduced inhibition may lead to high-risk sexual activity and a lowered likelihood of practicing safe sex (such as using a condom). Heavy drinkers are more likely to have multiple sex partners and to engage in other risky sexual behaviors. These behaviors are associated with increased risk of sexually transmitted disease and unplanned pregnancy.[24]

Violence is another problem associated with alcohol use. The National Crime Victimization Survey (NCVS) has consistently found that alcohol is more likely than any other drug to be associated with all forms of violence, including robbery, assault, rape, domestic violence, and homicide. Women who binge drink or date men who binge drink are at increased risk for sexual exploitation (rape and other forms of nonconsensual sex).[25]

Consumer Clipboard

Malternatives: "Starter" Beverages for Young Drinkers

A new kind of beverage hit the shelves of convenience stores and liquor outlets in the mid-1990s—fruit-flavored alcoholic beverages with names like Skyblue, Smirnoff Ice, Tequiza, Snakebite, Moscow Mule, Hard Lemonade, and Wild Brew. Called "malternatives" or "alcopops," these drinks are malt based and contain 5 to 7 percent alcohol, about the same as beer.

Although alcohol manufacturers claim they market these beverages to 18- to 25-year-olds, the popularity of malternatives peaks for consumers between ages 13 and 16. Forty-one percent of teens say they have tried malternatives. Manufacturers use vibrant colors, rebellious or sexy names, and cartoon characters to target youth. Teens find malternatives appealing because they are more refreshing, taste less like alcohol, and are easy to get and cheap. (What they may not know is that malternatives are loaded with calories; most contain more calories than a Krispy Kreme donut.) Young people are much less likely to have experienced or understand the potentially harmful effects of alcohol on the body, especially the maturing brain. As teens get older, they tend to switch to more mature types of alcoholic beverages.

Why should we be concerned about malternatives? Alcohol is the leading drug problem in the United States, killing six times as many teenagers as are killed by the use of illicit drugs. People who drink before age 15 are four times more likely to develop alcohol dependence than are those who wait until age 21. The U.S. Department of Justice estimates that underage drinking costs more than $53 billion every year by contributing to injuries, violence, rape, and other crime.

Health authorities are calling for tighter regulation of these "starter" alcoholic beverages. They want to make them less appealing to teenagers by revising names, packaging, and labeling so that they more closely resemble other alcoholic drinks. Labels would clearly and conspicuously identify them as alcoholic beverages and disclose their alcohol content. Consumer organizations have petitioned the Alcohol and Tobacco Tax and Trade Bureau to require "Alcohol Facts" labels on every alcoholic beverage container, including alcopops.

Source: "Alcohol Policies Project Issue: Alcopops," Center for Science in the Public Interest, retrieved April 20, 2008, from www.cspinet.org/booze/iss_alcopops.htm.

The relationship between alcohol and risk of injury has been established for a variety of circumstances, including automobile crashes, falls, and fires. Reduced cognitive function, impaired physical coordination, and increased risk-taking behavior (impulsivity) are the alcohol-related factors that lead to injury.

Alcohol use is also a factor in about one-third of suicides, and it is second only to depression as a predictor of suicide attempts by youth.[19] The relationship between alcohol and depression is very strong. Estimates are that 20–36 percent of people who commit suicide were drinking shortly before their suicide or had a history of alcohol abuse.[26] Alcohol-associated suicides tend to be impulsive rather than premeditated acts.

is associated with more deaths from injuries and accidents. It is not recommended that anyone begin drinking or drink more frequently because of anticipated health benefits.

ALCOHOL MISUSE, ABUSE, AND DEPENDENCE

Alcohol misuse refers to the consumption of alcohol to the point where it causes physical, social, and moral harm to the drinker. **Problem drinking** is a pattern of alcohol use that impairs the drinker's life, causing personal difficulties and difficulties for other people. For college students, such difficulties might be missed classes or poor academic performance. **Alcohol abuse** is defined as the continued use of

Alcohol is more likely than any other drug to be associated with **all forms of violence.**

ANOTHER VIEW: HEALTH BENEFITS

Moderate alcohol consumption appears to be associated with a lowered risk of heart disease. Scientists speculate that consumption at moderate levels increases high-density lipoproteins (HDL, also called "good cholesterol"), has an anti-clotting effect on the blood, and reduces stress.[27] The beneficial effects of alcohol on HDL levels and blood clotting may be only temporary, lasting perhaps 24 hours, so that people who drink moderately every day maintain optimal protection against heart disease. It is apparently the pattern of drinking, not the type of alcoholic beverage, that confers benefits. People who drink wine, for example, tend to do so in small amounts every day rather than in large amounts. Binge drinking does not serve as a protective factor and can actually increase the risk for heart disease.[4] In women, the beneficial effects may be offset by an increased risk of breast cancer.

The *Dietary Guidelines for Americans* advises that moderate alcohol consumption— one drink a day for women and two drinks a day for men—can be beneficial for middle-aged and older adults, the age groups most susceptible to coronary heart disease. In younger adults, however, alcohol appears to have fewer, if any, health benefits, and it

alcohol despite negative consequences. It is a pattern of drinking that leads to impairment in the person's ability to fulfill major obligations at home, work, or school or to legal or social problems.[28]

Alcohol dependence is characterized by a strong craving for alcohol. People who are dependent on alcohol use it compulsively, and most will eventually experience physiological changes in brain and body chemistry as a result of alcohol use. As described in Chapter 3, one indicator of dependence is the development of *tolerance*, reduced sensitivity to the effects of a drug so that larger and larger amounts are needed to produce the same effects.[19] Another indicator is experiencing *withdrawal*, a state of acute physical and psychological discomfort, when alcohol consumption stops abruptly.

Alcohol dependence is also known as **alcoholism**, defined as a chronic disease with genetic, psychosocial, and environmental causes.[28] It is often progressive and fatal. About one in four heavy drinkers or at-risk drinkers is defined as an alcoholic or alcohol abuser. The manifestations of alcoholism include lack of control over drinking, preoccupation with alcohol, use of alcohol despite adverse consequences, and distortions in thinking (most notably denial).

problem drinking
Pattern of alcohol use that impairs the drinker's life, causing difficulties for the drinker and for others.

alcohol abuse
Pattern of alcohol use that leads to distress or impairment, increases the risk of health and/or social problems, and continues despite awareness of these effects.

alcohol dependence
Disorder characterized by a strong craving for alcohol, the development of tolerance for alcohol, and symptoms of withdrawal if alcohol consumption stops abruptly.

alcoholism
A primary chronic disease characterized by excessive, compulsive drinking.

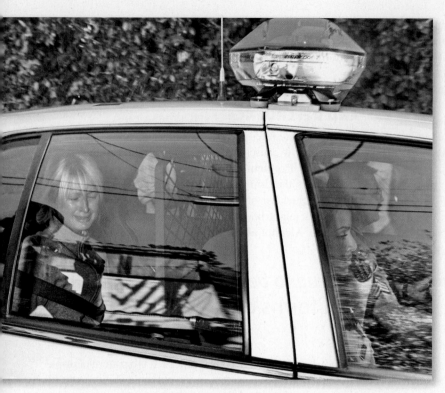

■ Paris Hilton was arrested in 2006 on charges of driving under the influence of alcohol. She pled no contest and was sentenced to three years' probation, paid a $1,500 fine, and had to attend an alcohol education program. A typical DUI case can cost $10,000 once lawyer fees, insurance costs, and bail money are factored in.

This definition is similar to that of problem drinking, but there is a difference in degree. Alcohol becomes a problem when individuals are impaired by their drinking, but drinkers become alcoholics when they become dependent on alcohol.

Treatment Options

Treatment options for alcohol-related disorders include brief interventions, inpatient treatment programs, outpatient treatment programs, and self-help approaches.

BRIEF INTERVENTIONS FOR HIGH-RISK YOUNG ADULT DRINKERS

Almost half of those individuals who develop alcohol dependence have alcohol abuse problems before age 21. Many colleges and universities focus their high-risk programs on freshmen, athletes, fraternity members, and, more recently, gay men, lesbians, and transgendered individuals. Programs are also directed at high-risk times and events such as spring break, fraternity rushing, homecoming, and pre-graduation events for seniors. See the box "Curbing College Drinking: What Needs to Change?" for more on campuswide efforts to control alcohol use.

The Alcohol Skills Training Program is a model brief intervention program adapted by many colleges and community-based organizations around the country. It is designed for college students and other young adults considered at risk for alcohol-related problems, such as poor class attendance and grades, accidents, sexual assault, and violence. It consists of a series of group sessions (usually six to eight) focusing on skills and knowledge development through lectures, discussion, and role plays.

The Brief Alcohol Screening and Intervention for College Students (BASICS) program is another brief intervention model for college students who drink heavily and have experienced or are at risk for alcohol-related problems. BASICS is conducted in two 50-minute interviews and includes personalized feedback on the effects and consequences of alcohol use, strategies for reducing risks and making better decisions, and options that can help students make changes. Students who receive BASICS report fewer consequences and more rapid changes in their alcohol-related behavior and consequences than at-risk drinkers who do not receive the intervention.[29]

INPATIENT TREATMENT

When alcohol-related problems are severe, individuals benefit from placement in a residential facility specializing in alcohol recovery. The first stage of treatment is detoxification, the gradual withdrawal of alcohol from the body. Withdrawal symptoms include profuse sweating, rapid heart rate, elevated blood pressure, nausea, headache, difficulty sleeping, depression, and irritability.[30] People who have been heavy drinkers for a long time and/or who have an underlying medical condition may experience more severe withdrawal symptoms, such as seizures and, rarely, a disturbance called **delirium tremens (DTs)** characterized by disorientation and hallucinations. An acute DT episode is a medical emergency requiring hospitalization.

delirium tremens (DTs)
Severe condition characterized by delirium, disorientation, and hallucinations, associated with withdrawal from alcohol.

The early phase of alcohol treatment may also include medications, such as anti-anxiety drugs and antidepressants. Another drug that may be prescribed is disulfiram (Antabuse). This drug causes a person to become acutely nauseated if any alcohol is consumed, although it does not reduce alcohol cravings.[19] Researchers are exploring drugs that increase levels of the neurotransmitter serotonin as a way to reduce cravings and relapse.[14] Naltrexone, for example, is a drug that lessens alcohol craving by blocking opioid receptors in the brain.

Highlight on Health

Curbing College Drinking: What Needs to Change?

Campuswide approaches to reducing high-risk drinking usually focus on either making the college community a less hospitable environment for drinking or changing student perception about alcohol use on campus.

Schools that have banned alcohol have not removed its presence entirely, but they have seen fewer students binge drink, and to a greater degree, nondrinking students have experienced fewer secondhand effects from others' drinking than at schools without alcohol bans.

One program, called "A Matter of Degree," has seen a small measure of success at campuses that have implemented its guidelines, although the program's approach, which does not seek to change student attitudes about drinking, remains controversial. Ten participating schools, including Florida State University and the Universities of Colorado and Wisconsin, implemented measures that sought to alter campus conditions that promoted heavy drinking, which included requiring keg registration, increasing oversight of fraternities and sororities and alcohol outlets, instituting parental notification policies, and offering more substance-free housing. The five schools that implemented the most components of the program saw small decreases in alcohol consumption and alcohol-related harm, but there was no change reported at the five schools that implemented fewer measures. Critics of the program say that measures need to focus on the students themselves, that drinking patterns cannot change unless students themselves change their habits and attitudes about drinking.

Some college campuses have tried to change students' misperceptions about how much their peers are drinking. Students often think that more drinking occurs on their campus than actually does, and as a result, students feel pressured to do more drinking themselves. One successful program targeted student athletes at an undergraduate college. Athletes received factual information about the amount of drinking done by their peers (such as "The majority (66%) of [this school's] student-athletes drink alcohol once per week or less often or do not drink at all") and their peers' attitudes about drinking (such as "88% of student-athletes at [this school] believe one should never drink to an intoxicating level that interferes with academics or other responsibilities") via posters, email, and other mediums. This specific program was found to be effective; there was a 30 percent reduction in high-quantity alcohol consumption and negative consequences of drinking among the athletes who had high exposure to the program. However, more generalized programs have not resulted in lowered rates of drinking.

The dichotomy between changing student perceptions and attitudes, on the one hand, and changing the alcohol-related campus culture, on the other, may be a false one. Ideally, the best solution may be to combine the two approaches, considering both individual factors and broader social and environmental factors. What approaches are used on your campus?

Sources: "What We Have Learned from the Harvard School of Public Health College Alcohol Study: Focusing Attention on College Student Alcohol Consumption and the Environmental Conditions That Promote It," by H. Wechsler and T.F. Nelson, 2008, Journal of Studies on Alcohol and Drugs 69 (4), pp. 481–490; "A Successful Social Norms Campaign to Reduce Alcohol Misuse Among College Student-Athletes," by H.W. Perkins and D.W. Craig, 2006, Journal of Studies on Alcohol, 67 (6), pp. 880–889.

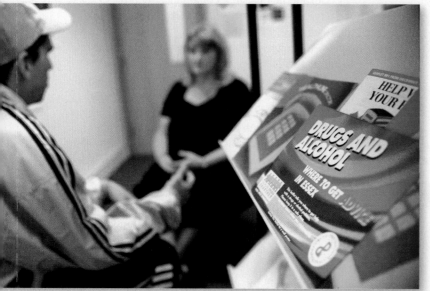

■ Brief intervention programs for high-risk young adult drinkers include counseling sessions that help individuals see the consequences of alcohol use and develop strategies for change.

Programs typically include education about alcohol and drugs, skills training, and group and individual counseling. Family members are often encouraged to participate in the recovery process.

OUTPATIENT TREATMENT

In outpatient programs, patients participate in a treatment program during the day and return home in the evening. Treatment typically includes individual counseling, group counseling, and marital or family counseling. Research suggests that outpatient programs are as effective as, or more effective than, inpatient programs.[6]

SELF-HELP PROGRAMS

The best-known self-help program is Alcoholics Anonymous (AA). The goal of AA is total abstinence from alcohol. A basic premise of AA is that an alcoholic is biologically different from a nonalcoholic and consequently can never safely drink any alcohol at all. Key components of AA are progression through a 12-step path to recovery, reliance on one's "higher power" (whatever the person considers to be a power greater than him- or herself, whether a divine being, nature, or even the AA community itself), and group support.

Some people are uncomfortable with AA's focus on spirituality, and alternative programs have been developed that do not have this focus. One such group is Rational Recovery, which focuses on self rather than spirituality. Another objection to AA is its perceived masculine orientation, and alternative programs have been developed by and for women, such as Women for Sobriety. Although AA dominates self-help programs for alcoholism, it has not been shown to be more effective than some of these alternative programs.[6]

Self-help programs have also been developed for family members and friends of alcoholics. Al-Anon is a support program whereby individuals can explore how they may have enabled the alcoholic's behavior (for example, by covering up or rationalizing) and how they can change their behavior. Alateen is a support program for young people who have been affected by someone else's drinking. Adult Children of Alcoholics is a program that provides a supportive environment where people can confront the potentially lifelong emotional effects associated with growing up in an alcoholic household.

RELAPSE PREVENTION

Recovery from alcoholism is a lifelong process. The difficulty of recovery is thought to be due to the changes that alcohol has produced in the brain. The brain's circuitry has been reprogrammed such that pleasure has become associated primarily with alcohol. Relapse prevention focuses on social skills training (stress management, assertiveness,

communication skills, self-control) and family and marital therapy. Despite a high relapse rate, those who participate in treatment programs do better than those who do not.

THE HARM REDUCTION APPROACH

The **harm reduction** approach to treatment focuses on reducing the harm associated with drinking, both to the individual and to society. An example of harm reduction is **controlled drinking**, which emphasizes moderation rather than abstinence.[31]

Some experts fear that making controlled drinking an option for alcoholism treatment will cause a stampede of patients away from abstinence programs, although research has not shown that this happens.[32] Most mental health experts agree that total abstinence is the most effective approach for recovery from alcoholism.[26] Controlled drinking is considered appropriate for early-stage problem drinkers.[33]

harm reduction
Approach to alcohol treatment that focuses on a broader range of drinking behaviors and treatments than those associated with abstinence programs.

controlled drinking
Approach to drinking that emphasizes moderation rather than abstinence.

PUBLIC POLICIES AND LAWS AIMED AT HARM REDUCTION

A variety of public policies and laws are aimed at reducing the harm caused by alcohol consumption. A prime example is the minimum drinking age.

Since 1984, all states have had laws prohibiting the purchase and public possession of alcohol by people under the age of 21. Despite inconsistent compliance with these laws, research suggests that they result in less underage drinking than occurred when the drinking age was 18.[34] Evidence also suggests that these laws result in less drinking after age 21.[6]

A practice that substantially increases compliance with drunk driving laws is the use of sobriety checkpoints. Law enforcement agents check drivers for intoxication with alcohol sensors and breath analyzer tests. Alcohol sensors are noninvasive tests that can detect the presence of alcohol on the breath when held in the vicinity of a driver. Breath analyzer tests measure the amount of alcohol exhaled in the breath.

One approach to reducing alcohol consumption involves restrictions on liquor sales and outlets. The more places there are to purchase alcohol within a

Breath analysis and sobriety checkpoints are public health measures designed to reduce the harm to self and others associated with alcohol use.

certain geographical area, the higher the rates of alcohol consumption and alcohol-related harm.[5] Some communities have worked for a more even distribution of alcohol outlets throughout their area to curb this problem. Although parents and other adults are the most common source for underage drinkers, they also buy alcoholic beverages at convenience stores, liquor stores, and bars.[35] Recently, the Internet has become a source for underage purchase of alcoholic beverages, although regulations are being put in place to curb this practice.

Another way to control alcohol consumption is by increasing taxation. Research suggests that an increase in the price of alcohol is met by a corresponding decrease in consumption per capita. Higher prices appear to reduce consumption by underage and moderate drinkers but not by heavy drinkers. Raising prices too much might also create a black market for alcoholic beverages.[6,34,35]

Finally, local communities have a variety of measures at their disposal for influencing alcohol consumption, including limiting drink specials at local bars, prohibiting out-of-sight sales (purchases made by one person for several others), imposing a minimum drink price, enforcing fines, revoking liquor licenses, and controlling house parties.[36] Research suggests that comprehensive community programs that unite city agencies and private citizens are effective in reducing drunk driving, related driving risks, and traffic deaths and injuries.[6]

Taking Action

Is alcohol a problem in your life? Do you wonder what you can do to reduce or prevent harm from alcohol-related activities? In this section we provide some suggestions for individual actions.

ARE YOU AT RISK?

Physicians sometimes use the CAGE questionnaire to identify individuals at risk for alcohol problems:

C: Have you ever tried to *cut down* on your drinking?

A: Have you ever been *annoyed* by criticism of your drinking?

G: Have you ever felt *guilty* about your drinking?

E: Have you ever had a morning *"eye-opener"*?

A yes answer to one or more of these question suggests that you may be at risk for alcohol dependence.

DEVELOPING A BEHAVIOR CHANGE PLAN

If you decide you would like to change your behavior around alcohol, you can develop a behavior change plan to do so. First, keep track of when, how much, and with whom you drink for 2 weeks, and then analyze your record to discover your drinking patterns. Do you drink mostly on weekends,

Challenges & Choices

Tips for Changing Your Alcohol-Related Behavior

- Stock your refrigerator with healthy beverages—juice, bottled water, milk, sports drinks, diet soda.

- If you want to have alcoholic beverages on hand, buy small quantities—one or two bottles of beer rather than a six-pack, for example.

- If you drink when you're upset, lonely, or stressed out, learn how to handle these feelings in a healthier way, such as by exercising, meditating, or talking with a friend or counselor.

- If you drink when you're with other people, learn how to socialize without alcohol; try hiking or playing sports with friends, or attend alcohol-free events.

- If others are pressuring you to drink, learn how to say no.

- When you are drinking, keep your BAC low by drinking slowly, drinking water and nonalcoholic beverages along with alcoholic ones, eating food, and staying within your limits; avoid mixed or carbonated drinks.

- When you are the host, provide food and nonalcoholic beverages, and make sure no one who drives away from your house at the end of the party is drunk or impaired.

or do you drink every day? Do you drink mostly with certain people, or do you drink alone? Do you drink when you're under stress? Information like this can help you get a sense of the role alcohol plays in your life.

If you decide you want to change your drinking behavior, set goals for yourself. Goals should be specific, motivating, achievable, and rewarding. "I'm going to drink less" is too vague a goal. "I'm going to drink only once a week and have no more than four drinks" is a more specific, measurable goal.

Then develop specific strategies to attain your goals. For example, if you drink in social situations or with certain people, learn to say no to some drinks. Tell people you feel better when you don't drink, and avoid people who can't accept that. Plan ahead what you will do when you're tempted to have a drink. Ask family and friends for their support. For more suggestions, see the box "Tips for Changing Your Alcohol-Related Behavior."

After a few weeks, evaluate the outcome of your behavior change plan. Did you achieve your goals? If not, what obstacles prevented you from succeeding? How can you overcome these obstacles? Periodically assessing your progress allows you to devise alternative strategies for reaching your goals.

BE AN ADVOCATE

If you are interested in addressing irresponsible alcohol consumption, you can join an advocacy organization or concerned citizens group on your campus or in your community. Mothers Against Drunk Driving (MADD) is a nationwide advocacy organization with hundreds of local chapters throughout North America. It was founded to educate citizens about the effects of alcohol on driving and to influence legislation on drunk driving. Students Against Destructive Decisions (SADD) initially focused on drunk driving by youth but has broadened its activities to include initiatives against underage drinking, illicit drug use, failure to use seat belts, and drugged driving.

Boost Alcohol Consciousness Concerning the Health of University Students (BACCHUS) is a nonprofit organization with hundreds of chapters across North America. It is run by student volunteers and promotes both abstinence and responsible drinking. Some BACCHUS chapters have joined with Greeks Advocating Mature Management of Alcohol (GAMMA) to provide a peer education network. This network program may be called BACCHUS or GAMMA on your college campus. The merging of BACCHUS and GAMMA has led to a broadening of approaches to health issues that affect college students.

Understanding Tobacco Use

Like alcohol, tobacco poses a problem for society. Adults are free to use it, but such use causes an array of health problems, both for users and for those around them. Tobacco use is the leading preventable cause of death in the United States, implicated in a host of diseases and debilitating conditions. The health hazards of tobacco use are well known, yet one in five Americans smokes, and nearly 4,000 young people under the age of 18 start smoking every day.[37]

WHO SMOKES? PATTERNS OF TOBACCO USE

About 20.6 percent of the adult population of the United States 18 years old or over are smokers. The percentage of Americans who smoke is down from a high of nearly 42 percent in 1965. The decline since then has occurred largely as a result of public health campaigns about the hazards of smoking. Although the prevalence of smoking in the United States continues to decline, the rate of decline has slowed since 1990.[38]

Smoking is more prevalent among men than women and rates of smoking are higher among young people than among older people. Most smokers get hooked in adolescence—more than 90 percent of smokers begin smoking before the age of 21.[37]

Currently, college students are more likely than the general population to smoke. Overall, however, cigarette smoking is negatively correlated with educational attainment. Adults with less than a high school education are three times as likely as those who graduate from college to smoke.[3]

Other psychosocial factors that increase the likelihood that a person will smoke include having a parent or sibling who smokes, associating with peers who smoke, being from a lower socioeconomic status family, doing poorly in school, and having positive attitudes about tobacco.

Smoking is more prevalent among the White population than among African Americans, Hispanics, or Asian Americans and Pacific Islanders.[8] The highest rates of smoking occur among American Indians and Alaska Natives.[39,40]

Smoking rates can vary tremendously among groups within broad ethnic categories. For example, despite low rates of smoking overall among Asian Americans and Pacific Islanders, rates are very high among some of the 50 distinct ethnic groups that fall under this umbrella label. Among

■ The vast majority of smokers start when they are teenagers, like actress Taylor Momsen, who was 16 years old when this photo was taken. Many young smokers don't realize they are addicted to nicotine until they try to quit.

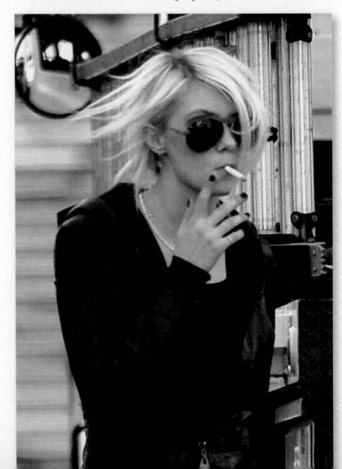

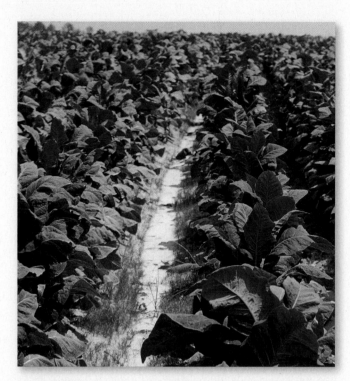

■ Tobacco use originated in the Americas, where it was used ceremonially and medicinally by native populations. By 1600, it was being exported to Europe and Asia. Today, tobacco is still an important crop in Virginia, Kentucky, North and South Carolina, and other southeastern states.

Cambodian American men, for example, the smoking rate is 71 percent. Clearly, behaviors like smoking are influenced by sociocultural factors, including acculturation and access to health information and health care.

TOBACCO PRODUCTS

Tobacco is a broad-leafed plant that grows in tropical and temperate climates. Tobacco leaves are harvested, dried, and processed in different ways for the variety of tobacco products—rolled into cigars, shredded for cigarettes, ground into a fine powder for inhalation as snuff, or ground into a chewable form and used as smokeless tobacco.

Substances in Tobacco   When tobacco leaves are burned, thousands of substances are produced, and nearly 70 of them have been identified as carcinogenic (cancer causing). The most harmful substances are tar, carbon monoxide, and nicotine.

Tar is a thick, sticky residue that contains many of the carcinogenic substances in tobacco smoke. Tar coats the smoker's lungs and creates an environment conducive to the growth of cancerous cells. Tar is responsible for many of the changes in the respiratory system that cause the hacking "smoker's cough."

One of the most hazardous gaseous compounds in burning tobacco is carbon monoxide, the same toxic gas emitted from the exhaust pipe of a car. Carbon monoxide interferes with the ability of red blood cells to carry oxygen, so that vital body organs, such as the heart, are deprived of oxygen. Many of the other gases produced when tobacco burns are carcinogens, irritants, and toxic chemicals that damage the lungs.

Nicotine is the primary addictive ingredient in tobacco. It is carried into the body in the form of thousands of droplets suspended in solid particles of partially burned tobacco. These droplets are so tiny that they penetrate the alveoli (small air sacs in the lungs) and enter the bloodstream, reaching body cells within seconds.

Nicotine is both a poison (it is used as a pesticide) and a powerful psychoactive drug. The first time it is used, it usually produces dizziness, light-headedness, and nausea, signs of mild nicotine poisoning. These effects diminish as tolerance grows. Nicotine causes a cascade of stimulant effects throughout the body by triggering the release of adrenaline, which increases arousal, alertness, and concentration. Nicotine also stimulates the release of endorphins, the body's "natural opiates" that block pain and produce mild sensations of pleasure. (We discuss the effects of nicotine in greater detail later in the chapter.)

tar
Thick, sticky residue formed when tobacco leaves burn, containing hundreds of chemical compounds and carcinogenic substances.

nicotine
Primary addictive ingredient in tobacco; a poison and a psychoactive drug.

Cigarettes   By far the most popular tobacco product is cigarettes, followed by cigars and chewing tobacco. Cigarettes account for nearly 95 percent of the tobacco market in the United States.[38] Nicotine from a cigarette reaches peak concentration in the blood in about 10 minutes and is reduced by half within about 20 minutes, as the drug is distributed to body tissues. Rapid absorption and distribution of nicotine enable the smoker to control the peaks and valleys of nicotine absorption and effect. This process of control—absorption, distribution, elimination—makes cigarettes an effective drug-delivery system for nicotine.[41]

In 2009 the U.S. Congress passed the Family Smoking Prevention and Tobacco Control Act, which banned a variety of once-legal cigarettes. Fruit- and candy-flavored cigarettes are now prohibited due to concerns that they appealed particularly to children. Clove cigarettes, which contain higher levels of tar and nicotine than regular cigarettes, and bidis, small cigarettes made from unprocessed tobacco and which also contain higher levels of tar and nicotine than regular cigarettes, were also banned by the act.

The Electronic cigarette, or e-cigarette, is a newcomer to the market. It is a battery-powered device that provides inhaled doses of nicotine by heating a nicotine chemical solution into a vapor, which the smoker inhales. The vapor provides a flavor and physical sensation similar to that of inhaled tobacco smoke. Most e-cigarettes are reusable devices with replaceable and refillable parts. They produce no tar, burning, real smoke, or air pollution. They are virtually odorless and do not cause teeth discoloration as traditional cigarettes do. Although e-cigarettes are marketed as a safer alternative to regular cigarettes, they still contain tobacco-specific organic compounds, nicotine, and other potential carcinogenic chemicals. The Food and Drug Administration (FDA) disputes claims by manufacturers that e-cigarettes are safer than regular cigarettes and discourages their use, particularly since they do not bear health warnings and are often marketed to young adults and to people who have never smoked.[42] The legal status of e-cigarettes varies by country. Manufacturers of e-cigarettes have filed a lawsuit that challenges the authority of the FDA to regulate e-cigarettes.

Hookahs, or water pipes, have recently become popular among college students and other young adults as a supposedly safe alternative to cigarettes. Groups of smokers pass the mouthpiece around, inhaling *shisah*, a mixture of tobacco, molasses, and fruit flavors. The aromatic flavors of hookah tobacco and the smooth smoke produced by the water pipe, which is less irritating to the throat than cigarette smoke, have driven the perception that hookah use is safe. The World Health Organization and the CDC warn that hookah use can pose even greater dangers than cigarette smoking.

Cigars   Cigars have more tobacco and nicotine per unit than cigarettes do, take longer to smoke, and generate more smoke and more harmful combustion products than cigarettes do. The tobacco mix used in cigars makes it easier for cigar smoke to be absorbed through the mucous membranes of the oral cavity than is the case with cigarettes. Nicotine absorbed via this route takes longer to reach the brain than nicotine absorbed in the lungs and has a less intense but longer lasting effect.

Cigar smokers who do not inhale have lower mortality rates than cigar smokers who do.[16] Inhalation substantially increases the cigar smoker's exposure to carcinogenic chemicals and increases the risk for lung cancer and chronic respiratory disease.[43]

Whether or not smoke is inhaled, cigar smoking exposes the oral mucosa to large amounts of carcinogenic chemicals; consequently, cigar smokers have a higher risk than cigarette smokers for oral cancers.

Black & Mild is a brand of "little cigars" or cigarillos that are popular among teens and young adults. Black & Milds are long and thin like a cigarette but wrapped in tobacco leaf rather than paper, like a cigar. The difference in wrapping means they are not subject to certain cigarette regulations and taxes. Black & Mild little cigars contain more tobacco and more nicotine than cigarettes and are addictive if inhaled. Use of Black & Mild cigars is much higher among African Americans (54 percent) than in any other ethnic group.

Pipes   Pipe smoke has more toxins than cigarette smoke does and is more irritating to the respiratory system. Pipe smokers who do not inhale are at less risk for lung cancer and heart disease than cigarette smokers are. Like cigar smokers, however, pipe smokers are exposed to more toxins than cigarette smokers. Pipe smokers are just as likely as cigarette smokers to develop cancer of the mouth, larynx, throat, and esophagus.[44]

Smokeless Tobacco   *Snuff* is a powdered form of tobacco that can be inhaled through the nose or placed between the bottom teeth and lower lip. *Chewing tobacco* is used by lodging a cud or pinch of smokeless tobacco between the cheek and gum. It is available as loose leaf or as a plug (a compressed, flavored bar of processed tobacco). Smokeless tobacco is sometimes called *spit tobacco* because users spit out the tobacco juices and saliva that accumulate in the mouth.

Tobacco does not have to burn to cause health hazards. Spit tobacco contains at least 28 carcinogens, and use of spit tobacco is believed to cause about 10–15 percent of oral cancers, leading to about 6,000 deaths each year. When spit tobacco is kept in contact with the oral mucosa, it can cause *dysplasia*, an abnormal change in cells, and *oral lesions*, whitish patches on the tongue or mouth that may become cancerous. Spit tobacco also causes gum disease, tooth decay and discoloration, and bad breath.[45–48] The amount of nicotine absorbed from smokeless tobacco is two to three times greater than that delivered by cigarettes.

Snus is a smokeless tobacco that is being marketed as a safer alternative to cigarettes. It is made from tobacco mixed with water, salt, sodium carbonate, and aroma and is often packaged in small bags resembling teabags. It is produced and sold mainly in Sweden and Norway but is being

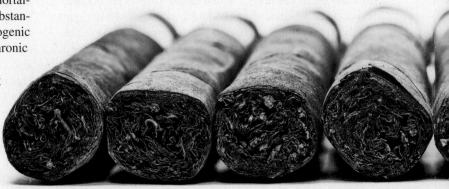

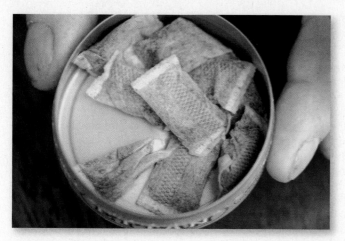

Snus is a form of smokeless tobacco produced in Sweden and Norway, where it is marketed as a safe way to enjoy tobacco. Users place one of the small prepackaged bags under the upper lip and leave it there for an extended period of time.

test-marketed in other countries, including the United States. Snus contains more nicotine than cigarettes but lower levels of other dangerous compounds, and since it isn't burned, there is no secondhand smoke. Users have lower rates of certain cancers, but snus may cause oral lesions, hypertension, and complications of pregnancy.[47]

Why Do People Smoke?

Tobacco use and its relationship to health are complex issues that involve nicotine addiction, behavioral dependence, and aggressive marketing by tobacco companies, among other factors.

NICOTINE ADDICTION

Nicotine is a highly addictive psychoactive drug—some health experts believe it is the most addictive of all the psychoactive drugs—and tobacco products are very efficient delivery devices for this drug. Once in the brain, nicotine follows the same pleasure and reward pathway that other psychoactive drugs follow (see Chapter 11). Increases in release of the neurotransmitter dopamine produce feelings of pleasure and a desire to repeat the experience. As noted earlier, nicotine also affects alertness, energy, and mood by increasing levels of endorphins and other neurotransmitters, including serotonin and norepinephrine.

With continued smoking, neurons become more sensitive and responsive to nicotine, causing *addiction*, or dependence on a steady supply of the drug; *tolerance*, or reduced responsiveness to its effects; and *withdrawal* symptoms if it is not present (see the box "Ramiro: An Occasional Smoker"). Nicotine withdrawal symptoms include irritability, anxiety, depressed mood, difficulty concentrating, restlessness, decreased heart rate, increased appetite, and increased craving for nicotine.

More than two-thirds of cigarette smokers who attempt to quit relapse within two days, unable to tolerate the period when withdrawal symptoms are at their peak. It takes about two weeks for a person's brain chemistry to return to normal. Withdrawal symptoms decrease and become more subtle with prolonged abstinence, but some smokers continue to experience intermittent cravings for years. Smoking tobacco may cause permanent changes in the nervous system, which may explain why some people who haven't smoked in years can become addicted again after smoking a single cigarette.[49–51]

BEHAVIORAL DEPENDENCE

People who smoke are not just physiologically dependent on a substance; they also become psychologically dependent on the habit of smoking. Through repeated paired associations, the effects of nicotine on the brain are linked to places, people, and events. Tobacco companies design their advertising to take advantage of these associations. Many smokers have a harder time imagining their future life without cigarettes than they do dealing with the physiological symptoms of withdrawal.

WEIGHT CONTROL

Nicotine suppresses appetite and slightly increases basal metabolic rate (rate of metabolic activity at rest). People who start smoking often lose weight, and continuing smokers gain weight less rapidly than nonsmokers. Weight control is one of the major reasons young women give for smoking, and weight gain can be a deterrent to quitting. People who quit smoking initially consume about 300 to 400 additional calories a day but only expend an additional 100 to 150 calories a day. Gaining 7 to 10 pounds is typical before the body adjusts to the absence of nicotine.[52] Once a person has successfully quit, this weight can be lost through exercise and sensible eating.

TOBACCO MARKETING AND ADVERTISING

Every day, the tobacco industry loses 4,600 smokers, either to quitting or to death.[49] These users have to be replaced if tobacco companies are to stay in business. Because most smokers get hooked in adolescence, children and teenagers are prime targets of tobacco advertising. Tobacco advertising aimed at children associates smoking with cartoon characters, and advertising aimed at teenagers associates smoking with alcohol, sex, and independence. Judging by the number of people who take up tobacco use every year, tobacco advertising and marketing are extremely effective. Although the industry continues to claim that it does not market its products to children, research suggests otherwise.[49,53]

Ramiro: An Occasional Smoker

Ramiro had tried a cigarette when he was 15 and a sophomore in high school. A group of friends he was hanging out with after a basketball game were smoking, and he asked to take a hit off his friend's cigarette, just out of curiosity. He was embarrassed that he started coughing as he inhaled the first drag, but tried a few more puffs and felt dizzy and a little bit high—kind of good. But Ramiro's parents were vehemently opposed to smoking. Ramiro respected them and also knew that it would be impossible to get away with smoking behind their backs, so he didn't try cigarettes again.

About two months into his freshman year at a college in another state, Ramiro was at a party and started talking to a friend from one of his classes. His friend pulled out a pack of cigarettes and lit up. The smell of the smoke distracted Ramiro and reminded him of his first time smoking. His friend noticed him staring at her cigarette and offered him one. He hesitated, but he was opening up to a lot of new experiences, and his parents' rules seemed part of his distant past. He didn't see the harm of having just one, so he accepted the cigarette and lit up. He felt the same dizzy and high feelings he had had with his first cigarette. Later in the evening he had a second cigarette and the following weekend he bummed a few cigarettes from someone at a party.

On Sunday, feeling independent, he bought a pack of cigarettes of his own. He told himself he would have only a few, maybe one or two, and would smoke only occasionally, in social situations. But later that day, after finding out on Facebook that a friend was dating a girl he was interested in, he went downstairs and smoked a cigarette outside his dorm. It helped him calm down and not think about his troubles.

Over the next two months, Ramiro gradually started smoking more. He allowed himself a cigarette to celebrate a good grade on a paper or to get over a disagreement with a roommate. He no longer felt high when he smoked, but he still enjoyed it. He knew he was smoking more, but he knew several other people with smoking patterns similar to his. None of them really considered themselves smokers—they just smoked occasionally and could quit at any time.

When he went home for winter vacation, Ramiro thought it would be a good idea to take a break from cigarettes, and he didn't want his parents to know he was smoking. After being at home for two days, he felt unusually irritable and unfocused. He wanted a cigarette to calm down and clear his mind, and the more he tried not to think about it, the more he wanted one. That night after everyone had gone to bed, he pulled out his cigarettes from where he had hidden them in his backpack, sneaked out of the house, and lit up. He instantly felt better. At the same time, he realized that what he had just gone through was an indication that he had gotten hooked. Although he enjoyed smoking, he didn't want to be addicted. He decided that he had to quit and find better ways to reward himself, deal with stress, and socialize.

connect ACTIVITY

Effects of Tobacco Use on Health

Tobacco use is also a causal factor in heart disease, respiratory diseases, and numerous other debilitating conditions. Overwhelming evidence confirms that smoking is the single

points,[55] and body temperature in the fingertips to decrease by a few degrees.

The tar and toxins in tobacco smoke damage cilia, the hairlike structures in the bronchial passages that prevent toxins and debris from reaching delicate lung tissue. Researchers believe that chemicals in tar, such as benzopyrene, switch

Overwhelming evidence confirms that **smoking is the single greatest preventable cause of illness and premature death** *in North America.*

greatest preventable cause of illness and premature death in North America.[49] Even people who are only occasional smokers, or "chippers," face health risks.[54]

SHORT-TERM EFFECTS

Smoking affects virtually every system in the body (Figure 10.4). When a smoker lights up, nicotine reaches the brain within 7 to 10 seconds, producing both sedating and stimulating effects. Adrenaline causes heart rate to increase by 10 to 20 beats per minute, blood pressure to rise by 5 to 10

on a gene in lung cells that causes cell mutations that can lead to cancerous growth.[56] These chemicals may also damage a gene with a role in killing cancer cells.

Carbon monoxide in tobacco smoke affects the way smokers process the air they breathe. Normally, oxygen is carried through the bloodstream by hemoglobin, a protein in red blood cells. When carbon monoxide is present, it binds with hemoglobin and prevents red blood cells from carrying a full load of oxygen. Heavy smokers quickly become winded during physical activity because the cardiovascular system cannot effectively deliver oxygen to muscle cells.[41]

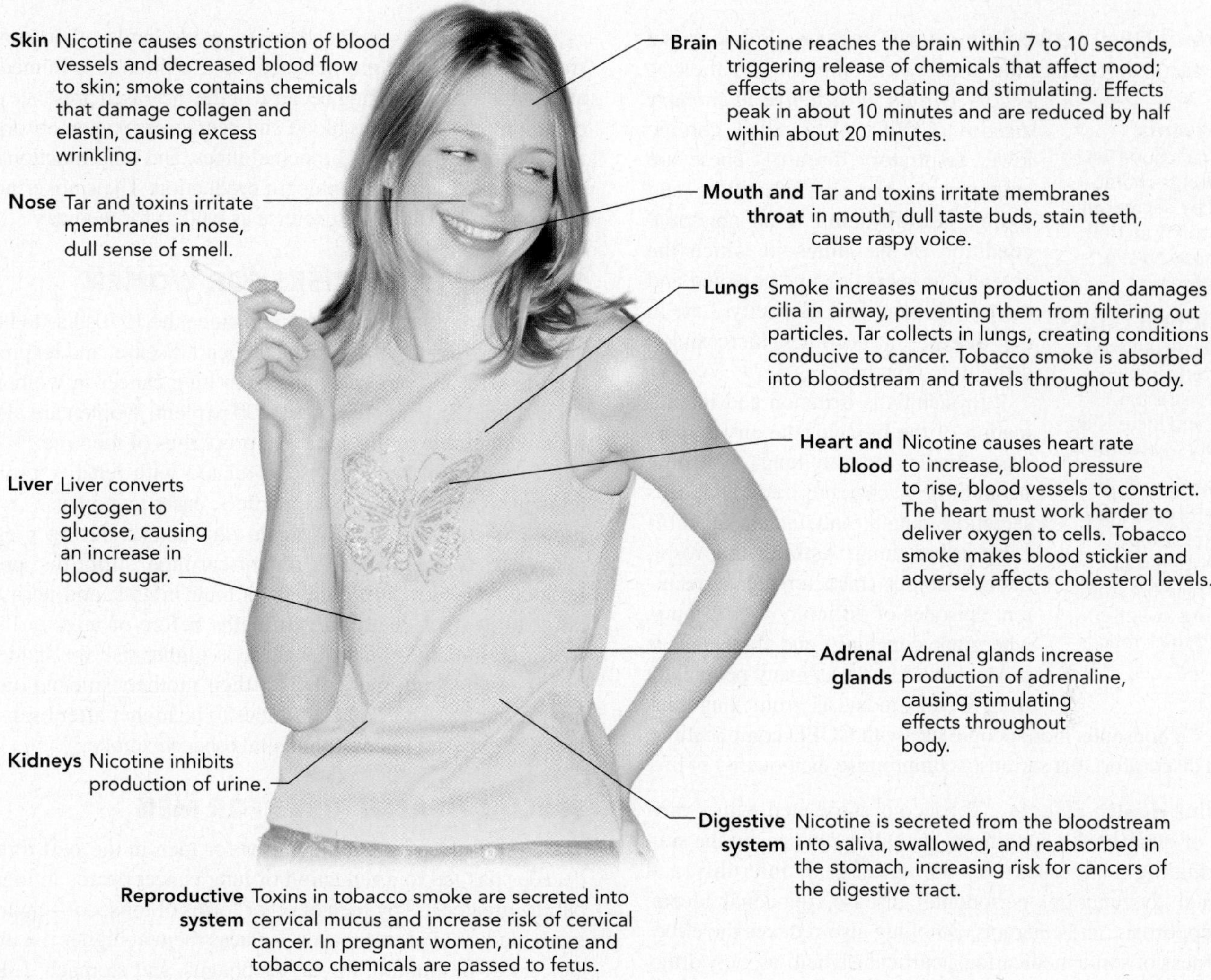

Skin Nicotine causes constriction of blood vessels and decreased blood flow to skin; smoke contains chemicals that damage collagen and elastin, causing excess wrinkling.

Nose Tar and toxins irritate membranes in nose, dull sense of smell.

Liver Liver converts glycogen to glucose, causing an increase in blood sugar.

Kidneys Nicotine inhibits production of urine.

Reproductive system Toxins in tobacco smoke are secreted into cervical mucus and increase risk of cervical cancer. In pregnant women, nicotine and tobacco chemicals are passed to fetus.

Brain Nicotine reaches the brain within 7 to 10 seconds, triggering release of chemicals that affect mood; effects are both sedating and stimulating. Effects peak in about 10 minutes and are reduced by half within about 20 minutes.

Mouth and throat Tar and toxins irritate membranes in mouth, dull taste buds, stain teeth, cause raspy voice.

Lungs Smoke increases mucus production and damages cilia in airway, preventing them from filtering out particles. Tar collects in lungs, creating conditions conducive to cancer. Tobacco smoke is absorbed into bloodstream and travels throughout body.

Heart and blood Nicotine causes heart rate to increase, blood pressure to rise, blood vessels to constrict. The heart must work harder to deliver oxygen to cells. Tobacco smoke makes blood stickier and adversely affects cholesterol levels.

Adrenal glands Adrenal glands increase production of adrenaline, causing stimulating effects throughout body.

Digestive system Nicotine is secreted from the bloodstream into saliva, swallowed, and reabsorbed in the stomach, increasing risk for cancers of the digestive tract.

figure 10.4 **Short-term effects of smoking on the body.**

LONG-TERM EFFECTS

The greatest health concerns associated with smoking are cardiovascular disease, cancer, and chronic lower respiratory diseases.

Cardiovascular Disease The increased heart rate, increased tension in the heart muscle, and constricted blood vessels caused by nicotine lead to hypertension (high blood pressure), which is both a disease in itself and a risk factor for other forms of heart disease, including coronary artery disease, heart attack, stroke, and peripheral vascular disease. Nicotine also makes blood platelets stickier, increasing the tendency of blood clots to form. It raises blood levels of low-density lipoproteins ("bad cholesterol") and decreases levels of high-density lipoproteins ("good cholesterol").[49] People who smoke more than one pack of cigarettes per day have three times the risk for heart disease and congestive heart failure that nonsmokers have.[50] People who smoke only one to four cigarettes a day still double their risk of heart disease.[54]

Cancer Smoking is implicated in about 30 percent of all cancer deaths. It is the cause of 87 percent of deaths from lung cancer, and it is associated with cancers of the pancreas, kidney, bladder, breast, and cervix. Smoking and using smokeless tobacco play a major role in cancers of the mouth, throat, and esophagus. Oral cancers caused by smokeless tobacco tend to occur early in adulthood. The use of alcohol in combination with tobacco increases the risk of oral cancers.[56]

Every day, the tobacco industry loses 4,600 smokers, either to quitting or to death. **These users have to be replaced if tobacco companies are to stay in business.**

Chronic Obstructive Pulmonary Disease   Smoking is a key factor in causing the diseases encompassed by the catgegory *chronic obstructive pulmonary disease* (COPD, also called chronic lower respiratory disease). These are emphysema, chronic bronchitis, and asthma. **Emphysema** is an abnormal condition of the lungs in which the alveoli (air sacs) become enlarged and their walls lose their elasticity. Late in the disease, it becomes increasingly difficult to breathe.

Bronchitis is irritation and inflammation of the bronchi, the airway passages leading to the lungs. **Chronic bronchitis** is characterized by mucus secretion, cough, and increasing difficulty in breathing. **Asthma** is a respiratory disorder characterized by recurrent episodes of difficulty in breathing, wheezing, coughing, and thick mucus production. Almost as many people die from COPD today as from lung cancer.[49] Thousands more people live with COPD complications and discomfort that seriously compromise their quality of life.

emphysema
Abnormal condition of the lungs characterized by decreased respiratory function and increased shortness of breath.

chronic bronchitis
Respiratory disorder characterized by mucus secretion, cough, and increasing difficulty in breathing.

asthma
Respiratory disorder characterized by recurrent episodes of difficulty in breathing, wheezing, coughing, and thick mucus production.

Other Health Effects   Tobacco is associated with a variety of other health conditions, including changes in the skin (wrinkling), increased risk during surgery, infertility and sexual dysfunction, periodontal disease, duodenal ulcers, osteoporosis, and cataracts. Smoking also reduces the effectiveness of some medications, particularly anti-anxiety drugs and penicillin.

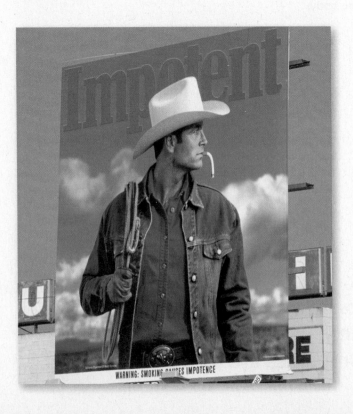

WARNING: SMOKING CAUSES IMPOTENCE

Athletes who smoke have to work harder than nonsmokers in the same physical activity. Respiration is immediately affected by smoking because of the increased presence of carbon monoxide in the blood and decreased oxygen absorption. Nicotine constricts bronchial tubes, and lung function is compromised further by phlegm production. The smoker has less oxygen available for exercise as well as for recovery.

SPECIAL HEALTH RISKS FOR WOMEN

Increased smoking among women since the 1970s has led to an increase in rates of lung cancer, heart disease, and respiratory disease in women; deaths from lung cancer in women, for example, have increased by 400 percent. Women are also more vulnerable to the addictive properties of nicotine.[57,58]

In addition, smoking is associated with fertility problems in women, menstrual disorders, early menopause, and problems in pregnancy. Women who smoke during pregnancy are at increased risk for miscarriage, stillbirths, preterm delivery, low birth weight in their infants, and perinatal death (infant death a few months before or after birth). Research indicates that infants are at higher risk for sudden infant death syndrome (SIDS) if their mothers smoked during pregnancy. Their risk continues to be higher after birth if they are exposed to environmental tobacco smoke.[59]

SPECIAL HEALTH RISKS FOR MEN

The overall drop in smoking rates for men in the past three decades has led to a reduction of lung cancer deaths in men, but the greater use by men of other forms of tobacco—cigars, pipes, and smokeless tobacco—places them at higher risk for cancers of the mouth, throat, esophagus, and stomach. Like women, men who smoke experience problems with sexual function and fertility. Smoking adversely affects blood flow to the erectile tissue, leading to a higher incidence of erectile dysfunction (impotence); it also alters sperm shape, reduces sperm motility, and decreases the overall number of viable sperm.[60]

SPECIAL HEALTH RISKS FOR ETHNIC MINORITY GROUPS

Mortality rates from several diseases associated with tobacco use, including cardiovascular disease, cancer, and SIDS, are higher for ethnic minority groups than for Whites.[26] For example, African American men and women are more likely to die from lung cancer, heart disease, and stroke than are members of other ethnic groups, despite lower rates of tobacco use. Reductions in smoking among African Americans since the mid-1980s have led to a decline in lung cancer for African American men and a leveling off in African American women. Reduced smoking rates have also led to a decrease in lung cancer deaths in Hispanic men.[39]

■ Sexual dysfunction is one of the lesser known health effects of tobacco use for both men and women. This billboard is part of an antismoking campaign warning that "smoking causes impotence."

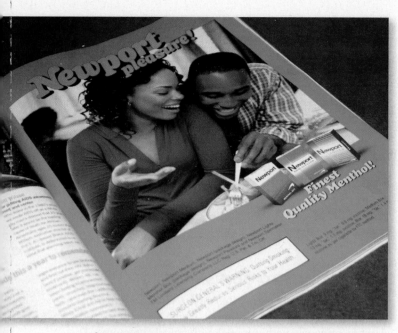

■ African Americans have higher mortality rates from smoking-related illnesses despite lower rates of smoking. Tobacco manufacturers deny that they promote certain products and brands to minority populations and other segments of the general population.

BENEFITS OF QUITTING

Smokers greatly reduce their risk of many health problems when they quit. Health benefits begin immediately and become more significant the longer the individual stays smoke free. Respiratory symptoms associated with COPD, such as smoker's cough and excess mucus production, decrease quickly after quitting. Recovery from illnesses like colds and flu is more rapid, taste and smell return, and circulation improves.

In addition to reducing risk of diseases, quitting also increases longevity. Individuals who quit before the age of 50 cut their risk of dying within the next 15 years in half. Men who quit between ages 35 and 39 add an average of 5 years to their lifespan, and women add 3 years. Even quitting after the age of 70 substantially lowers the risk of dying and improves the quality of life (see the box "When You Quit Smoking: Health Benefits Timeline").

EFFECTS OF ENVIRONMENTAL TOBACCO SMOKE

You don't have to be a smoker to experience adverse health effects from tobacco smoke. Abundant evidence shows that inhaling the smoke from other people's tobacco products—called **environmental tobacco smoke (ETS)**, secondhand smoke, or passive smoking—has serious health consequences. Even 30 minutes of daily secondhand smoke exposure causes heart damage similar to that experienced by a habitual smoker. People who are exposed daily to secondhand smoke have a 30 percent higher rate of death and disease than nonsmokers.

environmental tobacco smoke (ETS)
Smoke from other people's tobacco products; also called *secondhand smoke* or *passive smoking.*

In 1993 the Environmental Protection Agency designated ETS a Class A carcinogen—an agent known to cause cancer in humans—and in 2000 the U.S. Department of Health and

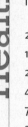

Highlight on Health

When You Quit Smoking: Health Benefits Timeline

Immediately	You stop polluting the air with secondhand smoke; the air around you is no longer dangerous to children and adults.
20 minutes	Blood pressure decreases; pulse rate decreases; temperature of hands and feet increases.
12 hours	Carbon monoxide level in blood drops; oxygen level in blood increases to normal.
24 hours	Chance of heart attack decreases.
48 hours	Nerve endings start to regrow; exercise gets easier; senses of smell and taste improve.
72 hours	Bronchial tubes relax, making breathing easier; lung capacity increases.
2–12 weeks	Circulation improves; lung functioning increases up to 30 percent.
1–9 months	Fewer coughs, colds, and flu episodes; fatigue and shortness of breath decrease; lung function continues to improve.
1 year	Risk of smoking-related heart attack is cut by half.
5 years	Risk of dying from heart disease and stroke approaches that of a nonsmoker; risk of oral and esophageal cancers is cut by half.
10 years	Risk of dying from lung cancer is cut by half.
10–15 years	Life expectancy reaches that of a person who never smoked.

Source: Health Canada: On the Road to Quitting, www.hc-sc.gc.ca. Copyright © 2008 Health Canada. Reproduced with the permission of the Minister of Public Works and Government Services Canada, 2008.

Human Services added it to their list of known human carcinogens. In 2006, the U.S. surgeon general stated that there is *no* safe level of ETS exposure.

Because of their smaller body size, infants and children are especially vulnerable to the effects of ETS. Children exposed to ETS experience 10 percent more colds, flu, and

are quitting, because alcohol interacts with nicotine in complex ways and can make quitting more difficult. Dieting is not recommended while trying to quit, despite the potential for weight gain. Combining exercise with smoking cessation appears to be the most effective approach to managing the potential for weight gain. Another element is social support

Even 30 minutes of **daily secondhand smoke exposure causes heart damage** *similar to that experienced by a habitual smoker.*

other acute respiratory infections than do those not exposed. ETS aggravates asthma symptoms and increases the risk of SIDS.[61] Legislation is also needed to protect children from secondhand smoke in public housing projects, where rates of smoking tend to be much higher than they are among the general population. Some states, including California, Arkansas, and Louisiana, have moved to ban smoking in cars when children under the age of 6 are present.

Quitting and Treatment Options

Once a person becomes an established smoker, quitting is exceptionally difficult. Nearly four of every five smokers want to quit smoking. Only about 7 percent of smokers who quit are successfully abstaining a year later. Even among smokers who have lost a lung or undergone major heart surgery, only about 50 percent stop smoking for more than a few weeks.[40,50,61]

The good news is that smokers who quit for a year have an 85 percent chance of maintaining their abstinence. Those who make it to 5 years have a 97 percent chance of continued success. Most people don't succeed the first time they try to quit—in fact, the average number of attempts required for successful smoking cessation is seven—but many succeed on subsequent attempts.[50]

TREATMENT PROGRAMS TO QUIT SMOKING

Treatment programs can be quite effective; 20–40 percent of smokers who enter good treatment programs are able to quit smoking for at least a year.[49,62] In some cases, smokers choose an intensive residential program; such a program might include daily group and individual therapy, stress reduction techniques, nutrition information, exercise, and a 12-step program similar to Alcoholics Anonymous.

Many programs encourage smokers to limit or eliminate their consumption of alcohol while they

and encouragement from important people in the smoker's life.

MEDICATIONS TO QUIT SMOKING

In **nicotine replacement therapy (NRT)**, a controlled amount of nicotine is administered, which gradually reduces daily nicotine use with minimal withdrawal symptoms. The transdermal patch and nicotine gum are the most common delivery systems, but also available are a nicotine inhaler, a nicotine spray, a nicotine lozenge, and a nicotine hand gel. The gel, sold under the name Nicogel, is marketed as a product for tobacco users who find themselves in situations where they can't smoke. A quick-evaporating hand gel made from tobacco extracts, Nicogel can reduce nicotine cravings for up to 4 hours.

nicotine replacement therapy (NRT) Treatment for nicotine addiction in which a controlled amount of nicotine is administered to gradually reduce daily nicotine use with minimal withdrawal symptoms.

Although nicotine is addictive no matter how it is administered, NRT products contain none of the carcinogens or toxic gases found in cigarette smoke, so they are a safer form of nicotine delivery.[63] Using one or more of the NRT products doubles a person's chances of success in quitting. NRT is beneficial when used as part of a comprehensive physician-promoted cessation program. It can help control withdrawal symptoms and craving while the individual is learning new behavioral patterns.[61,63,64]

Other smoking cessation aids work not by replacing nicotine but by acting on the neurotransmitter receptors in the brain that are affected by nicotine. Bupropion is a prescription smoking cessation drug that acts in this way. It was

■ Zyban and Chantix belong to a newer category of smoking cessation aids that work by acting on neurotransmitter receptors in the brain rather than replacing nicotine. However, both carry black-box warnings about potential side effects, such as depression and suicidal thinking.

approved in 2001 by the FDA and is marketed under the trade name Zyban. Bupropion is also prescribed as an antidepressant under the name Wellbutrin; Zyban and Wellbutrin should not be taken together.

Varenicline (marketed in the United States as Chantix) is another smoking cessation drug that acts on neurotransmitter receptors. It was approved by the FDA in 2006. Clinical studies found that more than one in five people using varenicline quit smoking for at least 1 year, a significant improvement over rates for other smoking cessation drugs.

Both Chantix and Zyban now carry black-box warnings due to the potential risks of psychiatric problems associated with their use, particularly depression and suicidal thinking. Black-box is the strictest drug warning imposed by the FDA. Additionally, the FDA mandated that these drugs include more prescription information on the drug label and new information for patients that explains the potential mental health risks and their symptoms.[65]

NicVax is an experimental nicotine vaccine that blocks the pleasurable effects of smoking. It works by eliciting the production of antibodies that bind with nicotine molecules in the bloodstream, preventing them from entering nicotine receptors in the brain. NicVax has not been approved by the FDA, but early studies have been encouraging.

QUITTING ON YOUR OWN: DEVELOPING A BEHAVIOR CHANGE PLAN

Despite the hardships of withdrawal and the challenges of behavior change, quitting smoking is worth it, and the majority of people who quit do so on their own.

One approach is to develop a behavior change plan similar to the one described for cutting back on alcohol consumption. A first step is determining your readiness to quit. As discussed in Chapter 1, trying to change a behavior when you are not ready to change is pointless and counterproductive. It will only lead to failure and discouragement. Refer to the box "Assessing Your Stage of Change" in Chapter 1 (p. 10) for a quick evaluation of your own stage of change in regard to quitting smoking. If you are in the contemplation or action stage, you can develop a behavior change plan by following the steps described next.

Record and Analyze Your Smoking Patterns First, keep track of your smoking for two weeks, noting when, where, and with whom you smoke. Note the triggers or cues for smoking and your thoughts and feelings at the time. Then analyze your record to get a sense of your smoking patterns. Understanding these patterns can help you develop strategies for avoiding or dealing with the most challenging times and situations.

Establish Goals Set a specific date to quit. Choose a time when you will be relatively stress free—not during exams, for example—so that you will have the needed energy, attention, and focus. Experts recommend aiming for some time within two weeks of when you begin to plan. Plan to quit

completely on that date; tapering off rarely works because it only prolongs withdrawal.

Prepare to Quit Your most important asset in quitting is your firm commitment to do so. At the same time, you can take specific, concrete steps to increase your chances of success. Consider these questions:

- Why do you want to quit? Make a list of your reasons and post them on your refrigerator or in another prominent place in your home.

- If you tried to quit in the past, what helped and what didn't? Learn from your mistakes.

- What situations are going to be the most difficult? How can you plan ahead to handle them? To the extent you can, reorganize your life to avoid situations in which you were accustomed to smoking.

- What pleasures do you get from smoking? How can you get those pleasures from life-enhancing activities instead of smoking?

- Who can help you? Tell your family and friends you are planning to quit and ask for their support. Find out if your state has a telephone quitline.

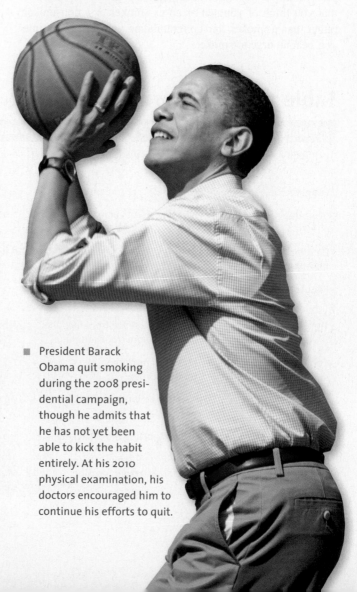

- President Barack Obama quit smoking during the 2008 presidential campaign, though he admits that he has not yet been able to kick the habit entirely. At his 2010 physical examination, his doctors encouraged him to continue his efforts to quit.

Implement Your Plan   Be prepared to experience symptoms of withdrawal and have a plan for handling them, even if it's just "toughing it out." Exercise will help ease cravings for nicotine and elevate your mood, so make sure you exercise daily. Exercise will also improve sleep and help you limit weight gain. Drink plenty of fluids; they help flush nicotine from your body.

Prevent Relapse   Symptoms of nicotine withdrawal last from two to three weeks, although the most acute symptoms may last only a few days. See Table 10.2 for a summary of symptoms, their causes, and suggested relief strategies.

Abstinence becomes easier with time, although it can still be difficult. Most relapses occur within the first three months.[66] There are two main lines of defense for maintaining prolonged abstinence. First, avoid high-risk situations, and second, develop coping mechanisms. Relapses are prompted by stress, anger, frustration and depression.[39] Make sure you have strategies to deal with these feelings, whether relaxation techniques, exercise, social support, or cognitive techniques. Examples of cognitive techniques are reminding yourself of why you quit, thinking about the people you know who have quit, adjusting your self-image so that you think of yourself as an ex-smoker or a nonsmoker rather than a smoker, and congratulating yourself every time you beat an urge to smoke.

Confronting the Tobacco Challenge

Given the cost of tobacco use, why are the manufacture and sale of tobacco products legal in this country? The answer to this question is complex. Tobacco has been part of the economy of the country since colonial times, and today it is a multibillion-dollar industry with tremendous lobbying power and a huge impact on the nation's economic health. Many state economies depend on tobacco, and elected representatives from those states make sure tobacco interests are protected at the federal level. Because smoking is viewed as a personal decision, there are many constraints on the government's ability to protect citizens and consumers from the hazards of tobacco use. Still, significant inroads have been made in confronting the challenge posed by tobacco, and the tobacco industry is facing tremendous pressure on many fronts. Successes in the United States, however, have caused tobacco companies to turn to foreign markets to sell their products (see the box "Smoking: A Global Challenge").

THE NONSMOKERS' RIGHTS MOVEMENT AND LEGISLATIVE BATTLES

Beginning in the 1970s, a nonsmokers' rights movement took shape as a result of growing public awareness of the

Table 10.2   What to Expect When You Quit

Symptom	Reason	Duration	Relief
Irritability	Body craves nicotine.	2–4 weeks	Take walks, hot baths; use relaxation techniques.
Fatigue	Nicotine is a stimulant.	2–4 weeks	Take naps; don't push yourself.
Insomnia	Nicotine affects brain waves.	2–4 weeks	Avoid caffeine after 6:00 p.m.; use relaxation techniques.
Coughing, dry throat, nasal drip	Body is getting rid of excess mucus.	A few days	Drink fluids; try cough drops.
Poor concentration	Nicotine is a stimulant, boosts concentration.	1–2 weeks	Get enough sleep; exercise; eat well.
Tightness in chest	Muscles are tense from nicotine craving or sore from coughing.	A few days	Use relaxation techniques, especially deep breathing; take hot baths.
Constipation, gas, stomach pain	Intestinal movement decreases for brief time.	1–2 weeks	Drink fluids; add fiber to diet (fruits, vegetables, whole grains).
Hunger	Nicotine craving can feel like hunger.	Up to several weeks	Drink water or low-calorie drinks; have low-calorie snacks on hand.
Headaches	Brain is getting more oxygen.	1–2 weeks	Drink water; use relaxation techniques.
Craving for a cigarette	Withdrawal from nicotine.	Most acute first few days; can recur for months	Wait it out; distract yourself; exercise; use relaxation techniques.

Source: www.quitnet.com.

Public Health in Action

Smoking: A Global Challenge

Public health measures like educational campaigns, tobacco taxes, and advertising restrictions have helped decrease rates of smoking among Americans from a peak of 40 percent in 1965 to about 21 percent in 2009. However, with a shrinking market in the United States, tobacco companies have aggressively pursued new markets overseas, especially in developing countries. These countries are more likely to have populations who are unaware of the risks associated with smoking, governments in need of tax revenue generated by tobacco sales, and fewer educational and public health measures designed to curb smoking and minimize its health effects. Tobacco use in Pakistan has increased 42 percent since 2001, and consumption in Ukraine has increased 36 percent since that same year. Deaths from tobacco are increasing at a faster rate in developing countries than in developed countries. By 2030, it is expected that 70 percent of the world's tobacco-related deaths will occur in developing countries.

In 2003, the World Health Organization (WHO) attempted to push back the tobacco companies' advances in developing nations by gathering countries to sign the WHO Framework Convention on Tobacco Control. Countries that signed the treaty agreed to implement specific demand- and supply-reduction measures, including regulation of package labeling and advertising. The treaty went into effect in 2005 and has 168 signatory countries.

However, the treaty has not completely thwarted the tobacco industry's advances. In 2008, Philip Morris split its international corporation from its domestic corporation in order to exempt its international sales from legal restrictions in the United States. This split allowed the

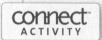
connect
ACTIVITY

company to develop a range of products targeted for markets in developing countries, such as sweet-smelling cigarettes, extra-thick cigarettes, and cigarettes that contain twice as much tar and nicotine as cigarettes sold in the United States. Philip Morris International, whose sales volume is approximately four times that of Philip Morris USA, is targeting markets in eastern Europe, China, Indonesia, and other Asian and Southeast Asian countries. PMI has developed tobacco products that appeal to the specific tastes and preferences of each population.

In 2009 the WHO assessed the progress of the countries who signed on to the Framework Convention on Tobacco Control and found that some parts of the treaty were more successfully implemented than others. Fewer than half of the signatories had been able to keep the tobacco industry from interfering with their tobacco-control policies. Just over half had been able to implement a comprehensive ban on tobacco advertising, sponsorship, and promotion. However, workplace smoking restrictions had been implemented by 85 percent of the countries, and smoking restrictions on public transportation had been implemented by 88 percent. The WHO is optimistic that the global tobacco epidemic can be overcome. In the coming years it will continue to facilitate the implementation of the treaty provisions and to collect data on member countries' progress. As public health initiatives are implemented in developing countries, populations around the world will benefit from the same awareness and protections that have decreased tobacco use in the United States and other developed countries.

Sources: "Philip Morris Readies Aggressive Global Push," by V. O'Connell, 2008, The Wall Street Journal, retrieved April 15, 2010, from http://online .wsj.com/article/SB120156034185223519.html; "2009 Summary Report on Global Progress in the Implementation of the WHO Framework Convention on Tobacco Control," World Health Organization, 2009, retrieved April 15, 2010, from http://www.who.int/fctc/FCTC-2009-1-en.pdf; "History of the WHO Framework Convention on Tobacco Control," World Health Organization, 2009, retrieved April 15, 2010, from http://whqlibdoc.who .int/publications/2009/9789241563925_eng.pdf.

damage inflicted by tobacco. Smoking came to be seen as both a public health problem and a problematic behavior.[67]

By 2003, thousands of local laws and ordinances were in place across the country, creating smoke-free workplaces, restaurants, bars, and public places. Some tobacco control laws have also been passed at the state level. California has had a ban on smoking in workplaces since 1994 and on smoking in bars since 1998. The federal government also has tobacco control measures in place, such as the ban on smoking on domestic airline flights.

LAWSUITS AND COURT SETTLEMENTS

In the 1990s, tobacco companies began to face class action suits, cases representing claims of injury by hundreds or thousands of smokers. In addition, states began suing

tobacco companies for losses incurred by state health insurance funds used to pay for tobacco-related diseases.

These pressures led to the 1998 Master Settlement Agreement (MSA), in which the tobacco industry agreed to pay $206 billion to 46 states over a 25-year period in exchange for protection from future lawsuits by the states and other public entities. Other provisions of the MSA included a ban on billboard advertising and restrictions on advertising aimed at children. The settlement money from the MSA was to be used by the states primarily to fund tobacco education and prevention programs.

Some of the money went to the American Legacy Foundation's "Truth" campaign, a nationwide effort to tell the truth about tobacco products to youth. Studies indicate that this campaign was successful in deterring children and teenagers from taking up smoking.[68] Still, the campaign's annual spending pales in comparison with the billions spent by tobacco companies on advertising and promoting tobacco products.

REGULATION AND TAXATION: HARM REDUCTION STRATEGIES

The U.S. government doesn't prohibit tobacco use by adults or force individuals to stop smoking, but it does take actions aimed at reducing the harm associated with the use of tobacco products by those who continue to smoke. A *harm reduction* approach to tobacco use focuses on reducing a smoker's exposure to nicotine, tar, and carbon monoxide. One way to achieve this is by limiting access to tobacco products, such

and nicotine by taking more puffs per cigarette, inhaling more deeply, and smoking more cigarettes per day.[73] Large studies of mortality risks have found no evidence that lower tar cigarettes reduce health risks.[74] The truth is that there is no such thing as a safe cigarette.

EDUCATION AND PREVENTION: CHANGING THE CULTURAL CLIMATE

In the 1950s, cigarette smoking was an accepted part of everyday life. People smoked in restaurants, movie theaters, concert halls, college classrooms, offices, and airplanes, and smoking was depicted in a positive light on television and in movies.

Tobacco has been a part of the country's economy since colonial times, and today it is a **multibillion-dollar industry** *with tremendous lobbying power and a huge impact on the nation's economic health.*

as by increasing the price through taxes.[69] Another way, one promoted by tobacco companies, is the use of "low-tar" and "low-nicotine" cigarettes. The latter approach has proved to be just another way to dupe consumers.

Limiting Access to Tobacco Access to tobacco can be limited by increasing cost, reducing physical availability, and regulating tobacco marketing campaigns. When taxes on tobacco products are increased, raising their price, sales and use decline. Cigarette tax increases have been particularly effective in discouraging people from starting smoking.[70]

Physical availability of tobacco products is reduced when the laws restricting sales to minors are enforced. States are required to conduct random, unannounced inspections of places where tobacco is sold, and reports detailing results of these inspections must be submitted to the federal government each year.

Restrictions on tobacco advertising may affect access to tobacco as well.[71] Tobacco companies argue that their advertising efforts are aimed solely at creating brand loyalty, not at attracting new smokers. Antitobacco activists draw from extensive research to refute this claim. Tobacco marketing campaigns appear to be specifically directed at children, women, and minorities. Children as young as age 6 have reported familiarity with cigarette ads using cartoon characters.[71]

The Scam of "Low-Tar" and "Low-Nicotine" Cigarettes
"Low-tar" and "low-nicotine" cigarettes with lower levels of tar and nicotine have been promoted by the tobacco industry as safer than regular cigarettes. However, lower tar cigarettes are not safer than regular cigarettes.[72] Smokers who switch to these cigarettes compensate for reduced yields of tobacco

Those days are gone, along with the social norms that made smoking a socially acceptable behavior. Awareness of the health hazards of smoking and ETS and increased willingness on the part of nonsmokers to assert their rights have contributed to changes in the cultural climate surrounding tobacco use.

Clearly, however, there is more to do. Antismoking campaigns that focus on the risks of smoking fail to counter the positive images that are conveyed by movies, media, and advertising and that motivate young people to take up smoking.[75]

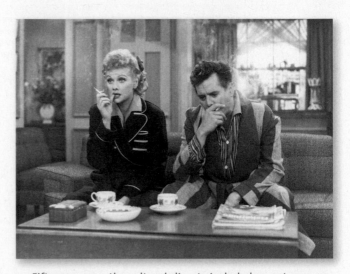

■ Fifty years ago, the cultural climate included acceptance and normalization of smoking in virtually all settings. Lucille Ball and Desi Arnaz were just two of the many TV actors and celebrities who modeled smoking for the public.

One recommendation by health experts is that anti-smoking campaigns use some of the same strategies that have worked for the tobacco companies.[74] For example, they should target specific market segments, focusing on young people and their attitudes, values, and lifestyles. Messages should be delivered repeatedly over long periods of time in a multitude of formats, and they should be varied to appeal to the age and ethnic/cultural identity of the intended audience.

Community interventions are also recommended, working through schools, local government, civic organizations, and health agencies. Many colleges and universities are now smoke-free environments. All of these efforts have the potential to create a fundamental change in social norms and in public attitudes toward tobacco use. Such a change, in turn, has the potential to close the pipeline of new smokers and motivate current smokers to quit.

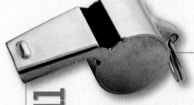

You Make the Call

Should the National Drinking Age Be Lowered?

In 2008, a collection of college and university presidents and chancellors formed an organization called the Amethyst Initiative to spark a national debate about whether our current legal drinking age of 21 is actually an effective way to keep teens from binge drinking. Members of the Amethyst Initiative believe that lowering the drinking age is a practical and sensible way to confront binge drinking problems among young people. As of 2010, 135 college presidents from schools that include Dartmouth and Virginia Tech have signed the Amethyst Initiative. The initiative's call to rethink the current drinking age has received national attention and considerable controversy, particularly from Mothers Against Drunk Driving (MADD), the Institute for Highway Safety, and the American Medical Association, who all oppose the idea.

As mentioned in the chapter, the drinking age of 21 was enacted by Congress in 1984 under the National Minimum Drinking Age Act with the goal of reducing drunk driving. States that failed to increase the drinking age to 21 were threatened with the loss of 10 percent of their annual federal highway appropriation. Since the law has gone into effect, the National Highway Traffic Safety Administration estimates that the act has reduced the number of fatal car crashes involving drivers 18 to 20 by 13 percent. Opponents of lowering the drinking age point to these data as evidence that the act has been successful and should be kept.

However, signatories of the Amethyst Initiative argue that today, more than 25 years since the passage of the National Minimum Drinking Age Act, we are much more aware of the risks associated with drinking and driving. Public advocacy organizations like MADD have been very successful in educating the public about these risks. Mandatory seat belt laws and airbags, designated drivers, sobriety checkpoints, and stiff civil and criminal policies for driving under the influence are largely responsible for the decrease in alcohol-related fatalities in motor vehicle crashes since 1984. According to signatories, the principal problem is no longer drunk driving but clandestine binge drinking, especially by college students. Thirty percent of college students abuse alcohol and 6 percent are alcohol dependent. On college campuses, they argue, students can bypass the legal drinking age and obtain alcohol from their friends and consume it in a dorm room or apartment.

Supporters of the Amethyst Initiative also argue that the current law sends an ineffective message to young people. Prohibiting people under 21 from drinking requires that they abstain completely from alcohol, which is not a realistic approach, they contend. A more effective approach to the problem of binge drinking would be to prepare young adults to drink responsibly through education and licensing. Full drinking privileges would be granted only to young adults who demonstrated their ability to observe the law.

Some states have also considered lowering the legal drinking age, but for different reasons. Legislators in Kentucky, Wisconsin, and South Carolina have contended that if 18-year-olds are deemed mature and responsible enough to join the army, they should also be able to buy alcohol. Opponents argue that teens' brains have not matured enough to safely drink alcohol. They point to scientific evidence that the human brain is not fully developed until the early 20s, possibly until age 25. Excessive alcohol exposure during brain development years may permanently alter a person's mental, emotional, and cognitive development.

Proponents of lowering the drinking age argue that the law currently in place has failed to curb excessive drinking and is no longer needed to reduce the incidence of drunk driving. Opponents say that the law is still needed. What do you think?

PROS

- The problem today is not drunk drivers under 21. It is reckless alcohol consumption with the intention to get drunk that occurs in "underground" locations like dorm rooms and apartments.

- Binge-drinking rates for college-aged men have not changed since 1979 and they have increased by 40 percent among college women; current laws have not been effective in reducing binge drinking.

- The current law does not say to drink responsibly or only in moderation—it says don't drink at all. This is prohibition, which has been historically shown not to work. A more effective action would be to prepare young adults to drink responsibly through education and licensing.

CONS

- The implementation of a legal drinking age of 21 years has saved lives by reducing the number of fatal car crashes involving drivers 18 to 20 by 13 percent.

- The human brain is not fully developed until a person is in the early 20s. Exposure to alcohol during the brain's formative years could have permanent negative consequences.

- Colleges do and should take their own actions to curb excessive drinking on campus. Lowering the drinking age would undercut these efforts.

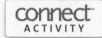

Sources: Amethyst Initiative Organization, www.amethystinitiative.org; "Commentary: Drinking Age of 21 Does Not Work," by J.M. McCardell, Jr., 2009, retrieved April 7, 2010, from www.cnn.com/2009/POLITICS/09/16/mccardell.lower.drinking.age; "States Weigh Lower Drinking Age," by J. Keen, 2008, retrieved April 7, 2010, from www.usatoday.com/news/nation/2008-03-20-drinkingage_N.htm.

IN REVIEW

Why do people drink, and why do some people develop problems with alcohol?

People ingest psychoactive substances like alcohol for a wide range of reasons, from wanting to enhance positive feelings to wanting to numb negative feelings. A complex interplay of individual and environmental factors leads some people who drink to develop problems with alcohol, including alcohol dependence.

What are the health risks of alcohol consumption?

Over the long term, alcohol consumption can cause cardiovascular disease, liver disease, cancer, brain damage, and unhealthy changes in body weight and food absorption. Alcohol use is also associated with high-risk sexual activity, violence, injury, and suicide.

Who smokes, and why is it a problem?

About 20 percent of the U.S. adult population are smokers, with higher rates of smoking among men than women and among college students than the general population. Tobacco use is the leading preventable cause of death in the United States.

What are the main tobacco products?

Cigarettes are by far the most commonly used tobacco products, trailed by cigars, pipes, and smokeless (chewing) tobacco. Other products (for example, tobacco for water pipes, little cigars, snus) are marketed as safer alternatives, but nearly all contain nicotine, and, when burned, produce thousands of toxic substances. Electronic cigarettes deliver nicotine through inhaled vapor but still contain potentially harmful chemicals.

Web Resources

Alcoholics Anonymous (AA) World Services: This organization provides information on Alcoholics Anonymous, including the philosophy of its 12-step program. It features a preventive approach to alcohol abuse.
www.alcoholics-anonymous.org

American Lung Association: See the Quit Smoking feature of the association's Web site for news articles, resources for support, information on legislation, and fact sheets.
www.lungusa.org

Americans for Nonsmokers' Rights: This organization offers information on environmental smoke; how to protect yourself from smoke at home, at work, and in the community; legal issues related to smoking; and special concerns for youth.
www.no-smoke.org

BACCHUS and GAMMA Peer Education Network: Made up of college and university students, this organization promotes peer education programs designed to prevent alcohol abuse.
www.bacchusgamma.org

CDC's Tobacco Information and Prevention Sources (TIPS): Everything from the surgeon general's reports to Celebrities Against Smoking and community action programs can be found here.
www.cdc.gov/tobacco

National Institute on Alcohol Abuse and Alcoholism (NIAAA): NIAAA is dedicated to public education on alcohol abuse and alcoholism.
www.niaaa.nih.gov

Smokefree.Gov: The online guide to quitting smoking offered at this site includes practical steps for preparing to quit, quitting, and "staying quit." You can also instant-message an expert or get telephone support.
www.smokefree.gov

Substance Abuse and Mental Health Services Administration: The U.S. government site features a wide range of resources on substance abuse and closely related issues, such as mental health, homelessness, and AIDS/HIV.
www.samhsa.gov

11 Drugs

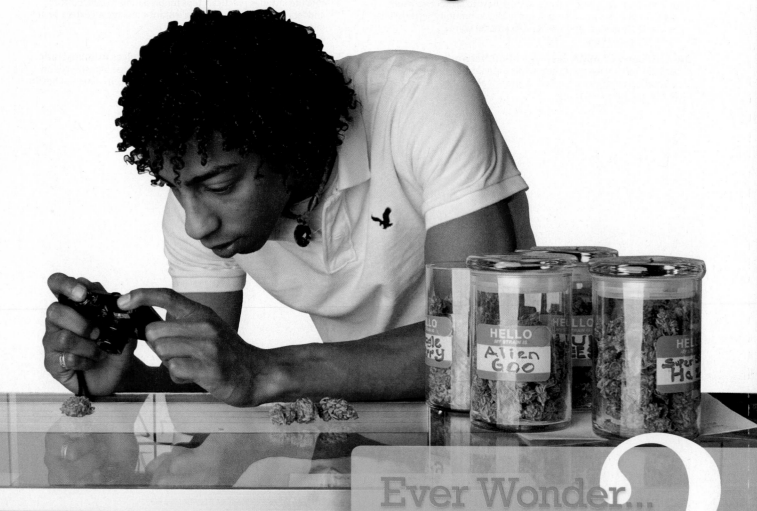

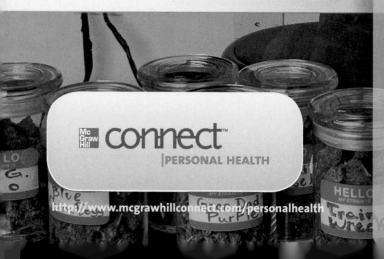
Ever Wonder...

- which drugs have the highest potential for physical and psychological dependence?

- why some people can't seem to stop using drugs?

- how to know if someone is starting to have a problem with drugs?

Like alcohol, drugs have a pervasive presence in American life. We use them for headaches, insomnia,

anxiety, stress—and some of us use them for fun. In 2008 an estimated 20.1 million Americans aged 12 or older were current users of illicit (illegal) drugs, representing 8 percent of the population (Table 11.1).[1] Although these numbers seem large, it's worth noting the other side of the picture, namely, that 92 percent of the population aged 12 or older—more than 200 million people—do not use illicit drugs.

Drugs are used by different people for different reasons. Many people take drugs as a recreational activity—to alter their state of consciousness, to relax and feel more sociable, to experience euphoria, to get high. Some people take drugs to rebel, and others take them to fit in. For some people, drug use is a way to cope with stress, pain, or adversity, and for some, it is a way of life, a behavior they can no longer control.

Who Uses? Patterns of Illicit Drug Use

Rates of illicit drug use vary by age, gender, race and ethnicity, education, employment status, and geographical region (see Figure 11.1 and the box "Rates of Illicit Drug Use"). Among Americans aged 12 or older, more than 45 percent report having used an illicit drug in their lifetime (see Table 11.1). The most commonly used drug is marijuana, with over 15 million current users among Americans aged 12 or older.[1] An estimated 6.2 million Americans use prescription-type drugs nonmedically, including pain relievers, tranquilizers, stimulants, and sedatives.[1]

Among young adults aged 18–25, the most commonly used drugs are marijuana, prescription-type drugs used nonmedically, hallucinogens, and cocaine. Marijuana use and overall illicit drug use generally remained stable for this age group from 2002 to 2007. However, in the larger scope of time prescription drug abuse stands out as a relatively recent

Table 11.1 Illicit Drug Use in Lifetime and Past Year Among Persons Aged 12 or Older: Percentages, 2008

Drug	Time Period	
	Lifetime	Past year
Any illicit drug	47.0	14.2
Marijuana and hashish	41.0	10.3
Cocaine	14.7	2.1
Crack	3.4	0.4
Heroin	1.5	0.2
Hallucinogens	14.4	1.5
LSD	9.4	0.3
PCP	2.7	0.0
Ecstasy	5.2	0.9
Inhalants	8.9	0.8
Nonmedical use of any prescription drug	20.8	6.1
Pain relievers	14.0	4.8
OxyContin	1.9	0.6
Tranquilizers	8.6	2.0
Stimulants	8.5	1.1
Sedatives	3.6	0.2

Source: Results from the 2008 National Survey on Drug Use and Health: National Findings, Substance Abuse and Mental Health Services Administration, 2009, Rockville, MD: Office of Applied Studies.

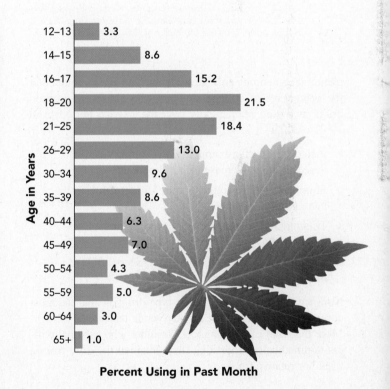

Percent Using in Past Month

figure **11.1** **Percent of people aged 12 or older who reported illicit drug use in the past month.**

Source: Results from the 2009 National Survey on Drug Use and Health: National Findings, Substance Abuse and Mental Health Services Administration, 2009, Rockville, MD: Office of Applied Studies.

Who's at Risk?

Rates of Illicit Drug Use

- **Age.** The highest rates of illicit drug use occur among young adults aged 18–20 (Figure 11.1), with these rates remaining stable from 2002 to 2008. Among teenagers, rates decreased during this period, from 11.6 to 9.3 percent. Among those aged 55–59, rates of illicit drug use more than doubled between 2002 and 2008, from 1.9 percent to 5.0 percent, perhaps reflecting the aging of the baby boomers, whose lifetime use of illicit drugs is higher than that of older cohorts.

- **Gender.** Males are more likely to use drugs than females, at rates of 9.9 percent versus 6.3 percent among persons aged 12 or older. The rate of marijuana use is higher among males than females (7.9 percent versus 4.4 percent), but rates are similar for stimulants, Ecstasy, sedatives, OxyContin, LSD, and PCP. Rates for all of these drugs are less than 1 percent.

- **Race/ethnicity.** Rates are highest among persons reporting two or more races (14.7 percent), and lowest among Asian Americans (3.6 percent), with rates for Blacks (10.1 percent), American Indian/Alaskan Natives (9.5 percent), Whites (8.2 percent), Native Hawaiians

  or Other Pacific Islanders (7.3 percent), and Hispanics (6.2 percent) falling in between.

- **Education.** Rates are lower among college graduates than among those with some college education, high school graduates, and those who did not graduate from high school. However, adults who had graduated from college were more likely than adults who had not completed high school to have tried illicit drugs in their lifetime.

- **Employment.** Rates are higher for adults who are unemployed than for those who are employed either full-time or part-time. However, 72.7 percent of drug users are employed. Of the 17.8 million adults aged 18 or older who used illicit drugs in 2008, 12.9 million were employed.

- **Geographical region.** Among persons aged 12 or older, rates are highest in the West (9.8 percent) compared with the Northeast (8.2 percent,) the Midwest (7.6 percent), and the South (7.1 percent). For methamphetamine use, however, rates are higher in the West and the South than in the Northeast or Midwest.

Source: Results from the 2008 National Survey on Drug Use and Health: National Findings, Substance Abuse and Mental Health Services Administration, 2009, Rockville, MD: Office of Applied Studies.

phenomenon among college students. One survey found that the percentage of college students who abuse prescription drugs increased dramatically over the 12-year period from 1993 to 2005:[2]

- Pain relievers (for example, OxyContin, Vicodin, Percocet): Use increased by 343 percent
- Stimulants (for example, Ritalin, Adderall): Use increased by 93 percent
- Tranquilizers (for example, Xanax, Valium): Use increased by 450 percent
- Sedatives (for example, Nembutal, Seconal): Use increased by 225 percent

Nonmedical use of prescription-type drugs is also the most common form of drug use among young teens aged 12–13.[1] More than half of those aged 12 or older who used painkillers nonmedically report that they obtained the drug from a friend or relative for free.[1]

What Is a Drug?

A **drug** is a substance other than food that affects the structure or the function of the body through its chemical action. Alcohol, caffeine, aspirin, and nicotine are all drugs, as are amphetamines, cocaine, hallucinogens, sedatives, and inhalants. The drugs discussed here are *psychoactive*

drugs—substances that cause changes in brain chemistry and alter consciousness, perception, mood, and thought. This state is known as *intoxication*.

Psychoactive drugs are used for both medical and nonmedical (recreational) purposes. For example, Ritalin, a central nervous system (CNS) stimulant with effects similar to those of amphetamine, is prescribed to treat hyperactivity in children—a medical use. Cocaine, another CNS stimulant, is used recreationally to cause a burst of pleasurable sensations and to increase energy and endurance—a nonmedical use. When a medical drug is used for nonmedical (recreational) purposes, or when a drug has no medical uses, it is referred to as a **drug of abuse**.

All drugs have the potential to be toxic, that is, poisonous, dangerous, or deadly. Central nervous system depressants, such as alcohol, barbiturates, tranquilizers, and opium-derived drugs such as morphine and heroin can cause death if used in sufficient amounts to suppress vital functions like respiration. At the other extreme, CNS stimulants such as cocaine can cause sudden death by speeding up heart rate, elevating blood pressure, and accelerating other body functions to the point that systems are overwhelmed and collapse.

drug
Substance other than food that affects the structure or function of the body through its chemical action.

drug of abuse
Medical drug used for nonmedical (recreational) purposes or a drug that has no medical uses.

Consumer Clipboard

Taking a Smart Approach to Self-Medication

More than 700 products sold over the counter today include ingredients or dosage strengths that were available only by prescription just 30 years ago. With this wide range of products to choose from, self-medication has become common. Helpful as these products may be, they need to be approached with caution and common sense. When choosing to use over-the-counter drugs, keep these points in mind:

- Read the label each time you purchase an OTC medication. The format for OTC drug labels is set by the FDA and includes ingredients, uses, warnings, directions, and additional information, including a phone number to call for questions or comments.

- Do not exceed the recommended dose or take the medication for a longer period of time than recommended. If your condition does not improve, you need to see a physician.

- Be alert for possible interactions with other drugs you may be taking. Here are a few cautions:
  - Avoid alcohol if you're taking antihistamines, cough or cold products that contain dextromethorphan, or drugs used to treat sleeplessness.
  - Don't use drugs for sleeplessness if you're taking prescription sedatives or tranquilizers.

- If you're taking a prescription blood thinner, or if you have diabetes or gout, check with your physician before taking any product that contains aspirin.
- Unless your physician has instructed you to do so, don't use a nasal decongestant if you're taking a prescription drug for high blood pressure or depression, or if you have thyroid disease, diabetes, or prostate problems.

- Dietary supplements are not regulated by the FDA, so the ingredient amounts listed on the label are not always accurate. In addition, the manufacturer's claims about the safety and effectiveness of their products are not always backed up by solid research.

- If possible, select a medication with a single ingredient targeted at your symptoms rather than a combination of ingredients. You may not have all the symptoms treated by the multiple ingredients and may expose yourself to side effects unnecessarily.

- Choose a generic product over a brand-name product to save money. The active ingredients are the same.

- If the product has an expiration date, it refers to how long the drug will be active in an unopened package. Once the package is opened, the drug will probably be good for about a year.

Source: Data from "Over-the-Counter Medicines: What's Right for You?" 2005, U.S. Food and Drug Administration, www.fda.gov.

The American Psychiatric Association (APA) uses the term **substance** to refer to a drug of abuse, a medication, or a toxin.[3] In this chapter we use the terms *drug* and *substance* interchangeably.

substance
Drug of abuse, a medication, or a toxin; the term is used interchangeably with *drug*.

pharmaceutical drugs
Drugs developed for medical purposes, whether over-the-counter or prescription.

illicit drugs
Drugs that are unlawful to possess, manufacture, sell, or use.

TYPES OF DRUGS

Drugs are classified in several different ways. A basic distinction is often made between legal drugs and illicit (illegal) drugs. *Legal drugs* include medications prescribed by physicians, over-the-counter (OTC) medications, and herbal remedies. Drugs developed for medical purposes, whether OTC or prescription, are referred to as **pharmaceutical drugs**.

OTC medications can be purchased easily by consumers without a prescription. They include common remedies for headache, pain, colds, coughs, allergies, stomach upset, and other mild symptoms and complaints. Herbal remedies are usually botanical in origin; there are hundreds of substances in this group. At this time, the federal government's Food and Drug Administration (FDA) does not regulate herbal remedies before they are brought to market the way it regulates the development and approval of pharmaceutical drugs.

The FDA does have the power to remove an herbal remedy from the market if it has proven harmful. This was the case with the dietary supplement ephedra, a stimulant used for weight loss and body building, which the FDA banned after it was linked with more than 100 deaths from heart attack and stroke (see the box "Taking a Smart Approach to Self-Medication").

Prescription drugs can be ordered only by a specific health care provider. They must undergo a rigorous testing and approval process by the FDA. Today the pharmaceutical industry is one of the largest and most profitable industries in the United States, with sales well over $100 billion a year. Despite these astronomical sales, however, more than half of all prescriptions are filled with only 200 drugs.

Illicit drugs are generally viewed as harmful, and it is illegal to possess, manufacture, sell, or use them. Many drugs that are available by prescription are legal when obtained through a physician but illicit when manufactured or sold outside of the regulated medical system. Tobacco and alcohol are illegal drugs in the hands of minors, but they are usually not considered illicit because of their widespread availability to adults.

DRUG MISUSE AND ABUSE

The term **drug misuse** generally refers to the use of prescription drugs for purposes other than those for which they were prescribed or in greater amounts than prescribed. The term can also refer to the use of nonprescription drugs or chemicals such as glues, paints, or solvents for any purpose other than that intended by the manufacturer.

Injection The injection route involves using a hypodermic syringe to deliver the drug directly into the bloodstream (intravenous injection), to deposit it in a muscle mass (intramuscular injection), or to deposit it under the upper layer of skin (subcutaneous injection). With an intravenous (IV) injection ("mainlining"), the drug enters the bloodstream directly; onset of action is more rapid than with oral administration or other means of injection.

Inhalation The inhalation route is used for smoking tobacco, marijuana, and crack cocaine and for "huffing"

Although the number of people who use illicit drugs seems high, it's worth noting the other side of the picture, namely, that 92 percent of the population aged 12 or older— more than 200 million people—do not use illicit drugs.

The term **drug abuse** generally means the use of a substance in amounts, situations, or a manner such that it causes problems, or greatly increases the risk of problems, for the user or for others. The APA's *Diagnostic and Statistical Manual of Mental Disorders* (*DSM-IV-TR*) defines *substance abuse* as a maladaptive pattern of use leading to impairment or distress that continues despite serious negative consequences.

Drug abuse is not the same as drug dependence; a person can abuse a drug—for example, by binge drinking— without being dependent on it. We discuss drug dependence later in the chapter.

Effects of Drugs on the Body

All psychoactive drugs have an effect on the brain, and they reach the brain by way of the bloodstream. Like alcohol, some psychoactive drugs are consumed by mouth, but other routes of administration are used as well.

ROUTES OF ADMINISTRATION

Psychoactive drugs can be taken by several methods: orally (by mouth), injection, inhalation, application to the skin, or application to the mucous membranes. The speed and efficiency with which the drug acts are strongly influenced by the route of administration (Table 11.2).

Oral Most drugs are taken orally. Although this is the simplest way for a person to take a drug, it is the most complicated way for the drug to enter the bloodstream. A drug in the digestive tract must be able to withstand the actions of stomach acid and digestive enzymes and not be deactivated by food before it is absorbed. Drugs taken orally are absorbed into the bloodstream in the small intestine.

gasoline, paints, and other inhalants. An inhaled drug enters the bloodstream quickly because capillary walls are very accessible in the lungs.

Application to Mucous Membranes Application of a drug to the mucous membranes results in rapid absorption, because the mucous membranes are moist and have a rich blood supply. People who snort cocaine absorb the drug quickly into the bloodstream through the mucous membranes of the nose. People who chew tobacco absorb nicotine through the mucous membranes lining the mouth. Rectal and vaginal suppositories are also absorbed quickly, although these methods are less commonly used.

Application to the Skin Application to the skin is a less common method of drug administration. Most drugs are not well absorbed through the skin. *Dermal absorption* occurs when an oil or ointment is rubbed on the skin, producing a topical, or local, effect. *Transdermal absorption* occurs when a longer lasting application produces a systemic effect, such as when a patch delivers estrogen or nicotine. The advantage of the transdermal route is that it affords slow, steady absorption over many hours, producing stable levels of the drug in the blood.

drug misuse
Use of prescription drugs for purposes other than those for which they were prescribed or in greater amounts than prescribed, or the use of nonprescription drugs or chemicals for purposes other than those intended by the manufacturer.

drug abuse
Use of a substance in amounts, situations, or a manner such that it causes problems, or greatly increases the risk of problems, for the user or for others.

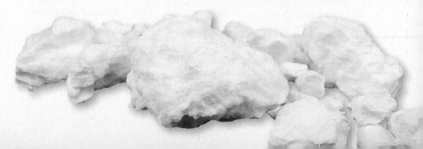

Table 11.2   Routes of Administration

Route	Time to Reach Brain	Drug Example	Potential Adverse Effects
Inhalation Smoking Huffing	7–10 seconds	Marijuana Crack cocaine Tobacco Inhalants	Irritation of lungs
Injection Intravenous Intramuscular Subcutaneous	15–30 seconds 3–5 minutes 5–7 minutes	Heroin Cocaine Methamphetamine	Danger of overdose Collapsed veins Infection at injection site Blood infection Transmission of HIV, hepatitis C, and other pathogens
Mucous membranes Snorting	3–15 minutes	Cocaine Methamphetamine Heroin	Irritation or destruction of tissue Difficulty controlling dose
Oral ingestion Eating, drinking	20–30 minutes	Alcohol Pills	Vomiting
Skin contact Dermal Transdermal	1–7 days	Oils, ointments Nicotine patch	Irritation of skin

FACTORS INFLUENCING THE EFFECTS OF DRUGS

The effect a drug has on a person depends on a number of variables, including the characteristics of the drug, the characteristics of the person, and the characteristics of the situation.

The first of these categories includes the chemical properties of the drug and its actions. Depending on the drug's chemical composition, it may speed up body processes or slow them down, produce a mild high or acute anxiety, or cause disorientation or hallucinations. These effects also depend on how much of the drug is taken, how often it is taken, and how recently it was taken.

Characteristics of the person include age, gender, body weight and mass, physical condition, mood, experience with the drug, and expectations. Generally speaking, the same amount of a drug has less effect on a 180-pound man than on a 120-pound woman. If a person has taken other drugs, the interactions of the chemicals can influence outcomes, as when one CNS depressant intensifies the effect of another.

The effects of drugs are also influenced by the characteristics of the situation or the environment. Taking a drug at home while relaxing with a group of friends may produce a different experience than will taking the same drug at a crowded, noisy bar or club, surrounded by strangers.

DRUG DEPENDENCE

As we saw in the case of alcohol, continued use of a drug can lead to *dependence* (or *addiction*), a condition characterized by a strong craving for a drug and by compulsive use of the drug despite serious negative consequences. Dependence usually means that physiological changes have taken place in brain and body chemistry as a result of using the drug. As described in Chapter 3, the main two indicators of physiological dependence are the development of *tolerance*, reduced sensitivity to the effects of the drug, and *withdrawal*, the experience of uncomfortable feelings when drug use stops.

Withdrawal symptoms are different for different drugs. For example, withdrawal from amphetamines is marked by intense feelings of fatigue and depression, increased appetite and weight gain, and sometimes suicidal thinking. Withdrawal from heroin causes nausea, vomiting, sweating, diarrhea, yawning, and insomnia.

EFFECTS OF DRUGS ON THE BRAIN

What accounts for the phenomenon of drug dependence? Scientists studying the effects of drugs on the brain have found that many addictive drugs, including cocaine, marijuana, opioids, alcohol, and nicotine, act on neurons in three brain structures—the ventral tegmental area (VTA) in the midbrain, the nucleus accumbens, and the prefrontal cortex.[4] Neurons in these three structures form a pathway referred to as the **pleasure and reward circuit** (Figure 11.2).

Under normal circumstances, this network of neurons is responsible for the feelings of satisfaction and pleasure when a physical, emotional, or survival need is met (for example, hunger, thirst, bonding, sexual desire). When it is activated, the circuit powerfully reinforces the behavior that satisfied the need (for example,

pleasure and reward circuit
Pathway in the brain involving three structures—the ventral tegmental area, the nucleus accumbens, and the prefrontal cortex—associated with drug dependence.

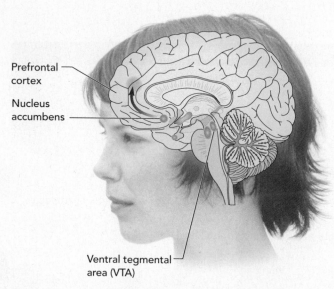

Prefrontal cortex

Nucleus accumbens

Ventral tegmental area (VTA)

figure 11.2   The pleasure and reward circuit in the brain.

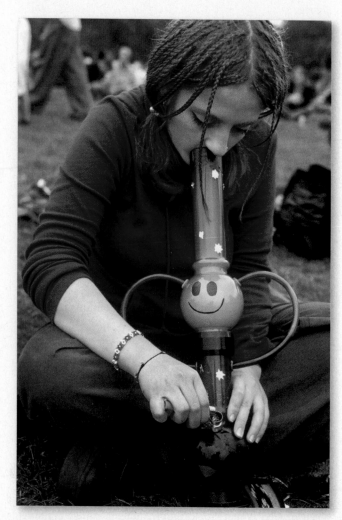

■ The most commonly used illicit drug in the United States is marijuana. Over 14 million Americans are current users.

eating), sending the message to "do it again." Neurons in the VTA increase production of dopamine, a neurotransmitter associated with feelings of pleasure. The VTA neurons pass messages to clusters of neurons in the nucleus accumbens, where the release of dopamine produces intense pleasure, and to the prefrontal cortex, where thinking, motivation, and behavior are affected.

Addictive psychoactive drugs activate this same pathway, causing an enormous surge in levels of dopamine and the associated feelings of pleasure. The nucleus accumbens sends the message to repeat the behavior that produced these feelings, and using the drug begins to take on as much importance as normal survival behaviors. Because the drug produces such huge surges of dopamine, the brain responds by reducing normal dopamine production. Eventually the person is unable to experience any pleasure, even from the drug, due to the disrupted dopamine system. Parts of the brain involved in rational thought and judgment are also disrupted, leading to loss of control and powerlessness over drug use. The very parts of the brain needed to make good life decisions are "hijacked" by addiction. Nonaddictive drugs do not cause these changes.

All or nearly all addictive drugs, whether "uppers" or "downers," operate via the pleasure and reward circuit, but some also operate via additional mechanisms. An example is the opioids (opium and its derivatives, morphine, codeine, and heroin). The brain has neurons with receptors for **endorphins**, its own "natural opiates"—brain chemicals that block pain when the body undergoes stress, such as during extreme exercise or childbirth. The structure of drugs in the opium family is similar to the structure of endorphins, so opioids readily bind to endorphin receptors, reducing pain and increasing pleasure. These effects occur in addition to the dopamine-related changes in the pleasure and reward circuit.

endorphins
Natural chemicals in the brain that block pain during stressful or painful experiences.

Individuals trying to recover from addiction are disadvantaged by their altered brain chemistry, drug-related memories, and impaired impulse control. Recovery is not simply a matter of willpower, nor does it involve abstinence from substances alone. Rather, multiple areas of the person's life have to be addressed—emotional, psychological, social, occupational, and so on. As a chronic, recurring disease, addiction typically involves repeated relapses and treatments before the person achieves recovery and return to a healthy life.

Drugs of Abuse

Drugs of abuse are usually classified as stimulants, depressants, opioids, hallucinogens, inhalants, and cannabinoids (Figure 11.3). For an overview of commonly abused drugs, their trade and street names, their intoxication effects, their potential for physical and psychological dependence, their potential health consequences, and their withdrawal effects, see Table 11.3.

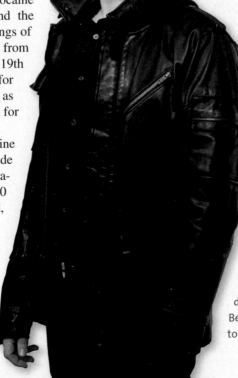

figure **11.3**   **Classification of psychoactive drugs.**

CENTRAL NERVOUS SYSTEM STIMULANTS

Drugs that speed up activity in the brain and sympathetic nervous system are known as **stimulants**. Their effects are similar to the response evoked during the fight-or-flight reaction (see Chapter 3). Heart rate accelerates, breathing deepens, muscle tension increases, the senses are heightened, and attention and alertness increase. These drugs can keep people going, mentally and physically, when they would otherwise be fatigued. The drugs may stimulate movement, fidgeting, and talking, and they may produce intense feelings of euphoria and create a sense of energy and well-being (see the box "Signs of Drug Use: CNS Stimulants"). Although stimulants do not meet the strict definition for physical dependence, users can develop tolerance and experience serious withdrawal effects.

stimulants
Drugs that speed up activity in the brain and the sympathetic nervous system.

Cocaine   A powerful CNS stimulant, cocaine heightens alertness, inhibits appetite and the need for sleep, and provides intense feelings of pleasure. Pure cocaine was first extracted from the leaves of the coca plant in the mid-19th century; it was introduced as a remedy for a number of ailments and used medically as an anesthetic.[5] Cocaine has high potential for abuse.

The most common form of pure cocaine is cocaine hydrochloride powder, made from coca paste. Snorting produces a relatively quick effect that lasts from 15 to 30 minutes; IV injection produces a rapid, powerful, and brief effect.

Two other methods of use are freebasing and smoking crack cocaine. Freebasing involves heating cocaine hydrochloride with a volatile solvent such as ether or ammonia and smoking it. This practice is dangerous because the solvent can ignite and burn the

■ Adam "DJ AM" Goldstein grew up in a home where drugs were abused. He battled his own addiction to crack cocaine in his 20s, was sober for more than 11 years, but fell back into drug use after surviving a plane crash in which several of his friends were killed. He was found dead on August 28, 2009, due to an accidental overdose from a combination of cocaine, oxycodone, Vicodin, Ativan, Klonopin, Xanax, Benadryl, and Levamisole, a substance used to dilute cocaine.

Table 11.3   Commonly Abused Drugs

Category & Name	Trade Names/Street Names	Potential for Physical Dependence	Potential for Psychological Dependence	Intoxication Effects	
CNS Stimulants				**Increased heart rate, blood pressure, metabolism; feelings of exhilaration, increased mental alertness**	
Cocaine	*Cocaine hydrochloride*/Coke, blow, crack	P	√√√	Also: Increased body temperature	
Amphetamine	*Biphetamine, Dexedrine*/Bennies, uppers, black beauties	P	√√√	Also: Rapid breathing, hallucinations	
Methamphetamine	*Desoxyn*/Meth, speed, crystal, ice	P	√√√	Also: Aggression, violence, psychotic behavior	
MDMA	Ecstasy, X, XTC	N	√√	Also: Mild hallucinogenic effects, increased tactile sensitivity, empathic feelings	
CNS Depressants				**Reduced pain and anxiety, feeling of well-being, lowered inhibitions, slowed pulse and breathing, lowered blood pressure**	
Barbiturates (sedatives)	*Amytal, Nembutal, Seconal, Phenobarbital*/Barbs, reds, yellows	√√	√√	Also: Sedation, drowsiness	
Benzodiazepines (tranquilizers)	*Ativan, Librium, Valium, Xanax*/Downers, tranks	√√	√√	Also: Sedation, drowsiness	
Flunitrazepam	*Rohypnal*/Roofies, forget-me pill, Mexican Valium	√√	√√		
GHB	*Gamma-hydroxybutyrate*/G, Georgia home boy, grievous bodily harm	√√	√√		
Opioids (Narcotics)				**Pain relief, euphoria, drowsiness**	
Morphine	*Roxanol, Duramorph*/M, Miss Emma, monkey	√√√	√√√		
Heroin	*Diacetyl-morphine*/H, junk, smack	√√√	√√√	Also: Staggering gait	
Synthetic opioids	*OxyContin, Vicodin, Percodan, Percocet, Demerol, Darvan*/Hillbilly heroin, percs, demmies	√√√	√√√		
Hallucinogens				**Altered states of perception and feeling, nausea**	
LSD	*Lysergic acid diethylamide*/Acid, blotter, boomers	N	?	Also: Increased body temperature, heart rate, blood pressure; loss of appetite; sleeplessnesss; tremors	
PCP	*Phencyclidine*/Angel dust, boat, love boat	P	√√√	Also: Increased heart rate and blood pressure; impaired motor function; panic, aggression, violence	
Inhalants	*Solvents, gases, nitrites*/Laughing gas, poppers, snappers	?	√–√√√	**Stimulation; loss of inhibition, headache, nausea, vomiting, slurred speech, loss of motor coordination**	
Cannabinoids				**Euphoria, slowed thinking and reaction time, confusion, impaired balance and coordination**	
Marijuana	Pot, weed, ganja, Mary Jane, reefer	?	√√		
Hashish	Hash, hemp, boom	?	√√		

Key:
N = None   P = Possible   √√ = Moderate
? = Unknown   √ = Low   √√√ = High

Source: "Commonly Abused Drugs," National Institute on Drug Abuse, retrieved April 9, 2010, from www.nida.nih.gov/DrugPages/DrugsofAbuse.html; "Drugs of Abuse/Uses and Effects," United States Drug Enforcement Administration, retrieved April 9, 2010, from www.justice.gov/dea/pubs/abuse/chart.htm.

Potential Health Consequences	Withdrawal Effects
Rapid or irregular heart rate, reduced appetite, weight loss, heart failure	Apathy, long periods of sleep, irritability, depression, disorientation
Also: Chest pain, respiratory failure, strokes, seizures, headaches, malnutrition	Also: Fatigue, increased appetite
Also: Tremor, irritability, anxiety, impulsivity, aggressiveness, restlessness, panic, paranoia	Also: Suicidal thoughts
Also: Memory loss, cardiac and neurological damage	
Also: Impaired memory and learning, hyperthermia, renal failure	Also: Muscle aches, drowsiness, depression
Fatigue; confusion; impaired memory, judgment, coordination; respiratory depression and arrest	Anxiety, insomnia, tremors, delirium, convulsions, possible death
Also: Depression, fever, irritability, poor judgment, dizziness, slurred speech	
Also: Dizziness	
Memory loss for time under the drug's effects, visual and gastrointestinal disturbances, urine retention	
Drowsiness, nausea, vomiting, headache, loss of consciousness, loss of reflexes, seizures, coma, death	
Nausea, constipation, confusion, sedation, respiratory depression and arrest, unconsciousness, coma, death	Watery eyes, runny nose, yawning, loss of appetite, irritability, tremors, panic, cramps, nausea, chills and sweating
Persisting perception disorder (flashbacks)	
Also: Persisting mental disorders	None
Also: Memory loss, numbness, nausea, vomiting, loss of appetite, depression	Also: Drug-seeking behavior
Unconsciousness, cramps, weight loss, muscle weakness, depression, memory impairment, damage to cardiovascular and nervous systems, sudden death	Agitation, trembling, anxiety, insomnia, vitamin deficiency, confusion, hallucinations, convulsions
Cough, frequent respiratory infections, impaired memory and learning, increased heart rate, anxiety, panic attacks	Occasional reports of insomnia, hyperactivity, decreased appetite
Also: Chronic bronchitis	

user. Crack is a form of cocaine that has been processed to make a rock crystal. It appeared in the mid-1980s and led to an epidemic of cocaine use in the United States. When smoked, crack cocaine produces the highest rate of dependence. Cocaine mixed with heroin produces a drug called a "speedball."

Cocaine is still used as a local anesthetic, often for surgeries in the areas of the nose and throat. Most uses, however, are recreational. Like other CNS stimulants, cocaine causes acceleration of the heart rate, elevation of blood pressure, dilation of the pupils, and an increase in alertness, muscle tension, and motor activity. It produces feelings of euphoria, often accompanied by talkativeness, sociability, and a sense of grandiosity. These effects appear almost immediately after a single dose and usually last for 15 minutes to an hour. When the effects wear off, the user typically wants to repeat the experience. Dependence can occur after only a few uses. Withdrawal after prolonged use is characterized by a depressed mood, fatigue, sleep disturbances, unpleasant dreams, and increased appetite.

At higher doses, cocaine use can lead to cardiac arrhythmias, respiratory distress, bizarre or violent behavior, psychosis, convulsions, seizures, coma, and even death. Regular snorting can irritate the nasal passage and result in a chronic runny nose. Some users may become malnourished because the drug suppresses appetite.

Amphetamines   For centuries practitioners of Chinese medicine have made a medicinal tea from herbs called Ma-huang. In the 1920s a chemist working for the Eli Lilly Company identified the active ingredient in Ma-huang as the compound ephedrine. The actions of this compound include opening the nasal and bronchial passages, allowing people to breathe more easily. The drug quickly became an important treatment for asthma, allergies, and stuffy noses. Researchers worked to develop synthetic forms of this botanical product, and a few years later, amphetamine was synthesized. Nasal amphetamine inhalers quickly grew in popularity; consumers found that they not only cleared the bronchioles but also produced elation.

In the 1930s amphetamines were put to additional uses: helping patients with narcolepsy stay awake, suppressing appetite in people who wanted to lose weight, and treating depression. In the 1940s soldiers fighting in World War II took amphetamines to stay alert and combat drowsiness. By the 1960s amphetamines were so widely available that they were quickly swept up into the drug culture of that period.

Amphetamines are no longer recommended for depression or weight control. Particularly in the case of depression, a host of newer, more effective drugs are available. Amphetamines are still used to treat *attention deficit/hyperactivity disorder (ADHD)* in children and adults. Although they are stimulants, they have a paradoxical effect in individuals with ADHD, helping them gain control of their behavior. More than 1 million children in the United States now take Ritalin and other amphetamines to control hyperactivity.

Concerns about the use of amphetamines involve their effects on the heart, lungs, and many other organs. At low levels they may cause loss of appetite, rapid breathing, high blood pressure, and dilated pupils. Decision making can be impaired even at moderate dosage levels. At higher levels, amphetamines can cause paranoia, panic, fever, sweating, headaches, blurred vision, dizziness, and sometimes aggressiveness and violence. Very high doses may cause flushing, rapid or irregular heartbeat, tremors, and even collapse. Deaths due to heart failure and burst blood vessels in the brain have also been reported. Withdrawal symptoms after continued amphetamine use include a drop in energy, feelings of helplessness, and thoughts of suicide. The person may "crash" into depression or sleep for 24 hours. Some symptoms can continue for days or weeks.

Methamphetamine ("speed") has a chemical structure similar to that of amphetamine and produces similar but more intense effects. It is usually snorted. A very pure form of methamphetamine, called "ice" or "crystal meth," can be smoked, producing an intense rush of pleasure lasting a few minutes.

Methamphetamine is more addictive and dangerous than most other forms of amphetamine because it contains so many toxic chemicals. Aside from addiction and brain damage, health effects of meth use include severe weight loss, cardiovascular damage, increased risk of heart attack and stroke, extensive tooth decay and tooth loss ("meth mouth"), and oily skin. Users are also at risk for paranoia and violent behavior.

Rates of meth use have soared in the past decade, in part due to its easy manufacture in makeshift labs from relatively inexpensive and commonly available drugs and chemicals.[6]

One such drug is pseudoephedrine, a nasal decongestant used in some cold and allergy medications. In 2005 Congress passed the Combat Methamphetamine Epidemic Act requiring that over-the-counter drugs like pseudoephedrine be sold from behind the counter and subjected to additional regulations. Some law enforcement agencies consider meth the number one drug problem in the United States.

MDMA Also known as Ecstasy, MDMA has chemical similarities to those of both stimulants (such as methamphetamine) and hallucinogens (such as mescaline).[7] Thus it produces both types of effects. MDMA appears to elevate levels of the neurotransmitter serotonin, the body's primary regulator of mood, perhaps in a manner similar to the action of antidepressants. Users experience increased energy, feelings of euphoria, and a heightened sense of empathy with and closeness to those around them. Some users report enhanced hearing, vision, and sense of touch, but only a few report actual visual hallucinations.

In addition to the drug's euphoric effects, MDMA can cause increased heart rate, elevated body temperature (sometimes to dangerous levels), profuse sweating, dry mouth, muscle tension, blurred vision, and involuntary teeth clenching. Serious risks include dehydration, hypertension, and heart or kidney failure. MDMA use can lead to psychological problems, such as depression, anxiety, confusion, paranoia, and sleep disturbances. Findings from several studies show that long-term users of MDMA can suffer cognitive defects, including problems with memory. However, more research on the long-term effects of this drug is needed.

Caffeine The mild stimulant caffeine is probably the most popular psychoactive drug. Common sources of caffeine

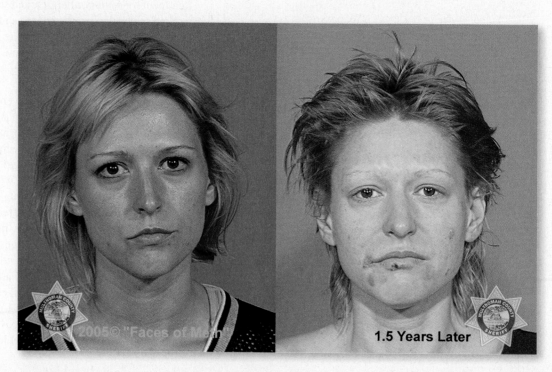

■ Faces of Meth is a project initiated by an Oregon sheriff to combat methamphetamine addiction in his county. The before-and-after photographs he compiled of methamphetamine users are shown in presentations to high school students. To see more photographs, go to www.facesofmeth.us.

1.5 Years Later

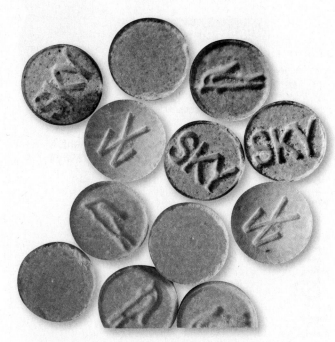

■ MDMA (Ecstasy) is frequently adulterated with a variety of other drugs and toxic substances. At some clubs, raves, and other dance events, pills can be screened by volunteers from DanceSafe, a harm reduction organization with services aimed at "non-addicted, recreational drug users."

include coffee, tea, soft drinks, headache and pain remedies like Excedrin, stay-awake products like No-Doz, and weight loss aids. Chocolate contains caffeine but at much lower levels than these sources.

At low doses caffeine increases alertness; at higher doses it can cause restlessness, nervousness, excitement, frequent urination, and gastrointestinal distress. At very high levels of consumption (1 gram a day, or 8–10 cups of coffee), symptoms of intoxication can include muscle twitching, irregular heartbeat, insomnia, flushed face, excessive sweating, rambling thoughts or speech, or excessive pacing or movement. People can develop tolerance to caffeine and experience withdrawal symptoms (usually irritability, headache, and fatigue) when cutting back on or eliminating it.

CENTRAL NERVOUS SYSTEM DEPRESSANTS

Central nervous system **depressants** slow down activity in the brain and sympathetic nervous system (see the box "Signs of Drug Use: CNS Depressants"). This category of drugs includes sedatives (for example, barbiturates), hypnotics (sleeping medications), and most anti-anxiety drugs. They can be deadly if misused, especially when mixed with one another or with alcohol (another CNS depressant). CNS depressants carry a high risk for dependence.

Barbiturates and Hypnotics   Barbiturates ("downers") are powerful sedatives that produce pleasant feelings of relaxation when first ingested, usually followed by lethargy, drowsiness, and sleep. Users experience impairments in judgment, decision making, and problem solving, as well as slow, slurred speech and lack of coordination. Dependence is common among middle-aged and older adults who use barbiturates as sleep aids. Withdrawal is difficult, and symptoms, including insomnia, anxiety, tremors, and nausea, can last for weeks; they can be mitigated by gradually tapering off the drug.

Hypnotics are prescribed for people with insomnia and other sleep disorders. They are also used to control epilepsy and to calm people before surgery or dental procedures.

Anti-Anxiety Drugs   The most widely prescribed CNS depressants fall into the group of anti-anxiety drugs known as the *benzodiazepines*; examples are Xanax, Valium, and Ativan. Also known as *tranquilizers*, the benzodiazepines are used to control panic attacks and anxiety disorders. Users are at risk for dependence and for increasing dose levels as they become tolerant.

Another concern is the **rebound effect**, which occurs when a person stops using a drug and experiences symptoms that are worse than those experienced before taking the drug. The rebound effect can make it difficult to stop taking a particular medication.

Rohypnol   A relatively new CNS depressant is flunitrazepam (Rohypnol); it started appearing in the United States in the 1990s. This powerful sedative has depressive effects and causes confusion, loss of memory, and sometimes loss of consciousness. It is especially dangerous when mixed with alcohol. Rohypnol is known as a "date rape drug" because men have slipped it into women's drinks in order to sexually assault them later. As of this time the drug's manufacturer has changed the formulation of this drug so that it will not remain colorless when dissolving in a drink.

depressants
Drugs that slow down activity in the brain and sympathetic nervous system.

rebound effect
Phenomenon that occurs when a person stops using a drug and experiences symptoms that are worse than those experienced before taking the drug.

Highlight on Health

Signs of Drug Use: CNS Depressants

Barbiturates, benzodiazepines
■ Reduced anxiety, euphoria
■ Relaxation, drowsiness, sedation

Flunitrazepam (Rohypnol)
■ Relaxation, sedation, lowered inhibitions, incapacitation
■ Disrupted memory, amnesia

GHB Another so-called date rape drug is gamma hydroxy-butyrate (GHB). This CNS depressant produces feelings of pleasure along with sedation and is a drug of choice among young people at bars, clubs, and parties. It can be produced in several forms, including a clear, tasteless, odorless liquid and a powder that readily dissolves in liquid. Like Rohypnol, it has been slipped into the drinks of women who later did not remember being sexually assaulted. It usually takes effect within 15 to 30 minutes and lasts from 3 to 6 hours. Besides sedation and amnesia, GHB can cause nausea, hallucinations, respiratory distress, slowed heart rate, loss of consciousness, and coma. Users are at risk for dependence with sustained use.

GHB, Rohypnol, and MDMA are sometimes referred to as *club drugs* because of their widespread use at clubs and parties. Their use is particularly dangerous because of the unpredictable setting in which they are usually taken. When GHB and Rohypnol are consumed with alcohol, the combined sedative effects can lead to life-threatening conditions. Additionally, all of these drugs are typically produced in basement labs, so dose and purity are uncertain.

OPIOIDS

Natural and synthetic derivatives of opium, a product harvested from a gummy substance in the seed pod of the opium poppy, are known as **opioids**. Opium originated in the Middle East and has a long history of medical use for pain relief and treatment of diarrhea and dehydration. Currently, opioids are prescribed as pain relievers, anesthetics, antidiarrheal agents, and cough suppressants.

■ Opium poppies are an important cash crop for subsistence farmers in developing countries around the world. Although there are legal medical uses for opium, virtually all of Afghanistan's opium poppy harvest is sold on the international market as heroin.

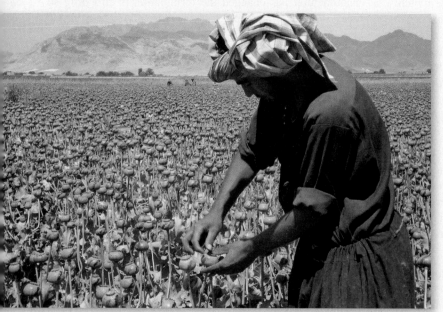

Drugs in this category include morphine, heroin, codeine, and oxycodone. Also known as *narcotics*, opioids are commonly misused and abused. They produce a pleasant, drowsy state in which cares are forgotten, the senses are dulled, and pain is reduced. They act by altering the neurotransmitters that control movement, moods, and a number of body functions, including body temperature regulation, digestion, and breathing.

opioids
Natural and synthetic derivatives of opium.

With low doses, opioid users experience euphoria, followed by drowsiness, constriction of the pupils, slurred speech, and impaired attention and memory (see the box "Signs of Drug Use: Opioids"). With higher doses, users can experience depressed respiration, loss of consciousness, coma, and death. When first used, opioids often cause nausea, vomiting, and a negative mood rather than euphoria. Chronic users usually experience dry mouth, constipation, and vision problems. Opioids have a high potential for dependence.

Morphine The primary active chemical in opium, morphine is a powerful pain reliever. Its first widespread use, facilitated by the development of the hypodermic syringe in the 1850s, was during the Civil War. So many soldiers became addicted that after the war, morphine addiction was called "the soldier's disease."[8] Because of the high risk of dependence, physicians prescribing morphine today do so conservatively.

Heroin   Heroin is three times more potent than morphine. It was developed in the late 19th century as a supposedly nonaddictive substitute for codeine (another derivative of morphine, useful for suppressing coughs). Just as Civil War veterans suffered from morphine addiction, many soldiers came home from the war in Vietnam addicted to heroin.

Whereas morphine has medical uses, heroin is almost exclusively a drug of abuse. Its use is associated with unemployment, divorce, and drug-related crimes. Users are at risk for such diseases as hepatitis, tuberculosis, and HIV infection from contaminated needles. Heroin abuse is associated with a variety of health conditions, particularly for those who inject it and do not practice safe use by using clean syringes. Among health conditions for which heroin users are at high risk are infectious diseases (including hepatitis and HIV/AIDS), various types of pneumonia, collapsed veins, liver and kidney disease, and permanent damage to various vital organs.[9] Babies born to women who used heroin during pregnancy are often drug dependent at birth.

Synthetic Opioids   Some of the most widely prescribed drugs in the United States are synthetic opioids, made from

■ Abuse of prescription painkillers has soared in the past 10 to 15 years, especially among teenagers and young adults. Overdoses from these central nervous system depressants now kill more people than overdoses from either heroin or cocaine.

oxycodone hydrochloride. Brand names include OxyContin, Vicodin, Demerol, Dilaudid, Percocet, and Percodan. Some people who start using these drugs for pain become addicted and misuse or abuse them (see the box "Diana: Pain, Stress, and Painkillers").

OxyContin, for example, provides long-lasting, timed-release relief for moderate to severe chronic pain when taken in tablet form. If the tablets are chewed, crushed and snorted, or dissolved in water and injected, they provide an

Life Stories

Diana: Pain, Stress, and Painkillers

Diana was a junior with dreams of becoming an athletic trainer after college. In high school she was overweight, but since coming to college she had taken up running and become healthy and fit. She had run two half-marathons and was training for a third. One day while she and her friend Ravi were out running, she landed wrong on her left foot and twisted her ankle. She collapsed in pain and with Ravi's help eventually got up and limped back to her car. Ravi drove her home and left to go to class, promising to return afterward. Diana called the health clinic and made an appointment for the next morning. Ravi returned and brought her a bottle of Percocet with a few pills left in it. He had been prescribed the drug last year after he had injured his back and hadn't finished the whole bottle. Diana's pain was intense, so she took one right away. Soon the pain vanished, and Diana began to feel blissful.

The next day she woke up in pain and took another Percocet. With crutches borrowed from a friend, she hobbled to her appointment. The nurse-practitioner who examined her took an X-ray of her foot to make sure she hadn't fractured her ankle. She hadn't, so he wrapped her ankle in an Ace bandage and told her to keep her weight off the foot, ice it, elevate it, and take ibuprofen for the pain. Diana lied that she had taken ibuprofen yesterday and that it hadn't helped. She asked him to prescribe something stronger. The nurse-practitioner agreed to write a five-day prescription for Vicodin—after a few days her pain should subside, he said.

Diana went through the Vicodin in three days. She was stressed about gaining weight now that she wouldn't be able to run for a while, and the high from the Vicodin, like that of the Percocet, helped her not think about it. On the fourth day, she had to take ibuprofen since her Vicodin had run out. It helped some with the pain, but not as much as the Vicodin had, and it didn't give her the same buzz. She returned to the health clinic the day after and met again with the nurse-practitioner. He examined her ankle and said that the swelling had gone down and that she was on the path to recovery. She told him that she needed more Vicodin because she was still in a lot of pain. He explained that for her type of injury—a simple sprain—Vicodin was not necessary and that the school also had specific guidelines for when synthetic opioids could be prescribed. He told her that prescription-strength ibuprofen should be sufficient.

Diana was upset and a little panicked as she left the appointment. She had been expecting to get more Vicodin. She called Ravi on her cell phone and asked if he could get a refill on his Percocet prescription. Ravi was surprised and concerned. He couldn't get a refill on a prescription that had expired a year ago. Was she okay? Diana said she was, and that she was sorry for having asked him. After she hung up, Diana felt embarrassed that she had asked Ravi to get her more pills. It wasn't like her to act this way. She realized that she was acting like a pill junkie—someone she didn't want to be. Taking stock of herself and putting her situation in perspective, she decided to face her current challenge without thinking she had to rely on drugs.

connect ACTIVITY

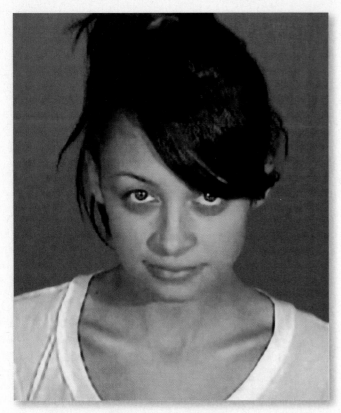

■ After trying to enter the wrong way onto a freeway in 2006, reality-TV star Nicole Richie was arrested for driving under the influence. She admitted to using marijuana and Vicodin prior to driving.

immediate, intense rush similar to that of heroin. One group particularly susceptible to opioid misuse is medical personnel with access to controlled substances.

HALLUCINOGENS

LSD, psilocybin, and mescaline are a few of the so-called **hallucinogens** (also called *psychedelics*). They differ chemically, but their effects are similar: They alter perceptions and thinking in characteristic ways. They produce intensification and distortion of visual and auditory perceptions as well as hallucinations (see the box "Signs of Drug Use: Hallucinogens and Inhalants"). Some hallucinogens are synthetic (for example, LSD), and others are derived from plants (for example, mescaline, from peyote, and psilocybin, from psilocybin mushrooms). They are Schedule I drugs with no current medical uses.[10]

hallucinogens
Drugs that alter perceptions and thinking, intensifying and distorting visual and auditory perceptions and producing hallucinations; also called *psychedelics*.

LSD   Lysergic acid diethylamide (LSD) is a synthetic hallucinogen that alters perceptual processes, producing visual distortions and fantastic imagery. Use of LSD peaked in the late 1960s and then declined, as reports circulated of

"bad trips," prolonged psychotic reactions, "flashbacks," self-injurious behavior, and possible chromosomal damage.

LSD is one of the most potent psychoactive drugs known. It is odorless, colorless, and tasteless, and a dose as small as a single grain of salt (about .01 mg) can produce mild effects. At higher doses (.05 mg to .10 mg), hallucinogenic effects are produced. Most users take LSD orally; absorption is rapid. Effects last for several hours and vary depending on the user's mood and expectations, the setting, and the dose and potency of the drug. It usually takes hours or days to recover from an LSD trip. Although LSD is thought to stimulate serotonin receptors in the brain, its exact neural pathway is not completely understood.

Besides visual distortion, LSD can produce auditory changes, a distorted sense of time, changes in the perception of one's own body, and *synesthesia*, a "mixing of senses," in which sounds may appear as visual images or a visual image changes in rhythm to music. Feelings of euphoria may alternate with waves of anxiety. In a bad trip, the user may experience acute anxiety or panic. LSD does not produce compulsive drug-seeking behaviors, and physiological withdrawal symptoms do not occur when use is stopped.

Phencyclidine (PCP)   First developed in the 1950s as an anesthetic, PCP was found to produce such serious side effects—agitation, delusions, irrational behavior—that its use was discontinued. Since the 1960s it has been manufactured illegally and sold on the street, often under the name "angel dust." It has fewer hallucinogenic effects than LSD and more disturbances in body perception. A drug with similar effects is ketamine.

PCP is a white crystalline powder that is readily soluble in water or alcohol. It can be smoked, snorted, or injected intravenously. At low doses it produces euphoria, dizziness, nausea, slurred speech, rapid heartbeat, high blood pressure, numbness, and slowed reaction time. At higher doses it causes disorganized thinking and feelings of unreality, and at very high doses it can cause amnesia, seizures, and coma. A person who has taken PCP is anesthetized enough to undergo surgery.

The drug is particularly associated with aggressive behavior, probably as a result of impaired judgment and disorganized thinking. Combined with insensitivity to pain, these effects can produce dangerous or deadly results.

INHALANTS

The drugs called **inhalants** are breathable chemical vapors that alter consciousness, typically producing a state of intoxication that resembles drunkenness. The vapors come from substances like paint thinners, gasoline, glue, and spray can propellant. The active ingredients in these products are chemicals like toluene, benzene, acetone, and tetrachlorethylene—all dangerously powerful toxins and carcinogens.[11]

inhalants
Breathable chemical vapors that alter consciousness, producing a state resembling drunkenness.

At low doses inhalants cause light-headedness, dizziness, blurred vision, slurred speech, lack of coordination, and feelings of euphoria. At higher doses they can cause lethargy, muscle weakness, and stupor. An overdose of an inhalant can result in a loss of consciousness, coma, or death. Inhalants can also cause behavioral and psychological changes, including belligerence, confusion, apathy, and impaired social and occupational functioning. Perhaps the most significant negative effect for chronic users is widespread and long-lasting brain damage.

Initial use of inhalants often starts early, with 15.7 percent of 8th graders having tried some type of an inhalant.

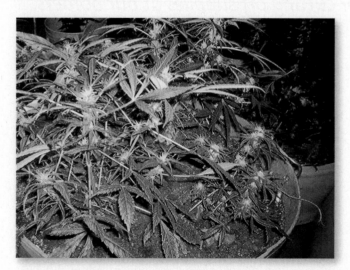

■ The *Cannabis* plant has a variety of uses, including as fiber (hemp), food, medications, and for its psychedelic effects. From its probable origin in China or central Asia, the plant spread to India, ancient Rome, Africa, Europe, and the Americas

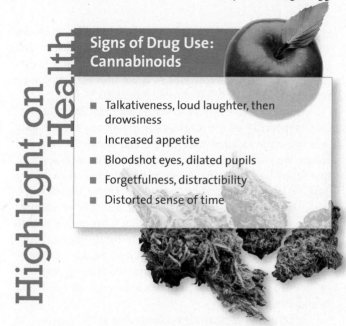

Highlight on Health

Signs of Drug Use: Cannabinoids

- Talkativeness, loud laughter, then drowsiness
- Increased appetite
- Bloodshot eyes, dilated pupils
- Forgetfulness, distractibility
- Distorted sense of time

Since 2001, the percent of 8th and 10th graders who see great risk in using inhalants has been steadily declining.[12]

CANNABINOIDS

The most widely used illicit drug in the United States is marijuana. In 2008 there were an estimated 14.4 million users among Americans aged 12 or older, and 13 percent of young people aged 12 to 17 had used marijuana at least once.[1]

Marijuana is derived from the hemp plant, *Cannabis sativa*, thus the name *cannabinoids*. The leaves of the plant are usually dried and smoked, but they can also be mixed in tea or food. Hashish is a resin that seeps from the leaves; it is usually smoked. The active ingredient in marijuana is delta-9-tetrahydrocannabinol (THC). The potency of the drug is determined by the amount of THC in the plant, which in turn is affected by the growing conditions. Since the 1960s, the amount of THC in marijuana sold on the street has increased from 1–5 percent to as much as 10–15 percent.

Marijuana use produces mild euphoria, sedation, lethargy, short-term memory impairment, distorted sensory perceptions, a distorted sense of time, impaired motor coordination, and an increase in heart rate (see the box "Signs of Drug Use: Cannabinoids"). Effects typically begin within a few minutes and last from three to four hours. Sometimes the drug causes anxiety or a negative mood. At high doses marijuana can have hallucinogenic effects, accompanied by acute anxiety and paranoid thinking. Chronic, heavy users of marijuana may develop tolerance to its effects and experience some withdrawal symptoms if they stop using it, but most dependence seems to be psychological.

Researchers have found that THC has a variety of effects on the brain. One effect is the suppression of activity in the information processing system of the hippocampus, perhaps accounting for some impairments in problem solving and decision making associated with being high on marijuana. Marijuana smoke has negative effects on the respiratory system; it contains more carcinogens than tobacco smoke and is highly irritating to the lining of the bronchioles and lungs. In addition to coughs and chest colds, users may experience more frequent episodes of acute bronchitis and may be more likely to develop chronic bronchitis.[13]

Many people claim that marijuana does have medical uses, especially as a treatment for glaucoma, for the pain and nausea associated with cancer and chemotherapy, and for the weight loss associated with AIDS. Research suggests that smoking marijuana is no more effective than taking THC in pill form for these purposes, but the use of marijuana for medical reasons has become a matter of political debate. Proponents of its use assert that it makes life livable for many people with painful and debilitating medical conditions and that there is no reason not to legalize it. Opponents argue that legalizing marijuana would imply approval of its use for recreational purposes and open the floodgates to abuse of all drugs.

Like alcohol, marijuana affects the skills required to drive a car safely, including concentration, attention, coordination, reaction time, and the ability to judge distance. Because it also impairs judgment, people who are high may not realize their driving skills are impaired.

It also appears that marijuana use during pregnancy affects both the likelihood of miscarriage and the health of the fetus.[13] Babies born to mothers who use marijuana may be smaller and more likely to develop health problems once they are born. During infancy and early childhood, these

specifically to Dilaudid use rose 309 percent during the same time period.[16]

Other economic costs of illicit drug use include social welfare costs, workplace accidents, property damage, incarceration of otherwise productive individuals, goods and services lost to crime, work hours missed by victims of drug-related crime, and costs of law enforcement.

Government approaches to the drug problem have traditionally fallen into two broad categories: supply reduction and demand reduction. A newer approach to the drug problem is harm reduction, an approach used in alcohol treatment programs as well.

SUPPLY REDUCTION STRATEGIES

Strategies to reduce the supply of drugs are aimed at controlling the quantity of illicit substances that enter or are produced in the United States. An example is *interdiction*, the interception of drugs before they enter the country, as when customs officials use dogs to sniff out drugs at airports or when the Coast Guard boards ships to search for drugs as they enter U.S. waters.

The U.S. government also puts pressure on governments in other countries to suppress the production and exportation of drugs. Unfortunately, the plants that yield drugs are important and profitable cash crops for peasant farmers in many countries, and the drug smuggling business is controlled by criminal interests that are often beyond the

Evidence indicates that **treatment is a more effective strategy for reducing drug use** *than locking up dealers or cutting off supplies at our borders.*

children may have more behavioral problems and cognitive deficits, and in school, they have more difficulty with tasks requiring memory, attention, and decision making.[14]

Approaches to the Drug Problem

Drug abuse and dependence have negative consequences affecting individuals, communities, and society. In addition to the human costs, illicit drug use and addiction cause considerable economic damage. An estimated $467.7 billion is drained from the U.S. economy by drug use annually, most of which is spent on health care and justice system costs. Only a very small percentage goes toward prevention and treatment.[15] In 2008 an estimated 4.4 million drug-related hospital emergency room visits were reported in the United States.[16] Visits related to synthetic opioid use increased 123 percent between 2004 and 2008, and visits related

control of the government. Efforts to reduce the drug supply at the international level have led to human rights abuses, an expansion of oppressive regimes, and increased corruption among police, government, and military personnel.

The government also attempts to prevent domestic production of drugs by raiding suspected underground drug labs or stamping out enterprises that grow marijuana on a large scale. Another domestic supply-side strategy is to obstruct the distribution of drugs, such as when a massive police presence is used in an area where drugs are sold.

DEMAND REDUCTION STRATEGIES

Demand-side strategies include penalizing users through incarceration; preventing drug use, primarily through education; and treating individuals once they have become dependent on drugs.

Incarceration for Drug-Related Crimes Penalizing users means enforcing the laws against drug possession,

Public Health in Action

Combating Teen Prescription Drug Abuse

*"Don't look at me, man.
Ain't my problem. I didn't do it."*

A drug dealer stands by a public phone complaining that he's losing his customers—they're now getting their drugs from their parents' medicine cabinets. This ad, called "Drug Dealer Testimonial," aired during Super Bowl XLII in 2008. It was the first ad in a media campaign launched by the federal government's Office of National Drug Control Policy (ONDCP) in conjunction with the Partnership for a Drug-Free America to educate parents about prescription and over-the-counter drug abuse by teenagers. Designed to reach more than 90 percent of parents a dozen times, the campaign has included TV ads, an Open Letter to Parents printed in national and regional newspapers, print ads in national magazines, online ads, and point-of-purchase messages in drugstores.

Although teen drug use is down overall, more teens abuse prescription drugs than any illicit drug except marijuana. In 2006 more than 2.1 million teenagers abused prescription drugs; the most commonly abused are painkillers (for example, OxyContin, Vicodin), depressants (for example, sleeping pills, anti-anxiety drugs), and stimulants (for example, Ritalin). Teens are also abusing over-the-counter drugs like cough and cold medications that contain the cough suppressant dextromethorphan, such as NyQuil and Robitussin.

Research suggests that teenagers believe that taking prescription medications is safer than using street drugs, not realizing the risks of addiction and overdose, especially if the medications are combined with alcohol or other drugs. Many parents are not aware of these dangers either, nor do they realize how much influence they have with their teenagers.

In 2009 the ONDCP evaluated the success of its "Drug Dealer Testimonial" campaign. After the airing of the first ad, traffic to the campaign's Web site, www.theantidrug.com, spiked more than 530 percent and remained high in the months afterward. By May 2008, 71 percent of parents were aware of advertising about prescription drug abuse prevention and those who had seen the ads were more likely to consider teen prescription drug use a serious problem and to have intentions to control the supply of prescription drugs at their home. Although the resulting impact of the campaign on teen prescription drug abuse is not known, the percentage of 12- to 17-year-olds who had used prescription drugs in the past month fell from 3.3 percent in 2007 to 2.9 percent in 2008. The campaign continues to produce new ads, which can be viewed at www.theantidrug.org.

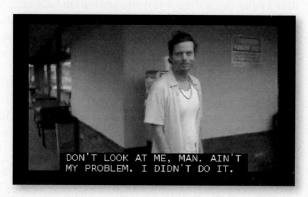

DON'T LOOK AT ME, MAN. AIN'T MY PROBLEM. I DIDN'T DO IT.

connect ACTIVITY

Sources: "ONDCP Launches First Major Initiative to Combat Teen Prescription Drug Abuse," Office of National Drug Control Policy, 2008, retrieved April 20, 2008, from www.mediacampaign.org/newsroom/press08/012408.html; Prescription for Danger: A Report on Prescription and Over-the-Counter Drug Abuse Among the Nation's Teens, Office of National Drug Control Policy, 2008, retrieved April 13, 2010, from http://theantidrug.com/pdf/prescription_report.pdf; "Effectiveness of a Mass Media Campaign for Parents on Teen Prescription Drug Abuse," Office of National Drug Control Policy, 2009, Drug Prevention + Social Marketing Brief, 4, pp. 1–4.

arresting offenders, and putting people in prison. The assumptions behind this approach are that incarceration will reduce drug-related crime by getting users off the streets and that the threat of punishment will deter others from using drugs. Most states mandate harsh prison terms for the possession or sale of relatively small quantities of drugs, regardless of whether the person is a first-time or repeat offender.

As a result, U.S. prisons are crowded with people convicted of drug-related crimes; in fact, more than half of the people in U.S. prisons are serving time for such offenses. The United States imprisons a larger percentage of its population than does any other nation. Elsewhere, low-level crimes like drug possession do not draw a prison sentence.

Since prisoners are a captive audience, it would make sense to provide treatment while they are in jail, but only a small percentage of prisoners who need drug treatment receive it. Incarceration does little to address the larger problem of drug use in our society.

Prevention Strategies   A second demand-side strategy is prevention through education. Prevention strategies focus on reducing the demand for drugs by increasing an individual's ability to decline drug use when confronted with an opportunity to experiment. Programs involve primary, secondary, or tertiary prevention, depending on their targeted audience. *Primary, or universal, prevention programs* are designed to reach the entire population without regard to individual risk factors. Public service commercials on television asking us to imagine a world without cigarettes or billboards referring to crystal meth as "crystal mess" are examples of primary prevention strategies (see the box "Combating Teen Prescription Drug Abuse").

Secondary, or selective, strategies focus on those subgroups that are at greatest risk for use or abuse, with the aim of increasing protective factors and decreasing potential risk factors. An example is a class that teaches problem-solving skills to adolescents.

Tertiary, or indicated, strategies target at-risk individuals rather than groups, again focusing on protective factors such as academic, interpersonal, social, or job skills. An example is a program that tutors individual students in ways to manage emotions and maintain self-esteem without drugs.

A prevention strategy used in the workplace is drug testing, usually random urine screening. The goal of drug testing is not to catch drug users and fire them but to create an environment in which it is clear that drug use is not condoned. Companies also want to limit their liability by reducing the likelihood that an employee will make a mistake that causes someone harm. Federal law requires that people in jobs involving transportation, such as air traffic controllers, train engineers, and truck drivers, undergo regular testing to ensure public safety. U.S. military personnel also undergo regular drug testing. Although some see the practice as an infringement of privacy rights, so far it has withstood judicial challenges.

On college campuses, a number of steps can be taken to prevent drug use and to reduce harm to those students who do use (see the box "Do you Know Someone With a Drug Problem?"). A comprehensive approach, known as

hot tip

The next time you vote in a presidential or congressional election, find out the candidates' positions on drug policy.

environmental management, can be implemented to modify an environment that often benignly accepts or overlooks drug use and experimentation during college. The most effective approaches seem to have a number of common factors:[2]

- Sending clear messages that drug use is not acceptable.
- Changing the climate of drug tolerance on campus, if it exists.
- Engaging parents.
- Identifying and intervening with at-risk students.
- Providing alternative activities.
- Involving students in the planning of prevention programs.

For those individuals who will experiment regardless of changes made on campus, harm reduction strategies are important. Implementing such strategies should not be seen as "giving permission" to students to use; rather, it reduces the likelihood that they will harm themselves or others. The following are some harm reduction strategies that have been implemented on college campuses:

- Providing containers in college buildings for the safe disposal of needles and syringes.
- Providing condoms so that students will not transmit infectious diseases if drug use leads to sexual activity.

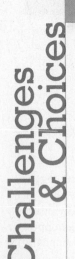

Challenges & Choices

Do You Know Someone With a Drug Problem?

College students turn to illicit drugs for a variety of reasons. They may want to experiment, relax, reduce stress, stay up late to study, or even self-medicate psychiatric problems. Some are continuing a pattern of drug use they began in high school, while others are experimenting with their new-found freedom away from home. Many young adults do not realize how easy it is to become dependent on a drug, whether physiologically or psychologically.

Most colleges identify alcohol abuse as their most pressing substance-related issue and focus their attention on alcohol-related programs. Very few schools report having programs specifically aimed at early identification of drug-related problems. Without formal programs, it is important that students take a role in the early identification of such problems in their friends, roommates, and fellow students. The following behaviors may indicate that someone is having a problem with drugs:

- A noticeable change in behavior, such as withdrawal or agitation.
- A change in sleep habits, needing either more or less.

- Nodding out during conversations or in class on a regular basis.
- Lack of interest in activities that used to be a source of enjoyment.
- An increase in physical complaints or pain.
- Preoccupation with a drug; activities scheduled around drug use.
- An increase in money borrowing.

If you notice these behaviors in a friend, you may want to express your concerns—keeping silent does nothing to help your friend acknowledge and address the problem. Be prepared to offer suggestions about where he or she might go to get help, such as the college counseling center, and also be prepared to be rebuffed in case your friend is in denial. The best thing you can do is continue to be supportive of your friend and look out for his or her best interest.

Source: Monitoring the Future: National Survey Results on Drug Use, 1975–2006: Volume II, College Students and Adults Ages 19–45 *(NIH Publication No. 07-6206), by L.D. Johnson, P.M. O'Malley, J.G. Bachman, and J.E. Schulenberg, 2007, Bethesda, MD: National Institute on Drug Abuse.*

- Making naloxone (Narcan) available in case of opioid overdose. Naloxone is an opiate antagonist that can counteract life-threatening depression of the respiratory system.

One of the best ways to understand and control your drug use is to first do a self-assessment to see the part drugs play in your life. Complete the self-assessment and questions in this chapter's Personal Health Portfolio to determine the impact drugs have on your life and whether you are in need of treatment by a professional.

Drug Treatment Programs   The third type of demand-side strategy is helping people to stop using drugs after they have started, that is, providing treatment. Evidence indicates that treatment is a more effective strategy for reducing drug use than locking up dealers or cutting off supplies at our borders.[17,18] As with alcohol, treatment is available in a variety of formats, ranging from hospital-based inpatient programs to self-help/mutual-help groups such as Narcotics Anonymous (NA).

Most experts agree that treatment is a long-term process, often marked by relapses and requiring multiple treatment episodes. The first step is acknowledging that there is a problem and getting into a program. No single treatment is appropriate for everyone; matching services to individual needs is important.

Treatment is more successful when the program lasts at least three months, includes individual counseling, and addresses all aspects of the client's life, including medical treatment, family therapy, living skills, and occupational skills. In counseling, clients work to increase motivation, build relapse prevention skills, improve problem-solving and interpersonal skills, and develop life-enhancing behaviors.

Participating in self-help support programs during and following treatment often helps maintain abstinence.

HARM REDUCTION STRATEGIES

As described in Chapter 10, harm reduction strategies are based on the idea that attempting to completely eliminate substance use is futile and that efforts should be focused on helping addicts reduce the harm associated with their substance use.[19–21]

Advocates of the harm reduction approach assert that drug users are in need of treatment rather than punishment. Examples of harm reduction strategies are needle exchange programs, in which addicts are provided with sterile needles in exchange for their used ones, and drug substitute programs, in which individuals are maintained on addictive but less debilitating drugs, such as methadone for heroin addicts.

Other harm reduction strategies include controlled availability (certain drugs are available through a government monopoly), medicalization (drugs are available by prescription but only to individuals who are already addicted to them), and decriminalization (the penalty for possession of certain drugs is reduced or eliminated if the quantity held is below a certain limit).

Proponents of harm reduction strategies claim that they represent a more realistic approach to the drug problem and would allow resources to be directed away from punishment, which is ineffective, and toward treatment, which is effective. Opponents of harm reduction strategies argue that they are thinly disguised forms of drug legalization and that any softening of a zero tolerance position would result in an epidemic of drug use. Although effective harm reduction programs are in place in England and Canada, harm reduction is rejected as an official policy by the U.S. government.

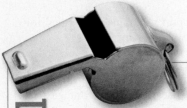

You Make the Call

Should Marijuana Be Legalized for Recreational Purposes?

Currently, 14 states have laws in place that legalize the use of marijuana for medical purposes, and many others are considering similar laws regarding medical marijuana. A somewhat different debate is also taking place—whether marijuana should be legalized for nonmedical use. This debate grew louder in 2010, when California became the first state to consider legalization of marijuana for adult recreational use.

Proponents of legalization contend that marijuana is safer than alcohol and tobacco. An estimated 76,000 people die each year due to excessive alcohol consumption, and more than 400,000 die each year from the effects of smoking. Marijuana has not been the primary cause of any recorded deaths and was a secondary cause in only 279 deaths during an eight-and-a-half-year period. Proponents cite statistics connecting alcohol with violence and point out that marijuana does not make people belligerent. Alcohol is involved in two-thirds of domestic violence cases, and an estimated 40 percent of rape and sexual assault perpetrators are under the influence of alcohol at the time of the crime. Opponents respond that we should not legalize another substance that will cause harm, even if it is relatively less harmful than alcohol or tobacco. They point to the negative health consequences of smoking marijuana, which include heart and respiratory problems, as evidence that marijuana is not a benign drug.

Proponents also argue that the legalization of marijuana would result in financial benefits for the government. The federal government would gain revenue from income taxes on profits made by marijuana businesses. States would no longer have to use money and resources to enforce current marijuana laws and would gain revenue from taxes on the sale of marijuana. The California Legislative Analyst's Office estimates that the legalization of marijuana would result in $1.4 billion a year in additional tax revenue for the state. Some of these tax monies could even be used to bolster underfunded prevention and treatment programs, proponents say.

Opponents respond that the additional revenue would not result in a financial boon because states would have to spend more money on treatment programs, and individuals and society would have to bear the costs of marijuana-related health problems. Opponents argue that legalization would increase the number of young people using marijuana and likely lead to higher rates of use of more addictive drugs. The federal government currently classifies marijuana itself as a Schedule I drug, meaning that it has a high potential for abuse. More teens are in treatment for marijuana use than for any other drug, and increasing the availability of marijuana to adults would increase the opportunities for children and teens to obtain it for themselves, opponents say.

A 2010 poll conducted by the Pew Research Center found that 41 percent of Americans favor the legalization of marijuana. Although people who oppose legalization are in the majority, the percentage of those who favor it has increased over the past two decades—in 1990 only 16 percent of people supported legalization. Harmless fun or dangerous drug—what do you think?

PROS

- The number of states that have legalized medical marijuana and California's consideration of legalizing marijuana for recreational use show that public opinion is shifting favorably toward legalizing the drug.

- Marijuana is a relatively safe drug when compared to legal drugs like alcohol and tobacco.

- Legalizing marijuana will save money on law enforcement and generate tax revenue.

CONS

- Marijuana is not a harmless drug. It can cause many health problems, including heart, respiratory, and short-term memory problems.

- Legalization would make the drug more available to children and teens.

- Taxing the sale of marijuana would not result in a net increase in federal and state revenues.

connect ACTIVITY

Sources: "Deaths from Marijuana v. 17 FDA-Approved Drugs," ProCon.org, 2009, retrieved April 12, 2010, from http://medicalmarijuana .procon.org/view.resource.php?resourceID=000145; "Alcohol and Violence," The Marin Institute, 2006, retrieved April 12, 2010, from www .marininstitute.org/alcohol_policy/violence.htm; "Don't Legalize Marijuana," by S. Miller, The Los Angeles Times, 2010, from http://articles .latimes.com/2010/jan/28/opinion/la-oe-miller28-2010jan28.

IN REVIEW

Why do people use drugs, and what are current patterns of drug use?

As with alcohol, people use drugs to feel better, often as a recreational activity; however, some people become addicted and lose control of their drug use. The most commonly used illicit drug is marijuana, but the nonmedical use of prescription-type drugs has increased dramatically in recent years.

How do drugs affect the body?

As psychoactive substances, drugs affect the brain and central nervous system (CNS). Effects vary depending on the chemical properties of the drug, the characteristics of the person, and the environment. Drug dependence occurs when the drug causes changes in the brain, particularly the brain structures that make up the pleasure and reward circuit and those parts of the brain involved in rational thought and judgment.

What are the different categories of drugs?

Drugs are classified as CNS stimulants (for example, cocaine, methamphetamine), CNS depressants (barbiturates, benzodiazepines), opioids (heroin, oxycodone), hallucinogens (LSD), inhalants (paint thinner, glue), and cannabinoids (marijuana).

What are the main approaches to the drug problem?

The main approaches are supply reduction strategies (for example, interdiction), demand reduction strategies (incarceration, prevention through education, treatment), and harm reduction strategies (needle exchange programs). Because colleges are often focused more on alcohol-related problems than on drug-related problems, students may have to be more proactive in identifying and helping friends who are developing a drug problem.

Web Resources

ClubDrugs.Org: This Web site offers information on club drugs such as Ecstasy, GHB, and LSD, including trends and statistics for these and other drugs of abuse.
www.clubdrugs.org

Narcotics Anonymous (NA): NA resources include drug information, help lines, contact information, news features, publications, and links.
www.na.org

National Institute on Drug Abuse: This government site features in-depth information on various drugs of abuse, offering research reports and drug information along with many other helpful resources.
www.nida.nih.gov

Substance Abuse and Mental Health Services Administration (SAMHSA): SAMHSA offers information and resources on mental health, drug abuse prevention and treatment, and workplace issues.
www.samhsa.gov

U.S. Drug Enforcement Administration: Drugs of Abuse: This comprehensive resource includes fact sheets on drugs of abuse and briefs on drug-related topics.
www.dea.gov

12

Relationships and Sexual Health

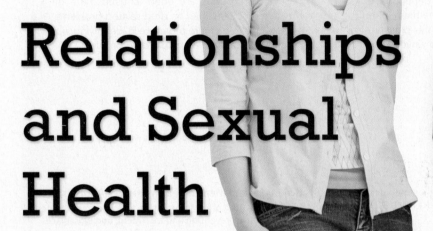

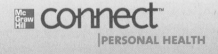

McGraw Hill **connect**™
|PERSONAL HEALTH

http://www.mcgrawhillconnect.com/personalhealth

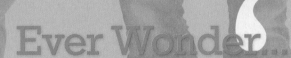

Ever Wonder...

- if you have the qualities of a good partner?

- why it's hard to communicate with someone of the other sex?

- how to talk to a prospective partner about your sexual histories?

Relationships are a vital part of wellness. People with a strong social support system have better mental and physical health, are more capable of dealing with stress and adverse life events, and may even live longer than those without such support. Similarly, sexuality is an important aspect of wellness. Studies show that an active sex life is associated with reduced risk of heart disease and depression, improved immune function, and lowered risk of death.[1] This chapter addresses some of the complexities of relationships and sexual health.

Relationships: Connection and Communication

Relationships are at the heart of human experience. We are born into a family; grow up in a community; have classmates, teammates, and colleagues; find a partner from among our acquaintances and friends; and establish our own family. Yet for all their importance in our lives, relationships are fraught with difficulties and challenges. About half of all marriages in the United States end in divorce, and many children grow up in a single-parent or blended family of one kind or another. Many people also live alone in the United States, either by choice or by chance. College students have less of an opportunity to experience real relationships on campuses where "hooking up"— having intimate experiences with no strings attached—is the norm (see the box "Who Hooks Up?").

HEALTHY RELATIONSHIPS

Three kinds of important relationships are the one you have with yourself, the ones you have with friends, and the ones you have with intimate partners. In each, certain qualities serve to enhance the relationship's positive effects.

A Healthy Sense of Self All your relationships begin with who you are as an individual. A healthy sense of self, reasonably high self-esteem, a capacity for empathy, and the ability both to be alone and to be with others are examples of such individual attributes. Many people develop these assets growing up in their families, but if you experience deficits in childhood, you can still make up for them later in life.

Relationships *are at the heart of* human experience.

Friendships and Other Kinds of Relationships Friendship is a reciprocal relationship based on mutual liking and caring, respect and trust, interest and companionship. We often share a big part of our personal history with our friends. Compared with romantic partnerships, friendships are usually more stable and longer lasting; in fact, some last a lifetime.

A recent survey found that despite experiencing very high levels of stress, 97 percent of Americans report having people in their lives whom they trust and can turn to when they need support.[2] The average American has four close social contacts, with most having between one and six.[3]

Along with family ties and involvement in social activities, friendships offer a psychological and emotional buffer against stress, anxiety, and depression. They help protect you against illness, and they help you cope with problems if you do become ill. Friendships and other kinds of social support increase your sense of belonging, purpose, and self-worth.[4]

Strengths of Successful Partnerships An intimate relationship with a partner has many similarities with friendships, but it has other qualities as well. Compared with friendships, partnerships are more exclusive, involve deeper levels of connection and caring, and have a sexual component. The following are some characteristics of successful partnerships:

■ The more mature and independent individuals are, the more likely they are to establish intimacy in their relationship. Independence and maturity often increase with age; in fact, the best predictor of a successful marriage is the age of the partners.

■ The partners have both self-esteem and mutual respect.

Who's at Risk?

Who Hooks Up?

In the past, the typical trajectory of a relationship was dating, becoming a couple, and then having sex. The pattern seems to have shifted among college students, where people hook up for sex without having dated or been in a relationship. Sex may or may not lead to becoming a couple—if it does, then dating follows. Although hooking up is usually discussed as a broad trend, there appear to be some common characteristics among students who are more likely to hook up for sex than others.

■ More males hook up for sex than do females

■ Females experience more negative psychological effects after hooking up for sex, such as regret, psychological distress, and depression

■ Students who are more likely to hook up for sex
  – are White
  – are non-religious
  – have divorced parents
  – have higher parental income
  – drink more alcohol than people who don't hook up
  – started having sex at an earlier age
  – like to take risks
  – like to be the center of attention
  – are rebellious
  – avoid attachment
  – have a "game playing" love style
  – are not very concerned about personal safety

■ Students who have never hooked up for sex
  – prefer not to be the center of attention
  – do not fear intimacy
  – are less likely to have a "game playing" love style
  – have more concern for personal safety

■ 81% of all college students have hooked up at least once

Sources: "Is Dating Really Dead? Emerging Evidence on the College Hookup Culture and Health Issues," by M. Bachtel, 2009, College Health in Action, 49 (2), pp. 1, 17–18; "No Strings Attached: The Nature of Casual Sex in College Students," by C. M. Grello, D. P. Welsh, and M. S. Harper, 2006, Journal of Sex Research, 43 (3), pp. 255–267.

■ The partners understand the importance of good communication and are willing to work at their communication skills. They know that listening to the other's feelings and trying to see things from the other's perspective are key in communication, even if they do not ultimately agree.

■ The partners have a good sexual relationship, one that includes the open expression of affection and respect for the other's needs and boundaries.

■ The partners enjoy spending time together in leisure activities, but they also value the time they spend alone pursuing their own interests.

■ The partners are able to acknowledge their strengths and failings and take responsibility for both.

■ The partners are assertive about what they want and need in the relationship and flexible about accommodating the other's wants and needs. They can maintain a sense of self in the face of pressure to agree or conform.

■ The partners know that disagreement is normal in relationships and that when conflict is handled constructively, it can strengthen the relationship.[5]

■ The partners are friends as well as lovers, able to focus unselfish caring on each other.

■ The couple has good relationships with family and friends, including in-laws, members of their extended family, and other couples.

■ The partners have shared spiritual values.

Developing and maintaining a successful intimate relationship takes time and effort, but it is a challenge worth pursuing (see the box "Healthy Vs. Unhealthy Relationships").

LOVE AND INTIMACY

How do we go about finding the right person for a successful partnership, and what is involved when we fall in love? Is it all about magic and

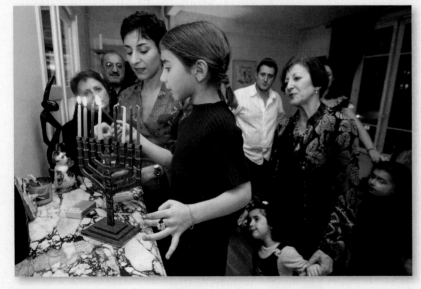

■ Relationships are more likely to be strong and lasting when partners share important values, including spiritual values.

Highlight on Health

Healthy Vs. Unhealthy Relationships

Being in a HEALTHY RELATIONSHIP means . . .	If you are in an UNHEALTHY RELATIONSHIP . . .
Loving and taking care of yourself, before and while in a relationship.	You care for and focus on the other person only and neglect yourself, or you focus only on yourself and neglect the other person.
Respecting individuality, embracing differences, and allowing each person to "be themselves."	You feel pressure to change to meet the other person's standards, you are afraid to disagree, and your ideas are criticized. Or you pressure the other person to meet your standards and criticize his or her ideas.
Doing things with friends and family and having activities independent of each other.	One of you has to justify what you do, where you go, and who you see.
Discussing things, allowing for differences of opinion, and compromising equally.	One of you makes all the decisions and controls everything without listening to the other's input.
Expressing and listening to each other's feelings, needs, and desires.	One of you feels unheard and is unable to communicate what you want.
Trusting and being honest with yourself and each other.	You lie to each other and find yourself making excuses for the other person.
Respecting each other's need for privacy.	You don't have any personal space and have to share everything with the other person.
Sharing sexual histories and sexual health status with a partner.	Your partner keeps his or her sexual history a secret or hides a sexually transmitted infection from you, or you do not disclose your history to your partner.
Practicing safer sex methods.	You feel scared about asking your partner to use protection, or he or she has refused your requests for safer sex. Or you refuse to use safer sex methods after your partner has requested, or you make your partner feel scared.
Respecting sexual boundaries and being able to say no to sex.	Your partner has forced you to have sex, or you have had sex when you don't really want to. Or you have forced or coerced your partner to have sex.
Resolving conflicts in a rational, peaceful, and mutually agreed-upon way.	One or both of you yells and hits, shoves, or throws things at the other in an argument.
Having room for positive growth and learning more about each other as you develop and mature.	You feel stifled, trapped, and stagnant. You are unable to escape the pressures of the relationship.

Source: Adapted from "Healthy Vs. Unhealthy Relationships," Copyright © Advocates for Youth. Reprinted with permission.

chemistry, or is there something more deliberate and purposeful about it?

Attraction People appear to use a systematic screening process when deciding whether someone could be a potential partner. According to one scholar, love is not blind, and we do not fall in love accidentally.[6] Some of the conscious and unconscious factors that affect this process include proximity, physical attractiveness, and similarity.

Proximity is an often overlooked but significant factor in how we find our romantic partners.[7] Simply being physically close to people makes it more likely that we will establish a relationship with them. Sometimes attraction is a function of familiarity, and proximity determines how often we are exposed to another person.

Of the people in proximity to us, we are most interested in those we find physically attractive. Only if we find a person attractive are we willing to consider his or her other traits, although "signaling" devices like coy looks and other flirtatious moves are also effective at garnering attention.[8] In general, people who are perceived as attractive in our society have an advantage. They are evaluated more positively by parents, teachers, and potential employers; make more money; and report having better sex with more attractive partners.

We are also drawn to people who are similar to ourselves, usually in characteristics such as age; physical traits such as height, weight, and attractiveness; educational attainment; family, ethnic, and cultural background; religion; political views; and values, beliefs, and interests. We are

Tips for Internet Dating

Know how to guard your safety, privacy, and emotional energy when dating through the Internet. Here are some tips:

- Allow for the "cyber exaggeration" factor. Most people lie a little about their age, looks, job, salary, or marital status. Some people lie a lot.

- Use your instincts. If you feel uncomfortable, discontinue the conversation and do not meet the person. Advise the dating service or bulletin board if you feel your experience with the person was threatening or dangerous.

- If you decide to meet someone in person, choose a public place and make it a coffee date. A person who insists on meeting for dinner or at a bar might be overeager or need to drink to feel comfortable.

- Tell a friend you are meeting someone you met on the Internet and say where and when. Print the profile of the person you are meeting and give it to your friend. Ask your friend to call you on your cell phone during the meeting to check in with you.

- Be aware that communication on the Internet can become intimate quickly and you may find yourself writing things you would never say to someone in person at an early stage of a relationship. When meeting in person, do not skip the usual steps in getting to know someone. Act in a manner appropriate to meeting a person for the first time, regardless of previous conversations or perceived closeness.

- Schedule a half-hour meeting at most. If it's not working out, be ready with a simple statement, such as "I've really appreciated meeting you, but I think I'm looking for a different match and I don't want to take more of your time. Thank you and good luck." Don't invent ridiculous excuses. Be polite and decisive.

- Limit your search to people who live within 30 or 40 miles of you. Otherwise, you may end up having a long-distance relationship, or the relationship will suffer from time and distance strains.

- Don't get discouraged. Ask your friends for their support and encouragement in your search.

---

attracted to people who agree with us, validate our opinions, and share our attitudes. Even though opposites may initially attract, partners who are like each other tend to have more successful relationships. The more differences partners have, the more important communication skills become.

The Process of Finding a Partner: Dating and More

Both in and out of college, many people prefer a more flexible approach to finding a life partner than traditional dating. For example, women often take the lead in asking men out and play a more assertive role in the development of the relationship. Although some people play "hard to get," research suggests that it is not an effective strategy.[8] Many people also search for partners on the Internet.

It makes sense to cast a wide net in the search for a partner. Even participating in such activities as social groups, volunteering, sports, and church may not bring you in contact with a broad range of people. Furthermore, most people lead busy lives, and these approaches to dating enhance your ability to be selective. Aside from dating and matchmaking sites, social networking sites like Facebook and Twitter now account for a large proportion of the time people spend connecting with others. Still, if

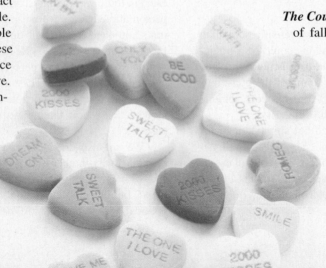

you decide to pursue a relationship with someone you meet over the Internet, be cautious because there can be much you do not know about the person. For some guidelines, see the box "Tips for Internet Dating."

What Is Love? Of all the people we are attracted to and all the potential mates we screen, what makes us fall in love with one or a few in a lifetime? Some theorists propose that we fall in love with people who are similar to us in important ways (*similarity theory*). Couples with more similarities seem to have not only greater marital harmony but also higher fertility rates. Other theorists suggest that falling in love and choosing a partner are based on the exchange of "commodities" like love, status, property, and services (*social exchange theory*). According to this view, we are looking for someone who fills not just our emotional needs but also our needs for security, money, goods, and more.

The Course of Love   The beginning stages of falling in love can feel like a roller-coaster ride, taking the lovers from the heights of euphoria to the depths of despair. They may actually become "lovesick" and find themselves unable to eat, sleep, or think of anything but the object of their desire. These early stages of a love relationship are typically romantic, idealistic, and passionate. The lovers are absorbed in each other and want to spend all their time together, sometimes to the exclusion of other people and everyday responsibilities.

Researchers think this experience of love involves increased levels of the neurotransmitter dopamine in the brain.[7] As we have seen in the context of psychoactive drugs (Chapter 11), dopamine is associated with the experience of pleasure. On the physiological level, this kind of love also causes arousal of the sympathetic nervous system, as evidenced by such physiological signs as increased heart rate, respiration, and perspiration. These responses gradually decrease as the relationship develops and progresses. Intense passion may subside as lovers become habituated to each other. In some cases, passion continues at a more bearable level and intimacy deepens; the relationship becomes more fulfilling and comes to include affection, empathy, tolerance, caring, and attachment. The partners are able to become involved in the world again, while maintaining their connection with each other. In other cases, the lessening of passion signals the ending of the relationship; the lovers drift apart, seeking newer, more satisfying partnerships.

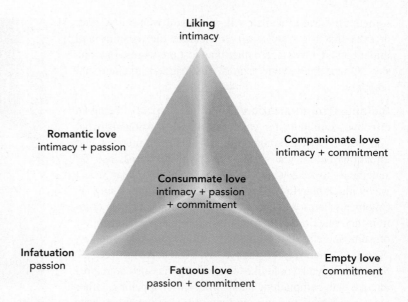

figure **12.1** **Sternberg's triangular theory of love.**

Source: "A Triangular Theory of Love," by Robert J. Sternberg, in Psychological Review, 93, pp. 119–135. Copyright © 1986. Reprinted by permission of Robert J. Sternberg.

intimacy
Emotional component of love, including feelings of closeness, warmth, openness, and affection.

passion
Sexual component of love, including attraction, romance, excitement, and physical intensity.

commitment
The decision aspect of a relationship, the pledge to stay with a partner through good times and bad.

nonverbal communication
Communication that takes place without words, mainly through body language.

metamessage
The unspoken message in a communication; the meaning behind the message, conveyed by nonverbal behavior and by situational factors such as how, when, and where the message is delivered.

Sternberg's Love Triangle Psychologist Robert Sternberg has proposed a view of love that can give us insight into its various aspects. In this view, love has three dimensions: intimacy, passion, and commitment. **Intimacy** is the emotional component of love and includes feelings of closeness, warmth, openness, and affection. **Passion** is the sexual component of love; it includes attraction, romance, excitement, and physical intensity. **Commitment** is the decision aspect of a relationship, the pledge that you will stay with your partner through good times and bad, despite the possibility of disappointment and disillusionment.[9]

Different combinations of these three components, represented metaphorically as a triangle, produce different kinds of love (Figure 12.1). When there is only intimacy, the relationship is likely to be a friendship. Passion alone is infatuation, the high-intensity early stage of a love relationship. Commitment alone is characteristic of a dutiful, obligatory relationship, one that many people would consider empty. When there is both intimacy and passion, the relationship is a romantic one; commitment may develop in time. When there is passion and commitment, the relationship has probably developed rapidly, without the partners getting to know each other very well; when passion fades, there may not be much substance to this type of relationship. When there is intimacy and commitment but no passion, the relationship may have evolved into more of a long-term friendship; Sternberg calls this relationship *companionate love*. Finally, when all three components are present, the couple has *consummate love*.[9] This type of relationship is what many dream of, but it's difficult to find and even harder to sustain. However love is conceptualized, it is something that enhances happiness and satisfaction in life.

COMMUNICATION

We establish, maintain, and nourish our relationships—or, alternatively, damage and destroy them—through communication. Clear, positive communication is a key to successful intimate relationships. Complete the activity in this chapter's Personal Health Portfolio to assess how well you communicate to people close to you.

Nonverbal Behavior and Metamessages A good deal of communication takes place as **nonverbal communication** through facial expressions, eye contact, gestures, body position and movement, and spatial behavior (how far apart people sit or stand). People tend to monitor their verbal behavior—what they say—much more carefully than their nonverbal behavior, yet nonverbal communication may convey their real message.

Nonverbal behavior is part of the **metamessage**—the unspoken message you send or get when you are communicating. The metamessage encompasses all the conscious and unconscious aspects of a message, including the way something is said, who says it, when and where it is said, or even that it is said at all. It includes the meaning and intent behind a message, rather than just the words someone says. Often, the metamessage is what triggers an emotional response.

Building Communication Skills   One aspect of being an effective communicator when you speak is knowing what you want to say. Examine your own feelings, motives, and intentions before you speak. When you do speak, use "I" statements to state what you feel or want in a clear, direct way without blaming or accusing the other person. Using "I" statements helps you take responsibility for your own emotions and reactions rather than trying to place responsibility on someone else. For example, it is more productive to say, "I feel . . . when you . . ." than to say, "You make me feel . . ." Saying what you would like to have happen is also more productive than complaining about what isn't happening. Other keys to positive, effective communication are avoiding generalizations, making specific requests, and remaining calm. If you feel yourself starting to get angry, take a time-out and come back to the conversation after you cool off.

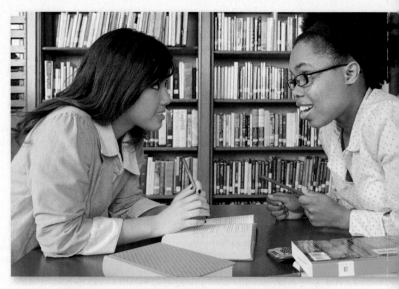

■ According to theories about gender differences in communication style, women are interested in sharing, finding similarities, and giving and receiving support when they interact with others.

People tend to monitor their verbal behavior—what they say— much more carefully than their nonverbal behavior, yet **nonverbal communication may convey their real message**.

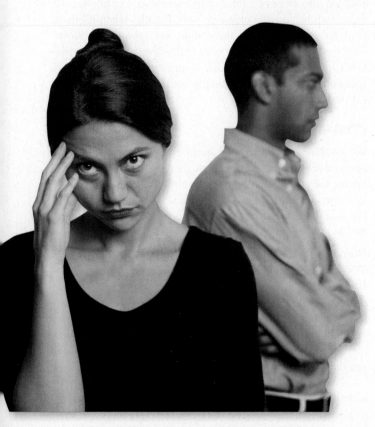

■ When words fail, body language speaks volumes.

When you are the listener, do just that—listen. Don't interrupt, give advice, explain, judge, analyze, defend yourself, or offer solutions. Give the other person the time and space to say fully what is on his or her mind, just as you would like when you are speaking. Attentive listening shows that you respect the other person and care about him or her. It is the cornerstone of good communication.

If you and your partner are experiencing conflict, good communication skills can help you resolve it constructively. Conflict is a normal part of healthy relationships. Often, it is a sign that partners are maintaining their right to be different people and to have different points of view; it can also indicate that the relationship is changing or growing.

assertiveness
The ability to stand up for oneself without violating other people's rights.

When you are trying to resolve a conflict with your partner, keep the topic narrow. Try not to generalize to other topics, incidents, or issues. Avoid being either passive or aggressive; **assertiveness** means speaking up for yourself without violating someone else's rights. Be prepared to negotiate and compromise, but don't give up something that is really important to you (for example, time to keep up your other friendships). If you feel that demands are being made on you that you cannot or do not want to meet, this may not be the right relationship for you. Communicating clearly about that is important, too.

Table 12.1   Gender Differences in Communication

Men	Women
Feel oppressed by lengthy discussions	Expect a decision to be discussed first and made by consensus
Do not want to have long discussions, particularly about what they consider to be minor decisions	Appreciate the discussion itself as evidence of involvement
Are inclined to resist what they perceive as someone telling them what to do; do not want to take orders	Are inclined to do what is asked of them
Think every question needs to be answered	Believe a question is not simply a question but the opening for a negotiation
Believe they are showing independence by not asking probing questions	Believe that when men change the subject they are showing a lack of interest and sympathy
Goal is to "fix" the problem	Goal is to share, develop relationships, and listen

Source: Adapted from You Just Don't Understand: Women and Men in Conversation, *by D. Tannen, 1990, New York: William Morrow.*

Gender Differences in Communication Styles   According to linguistics scholar Deborah Tannen, gender differences in communication patterns have a significant impact on relationships (see Table 12.1). Tannen suggests that men are more likely to use communication to compete and women are more likely to use communication to connect.[10]

Although these patterns are broad and general, they are sometimes at the root of misunderstandings between men and women. If you find yourself experiencing confusion or conflict in your communications with the other sex, consider whether gender differences may be involved. Neither style is right or wrong, better or worse—they are just different.

SEX AND GENDER

Most adult partnerships and intimate relationships include a sexual component. Sexuality encompasses not just sexual behavior but also biological, psychological, sociological, and cultural dimensions. In this section, we consider just two such dimensions—gender roles and sexual orientation.

Gender Roles   Although they are often used interchangeably, the terms *sex* and *gender* have different meanings. **Sex** refers to a person's biological status as male or female; it is usually established at birth by the appearance of the external genitals. A person with female genitals usually has XX chromosomes, and a person with male genitals usually has XY chromosomes.

Sex is not always clear-cut, however. As discussed in Chapter 2, chromosomes are sometimes added, lost, or rearranged during the production of sperm and ova, causing such conditions as Klinefelter syndrome (XXY) and Turner syndrome (XO).

sex
A person's biological status as a male or a female, usually established at birth by the appearance of the external genitals.

intersex
Condition in which the genitals are ambiguous at birth as a result of genetic factors or prenatal hormonal influences.

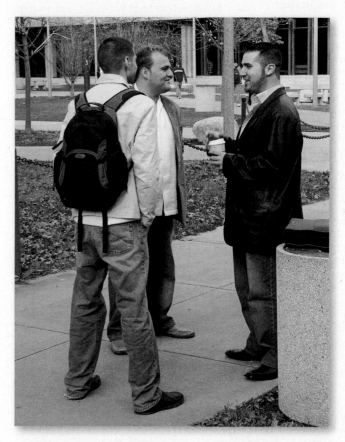

■ Men supposedly establish dominance in their interactions with others by showing off their knowledge and competence.

Sometimes, as a result of genetic factors or prenatal hormonal influences, a baby is born with ambiguous genitals—a condition referred to as **intersex**. Other times, a person experiences a sense of inappropriateness about his or her sex and identifies psychologically or emotionally with the other sex.

Gender refers to the behaviors and characteristics considered appropriate for a male or a female in a particular culture. "Masculine" and "feminine" traits are learned largely via the process of socialization during childhood. **Gender role** is the set of behaviors and activities a person engages in to conform to society's expectations. Gender role stereotypes suggest that a masculine man is competitive, aggressive, ambitious, power-oriented, and logical and that a feminine woman is cooperative, passive, nurturing, supportive, and emotional.

Today, we commonly assume that both genders are capable and can be successful in a variety of roles at home and at work. However, gender roles and gender stereotypes are learned in childhood and are hard to change, even when we are aware of them. For example, both men and women have been shown to play the stereotyped role assigned to their gender in order to appear romantically attractive to the other sex, and both men and women may be initially attracted to romantic partners because they fit the gender role stereotype.[11]

In long-term relationships, both sexes tend to prefer a partner who integrates so-called masculine and feminine traits. The term *androgynous* is applied to a person who displays characteristics or performs tasks traditionally associated with the other sex; sometimes it is also applied to a person who does not display overt characteristics of either sex.

Individuals who experience discomfort or a sense of inappropriateness about their sex (called *gender dysphoria*) and who identify strongly with the other sex are referred to as cross-gender identified, transsexual, or **transgender**. The term *transgender* can describe anyone whose **gender identity** differs from the sex of their birth. The *Diagnostic and Statistical Manual of Mental Disorders* includes gender identity disorder as a diagnostic category.

Many transgender individuals dress in the clothes of the other sex (*cross-dressing*) and live in society as the other sex. Some undergo surgery and hormone treatments to experience a more complete transformation into the other sex, and others do not. Transgender individuals have typically experienced gender dysphoria since earliest childhood, but there is controversy about using the gender identity disorder diagnosis with children.[12] Most children who do not fit the cultural stereotype of masculinity or femininity do not grow up to be transgender. According to the National Center for

Transgender Equality, fewer than 1 percent of the population in the United States (between 750,000 and 3,000,000 people) is transgender.

Sexual Orientation   **Sexual orientation** refers to a person's emotional, romantic, and sexual attraction to a member of the same sex, the other sex, or both. It exists along a continuum that ranges from exclusive heterosexuality through bisexuality to exclusive homosexuality. Although the role of genes in sexual orientation is not clearly understood (see Chapter 2), sexual orientation is known to be influenced by a complex interaction of biological, psychological, and societal factors, and these factors may be different for different people.

Sexual orientation involves a person's sense of identity. Most experts believe that it is not a choice and does not change (perhaps more so for men than for women). A person's sexual orientation may or may not be evidenced in his or her appearance or behavior, and the person may choose not to act on his or her sexual orientation.

gender
Masculine or feminine behaviors and characteristics considered appropriate for a male or a female in a particular culture.

gender role
Set of behaviors and activities a person engages in to conform to society's expectations of his or her sex.

transgender
Having a sense of identity as a male or female that conflicts with one's biological sex; transgendered individuals experience a sense of inappropriateness about their sex and identify strongly with the other sex.

gender identity
Internal sense of being male or female.

sexual orientation
A person's emotional, romantic, and sexual attraction to a member of the same sex, the other sex, or both.

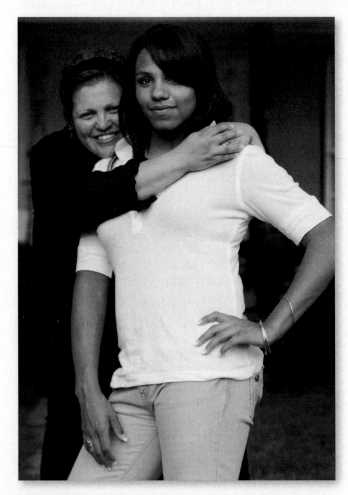

■ Rochelle Evans, shown here with her mom, is a transgender teen living in Texas. She started high school as Rodney Evans and fought a public battle to be allowed to wear women's clothes to school.

Heterosexuality is defined as emotional and sexual attraction to members of the other sex. Heterosexuals are often referred to as *straight*. Throughout the world, laws related to marriage, child rearing, health benefits, financial matters, sexual behavior, and inheritance generally support heterosexual relationships. **Homosexuality** is defined as emotional and sexual attraction to members of the same sex. In today's usage, homosexual men are typically referred to as *gay*, and homosexual women are referred to either as gay or as *lesbians*.

Homosexuality occurs in all cultures, but researchers have generally had difficulty determining exactly what proportions of the population are straight and gay. Sex researcher Alfred Kinsey estimated that about 4 percent of American males and 2 percent of American females were exclusively homosexual.[13,14] The popular media tend to place the combined figure for gays and lesbians at about 10 percent of the population.

Emotional and sexual attraction to both sexes is referred to as **bisexuality**. Bisexuals may date members of both sexes, or they may have a relationship with a member of one sex for a period of time and then a relationship with a member of the other sex for a period of time. After having relationships with members of both sexes, a bisexual may move toward a more exclusive orientation, either heterosexual or homosexual.

COMMITTED RELATIONSHIPS AND LIFESTYLE CHOICES

In this section we consider marriage, one of the most important social and legal institutions in societies throughout the world, along with other relationship and lifestyle choices that many people make today.

Marriage Marriage is not only the legal union of two people but also a contract between the couple and the state. In the United States, each state specifies the rights and responsibilities of the partners in a marriage. Although marriage has traditionally meant the union of a man and a woman, many same-sex couples are interested in marriage, and some states now issue marriage licenses to same-sex couples.

Although the percentage of Americans who marry and live together as married couples continues to decline, marriage still appears to be the most popular living arrangement. The decline in the number of married people may be accounted for by the increase in cohabiting couples, a decrease in the number of people getting married for a second time, and the choice made by many individuals to postpone marriage until they are older (Table 12.2).

Marriage confers benefits in many domains. Partnerships and family relationships provide emotional connection for individuals and stability for society. Married people live longer than single or divorced people, partly because they lead a healthier lifestyle. Married people report greater happiness than do single, widowed, or cohabiting people. Married couples have sex more frequently and consider their sexual relationship more satisfying emotionally and physically than do single people. Married people are more successful in their careers, earn more, and have more wealth. Children brought up by married couples tend to be more academically successful and emotionally stable.

What makes a marriage successful? One predictor of a successful marriage is positive reasons for getting married. Positive motivations include companionship, love and intimacy, supportive partnership, sexual compatibility, and interest in sharing parenthood. Poorer reasons for getting married, those associated with less chance of having a successful marriage, include premarital pregnancy, rebellion

heterosexuality
Emotional and sexual attraction to members of the other sex.

homosexuality
Emotional and sexual attraction to members of the same sex.

bisexuality
Emotional and sexual attraction to members of both sexes.

Table 12.2 Percentage of All Persons Aged 15 or Older Who Were Married, by Sex and Race, 1960–2009, United States

	Males			Females		
Year	Total*	Black	White	Total*	Black	White
1960	69.3	60.9	70.3	65.9	59.8	66.6
1980	63.2	48.9	65.0	58.9	44.6	60.7
2000	57.9	42.8	60.0	54.7	36.2	57.4
2009**	55.6	40.1	57.4	53.2	34.7	55.6

* Includes races other than Black and White.
** In 2003 the U.S. Census Bureau expanded its racial categories to permit respondents to identify themselves as belonging to more than one race. This means that racial data computations beginning in 2004 may not be strictly comparable with those of prior years.

Source: U.S. Census Bureau, Current Population Survey, March and Annual Social and Economic supplements, 2009 and earlier.

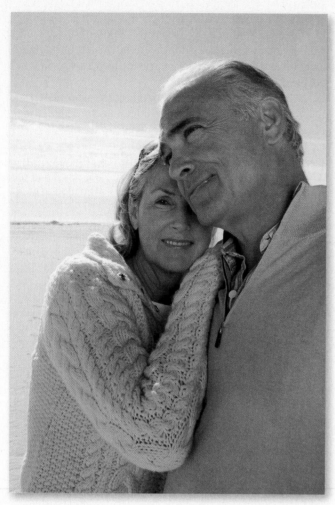

■ Some couples discover the secrets to a long and happy marriage.

against parents, seeking independence, seeking economic security, family or social pressure, and rebounding from another relationship.

Love alone is not enough to make a marriage successful. Research has found that the best predictors of a happy marriage are realistic attitudes about the relationship and the challenges of marriage; satisfaction with the personality of the partner; enjoyment of communicating with the partner; ability to resolve conflicts together; agreement on religious and ethical values; egalitarian roles; and a balance of individual and joint leisure activities. The characteristics associated with successful and unsuccessful marriages are typically present in a couple's relationship before they are married.[15]

Infidelity mars some marriages, though it does not necessarily end them. Men are twice as likely as women to have a sexual affair during marriage, but women are more likely to have an affair to end a bad marriage.[16] Men are more threatened if their partner has a sexual affair than if she falls in love with someone else, whereas women are more distressed if their partner falls in love with someone else.

Gay and Lesbian Partnerships Like heterosexual couples, same-sex couples desire intimacy, companionship, passion, and commitment in their relationships. Because they often have to struggle with "coming out" and issues with their families, gays and lesbians frequently have communication skills and strengths that are valuable in relationships. These qualities include flexible role relationships, the ability to adapt to a partner, the ability to negotiate and share decision-making power, and effective parenting skills among those who choose to become parents.[17,18]

Unfortunately, gays and lesbians often have to deal with discrimination and **homophobia** (irrational fear of homosexuality and homosexuals). Same-sex relationships do not receive the same level of societal support and acceptance as heterosexual relationships. The options of domestic partnership, civil union, and marriage have become available for same-sex partners in some states. The issue of gay marriage has become a hot political topic in the United States in recent years, with one side asserting that marriage must be defined as a union between a man and a woman and the other side arguing that denying marriage to gays and lesbians is a violation of their civil rights.[19]

homophobia
Irrational fear of homosexuality and homosexuals.

cohabitation
Living arrangement in which two people of the opposite sex live together as unmarried partners.

Cohabitation The U.S. government defines **cohabitation** as two people of the opposite sex living together as unmarried partners. Since the 1960s, cohabitation has become one of the most rapidly growing social phenomena in the history of our society. The rate of cohabitation has increased more than tenfold since the 1960s, when about half a million people were living together. In 2009 approximately 6.7 million couples, or 13.4 million men and women, were identified as cohabiting. About 20 percent of unmarried women between the ages of 20 and 24 are currently living with a partner.

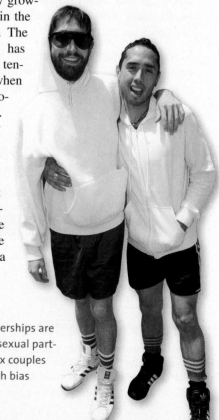

■ Gay and lesbian partnerships are very similar to heterosexual partnerships, but same-sex couples often have to deal with bias and discrimination.

Cohabitation seems to have become an accepted part of the process of finding a mate (see the box "Isabel and Paul: Living Together . . . Happily Ever After?"). Most couples today believe it is a good idea to live together in order to decide if they should get married, and more than 50 percent do live together before getting married. Yet an estimated 40 percent of these arrangements do not result in marriage.[20]

Divorce For a large percentage of couples, the demands of marriage prove too difficult, and the couple choose to divorce. The current divorce rate is nearly twice what it was in 1960, although it has declined since reaching its highest point in the 1980s. The lifetime probability of a couple in their first marriage experiencing divorce is between 40 and 50 percent.[20]

Because they often have to struggle with "coming out" and issues with their families, gay men and lesbians frequently have **communication skills and strengths that are valuable in relationships.**

Some studies have shown that cohabitation actually decreases the likelihood of success in marriage and increases the likelihood of divorce. Such findings are controversial, however, because of the difficulty in determining whether this effect results from the characteristics of those who choose to cohabit before marriage or from the experience of living together before marriage.[20,21]

Why do so many couples divorce in our society? Many couples simply cannot handle the challenges of married life. They may not have the problem-solving skills, or they may not be sufficiently committed to the relationship. Many people enter marriage with unrealistic expectations, and some people choose an unsuitable mate.

Life Stories

Isabel and Paul: Living Together . . . Happily Ever After?

Isabel and Paul were both 24 years old and had just graduated from a university in the Northeast. They had been in an exclusive relationship with each other for the past two years. They felt committed to each other but hadn't talked about their long-term plans or the future of their relationship. Neither of them had really thought about marriage. Paul was interviewing for jobs in New York City and hoping to move there. He asked Isabel to come live with him—she hadn't found a job yet, and it would be easier to find one in a big city rather than in the mid-sized city where their university was. They could save money by living together, he said, and besides, they cared about each other.

Isabel wasn't so sure. She hadn't planned to move to New York, but she didn't have any definite direction in her life yet. Paul was right that it would be easier to find a job there, and she wasn't sure what would happen to their relationship if she didn't move with him. She did love him, and the prospect of living in New York was exciting, so she said yes. They agreed to split rent and utilities in proportion to their earnings once they both found jobs.

Isabel turned out to really enjoy living in New York—and living with Paul. They bought furniture together and developed a social circle with old friends from school and new friends from work. A year passed quickly and Isabel found herself thinking about their future together. More and more of their friends were getting engaged. Isabel was ready to make a commitment to Paul. But when she brought up the subject of marriage or the future,

Paul always seemed to deflect the conversation. He said he didn't know what the rush was and didn't know why they needed to get married. They were still young and enjoying their life together—why change a good thing? He was happy just living with her.

Isabel felt hurt by his responses and began to wonder if he really wanted to spend his life with her. She knew that she wanted to be married—but did he? She wondered if he found living together convenient until something better came along. She thought about it more and more but felt reluctant to initiate further conversations about it for fear she would push him away. Because she didn't bring it up again, Paul thought that everything was fine between them.

Finally, Isabel felt she had to talk to someone about the growing distance she was experiencing in the relationship and decided to make an appointment with a therapist. When she told Paul she was going to see someone about "some issues," he was surprised and concerned and asked why she was going. She hesitantly told him. Paul had had no idea that she had so many doubts about their relationship and their future. He apologized for giving the appearance that he didn't want to talk about their future plans—he could now see that it was an important issue to her. He told her he knew he had some fears about marriage based on his parents' relationship and that he wasn't sure he felt ready to get married yet. Still, he said, he would be happy to go to counseling with her so that they could talk more about the issue in a healthy way.

connect ACTIVITY

Although divorce may seem to be a single event in a person's life, the termination of a marriage is almost always a traumatic process lasting months or years. Divorce is a leading cause of poverty, leaving many children in impoverished homes headed by a single parent, often the parent with the lower income. Most single-parent families cannot maintain the same lifestyle that they had before the divorce.

Divorce is one of the most stressful life events a person can experience. It is especially hard on children, leading to different kinds of problems for children of different ages. Counseling can help both children and adults deal with the stress of divorce and adjust to a new life. Children are best served by continuing to have contact with both parents as long as the adults can get along.

Blended Families   Many divorced people eventually remarry, and **blended families**, in which one or both partners bring children from a previous marriage, are becoming a common form of family.

Just as it takes time for a family to reorganize and stabilize itself after a divorce, it also takes time for a blended family to achieve some measure of cohesion after parents remarry. It can take 2 years or more for stepparents and stepchildren to build relationships. Adults should allow time for trust and attachment to develop before they take on a parenting role with their stepchildren. When children regularly see their noncustodial parent, they are better able to adjust to their new family. Children also adjust better if the parents in the blended family have a low-intensity relationship and if the relationships between ex-spouses are civil.

blended families
Families in which one or both partners bring a child or children from a previous marriage.

Singlehood   Although marriage continues to be a popular institution, a growing number of people in our society are unmarried. Many young adults are delaying marriage to pursue educational and career goals, but an increasing number of people view singlehood as a legitimate, healthy, and satisfying alternative to marriage. Some people, including some highly educated professionals and career-oriented individuals, prefer to remain unmarried. In singlehood they find the freedom to pursue their own interests, spend their money as they wish, invest time in their careers, develop a broad network of friends, have a variety of sexual relationships, and enjoy opportunities for solitude. For them, being single is a positive choice.

Keeping Your Relationships Strong and Vital   A characteristic of relationships—both partnerships and families—is that they change over time. No matter what specific challenges come up, three basic qualities seem to make

partnerships and families strong: cohesion, flexibility, and communication.[22]

Cohesion is the dynamic balance between separateness and togetherness in both couple and family relationships. Relationships are strongest when there is a balance between intimacy and autonomy. There are times when partners and family members spend more time together and other times when they spend more time apart, but they come back to a comfortably cohesive point.

Flexibility is the dynamic balance between stability and change. Again, relationships are strongest when there is a balance. Too much stability can cause rigidity; too much change can cause chaos. Communication is the tool that partners and families use to adjust levels of cohesion or flexibility when change is needed. It is important that communication with a partner include expressions of appreciation, healthy complaining, and the recognition of both partners' levels of sensitivity.[5]

When relationship problems persist for two or three months and the partners are not able to resolve them, the couple should probably seek help. Couples who receive help with difficulties before they become too severe have a better chance of overcoming the problems and developing a stronger relationship than do those who delay. Marriage and family therapists are specifically trained to help couples and families with relationship problems. Look for a therapist who is licensed by your state or who is a certified member of the American Association for Marriage and Family Therapists. Your physician or clergyperson may be able to recommend a qualified professional. A couples therapist can help you develop the strengths and resources you need to nourish and enhance this vital part of your life.

Sexual Health: Biology and Culture

Sexual health includes healthy sexual functioning across the lifespan, satisfying intimate relationships based on mutual respect and trust, and the ability and resources to procreate if so desired. It also includes knowledge about sexuality and access to the information needed to make responsible decisions.

Although sexual anatomy and physiology are similar in all human beings, sexual behavior and expression vary tremendously across societies, cultures, and eras. There are even differences in what is considered sexually pleasurable from one culture and time to another.

In the United States, sexual attitudes are marked by an ongoing tension between the two poles of sexual restrictiveness and sexual freedom. The so-called sexual revolution of

hot tip

Your partner cannot read your mind; ask (nicely) for what you want in your relationship.

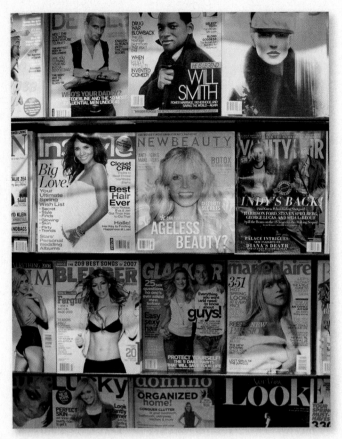

■ What we find sexually exciting, attractive, and acceptable is largely determined by the messages we get from our culture.

the 1960s gave way to a more conservative climate in the 1980s and 1990s. Prevailing attitudes toward sex and sexual pleasure in the early 21st century will be determined, in part, by college students and other young adults.

SEXUAL ANATOMY AND FUNCTIONING

Although sexuality serves many purposes in human experience, the biological purpose of sexuality is reproduction. In this section we explore some of the biological aspects of sexuality.

Sexual Anatomy   The male and female sex organs arise from the same undifferentiated tissue during the prenatal period, becoming male or female under the influence of hormones (discussed later in this section). In this sense, the sexual organs of males and females are very similar, and their purpose and functions are complementary. The female sex organs are responsible for the production of ova and, if pregnancy occurs, the development of the fetus. The male sex organs are responsible for producing sperm and delivering them into the female reproductive system to fertilize the ovum.

Female Sex Organs and Reproductive Anatomy   The external genitalia of the female are called the vulva and include the mons pubis, the labia majora and labia minora, the clitoris, and the vaginal and urethral openings (Figure 12.2). The mons pubis is a mound or layer of fatty tissue that pads and protects the pubic bone. The labia majora (major lips) and labia minora (minor lips) are folds of tissue that wrap around the entrance to the vagina. The labia minora form a protective hood, or prepuce, over the clitoris. The clitoris is a highly sensitive, cylindrical body about 3 centimeters in length that fills with blood during sexual excitement. Consisting of a glans, corpus, and crura, the clitoris is located at the top of the vulva between the lips of the labia minora.

The urethral opening, the passageway for urine from the urinary bladder, is located immediately below the clitoris. The hymen is a thin membranous fold, highly variable in appearance, which may partially cover the opening of the vagina. The hymen has no known biological function and is frequently absent. The perineum is the area between the

External Organs (Vulva)

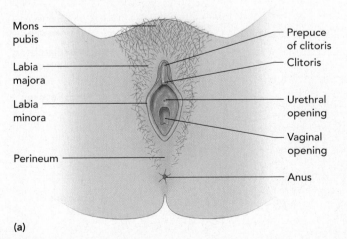

(a)

Internal Organs

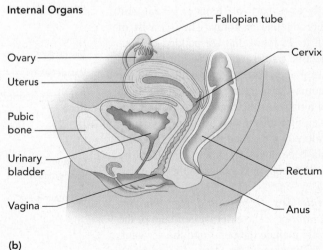

(b)

figure **12.2**   **Female sexual and reproductive anatomy.** (a) External structures; (b) internal structures.

bottom of the vulva and the anus. It contains many nerve endings.

The internal sex organs of the female include the vagina, cervix, uterus, fallopian tubes, and ovaries. The vagina is a hollow, muscular tube extending from the external vaginal opening to the cervix. The walls of the vagina are soft and flexible and have several layers. The existence of an area called the G-spot on the lower front wall of the vagina is a subject of debate; if it is present, it may feel like an elevated bump. Located on either side of the vagina under the labia are the crura, extensions of the clitoris.

The cervix is the lower part of the uterus; it extends into the vagina and contains the opening to the uterus. The cervix produces a mucus that changes with different stages of the menstrual cycle. The uterus is the organ in which a fertilized egg develops into an embryo and then a fetus. Approximately the size of a pear, the uterus is made up of several layers of muscle and tissue. The endometrium is the layer that is shed during menstruation.

The ovaries are the female reproductive glands that store and release the ova (eggs) every month, usually one at a time—the process of ovulation. They also produce the female sex hormones estrogen and progesterone. The ovaries are located on either side of the uterus. Extending from the upper sides of the uterus are the fallopian tubes (or oviducts), the passageways through which ova move from the ovaries into the uterus. Their openings are lined with fimbria, appendages with beating cilia that sweep the surface of the ovaries during ovulation and guide the ovum down into the tubes.

The mammary glands, or breasts, are also part of female sexual and reproductive anatomy. They consist of 15 to 25 lobes that are padded by connective tissue and fat. Within the lobes are glands that produce milk when the woman is lactating following the birth of a baby. At the center of each breast is a nipple, surrounded by a ring of darker colored skin called the areola. The nipple becomes erect when stimulated by cold, touch, or sexual stimuli.

Male Sex Organs and Reproductive Anatomy   The external genitalia of the male include the penis and the scrotum, which contains the testes (Figure 12.3). The penis, when erect, is designed to deliver sperm into the female reproductive tract. The shaft of the penis is

formed of three columns of spongelike erectile tissue that fill with blood during sexual excitement. The glans, or head of the penis, is an expansion of the corpus spongiosum (one of the three columns of erectile tissue in the penis shaft). The glans contains a higher concentration of nerve endings than the shaft and is highly sensitive.

The corona is a crownlike structure that protrudes slightly and forms a border between the glans and the shaft; it is also highly sensitive. The frenulum is a fold of skin extending from the corona to the foreskin. The foreskin, or prepuce, covers the glans, more or less completely. **Circumcision** involves removing this skin and leaving the head of the penis permanently exposed. The urethral opening, through which both

circumcision
Removal of the foreskin of the penis; a procedure often routinely performed on newborn male infants in the United States.

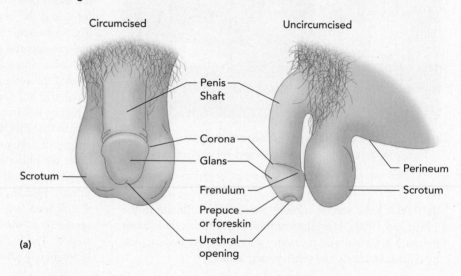

External Organs

Internal Organs

(a)

(b)

figure **12.3**   **Male sexual and reproductive anatomy.** (a) External structures; (b) internal structures.

urine and semen pass (at different times), is located at the tip of the penis in the glans. The urethra runs the length of the penis from the urinary bladder to the exterior of the body.

The scrotum, a thin sac composed of skin and muscle fibers, contains the testes. The scrotum is separated from the body to keep the testes at the lower temperature that is needed for sperm production. The area between the scrotum and the anus is the perineum; as in females, it contains many nerve endings.

The male internal reproductive organs include the testes; a series of ducts that transport sperm (the epididymis, vas deferens, ejaculatory ducts, and urethra); and a set of glands that produce semen and other fluids (the seminal vesicles, prostate gland, and Cowper's glands). The two testes, located in the scrotum, are the male reproductive glands; they produce both sperm and male sex hormones such as testosterone. Once sperm are produced in the testes, they enter the epididymis, a highly coiled duct lying on the surface of each testis. As they move along the length of the epididymis, immature sperm mature and develop the ability to swim.

When the male ejaculates, sperm are propelled from the epididymis into the vas deferens, another duct, which joins with ducts from the seminal vesicles to form the short ejaculatory ducts. The two seminal vesicles, located at the back of the bladder, produce about 60 percent of the volume of semen, the milky fluid that carries sperm and contains nutrients to fuel them. The sperm and semen travel through the ejaculatory ducts to the prostate gland, a doughnut-shaped structure that encircles the urethra and contributes the remaining volume of semen. The semen is then ejaculated through the urethra. The two Cowper's glands, located below the prostate gland, produce a clear mucus that is secreted into the urethra just before ejaculation. The volume of semen in one ejaculation is about 2 to 5 milliliters, containing between 100 and 600 million sperm.

Sexual Response   In order for reproduction to occur, ova and sperm have to be brought into close association with each other. The psychological and motivational mechanism for this is the human sexual response, which includes sex drive, sexual arousal, and orgasm.

Sex Drive   Sex drive—sexual desire, or libido—is defined as a biological urge for sexual activity. The principal hormone responsible for the sex drive in both males and females is testosterone, produced by the testes in males and by the adrenal glands in both sexes. Testosterone stimulates increased release of the neurotransmitters dopamine and serotonin in the brain; they are thought to be involved in making external stimuli arousing.

People usually seek to satisfy the sex drive through physical stimulation and release, either with a partner or through masturbation. Besides hormones, sex drive is also influenced by sexual imagery and sexual fantasies. It can be stimulated by sights, sounds, smells, tastes, and myriad other external stimuli, as well as by one's own thoughts and fantasies.

Sexual Arousal   Sexual arousal on the physiological level involves vasocongestion and myotonia. **Vasocongestion** is the inflow of blood to tissues in erogenous areas. In men, the arterioles supplying blood to the erectile tissue of the penis are normally constricted. Sexual arousal causes nerves in the penis to release nitric oxide, which in turn activates an enzyme that relaxes the arterioles and allows the penis to fill with blood. Engorgement compresses the veins in the penis and prevents blood from flowing out. In women, a similar process causes engorgement of the clitoris, labia, vagina, and nipples; vaginal lubrication also increases. **Myotonia** is a voluntary or involuntary muscle tension occurring in response to sexual stimuli. Both vasocongestion and myotonia build up during sexual excitement and decrease afterward.[23]

The Human Sexual Response Model
In the 1960s, sex researchers William Masters and Virginia Johnson conducted detailed studies of sexual activity and developed a four-phase model of the human sexual response (Figure 12.4) The four phases are excitement, plateau, orgasm, and resolution.[23]

The excitement stage begins with stimulation that initiates vasocongestion and myotonia. The first sign of excitement in men is penis erection. In women, signs include vaginal lubrication and, frequently, nipple and clitoral erection. Heart rate and respiratory rate generally increase in both men and women.

The plateau phase is a leveling-off period just before orgasm. Increased muscle tension continues during the plateau phase. The heart rate remains elevated and breathing is deep. The penis increases in size and length, and the upper two-thirds of the vagina widens and expands.

Orgasm is a physiological reflex in which a massive discharge of nerve impulses occurs in the nerves serving the genitals, usually in response to tactile stimulation, causing rhythmic muscle contractions in the genital area and a sensation of intense pleasure. In men, contractions occur in the penis, ducts, glands, and muscles in the pelvic and anal regions; orgasm is accompanied by the ejaculation of semen. In women, contractions occur in the uterus, vagina, and pelvic and anal regions.

Resolution is the return to an unexcited, relaxed state. Men enter a **refractory period**, lasting from minutes to hours, during which vasoconstriction of the arterioles supplying the erectile tissue causes the penis to become flaccid (soft) again. During the refractory period, the man is not able to have another orgasm. Most young men can have one to three orgasms in an hour, as can some older men.

sex drive
Biological urge for sexual activity; also called sexual desire or libido.

vasocongestion
Inflow of blood to tissues in erogenous areas.

myotonia
Voluntary or involuntary muscle tension occurring in response to sexual stimuli.

orgasm
Physiological reflex characterized by rhythmic muscle contractions in the genital area and a sensation of intense pleasure.

refractory period
Time following orgasm when a man cannot have another orgasm.

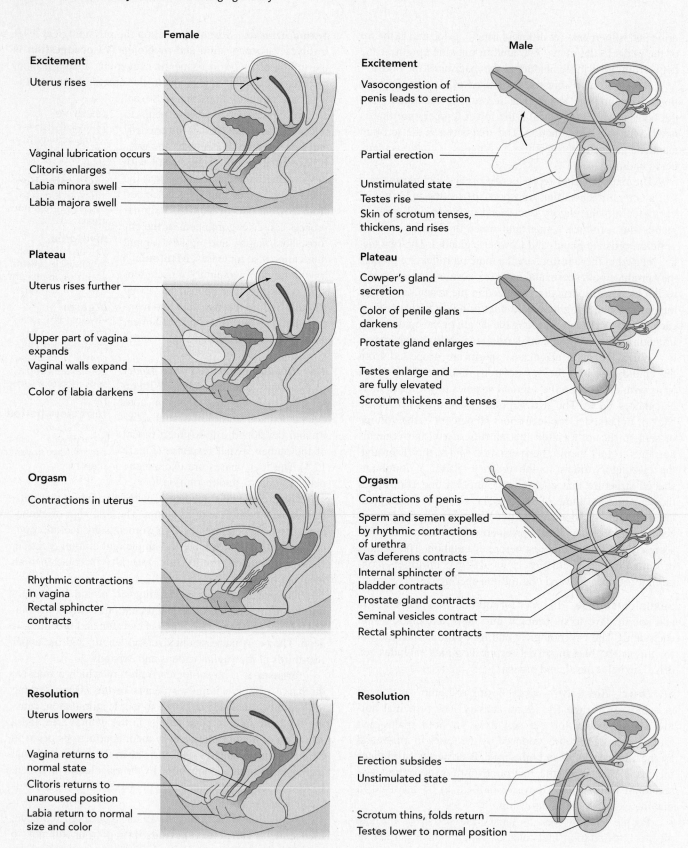

figure 12.4 **The human sexual response model.**

In women, orgasm is not followed by a refractory period, so women can experience multiple orgasms during a single sexual experience. Multiple orgasms may be experienced as part of the general climactic wave or as a series of orgasms as much as 5 minutes apart.

An alternative model suggests that many women, especially those in long-term relationships, may not experience sexual desire (conscious sexual urges) moving to sexual arousal. Instead, sexual arousal more commonly precedes sexual desire. Sexual desire occurs only after a sufficient period of sexual arousal and is more of a responsive event than a spontaneous event.[24] The choice to initiate sexual arousal is often more dependent on intimacy needs (needs for emotional closeness, bonding, love, affection) than on a need for physical sexual arousal or release. Intimacy benefits and appreciation for the sexual well-being of the partner serve as the motivational factors to move from sexual neutrality to sexual arousal.[24] This model may also apply to some men in long-term relationships.

The Experience of Orgasm Although orgasm is physically experienced in the genitals, it is also a mental and emotional event. The subjective experience of orgasm can be influenced by an infinite variety of physical, emotional, psychological, interpersonal, and environmental factors.

Most people experience a feeling of deep warmth or pressure when orgasm is imminent or inevitable. Orgasm is usually felt as waves of intense pleasure accompanied by contractions in the penis, vagina, or uterus. The sensations may be localized to the genitals, or they may be generalized over the whole body.

About a third of women reach orgasm from the sensations produced in the vagina by the thrusting of the penis, but many women need direct stimulation of the clitoris to reach orgasm.[25] Since most intercourse positions do not include such direct

■ Movie viewers watched Daniel Radcliffe, Emma Watson, and Rupert Grint transform from preteens to young adults as they played the lead roles in the Harry Potter movie series.

pressure or stimulation, intercourse alone may not be completely satisfying for a woman. Even women who reach orgasm regularly only climax about 50 to 70 percent of the time. Active stimulation of the clitoris with fingers or a vibrator can help women reach orgasm. When a woman is unable to reach orgasm, it is usually due to inhibition or lack of needed stimulation.

Sexual Development and Health Across the Lifespan The biology of sexual and reproductive development is directed by hormones, beginning in the womb. Male sex hormones, called **androgens**, are secreted primarily by the testes, and female sex hormones, called **estrogens** and **progestins**, are secreted by the ovaries. The adrenal glands also secrete androgens in both males and females. The pituitary gland and the hypothalamus in the brain both have roles in regulating levels and functions of the sex hormones.

During prenatal development, the presence of a Y chromosome causes the reproductive glands to develop into testes; the testes produce testosterone, which causes the undifferentiated reproductive structures to become male sex organs. If there is no Y chromosome, the glands develop into ovaries and the reproductive structures become female sex organs.

Hormones come into play again at puberty, when the secondary sex characteristics appear and the reproductive system matures. There is a growth spurt in both sexes (about 2 years earlier in girls than in boys), the sex organs become larger, and pubic and underarm hair appears. In boys, the voice deepens, facial hair begins to grow, and the onset of **ejaculation** occurs. Boys begin to experience **nocturnal emissions** (orgasm and ejaculation during sleep), and the testes start to produce sperm. In girls, breasts develop, body fat increases, and **menarche**, the onset of menstruation, occurs.

Every month between the ages of about 12 and about 50, except during pregnancy, women

androgens
Male sex hormones, secreted primarily by the testes.

estrogens
Female sex hormones; secreted by the ovaries.

progestins
Female sex hormones; secreted by the ovaries.

ejaculation
Emission of semen during orgasm.

nocturnal emission
Orgasm and ejaculation during sleep.

menarche
Onset of menstruation.

experience monthly menstrual periods. During the first half of the cycle, the lining of the uterus thickens with blood vessels in preparation for the possibility of pregnancy, and an ovum matures in one of the ovaries. About halfway through the cycle, the ovum is released (ovulation) and is carried into the uterus. If sperm are present, the ovum may be fertilized and begin to develop into an embryo. If sperm are not present, the uterine lining is shed, causing **menses**, and the cycle begins again.

menses
Flow of menstrual blood; the menstrual period.

menopause
Cessation of menstruation.

viropause
Changes in virility or sexual desire in middle-aged men.

celibacy
Continuous abstention from sexual activities with others.

Some girls and women experience uncomfortable physical symptoms during their periods, such as cramps and backache, and some experience physical and emotional symptoms before their periods, such as headache, irritability, and mood swings, referred to as premenstrual tension or premenstrual syndrome (PMS). If symptoms are severe and interfere with usual work, family, or social activities, the woman may be diagnosed with premenstrual dysphoric disorder (PMDD). The exact causes of PMS and PMDD are not known, but lifestyle changes, such as exercising, eating well, and avoiding alcohol, may help relieve symptoms. A physician may prescribe medications for more severe symptoms.

In middle age, hormonal changes cause a gradual reduction in ovarian functioning that culminates in **menopause**, the cessation of menstruation. Although the average age at

menopause in the United States is 52, a small percentage of women experience premature menopause before age 40.[26]

During the time leading up to menopause, a period of 3 to 7 years called *perimenopause*, many women experience symptoms caused by hormonal fluctuations, such as hot flashes, night sweats, irritability, and insomnia. A decrease in estrogen production can cause less visible symptoms as well, such as a reduction in bone density and changes in blood levels of cholesterol. These changes contribute to women's increased risk of osteoporosis and heart disease later in life.

Hormone replacement therapy (HRT) was a popular treatment for the symptoms of menopause and perimenopause until 2002, when the results of a large study led researchers to conclude that the risks of HRT far outweighed the benefits.[27] The risk of breast cancer rose more quickly for women on HRT after 4 years, and the risk of heart disease and blood clots increased each year for women on HRT.

Women who elect to use HRT are advised to take the lowest effective dose for the shortest possible time.[27] Uncomfortable symptoms of perimenopause and menopause can be improved in many cases by lifestyle changes like increased physical activity, stress management, and weight loss.

Men do not experience a dramatic change in reproductive capacity in midlife as women do; the testes continue to produce sperm throughout life. Some researchers believe, however, that middle-aged men experience a 5-to 12-year period during which their testosterone levels fluctuate.[28] The term **viropause** (pronounced VEER-o-pause) has been coined to refer to changes in virility or sexual desire in middle-aged men, analogous to menopause in women. The condition is also referred to as androgen decline in aging males. Besides changes in sexual functioning, common symptoms include irritability, sluggishness, mild to moderate mood swings, and a sense of declining vitality.[29]

For both men and women, however, biological changes in the sexual response phases have only a marginal effect on sexual interest and activity. There does tend to be a slow, steady decline in sexual activity over the course of life, caused by lower levels of sex hormones and physiological changes. The more sexually active a person is, the less effect these biological changes have.

VARIETIES OF SEXUAL BEHAVIOR AND EXPRESSION

Rather than thinking in terms of "normalcy," social scientists think in terms of behavior that is typical and behavior that is less typical (see the box "Sexuality and Disability").

Typical and Common Forms of Sexual Expression
Typical forms of sexual behavior and expression in U.S. society include celibacy, erotic touch, self-stimulation, oral-genital stimulation, and intercourse.

Celibacy Continuous abstention from sexual activities with others is called **celibacy**. People may be completely

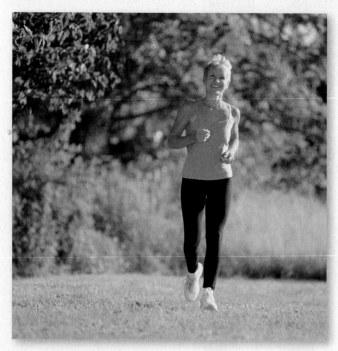

■ Exercise helps relieve many of the uncomfortable symptoms of menopause.

Sexuality and Disability

Although individuals with disabilities may experience limitations on their sexuality or may have to develop new or alternative forms of sexual activity, most people with disabilities can have a rewarding sex life. Information and education can help individuals with disabilities, as can counseling that focuses on building self-esteem;overcoming shame, guilt, fear, anger, and unrealistic expectations; and developing a holistic approach to sexuality that includes all activities that offer pleasure and intimacy. Information and education are also important for members of the general public, who too often fail to acknowledge the full humanity of individuals with disabilities, including their sexuality.

For people with physical limitations, different forms of sexual expression may be possible. A person with a spinal cord injury may or may not be able to have an orgasm, but he or she may be able to have intercourse, may experience sensuous feelings in other parts of the body, and may be able to have a child. As in any relationship, the key is nurturing emotional as well as sexual intimacy. When a partner in an established relationship is facing a disability, the couple may want to seek information and counseling on how the disability will affect their sexual functioning.

Changes in sexual functioning and desire can also be caused by chronic diseases, such as diabetes, arthritis, and cardiovascular disease, as well as by the medications used to treat them. For example, diabetes can cause nerve damage and circulatory problems that affect erectile functioning in men. Individuals and couples may have to make significant adjustments in their forms of sexual expression to accommodate such disabling conditions.

Sources: Human Sexuality, 6th ed., by B. Strong, W. Yarber, B. Sayad, and C. DeVault, 2008, New York: McGraw-Hill; The Sexual Male: Problems and Solutions, by R. Milsten and J. Slowinski, 1999, New York: W.W. Norton and Company.

Highlight on Health

celibate (do not engage in masturbation) or partially celibate (engage in masturbation). Moral and religious beliefs lead some people to choose celibacy. Lack of a suitable sexual partner or sexual relationship may be another reason for celibacy.[25]

Some people use the term *abstinence* interchangeably with *celibacy*, but **abstinence** usually means abstention only from sexual intercourse. As such, abstinence is promoted as a way to avoid sexually transmitted diseases and unintended pregnancy.

Erotic Touch Touch is a sensual form of communication that can elicit feelings of tenderness and affection as well as sexual feelings. It is an important part of **foreplay**, touching that increases sexual arousal and precedes sexual intercourse. Some areas of the body are more sensitive to touch than others. Skin in the nonspecific erogenous zones of the body (the inner thighs, armpits, shoulders, feet, ears, and sides of the back and neck) contains more nerve endings than do many other areas; these areas are capable of being aroused by touch. Skin in the specific *erogenous zones* (penis, clitoris, vulva, perineum, lips, breasts, and buttocks) has an even higher density of nerve endings, and nerve endings are closer to the skin surface.[25] The landscape of erotic touch includes holding hands, kissing, stroking, caressing, squeezing, tickling, scratching, and massaging.

Self-Stimulation The two most common self-stimulation sexual activities, called **autoerotic behaviors**, are sexual fantasies and masturbation. Sexual fantasies are mental images, scenarios, and daydreams imagined to initiate sexual arousal. They range from simple images to complicated erotic stories.

The fact that the body can become aroused when a person thinks about sex highlights the fact that the brain is a major player in sexual functioning. Fantasies are effective and harmless ways of exploring sexual fulfillment.

abstinence
Abstention from sexual intercourse, usually as a way to avoid conception or STDs.

foreplay
Touching that increases sexual arousal before sexual intercourse.

autoerotic behaviors
Self-stimulating sexual activities, primarily sexual fantasies and masturbation.

Pop star Lady Gaga, whose songs often feature provocative lyrics, surprised her fans in 2010 when she announced she was celibate, which she did in part to help promote HIV awareness among women. At a promotional event for MAC cosmetics' "Viva Glam" campaign to fight AIDS, she said "Even Lady Gaga can be celibate. You don't have to have sex to be loved."

Masturbation is self-stimulation of the genitals for sexual pleasure. It is usually done manually or with a vibrator or other sex toy. The stigma attached to masturbation is left over from a previous era, when it was considered sinful and dangerous to one's health, probably because its purpose was pleasure rather than procreation. Today, masturbation is better understood and more widely accepted as a natural and healthy sexual behavior. Masturbation is a part of sex therapy programs designed to help people overcome sexual problems, and mutual masturbation is promoted as a way to practice safer sex.[30]

Oral-Genital Stimulation **Cunnilingus** is the oral stimulation of the female genitals with the tongue and lips. **Fellatio** is the oral stimulation of the male genitals with the tongue, lips, and mouth. Oral stimulation can be part of foreplay, or it can be a sexual activity leading to orgasm. Some people find oral-genital stimulation very pleasurable; others refrain because of religious or moral beliefs. Oral sex is not an entirely safe form of sex because infections can be transmitted via the mouth. Using some form of protection during oral sex is recommended.

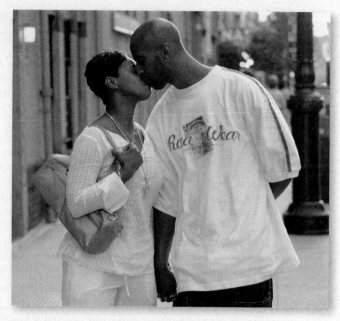

■ The lips are a highly sensitive part of the body, making kissing an intimate act.

The fact that the body can become aroused when a person thinks about sex highlights the fact that **the brain is a major player in sexual functioning**.

Anal Intercourse A small percentage of heterosexual couples and a larger percentage of gay male couples practice anal intercourse, the penetration of the rectum with the penis. The anal area has a high density of nerve endings and is sensitive to stimulation. Because the skin and tissue of the anus and rectum are delicate and can be easily torn, anal intercourse is one of the riskiest sexual behaviors for the transmission of infections, particularly HIV.[31] Condom use is strongly recommended during anal intercourse.

Sexual Intercourse Sexual intercourse, also known as coitus, is by far the most common form of adult sexual expression. It is a source of sexual pleasure for most couples. In sexual intercourse, a man typically inserts his erect penis into a woman's vagina and thrusts with his hips and pelvis until he ejaculates. A woman who is aroused responds with matching hip and pelvic thrusts, but she may or may not reach orgasm solely from penetration and thrusting, as mentioned earlier.

Sexual intercourse can be performed in a variety of positions. The most common is the so-called missionary position, in which the man lies on top of the woman. In this position, the penis can penetrate deeply into the vagina. When the woman lies on top of the man, penetration may not be as deep, but the woman has more control, an important psychological factor for some women. When the woman sits or kneels on top of the man, penetration is deeper and the woman can increase clitoral stimulation by rocking back and forth.[25]

In the rear-entry position, the woman lies face down and the man lies on top of her, or both lie on their sides. Although penetration is not as deep in this position, there is more opportunity for clitoral stimulation by either the woman or the man. Side-by-side positions may be popular for sexual partners with significant weight differences, pregnant women, partners with chronic pain disorders like arthritis, and partners who do not enjoy deep thrusting.[25]

Atypical Sexual Behaviors and Paraphilias Some sexual practices are much less common statistically in our society than those already described. If they are practiced between consenting adults and no physical or psychological harm is done to anyone, they are simply considered atypical. Examples are sex games in which partners enact sexual fantasies, use sex toys (vibrators, dildos), or engage in phone sex (talk about sex, describe erotic scenarios). Another kind of sex game is bondage and discipline, in which restriction of movement (using handcuffs or ropes, for example) or sensory deprivation (using blindfolds or masks) is employed for sexual enjoyment. Most sex games are safe and harmless, but partners need to openly discuss and agree beforehand on what they are comfortable doing.

masturbation
Self-stimulation of the genitals for sexual pleasure.

cunnilingus
Oral stimulation of the female genitals with the tongue and lips.

fellatio
Oral stimulation of the male genitals with the tongue, lips, and mouth.

Atypical sexual practices that do not meet the criteria described above (being consensual and causing no harm) are called paraphilias; they are classified as mental disorders, and many are illegal. Examples of paraphilias are exhibitionism (exposing one's genitals to strangers), voyeurism (observing others' sexual activity without their knowledge), and pedophilia (sexual attraction to and activity with children). Treatment focuses initially on reducing the danger to the patient and potential victims and then on strategies to suppress the behavior. Relapse prevention is essential since these behaviors are usually long-standing.[25]

SEXUAL DYSFUNCTIONS

At some point in their lives, many people experience some kind of **sexual dysfunction**—a disturbance in sexual drive, performance, or satisfaction. Up to 50 percent of couples report having experienced sexual dissatisfaction or dysfunction.[32] Sexual difficulties may occur at any point in the sexual response, although lack of sexual desire is cited as the most frequent problem in marriage and long-term relationships.[33] Most forms of sexual dysfunction are treatable.

Female Sexual Dysfunctions Common sexual dysfunctions in women include pain during intercourse, sexual desire disorder, female sexual arousal disorder, and orgasmic dysfunction.

Pain During Intercourse Some women experience pain during intercourse as a result of **vaginismus**, intense involuntary contractions of the outer third of the muscles of the vagina that tighten the vaginal opening when penetration is attempted. The muscle spasm may range from mild, causing discomfort during intercourse, to severe, preventing intercourse altogether. Vaginismus may be caused by the physiological effects of a medical condition, such as a pelvic or vaginal infection, by psychological factors, such as fear of

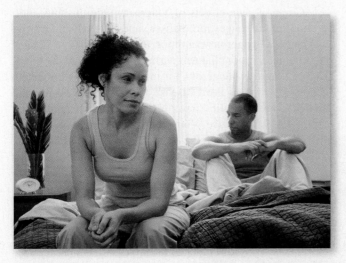

■ Sexuality has physical, psychological, emotional, and interpersonal dimensions. Although sexual problems can have medical or physical causes, they often occur because of relationship problems.

intercourse, or by lack of vaginal lubrication. A physician may recommend **Kegel exercises**, the alternating contraction and relaxation of pelvic floor muscles, to relieve vaginismus.

Sexual Desire Disorder Sexual desire disorder is characterized by lack of sexual fantasies and desire for sexual activity. Because individuals have different normal levels of sexual desire, a problem is considered to exist only if a person is dissatisfied with her own or her partner's level of sexual desire. Low sexual desire can have physical causes, such as medications or hormonal changes, or it can be caused by psychological, emotional, and relationship problems.

Female Sexual Arousal Disorder This disorder is characterized by an inability to attain or maintain the lubrication-swelling response of sexual arousal to the completion of sexual activity. The symptoms do not occur because of insufficient or misplaced sexual stimulation. Like sexual desire disorder, this disorder is considered a problem only if the individual experiencing it considers it a problem.

sexual dysfunction
Disturbance in sexual drive, performance, or satisfaction.

vaginismus
Intense involuntary contractions of the outer third of the muscles of the vagina that prevent penetration or make it uncomfortable.

Kegel exercises
Alternating contraction and relaxation of pelvic floor muscles, performed to help relieve vaginismus, among other effects.

Orgasmic Dysfunction Orgasmic dysfunction is defined as the persistent inability to have an orgasm following normal sexual arousal. Between 25 and 35 percent of women report having had difficulty with orgasm on one or more occasions, and 10–15 percent of women report that they have never had an orgasm.[34] Some women can achieve orgasm through masturbation or oral sex but not with penile penetration. Although orgasm is not necessary for conception or enjoyment of sex, difficulty achieving orgasm can become a frustrating experience.

Orgasmic dysfunction may be influenced by psychological and emotional factors, by lack of knowledge and experience, or by the person's beliefs and attitudes about sex.[35] Certain medications, including some antidepressants, also reduce the ability to reach orgasm. Therapy for orgasmic dysfunction focuses on encouraging women to experiment with their own bodies to discover what stimulates them to orgasm. They are then encouraged to transfer this learning to their sexual relationships.

Treatment of Female Sexual Dysfunctions Much of what is known about the neurophysiology of sexual arousal, desire, and orgasm has come from research on men and has been applied to women.[36] But women's sexuality is different from men's and much more complex than previously thought. Currently, there is a new interest in female sexuality on the part of scientists, sex therapists, and pharmaceutical companies, partly as a result of the success of Viagra in relieving men's sexual problems.

One approach to treatment of sexual problems in women is testosterone replacement therapy. As noted earlier, testosterone is responsible for sex drive in both men and women. Sensibly prescribed, medically necessary testosterone can increase a woman's sex drive, but possible side effects include increased risk of heart disease and liver damage.[26]

Viagra has been tried in women to treat low sexual desire, but results have been disappointing. A few studies suggest that Viagra combined with a low doses of testosterone replacement may have good results.[26] Despite setbacks, the drug market for treating female sexual dysfunction is likely to grow. In recent years, there has been an increase in personal lubricants targeted specifically for women (like Zestra), which may increase sexual arousal and orgasm by warming the clitoris.

Male Sexual Dysfunctions Male sexual dysfunctions include pain during intercourse, sexual desire disorder, erectile dysfunction, and ejaculation dysfunction.

Pain During Intercourse Penile pain usually results from infections from sexually transmitted diseases. Herpes can cause painful lesions on the penis, and gonorrhea and chlamydia cause a penile discharge and pain with urination or ejaculation for most men. Peyronie's disease, an abnormal curvature of the penis, can also make intercourse painful. Infections of the prostate and epididymis also cause pain and should be treated.

Sexual Desire Disorder Sexual desire disorders are frequently caused by emotional problems, including relationship difficulties, depression, guilt over infidelity, worry, stress, and overwork. Reduced sexual desire also can have some physical causes, such as changes in testosterone level.

erectile dysfunction (ED)
Condition in which the penis does not become erect before sex or stay erect during sex.

Erectile Dysfunction In men with **erectile dysfunction (ED)**, smooth-muscle cells constrict the local arteries and reduce blood flow into the penis to a trickle, preventing a buildup of blood. The penis remains flaccid if the smooth-muscle cells are contracted.

The causes of erectile dysfunction (formerly called impotence) can be psychological or physical or both. Less than 20 percent of ED cases have psychological causes.[25,37] Examples of such causes are

■ Male sexual problems have become a public topic as a result of the development of a new class of drugs that treat erectile dysfunction. Viagra is the most frequently prescribed drug in the United States.

anxiety about sexual performance and problems in the relationship with the partner.

Some of the physical causes of ED are low testosterone levels, medications (some antidepressants, blood pressure medications), drugs (alcohol, tobacco), injury, and nerve damage, such as from diabetes, injury, or prostate surgery (see the box "Sex and Alcohol").

Ejaculation Dysfunction Premature ejaculation, defined as ejaculation less than 2 minutes after the beginning of intercourse, is probably the most common type of ejaculation dysfunction.[37] (Men typically average 2 to 7 minutes before ejaculation.) About one-third of sexually active men experience premature ejaculation; gay men have lower rates of premature ejaculation.[37] Like ED, premature ejaculation often results from anxiety about sexual performance or unreasonable expectations. For example, a man might be worried about maintaining an erection and rush to a climax.[32]

An effective technique for preventing premature ejaculation is to stop before orgasm, slow down, and then start again. The stop-start method trains the body to lengthen the duration of the sexual arousal state and can increase enjoyment.

Treatment of Male Sexual Dysfunction Treatment of sexual dysfunction in men often relies on testosterone. Men with a low testosterone level may benefit from testosterone replacement therapy. It is not prescribed for men with normal testosterone levels because it can increase blood pressure, affect blood cholesterol levels, and possibly increase risk for prostate cancer.[32]

Viagra (Sildenafil) is the treatment of choice for ED. Taken an hour before sex, Viagra works by increasing the concentration of the chemical that allows smooth-muscle cells in the erectile tissue to stay relaxed so that the spongy chambers of the penis can remain filled with blood. Its effects last about 4 hours.

Common side effects of Viagra include flushing, indigestion, nasal congestion, nausea, and headaches. Overuse can cause a dangerous condition called priapism, a state of continuous erection that can permanently damage the penis. Use of Viagra is dangerous for men with preexisting health conditions such as heart disease, high blood pressure, and diabetes, and fatalities have been reported in connection with its use. Viagra is just one of several drugs now on the market for erectile problems. Levitra (Vardenafil) and Cialis (Tadolifil) are chemically similar to Viagra but more potent and efficient.

Drug approaches to sexual dysfunctions do not take into account the importance of relationships. They may offer a temporary confidence-builder, but they do not provide a long-term solution to issues that may lie behind sexual problems. Correcting unhealthy

Consumer Clipboard

Sex and Alcohol

Have you ever . . .

- Had regrets about sex the next day?
- Suspected that you might be pregnant because of unprotected sex?
- Had sex with someone you would not choose to have a relationship with?
- Been unable to remember the events from a previous night?
- Wondered whether you were victimized by a date rape drug?
- Been unable to perform sexually?

All of these concerns are much more likely to be on your mind if you consume excessive amounts of alcohol. Alcohol lowers sexual inhibitions and impairs judgment, decision making, effective listening, rational thinking, and the ability to assess risky behaviors and potentially dangerous situations. Alcohol consumption also reduces erectile response in men and vaginal lubrication in women. Heavy consumption of alcohol is even riskier, making it more difficult to maintain control. Psychoactive drugs like marijuana and Ecstasy also increase your risk of engaging in behavior you might regret later.

The physical consequences of sexual activity under the influence of alcohol are well known: increased risk for STDs, sexual assaults, and unwanted pregnancy. The emotional consequences are too often overlooked. Honesty, respect, trust, and communication are likely to be compromised under the influence of too much alcohol. Crossing sexual boundaries, acting against personal values, and rushing into sexual intimacy can cause awkwardness in an otherwise promising relationship.

To make sure you don't jeopardize your sexual health through alcohol consumption, you can take two simple precautions: first, know your alcohol limit and don't exceed it, and second, enlist a buddy when you go to a bar or party and look out for each other. Also, take time to clarify your values, attitudes, and standards about your own sexuality. Is your behavior consistent with your values? Are you influenced by media images and peer pressure, or are your decisions about sexual activity intentional and voluntary?

When you are going to be in a potentially sexual situation, consider these questions ahead of time: (1) Will I be sexually active and, if so, to what degree? (2) How does being sexually active fit with my personal values and beliefs? (3) If I choose to be sexually active, how can I ensure my physical and emotional safety? Along with all the sexual information and freedom available to people in our society comes the responsibility to make informed, healthy choices.

Source: "Drinking to Extremes to Celebrate 21," New York Times, April 8, 2008.

lifestyles, working on relationships, and cultivating a more realistic expectation of aging can improve mid- and late-life sexuality.

Misuse of ED Drugs by Young Men The misuse of Viagra and other ED drugs on college campuses has recently come to the attention of health experts. Viagra has been tagged the "thrill pill" on many campuses, where young men are taking it as a party drug at clubs, raves, and private parties. They mistakenly believe they will quickly and easily attain an erection that will allow them to have sex for hours. Erection drugs do not work unless nitric oxide is present in the penis, and nitric oxide is produced only in response to physical and mental stimulation. Any effect these drugs seem to have is more likely a placebo effect in healthy young men.

More important, the combination of ED drugs with alcohol or illicit drugs such as cocaine, amphetamines, or Ecstasy can be life-threatening. Even more dangerous is combining them with amyl nitrate ("poppers"). The combination of ED drugs with any stimulant drug dilates blood vessels, which can result in a sudden drop in blood pressure.[38]

safer sex
Sexual activities that do not include exchange of body fluids during sex.

condom
Thin sheath, usually made of latex, that fits over the erect penis during sexual intercourse to prevent conception and protect against STDs.

PROTECTING YOUR SEXUAL HEALTH

Safer sex practices prevent the exchange of body fluids during sex. Two safer sex practices are using condoms and having sex that does not involve genital contact or penetration. A third practice is abstinence, considered the only way to completely guarantee protection against STDs. Another key to safeguarding your sexual health is communicating about sex.

Using Condoms The **condom** (or *male condom*) is a thin sheath, usually made of latex, that fits over the erect penis during sexual intercourse. It provides a barrier against penile, vaginal, or anal discharges and genital lesions or sores. Although condoms do not provide complete protection against all STDs, they greatly reduce the risk of infection when used correctly (see Figure 13.2, in the next chapter). Latex condoms should

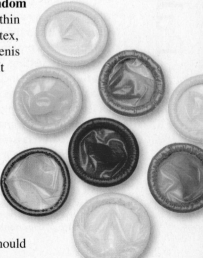

not be used with any oil-based lubricants (such as Vaseline or hand lotion) because such products cause latex to deteriorate. Plastic (polyurethane) condoms are also available and can be used by people who are allergic to latex. They are thinner, stronger, and less constricting than latex, and they are not eroded by oil-based lubricants. However, they are more expensive than latex condoms and have not been tested as fully for effectiveness.

Protection against STDs is also offered by the **female condom**, a soft pouch of thin polyurethane that is inserted into the vagina before intercourse. The female condom has a soft flexible ring at both ends. The ring at the closed end is fitted against the cervix, and the ring at the open end remains outside the body (see Figure 13.3, in the next chapter). The female condom covers more of the genital area, so it may provide more protection against an STD lesion or sore than the male condom does.

female condom
Soft pouch of thin polyurethane that is inserted into the vagina before intercourse to prevent conception and protect against STDs.

dental dams
Small latex squares placed over the vulva during oral sex.

Condoms and **dental dams** (a small latex square placed over the vulva) should be used during oral sex because bacteria and viruses can be transmitted in semen and vaginal fluids. Plastic wrap placed over the vulva, or a piece of latex cut from a latex glove, is an alternative to a dental dam. Protection is especially important if there are any cuts or sores in the mouth; even bleeding gums can increase the risk of getting an infection.

Sexual activities that do not involve genital or skin contact include hugging, massage, and erotic touching, stroking, and caressing with the clothes on.

Practicing Abstinence People practice abstinence for a variety of reasons. Abstinence is often promoted as a positive choice for young people; when this is the case, however, individuals should be provided with information and education about both contraception and STDs. Some unmarried couples choose to be abstinent until they are married, and some married couples use periodic abstinence as a contraceptive method. As noted earlier, abstinence is the only way that people can be completely certain they are not at risk for STDs and unintended pregnancy.

Public Health in Action

Sexting

While much of the concern about sexting has been centered on the unintended legal consequences that can occur, sexting can also have serious unintended psychological consequences. The case of 18-year-old Jessica Logan is especially tragic. In 2008, the Ohio high school student sent nude pictures of herself to her boyfriend. They broke up, and he sent the pictures to other girls at her school. The girls began harassing her, calling her names and throwing things at her. Jessica hanged herself shortly after going public with her story. Although someone who sends nude pictures of him- or herself to a "trusted" partner is not responsible for the actions that the recipient takes or the consequences that result from these actions, people do need to consider the risks.

Awareness of the problem is growing in the United States and is already in the public consciousness in other countries. Australia, for example, has implemented a country-wide program to raise awareness about the dangers of sexting. The program, called "Safe Sexting: No Such Thing," includes a fact sheet for parents and students that warns of the legal and psychological risks of sending nude pictures. Schools hold assemblies to address the issue, and discussions of sexting are incorporated into the classroom curriculum.

At the moment, state governments in the United States are focusing on changing their child pornography laws so that underage teens who send nude pictures of themselves—and those who receive them and pass them on—do not face the same serious legal consequences as convicted pedophiles and sex offenders. They are also beginning to get the word out to parents via public service announcements that parents need to talk with their kids about sexting and its consequences. One campaign targeting young texters was created by cell phone manufacturer LG in collaboration with James Lipton, the dramatic host of the TV series *Inside the Actor's Studio*. The campaign urges people to "Give it a ponder" before they text (www.giveitaponder.com). Comedic public service announcement videos feature James Lipton lending his infamous beard to would-be texters, who then think through their texting impulses. In one, Lipton's beard "saves" a young man from texting a picture of his "junk" to his Twitter-addicted girlfriend. In another, the beard gives a young woman the wisdom not to start a rumor about another girl. Posters show young people wearing Lipton's beard, which helps them to rethink potentially bad ideas. As states and schools catch up to the emerging trend of sexting, public service messages aimed at young people and their parents are likely to become more common.

connect
ACTIVITY

Sources: "Safe Sexting: No Such Thing," New South Wales Public Schools, 2009, retrieved April 22, 2010, from http://www.schools.nsw.edu.au/news/announcements/yr2009/may/sexting.php; "Her Teen Committed Suicide Over 'Sexting,'" by M. Celizic, 2009, The Today Show, retrieved April 22, 2010, from http://today.msnbc.msn.com/id/29546030/.

Life Stories

Madison: Hooking Up

Madison and Tomas were both sophomores and had been dating each other exclusively for a year. They met their freshman year and almost instantly bonded. Madison had had some sexual experiences before college, but Tomas was her first real boyfriend. Madison was shy and Tomas was outgoing—qualities that they both liked about each other. A lot of their friends hooked up with people at parties and had casual sex, but Madison and Tomas were happy with their exclusive relationship. Their friends thought they were a little boring and "old-fashioned" but also envied them for being satisfied with their relationship.

For spring semester of sophomore year, Tomas was planning to attend a study abroad program in Italy. A week before he was leaving, he told Madison that he wanted to be open to other relationships while they were apart. He said he cared about her but saw the trip as a chance to find out if they were "meant to be together." He wanted to have new experiences, including sexual experiences, if they came along, and he didn't want to feel as if he was cheating on her while he was away.

Madison was caught by surprise. She said okay, but only because she didn't know what else to say. She felt confused and rejected. After Tomas left, she figured she might as well use this time to explore new

relationships herself—at least it would help get her mind off Tomas. She started partying more with her friends and tried to cast off her shy persona. She would have a few drinks (or more) and make herself dance and flirt. She was surprised to find she got a lot of attention. It made her feel attractive and popular—and like she was getting back at Tomas. The first time a guy made it clear he wanted to hook up with her, she turned him down, but the next time she accepted. She found it exciting but also awkward, especially when the alcohol wore off. She enjoyed the sex but missed the intimacy she shared with Tomas—the talking, laughing, and sense of closeness and trust. She was also dismayed that the guy she hooked up with didn't call or email her. She felt rejected all over again and dreaded running into him on campus.

Tomas sent her messages on Facebook with upbeat descriptions of all the fun things he was doing and said that he missed her. Neither of them brought up the topic of seeing other people or hooking up. Reading messages from Tomas, Madison realized how much she missed him and how much hooking up was not helping her with her feelings. In fact, it was making her feel worse. She decided to ask Tomas to clarify his feelings about her so she could make some decisions about her own actions. She also decided that hooking up was not for her, at least not right now.

Communicating About Sex Conversations about sexual topics are important to your health, your partner's health, and the success of your relationship. If you are about to begin a sexual relationship, take the time to tell your partner your sexual health history and find out about his or hers. Here are some questions to guide your conversation:

- Are you having sex with anyone else? Are you willing to be monogamous with me?
- Have you ever had an STD? If so, how long ago, and what treatment did you get? Do you now have a clean bill of health?
- How many sexual partners have you had? As far as you know, did any of them ever have an STD?
- When was the last time you were tested for STDs? Would you be willing to get tested along with me?
- Are you willing to use condoms every time we have sex?

If you are not satisfied with the answers you get, take care of yourself by insisting on further conversations and behavioral changes before you begin a sexual relationship.

SEX AND CULTURE: ISSUES FOR THE 21ST CENTURY

While pornography and prostitution have been with us for centuries, advances in technology and changes in culture have created newer, complex issues that we face today. One is sex on the Internet, where people can find immediate, anonymous, and solitary sex without the complexities of relationships. Whether they are looking for it or not, people frequently encounter sexual images on the Internet, and they have access to pornography and sexually explicit Web sites. People access this explicit but virtual sex for many reasons—to obtain sexual gratification, to search for romance, to relieve boredom, to satisfy their curiosity. Issues arise over whether the availability of cybersex has harmful consequences, especially for children.

Some individuals are at risk for sex addiction, defined as compulsive, out-of-control sexual behavior that results in severe negative consequences. Sex addicts lose time every day to the isolating activities of fantasy and masturbation, and the Internet is a particularly seductive medium. Hours spent on the Internet are hours not spent on real-life activities, including time spent developing intimate relationships with real partners.

If you think you might be at risk for sex addiction, talk to a mental health professional at your campus counseling center. Sex addiction can cause serious physical, emotional, spiritual, family, financial, and legal problems, but treatment is available. You can also learn more about sex addiction at the Sexual Recovery Institute (www.sexualrecovery.com).

An emerging issue for teens is sexting—sending nude, sexually explicit messages (text, photo, or video) electronically, mostly by cell phone. The National Campaign to Prevent Teen and Unplanned Pregnancy estimates that 20 percent of 13- to 19-year-olds are sexting. Many young people are not aware of the potential serious legal consequences of sexting. Under federal and state laws, people who send nude or sexual images or video of minors may be subject to the possession, manufacturing, and distribution of child pornography. One 18-year-old male was sentenced to five years' probation and required to register as a sex offender for sending nude pictures of his 16-year-old girlfriend to dozens of her friends and family after an argument. Although photos or videos may be intended solely for a boyfriend or girlfriend, they may end up being shared with a much larger audience. People who sext—at any age—can also face emotional consequences including embarrassment, humiliation, and harassment from peers when their images are distributed without their knowledge or consent (see the box "Sexting"). The images they send leave a digital footprint that can last for years, potentially damaging their prospects for future relationships and careers.

A major issue on college campuses is the decline of traditional dating and the rise of the "hook-up" culture mentioned earlier that is devoid of emotional intimacy and romantic relationships. A national study of 20- to 29-year-olds found that only about one-third were in committed relationships.[31] Over 80 percent of college students have had an intimate physical encounter without any expectation of the development of a relationship—a hook-up.[39] Hooking up can constitute anything from kissing to sex. In a hook-up culture, students rarely go on formal dates. Instead, they frequent parties or bars in large groups, consume alcohol and/or drugs, and hook up with casual friends or strangers. The downside of the hook-up culture has been significant increases in sexually transmitted diseases and emotional and mental health issues, including sexual regret, negative or ambivalent emotional reactions, psychological distress, depression, and anxiety (see the box "Madison: Hooking

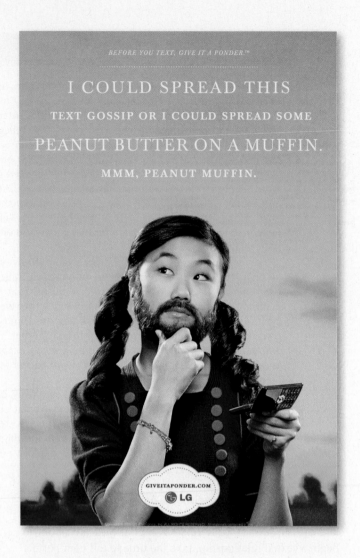

Up"). Women tend to suffer from these consequences more than men do. Perhaps the most costly consequence of a hook-up culture is the failure to develop the qualities that are essential for healthy, long-term relationships—trust, respect, admiration, honesty, caring, and communication.[39,40]

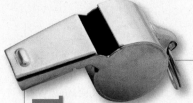

You Make the Call

Should Same-Sex Marriage Be Legal?

Although marriage has traditionally been defined as a religious and legal commitment between a man and a woman, many committed same-sex partners are challenging this definition and demanding the right to marry. In a few states, they have won some rights, and in Massachusetts, Connecticut, Iowa, Vermont, and New Hampshire, they have full marriage rights. Other states have passed "defense of marriage" acts, stating that marriage is a union between one man and one woman.

What is at stake in this issue? Proponents of same-sex marriage point out that the 14th Amendment to the U.S. Constitution prohibits the states from denying any citizen the equal protection of the laws, and many state constitutions protect equal rights for all. Proponents claim that same-sex couples are being discriminated against and denied equal rights by not being allowed to marry. Marriage gives heterosexual couples hundreds of legal, economic, and social benefits and rights, in areas such as child custody, joint ownership of property, taxation, health insurance, Social Security and pensions, medical decision making, inheritance, legal protection, and many others. Proponents argue that gay people are unfairly denied access to the same benefits that are available to heterosexual people.

Opponents of same-sex marriage argue that the Bible condemns homosexuality and that virtually all major religions consider gay relationships sinful or immoral. They further argue that a nation's laws should reflect the moral values on which it is founded and that many U.S. laws have their origin in religious teachings, such as the injunction against murder. Because laws imply moral approval of a behavior and shape the attitudes of society, legalizing same-sex unions condones behavior that the majority of people find unacceptable. Some but not all opponents with a religious orientation also argue that the purpose of marriage is procreation and because same-sex couples do not produce children, they are not entitled to be married.

Supporters of same-sex marriage respond to the religious argument by citing the U.S. Constitution. The First Amendment prohibits the establishment of a state religion, which is the basis for the separation of church and state in the United States. Laws based on religious views are not constitutional, nor is discrimination against an individual or a group on the basis of religious views. Even if certain churches do not want to perform same-sex marriages, marriage as a secular institution should be available to all.

Another argument against legalizing same-sex marriage is that doing so threatens the sanctity of marriage, one of society's most revered institutions. Marriage is the basis of the family, and one of the family's most important functions is raising and socializing children. Marriage is already in a precarious state in the United States, and legalizing gay marriage would further weaken it and cause it to lose respect, according to this view. Some opponents argue that if marriage is opened up to same-sex couples, it will lead down the "slippery slope" to marriage between multiple persons, marriage between friends for tax purposes, or even marriage to an animal. We need a firm definition of marriage to discourage such an explosion of possibilities, in the opinion of these opponents.

Supporters of same-sex marriage respond that society is changing and that sometimes the law has to take the lead in securing social justice for all. They point out that civil rights laws had to be passed to back up principles on which the United States was founded, such as that all people have equal rights. They note that interracial marriage was illegal in some states until the Supreme Court ruled otherwise in 1967. Prohibiting marriage between same-sex partners is a form of minority discrimination, as it would be if African American or Hispanic partners were not allowed to marry. Like interracial marriage, gay marriage is an idea whose time has come.

Proponents also say that allowing gay people to marry would only strengthen the institution of marriage, creating more families and environments for child rearing and promoting family values. They note that no research has ever shown that being raised by same-sex parents results in psychological or emotional harm or causes children to become gay or lesbian. They assert that the institution of marriage is far less threatened by gay marriage than by the social forces that have been eroding it for the past 50 years.

Some opponents say that same-sex partners who want to publicly declare their commitment to each other should be satisfied with the options of civil union or domestic partnership where available, leaving the institution of marriage to heterosexual couples. Proponents respond that these are second-class options, analogous to the "separate but equal" schools and facilities provided for African Americans until they were declared unconstitutional by the Supreme Court in 1954.

Should marriage be an option for everyone, or should it be limited to heterosexual couples? What do you think?

PROS

- All citizens are entitled to equal rights and equal protection under the law. When same-sex partners are prohibited from marrying, they are denied access to the many rights and benefits available to their fellow citizens who are heterosexual and thus allowed to marry. Prohibiting same-sex marriage is a form of discrimination.

- Prohibiting gay marriage on religious grounds is unconstitutional, as is discrimination based on religious views.

- Society is changing, and sometimes law and society have to lead the way in areas of social justice, setting a standard that encourages people to reconsider their prejudices. This was the case with many civil rights laws. Gay marriage is an idea whose time has come.

- Gay people form the same kind of loving, committed relationships as heterosexual people and have the same right to formalize their relationships in the eyes of society and the law.

- Gay marriage increases the number of committed relationships and families in society and promotes family values.

- Domestic partnerships and civil unions provide couples some rights at the state level, but many of the rights and benefits of marriage are conferred at the federal level, as, for example, in tax laws. Thus, these options are not the same as marriage.

CONS

- Virtually all major religions consider homosexuality sinful or immoral; this value should be reflected in the nation's laws. Legalizing gay marriage would condone behavior that the majority of people consider immoral or unacceptable.

- Legalizing gay marriage weakens the institution of marriage and threatens its sanctity. Opening up marriage to same-sex partners would lead to new definitions of marriage and family, contributing to a further devaluation of marriage and a decline in family values.

- The purpose of marriage is procreation. Since same-sex couples do not procreate, they do not need the protection or validation of marriage.

- Marriage is one of the most important traditional social institutions, and in nearly all societies it is considered to be a union between one man and one woman.

connect™
ACTIVITY

IN REVIEW

Why are relationships important for health?
People are social beings and need connections with others to live fully functioning lives. People with strong social support networks tend to enjoy better health than do those with fewer connections, although the mechanisms behind this difference are not fully known.

What kinds of relationships are important?
Two important kinds of relationships are friendships and intimate partnerships. Friendships are reciprocal relationships based on mutual liking; intimate partnerships have additional qualities, usually including exclusivity, commitment, and sexuality. Healthy relationships allow people to be themselves and to grow.

What sexuality-related attitudes and behaviors are prevalent in our society?
American attitudes are marked by tension between the poles of sexual restraint and sexual permissiveness. Most Americans are engaged in committed, monogamous relationships, and marital infidelity is relatively uncommon. Statistically speaking, men have about 13 years of premarital sexual activity and women have about 10 years.

What are the best ways to protect your sexual health?
Using condoms, practicing abstinence, avoiding alcohol in sexual situations, and practicing good communication skills are the best ways to protect your sexual health.

Web Resources

American Association for Marriage and Family Therapy: At this Web site, you can view FAQs about marriage and family therapy, read updates on family problems, locate a family therapist in your area, and find listings of resources.
www.aamft.org

American Psychological Association Help Center: The Families and Relationships section of this site features a wide variety of information, such as communication tips, psychological tasks for a good marriage, stepfamily issues, and social life problems.
www.apahelpcenter.org

Go Ask Alice: This Columbia University site features questions and answers of interest to young adults, including sexuality and sexual health.
www.goaskalice.columbia.edu

National Sexuality Resource Center: This organization addresses issues in contemporary sexuality. Its sexual literacy campaign is designed to counteract negative messages about sexuality and promote healthy attitudes toward sexuality.
http://nsrc.sfsu.edu

Prepare-Enrich / Life Innovations: This site offers a stronger-marriage inventory, a quiz for couples, information on finding a marriage counselor, and other resources for couples.
www.prepare-enrich.com

Sexuality Information and Education Council of the United States: This organization's Web site includes FAQs, information updates, fact sheets on sexuality at different life stages, gay and lesbian issues, and approaches to sex education.
www.siecus.org

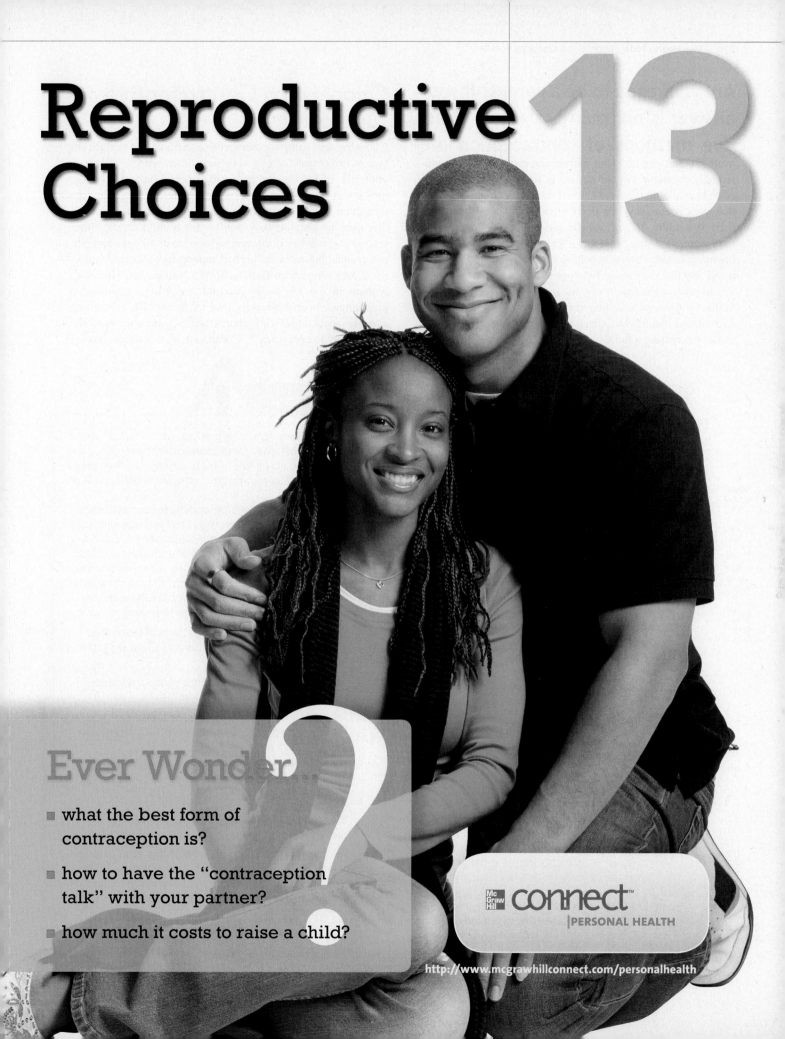

Reproductive Choices

13

Ever Wonder...

- what the best form of contraception is?
- how to have the "contraception talk" with your partner?
- how much it costs to raise a child?

McGraw Hill **connect** | PERSONAL HEALTH

http://www.mcgrawhillconnect.com/personalhealth

Are you ready to be a parent? If your answer is no, many safe and effective methods of contraception are

available that you and your partner can use to avoid an unintended pregnancy. If your answer is yes, a wealth of knowledge is available that you can use to increase the likelihood that your pregnancy is a positive experience and that your baby is healthy. If you want to have children sometime in the future, planning for it now—by using contraception and choosing healthy lifestyle behaviors—can give you peace of mind and the knowledge that you are doing everything you can to protect the health of your future family. This chapter builds on the topics discussed in Chapter 12—relationships and sexual health—to discuss reproductive choices and issues in creating a family.

Choosing a Contraceptive Method

Choosing and using a contraceptive method that is right for you is important for one very significant reason: It lowers your risk of unintended pregnancy. About half of all pregnancies in the United States are unintended, and many are unwanted, either because the couple don't want a child at this time or because they don't want a child at all. Unintended pregnancies occur among women of all ages and ethnic groups, but rates are highest among low-income, minority (Black, American Indian, Alaska Native, and Hispanic) women in the 18- to 24-year-old age group. Unintended pregnancies nearly always cause stress and life disruption and are associated with poorer health outcomes (see the box "Teen Pregnancies"). Compared with women having

Who's at Risk?

Teen Pregnancies

When teenagers get pregnant and give birth, their future prospects decline, as do those of their children. Compared with non-teenage mothers, teen mothers are less likely to finish high school or attend college, less likely to marry or stay married, and more likely to require public assistance. They are less likely to receive prenatal care and more likely to smoke, factors associated with poor birth outcomes.

About one-third of girls in the United States get pregnant before age 20. More than 80 percent of these pregnancies are unintended. In 2007 more than 445,000 infants were born to mothers aged 15–19 years, a birth rate of 42.5 live births per 1,000 females in this age group. Birth rates for girls aged 15–19 years declined from 1991 to 2005, but since then they have been on the increase.

Major disparities exist in pregnancy and birth rates. In 2007, Mississippi, New Mexico, and Arkansas had the highest teen birth rates, followed by Oklahoma and South Carolina. Massachusetts and New Jersey had the lowest teen birth rates. The highest birth rate in 15- to 19-year-olds was among Latinas; the rate was 82 live births per 1,000 females, nearly twice the overall rate. Among non-Hispanic Black females in this age group, the rate was 64; among American Indian or Alaska Native females, 59; and among non-Hispanic White females, 27.

Socioeconomic status appears to be a major factor in different rates. Teens living in poverty, with lower educational opportunities and fewer job opportunities, are at greater risk of having a child before the age of 20. Two-thirds of teen moms live at or below the poverty line when they give birth. They are more likely to initiate sex at a slightly earlier age, less likely to use contraception during their first sexual encounter, and less likely to successfully use contraceptives in ongoing relationships.

Reduced access to contraceptives, ambivalence about pregnancy, and lower motivation to avoid pregnancy are all believed to play a role in these differences. Teen pregnancy among low-income girls contributes to the cycle of poverty.

Health organizations are working to promote healthy decision making among teenagers and young adults, such as reducing numbers of partners, delaying initiation of sex, and increasing contraception and condom use. More work is needed, however, to identify interventions that speak to the social, cultural, economic, and environmental influences on unintended pregnancy. The National Campaign to Prevent Teen Pregnancy has these suggestions:

- Involve parents and encourage them to teach their children about sex, love, relationships, and expected behavior.
- Stop fighting about "abstinence versus contraception"—more of both are needed.
- Intensify efforts in communities with especially high rates of teen pregnancy, particularly Latinas and African American girls.
- Increase the focus on the role of boys and men in unintended pregnancy prevention.
- Target younger teens.
- Take advantage of ever-advancing technology to prevent teen pregnancy.

Perhaps most important is providing economic and educational opportunities and mentoring so today's youth have a hope for the future and a reason to plan for and delay childbearing until they are prepared.

Sources: "Births: Preliminary Data for 2007," by B.E. Hamilton, J.A. Martin, and S.J. Ventura, 2009, National Vital Statistics Reports, 57 (12); "Socioeconomic Disadvantage and Adolescent Women's Sexual and Reproductive Behavior: The Case of Five Developed Countries," by S. Singh, J.E. Darroch, J. J. Frost, et al., 2001, Family Planning Perspectives, 33 (6), Nov/Dec.

planned pregnancies, women with unintended pregnancies are less likely to receive adequate **prenatal care**, are more likely to drink alcohol and smoke, and are more likely to have babies with **low birth weight** (less than 5.5 pounds).[1]

Advances in reproductive technology have led to the development of many acceptable and reliable contraceptive methods. In this section we take a look at several of these methods. Complete the activities in this chapter's Personal Health Portfolio to determine which contraceptive method may best suit your needs.

prenatal care
Regular medical care during pregnancy, designed to promote the health of the mother and the fetus.

low birth weight
Birth weight of less than 5.5 pounds, often as a result of preterm delivery.

intrauterine device (IUD)
Small T-shaped device that when inserted in the uterus prevents conception.

COMMUNICATING ABOUT CONTRACEPTION

If you are in a serious relationship, you and your partner should decide together how to best protect each other from sexually transmitted diseases (STDs) and unintended pregnancy. If you have casual sex or hook up with people you do not know well, it may be more of a challenge to have this discussion. If this is the case for you, you may want to consider abstinence from intercourse until you are in a relationship where the conversation is possible.

How do you have the conversation? First, consider which method you think is best for you and your type of relationship. It will be easier to discuss if you feel educated and confident about what you want to use. Next, prepare yourself for the conversation. If you are comfortable, role-play the discussion with a friend. Consider how you will start the conversation, and think about your partner's potential responses.

When you have the conversation, talk about the relationship. Do you both have the same expectations about your relationship status—are you going to be monogamous, or does either of you plan to be sexually involved with other people? It is also important to discuss what you would want to do if your birth control fails. Can you agree on a contingency plan in the event of a pregnancy?

When do you have the conversation? Ideally, you should have this conversation prior to the initiation of any sexual contact! This requires being honest with yourself and your partner(s) about what you expect from a relationship in advance. In a recent study on hooking up, half of college students reported being carried away in the moment. Looking back on it, they did not understand how they became so sexually involved. Lack of planning is associated with a higher risk of unprotected sex.[2]

Don't underestimate the risk of pregnancy, and don't make assumptions about whether your partner is using contraception. Talking about birth control is a sign of respect for yourself and your partner. Contraception is not just a "woman's responsibility." The unintended consequences impact men and women alike, and thus the responsibility should be shared. If you cannot agree on a method to use or have very different beliefs regarding what you would do if you or your partner became pregnant, take time before starting a sexual relationship.

WHICH CONTRACEPTIVE METHOD IS RIGHT FOR YOU?

Given all the options available for contraception and the number of variables that have to be taken into account in choosing a method—effectiveness, cost, convenience, permanence, safety, protection against STDs, and consistency with personal values—deciding which method is the best one for you can be difficult. (For an overview of methods, see Table 13.1.) Here are some questions to consider:

- Is your main concern preventing pregnancy? Or do you also need to worry about sexually transmitted diseases? If you are concerned about STDs, you need to use condoms. If you are in a mutually faithful, monogamous relationship and neither you nor your partner has an STD, then a barrier method may not be necessary. You may want to consider birth control pills, an injectable contraceptive, or an **intrauterine device (IUD)**.

- Do you sometimes have sex under the influence of alcohol or drugs? Do you hook up with partners and not always know their sexual history? In these situations, you are at risk for both STDs and pregnancy. The best option is dual contraception—a barrier method plus a hormonal method. Condoms are the best way to reduce risk for STDs (discussed in Chapter 14). A hormonal contraceptive is important because its efficacy does not rely on your decision-making abilities at the time of intercourse.

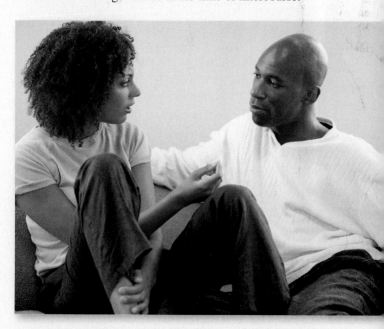

- Having a talk about contraception may be uncomfortable at first, but you and your partner will both be glad you had it. Think about what you want to say ahead of time and use good communication skills.

Table 13.1 Overview of Contraceptive Methods

| Method of Birth Control | Failure Rate (%) | | Advantages | Disadvantages | Cost | STD Protection | Rate of User Continuation (%) |
	Perfect Use	Actual Use					
No method	85	85		No protection against pregnancy	*	None	?
Abstinence	0	?	Available to all	Requires control; interrupts sexual expression Must agree on definition	None	++	?
Oral contraceptives (birth control pills)	0.3	8	Easy to use Does not interrupt intercourse Safe for most women Noncontraceptive benefits	Possible side effects/rare serious health problems Must be taken daily Prescription required	$$	None	68
Transdermal patch (Ortho Evra Patch)	0.3	8	Easy-to-use weekly application Does not interrupt intercourse Safe for most women Noncontraceptive benefits	Possible side effects/rare serious health problems Greater risk of blood clots than with pill or other hormonal methods Prescription required	$$	None	68
Vaginal contraceptive ring (NuvaRing)	0.3	8	Easy-to-use monthly application Does not interrupt intercourse Safe for most women Noncontraceptive benefits	Possible side effects/rare serious health problems Prescription required	$$	None	68
Injection (Depo-Provera)	0.3	3	Very effective Contains no estrogen Requires action only every 3 months	Possible side effects/rare serious health problems Visit to provider every 3 months Weight gain May decrease bone density over time	$$	None	56
Implant (Implanon)	0.05	0.05	Very effective Contains no estrogen Lasts 3 years	Similar to injection but without ongoing provider visits Minor procedure to remove	$$	None	70
Emergency contraception pills			Reduces risk of pregnancy in case of rape, unprotected sex, or failure of barrier Available over the counter for those aged 18 or older	Must be used within 5 days of unprotected intercourse Nausea/vomiting May alter menstrual cycle Not intended for regular use	$**	None	Not intended for ongoing use
Spermicides	18	29	Available over the counter Increase effectiveness of barriers Female involvement only	May cause allergic reaction Must be inserted with every act of intercourse May increase transmission of HIV	$	None	42
Male condom	2	15	Accessible, inexpensive, easily carried, over the counter Male involvement Reduces risk of STD transmission	Requires interruption of intercourse Male involvement Possible embarrassment Possible breakage	$	+/++	53

Method of Birth Control	Failure Rate (%)		Advantages	Disadvantages	Cost	STD Protection	Rate of User Continuation (%)
	Perfect Use	Actual Use					
Female condom	5	21	No male involvement Can insert before intercourse Accessible, easily carried, over the counter	Difficult for some women to insert Not as readily available More expensive	$$	+	49
Diaphragm	6	16	May reduce risk of some STDs May be inserted prior to onset of sexual activity	Requires provider appointment/prescription May cause allergic reaction Rarely associated with toxic shock syndrome Must be used with every act of intercourse	$$	+	57
Cervical cap (FemCap) w/o prior pregnancy	4	14	Same as for diaphragm	Same as for diaphragm	$$	+	57
Sponge w/o prior pregnancy	9	16	Over the counter Immediately effective upon insertion	May cause allergic reaction Rarely associated with toxic shock syndrome Must be used with every act of intercourse	$	+	57
Fertility awareness-based methods	3–5	25	Requires knowledge of fertility cycle Male involvement No serious side effects	Requires knowledge of fertility cycle Male involvement Variations in cycle may make methods difficult for some women	None	None	51
Withdrawal***	4	27	Available to all	Requires control Interrupts sexual expression	None	None	?
IUD—copper (ParaGard)	0.6	0.8	Always in place Effective for 10 years Very effective but reversible	May have pain/heavy menstrual flow Requires provider visit Possible complications	$$$	None	80
IUD— progesterone (Mirena)	0.2	0.2	Always in place Effective for 5 years Very effective but reversible Decreased menstrual flow	Requires provider visit Possible complications	$$$	None	80
Sterilization (female)	0.5	0.5	Highly effective No further action needed No significant long-term side effects	Difficult to reverse Requires surgery/ anesthesia Risk of ectopic pregnancy if failure	$$$	None	Permanent
Sterilization (male)	0.1	0.15	Highly effective No further action needed No significant long-term side effects Male involvement	Difficult to reverse Requires local anesthesia and minor surgery	$$$	None	Permanent

Cost: none; $ (low), $$ (low/moderate), $$$ (high).
Sexually transmitted disease (STD) protection: none; + (low—may offer some protection); ++ (high).
* "No method" has no initial cost but carries with it a high risk of pregnancy and associated costs.
** Emergency contraception pills are inexpensive for single use but expensive for regular use.
*** Many do not consider withdrawal a form of contraception. See text discussion.

Sources: Adapted from Contraceptive Technology, *19th rev. ed., by R.A. Hatcher, J. Trussell, F. Stewart, et al., 2007, New York: Ardent Media; "The Contraceptive Efficacy of Implanon: A Review of Clinical Trials and Marketing Experience," by O. Graesslin and T. Korver, 2008,* European Journal of Contraceptive & Reproductive Healthcare, *13 (Suppl. 1), pp. 4–12.*

- Are you planning to have children with this partner at some time in the future? The male and female condoms, the diaphragm, the cervical cap, and the contraceptive sponge are all safe, nonpermanent methods.

- Do you already have children and know that you do not want any more? Surgical sterilization is a highly effective method with no hassles after the initial procedure.

- How much can you afford to pay for contraception? There are several factors to consider here. For example, how often do you need contraception? If you have sex daily, the cost of buying condoms for every time can quickly add up, whereas the one-time cost of an IUD or sterilization may be less. If you have sex once a month or less, the opposite may be true. If you need to use two forms of contraception, one to prevent STDs and one to decrease your chances of pregnancy, again, the costs can add up. Don't forget to take into account the cost if you or your partner gets pregnant with the form of contraception you select. It might be the cost of having an abortion, or it might be the cost of raising a child.

- Are you worried about the safety and health consequences of contraception? These are important concerns, but people are often surprised to learn how safe all the contraceptive options available today have become. To put the risks in perspective, consider that the risk of being killed in a car crash in a given year is 1 in 5,900; the risk of dying from a pregnancy carried past 20 weeks is 1 in 10,000; and the risk of dying from the use of birth control pills in a nonsmoking woman aged 15 to 44 years is 1 in 66,700.[3]

- Is your choice influenced by your religious, spiritual, or ethical beliefs? Some people are not comfortable with any method that interferes with natural processes. Abstinence, periodic abstinence, or the fertility awareness method may be the right choice.

ABSTINENCE

The only guaranteed method of preventing pregnancy and STDs is *abstinence*. As noted in Chapter 12, abstinence is usually defined as abstention from sexual intercourse; that is, there is no penile penetration of the vagina. In heterosexual couples who have vaginal intercourse and use no contraceptive method, 85 percent of the women will become pregnant in one year.[3]

Abstinence requires that both partners feel empowered and free from sexual coercion. It requires control and commitment—that is, the ability or the determination not to change one's mind in the heat of the moment, especially in situations where one or both partners are intoxicated.

HORMONAL CONTRACEPTIVE METHODS

Hormonal methods come in a variety of forms—pills, injections, patches, and vaginal rings—and work by preventing ovulation. They also alter cervical mucus, making it harder for sperm to reach ova, and they affect the uterine lining so

that a fertilized egg is less likely to be implanted. They are prescribed or administered by a physician. The advantages of hormonal methods include their effectiveness, their ease of use, their limited side effects, and the fact that they do not permanently affect fertility. They do not require any action at the time of intercourse. In addition, they offer some general health benefits. They reduce menstrual cramping and blood loss, premenstrual symptoms, ovarian cysts, endometriosis, and the risk of endometrial and ovarian cancer. They can also improve acne.

A major disadvantage associated with hormonal contraceptives is that they offer no protection against STDs. In some women, they can cause some minor side effects, including symptoms of early pregnancy (nausea, bloating, weight gain, and breast tenderness), mood changes, lowered libido, and headaches. Serious side effects are rare and more common in women who are older and who smoke (Figure 13.1). Hormonal contraceptives require a visit to a health care provider to determine which method is best for you and to ensure you do not have a contraindication for use.

Birth control pills (*oral contraceptives*) are the most popular reversible form of contraception. They usually contain a combination of estrogen and progesterone. A pack of birth control pills typically contains a month's worth of pills (see the box "Do Women Need to Menstruate Monthly?"). Some formulations contain only progesterone; they are

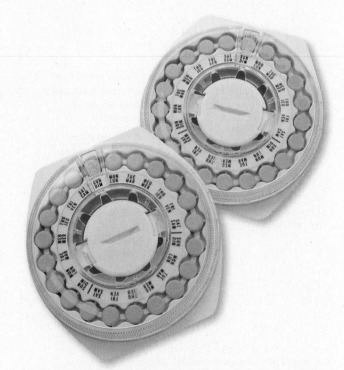

- The development of "the pill" and its approval by the FDA in 1960 ushered in an era of more relaxed sexual attitudes and behaviors—the so-called sexual revolution. Today, birth control pills remain the most popular form of contraception among unmarried women.

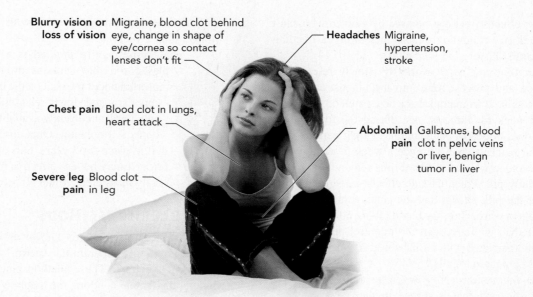

Blurry vision or loss of vision Migraine, blood clot behind eye, change in shape of eye/cornea so contact lenses don't fit

Headaches Migraine, hypertension, stroke

Chest pain Blood clot in lungs, heart attack

Abdominal pain Gallstones, blood clot in pelvic veins or liver, benign tumor in liver

Severe leg pain Blood clot in leg

figure **13.1** **Serious side effects of hormonal contraceptives.** Serious side effects are very rare, but if you are taking hormonal contraceptives, you need to be aware of the warning signs.

Highlight on Health

Do Women Need to Menstruate Monthly?

For a woman who is not taking hormonal contraceptives, the absence of a monthly period can mean that her hormones are not in balance. Hormone imbalance can be caused by many factors, including weight gain or loss, stress, high levels of exercise, pregnancy, and some health conditions. In addition, if the endometrium builds up in response to estrogen but is not shed regularly due to lack of ovulation, a woman has an increased risk for endometrial cancer. A woman who stops having her period for no apparent reason should consult with her physician.

So does a healthy woman *need* to menstruate every month? Perhaps not, if she is on contraceptive hormones. When they were first introduced, contraceptive hormones were designed to mimic the typical menstrual cycle to increase women's comfort with using them. Pill packages included three weeks of "active" pills (estrogen and progesterone) and a week of "placebo" pills (pills without hormones). When a woman takes the placebo pills, the uterine lining sheds in response to the drop in hormone levels. If a woman skips the placebo pills and continues taking the active pills, she does not menstruate.

As use of contraceptive hormones has become more widespread, the idea of not having periods has become popular among women. Almost 60 percent report they would be interested in not menstruating monthly, and 30 percent say they would choose to never have a period again. Some types of oral contraceptives (Seasonale and Seasonique) have been developed to give a woman a period only four times a year (an *extended cycle*), and one (Lybrel) contains only active pills, meaning that a woman does not get a period at all. Many other oral contraceptives, the contraceptive patch, and the vaginal ring can be used continuously or in an extended cycle.

Extended-cycle pills do appear to cause more irregular spotting or bleeding during the first 6 months of use than a monthly pill; however, by 12 months of use, 80 percent of women report no spotting. For women who have mild nausea or breast pain associated with pill use, extended-cycle pills appear to have more minor effects in comparison to monthly cycle pills. In addition, the extended-cycle pills may suppress ovulation more than monthly cycle pills, perhaps making them even better at preventing pregnancy. The balance of estrogen and progesterone in extended-cycle pills prevents excessive buildup of the uterine lining and therefore does not appear to increase risk for endometrial cancer.

There are two unanswered questions regarding long-term risk of extended-cycle pills. First, it is unclear if continuous hormone use has a negative effect on bone density, as estrogen is important in bone development. One recommendation is that extended-cycle hormone use may not be good for adolescents, who are at the peak time for building their bone density. Second, women on continuous pills receive 13 additional weeks of hormones in comparison to women taking placebo pills for one week each month. The long-term impact of continuous hormone use on a woman's risk of breast cancer, stroke, and heart attack remains unknown. Short-term data suggest the risk is low. More research is needed to answer both of these important questions.

Sources: "Continuous, Daily Levonorgestrel/Ethinyl Estradiol Vs. 21-Day, Cyclic Levonorgestrel/Ethinyl Estradiol: Efficacy, Safety, and Bleeding in a Randomized, Open-Label Trial," by A.L. Teichmann, D. Apter, J. Emerich, et al., 2009, Contraception, 80 (6), pp. 504–511; "Extended Regimens of the Vaginal Contraceptive Ring: Cycle Control," by C.A. Guazzelli, F. A. Barreiros, R. Barbosa, et al., 2009, Contraception, 80 (5), pp. 430–435.

slightly less effective but can be used by women who can't take estrogen (for example, because they are breastfeeding or have a family history of blood clots).

The *transdermal patch* works by slowly releasing estrogen and progesterone into the bloodstream through the skin. A woman places a new patch on her skin every week for three weeks; during the fourth week, she does not use a patch and has a light period. Because the patch is changed once a week, it can be useful for women who have a hard time remembering to take a daily pill. Potential side effects are similar to those of the pill, except that the patch results in higher levels of estrogen in the blood (about 60 percent higher than with a typical birth control pill) and may be associated with an increased risk of blood clots compared to pills.[4]

The *vaginal contraceptive ring* is a soft, flexible plastic ring that is placed in the vagina and slowly releases estrogen and progesterone. It is left in place for 21 days and then removed. After 7 days, a new ring is inserted. Women and their partners report that they rarely feel the ring during intercourse. The advantage of the ring is the monthly application; side effects are similar to those of birth control pills.

The *injectable contraceptive* currently available in the United States is Depo-Provera. A progesterone-only injection, it is administered as a shot in a health care provider's office every 3 months. It is highly effective and requires little action on the part of a woman except regular visits to the provider. Depo-Provera can cause menstrual changes with irregular bleeding early on and amenorrhea (no periods) in 50 percent of women after 1 year. Most women consider this an advantage. Disadvantages specific to Depo-Provera include weight gain (about 5.4 pounds on average in the first

hot tip
Don't be afraid to ask your partner to help pay for contraception.

year) and decreased bone density with prolonged use (longer than 2 years).

A *contraceptive implant* is a small, flexible plastic rod that contains progesterone. It is inserted under the skin on the inner side of the upper arm and slowly releases hormones. The only implant currently available in the United States is Implanon. Once inserted, it can be left in place for 3 years, thus eliminating user error. It may be less effective for women with a body mass greater than 30 percent of ideal.

BARRIER METHODS

Contraceptive methods known as **barrier methods** physically separate the sperm from the female reproductive tract. These methods include the male condom, the female condom, the diaphragm, the cervical cap, and the contraceptive sponge. To increase their effectiveness, the diaphragm and cervical cap should be used with **spermicide**, chemical agents that kill sperm. Spermicide usually comes in a foam or jelly and can be purchased at a grocery store or drugstore.

The chance of becoming pregnant while using a barrier method is low if the method is used consistently and correctly (the barrier is used 100 percent of the time and spermicide is correctly applied). Unfortunately, this is often not the case.

Condoms—Male and Female   The only form of contraception proven to decrease the risk of contracting an STD is the male condom. As described in Chapter 12, the *male condom* is a thin sheath, usually made of latex, that is rolled down over the erect penis before any contact occurs between the penis and the partner's genitals. The correct application of a condom is illustrated in Figure 13.2. Male condoms come with or without spermicide. There is no evidence that spermicide is necessary to reduce the risk of pregnancy, and spermicide can cause irritation for some users. Condoms can be purchased over the counter in grocery stores and drugstores (see the box "Buying and Using Condoms"). They are often given out free at health clinics.

Also as described in Chapter 12, the *female condom* is a pouch of thin polyurethane that is inserted into the vagina before intercourse (Figure 13.3).

Female Barrier Methods   The vaginal **diaphragm** is a circular rubber dome that is inserted in the vagina before intercourse; correct placement is shown in Figure 13.4. It fits between the pubic bone and the back of the vagina and covers the cervix. Spermicidal jelly or foam is placed in the dome, or cup, of the diaphragm before it is inserted; thus

barrier methods
Contraceptive methods based on physically separating sperm from the female reproductive tract.

spermicide
Chemical agent that kills sperm.

diaphragm
Circular rubber dome that is inserted in the vagina before intercourse to prevent conception.

■ The advantages of condoms are that they are portable, available over the counter, and inexpensive. Male condoms provide some protection against STDs, including HIV.

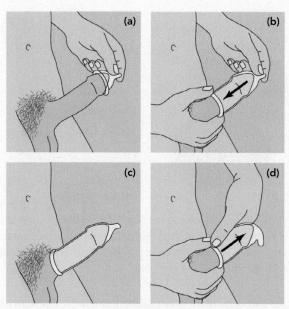

figure 13.2 Use of the male condom.
(a) Place the rolled condom over the head of the erect penis. Hold the top one-half inch of the condom with one hand, and squeeze the air out to allow space for semen. (b) With the other hand, unroll the condom downward, smoothing out any air bubbles. (c) Continue unrolling the condom down to the base of the penis. (d) After ejaculation, hold the condom around the base of the penis until the penis has been withdrawn completely to avoid any leakage of semen.

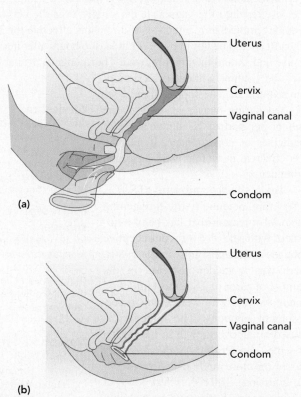

figure 13.3 Use of the female condom.
(a) Take the smaller ring of the condom and flex it gently to fit into the vaginal canal. Follow the manufacturer's detailed instructions for insertion. (b) When the condom is in place, the smaller ring covers the cervix and the larger ring remains outside the vagina.

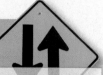

Challenges & Choices

Buying and Using Condoms

Condoms are effective in protecting against STDs and moderately effective in protecting against unintended pregnancy. Here are some tips to ensure the lowest risk of an unwanted outcome:

- Buy latex condoms if you are not allergic to them. Latex is the best material for preventing the transmission of STDs.

- Check the expiration date before buying or using condoms. Outdated condoms are more likely to break during use.

- Condoms are available with or without spermicide. The most commonly used spermicide is nonoxynol-9. Because of recent evidence that this product can cause skin irritation, it is currently recommended that condoms without spermicide be purchased.

- Don't remove the condom from its wrapper until you are ready to use it.

- Don't leave condoms in place where they will be exposed to heat. Temperature extremes weaken the condom and make it more likely to break.

- Use only water-based lubricants. Oil-based products quickly cause latex to deteriorate, leading it to leak or break.

- If you are buying a female condom, check the expiration date and make sure it includes directions. Practice inserting the condom before you actually use it. During use, make sure the man's penis is inserted inside the condom.

- Correct use of condoms means not only that they are placed on the penis correctly before intercourse and removed correctly afterward but also that they are used for every occasion of sexual intercourse and do not leak or break. Most failures occur because of incorrect or inconsistent use.

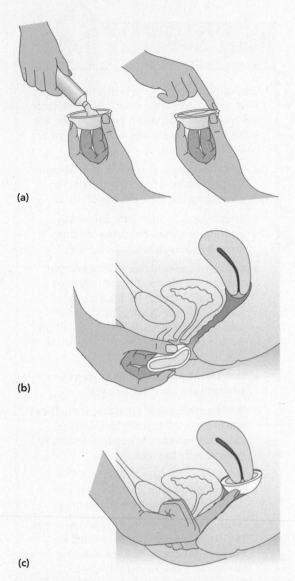

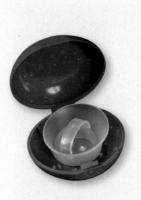 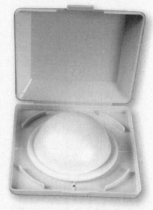

■ The FemCap cervical cap (left) and the diaphragm (right) work by creating a physical barrier at the cervical opening, preventing sperm from entering the uterus. Both are used with spermicidal cream or jelly.

figure 13.4 **Use of the diaphragm.** (a) With clean hands, place about 1 tablespoon of spermicide (jelly or cream) in the diaphragm, spreading it around the diaphragm and its rim. (b) Using the thumb and forefinger, compress the diaphragm. Insert it into the vagina, guiding it toward the back wall and up into the vagina as far as possible. (c) With your index finger, check the position of the diaphragm to make sure that the cervix is covered completely and the front of the rim is behind the pubic bone.

the spermicide covers the cervix, where it provides the best protection. Spermicide must be reapplied into the vagina if a second act of sex occurs. The diaphragm is removed 6 to 12 hours after sex.

A woman has to be fitted with the correctly sized diaphragm by a health care provider and shown how to insert and remove it. Diaphragm use has been associated with an increased risk for urinary tract infections.

The **cervical cap** is a small, cuplike device that covers the cervix and prevents sperm from entering the uterus. As with a diaphragm, the cervical cap requires a fitting by a

health care provider; it is replaced annually. Currently the FemCap is the only available model. It is made of nonallergenic silicone and comes in three sizes. A small amount of spermicide is placed in a groove on the vaginal side of the cap prior to insertion. It should be left in place for 6 to 48 hours after intercourse.[3]

The Today **contraceptive sponge** is a small, polyurethane foam device that is presaturated with 1 gram of the spermicide nonoxynol-9. The sponge is moistened with water and inserted into the vagina. It fits snugly over the cervix, becomes immediately effective, and remains effective for 24 hours. It should be left in place for at least 6 hours after intercourse and should then be removed. The sponge is available over the counter without prescription; one size fits all. The sponge should not be used during menstruation or if the user or her partner is allergic to sulfa medicines or polyurethane. It may be less effective in women who have had a pregnancy.

Toxic shock syndrome (TSS) is a very rare, potentially life-threatening bacterial infection that has been associated with the use of contraceptive sponges and diaphragms. In the 1980s, there was a sudden increase in the number of cases of TSS, most affecting young women who were using superabsorbent tampons. The infection is caused by an overgrowth in the vagina of the bacterium *Staphylococcus aureus* (or more rarely with *Streptococcal* infection). The risk is very low, but to reduce risk further, women should change tampons frequently (at least every 4 to 8 hours) and should not leave female barrier methods of contraception in place beyond the recommended

cervical cap
Small, cuplike rubber device that covers only the cervix and is inserted in the vagina before intercourse to prevent conception.

contraceptive sponge
Small polyurethane foam device presaturated with spermicide that is inserted in the vagina before intercourse to prevent pregnancy.

toxic shock syndrome (TSS)
A rare, life-threatening bacterial infection in the vagina associated with the use of tampons and female barrier contraceptive methods.

time. Symptoms of TSS include sudden high fever, vomiting or diarrhea, muscle aches, headache, seizures, and a rash that looks like a sunburn and eventually leads to peeling of the skin on the hands and feet.

THE IUD

Two types of IUD are available in the United States, the copper IUD and the progesterone IUD. Both are small, T-shaped devices that a health care provider inserts through the cervix into the uterus. A correctly placed IUD is shown in Figure 13.5.

The IUD is believed to work by altering the uterine and cervical fluids to reduce the chance that sperm will move up into the fallopian tubes, where they can fertilize an ovum. In addition, some women using the progesterone-containing IUD do not ovulate.

IUDs are highly effective and require little maintenance after they are in place. Once inserted, the copper IUD can be left in place for 10 years and the progesterone IUD can be left in place for five years. Because the IUD can move or fall out of the uterus, the woman must learn how to check to make sure the device is still properly located each month. Women may experience a change in menstrual patterns with use. The copper IUD is associated with heavier periods and cramping; the progesterone IUD is associated with irregular spotting initially and then the cessation of periods at one year for 20 percent of women. Neither appears to increase the risk of pelvic inflammatory disease unless a woman is infected with gonorrhea or chlamydia at the time of insertion. Both can be used in women who have not previously conceived. IUDs are becoming increasingly popular among college-age women.

THE FERTILITY AWARENESS–BASED METHODS

Women can usually become pregnant in a window of time around ovulation (release of an ovum). **Fertility awareness–based methods** rely on the identification of the fertile days

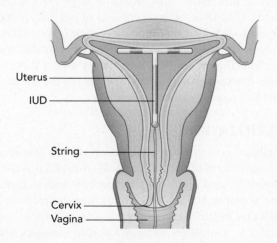

figure 13.5   **T-shaped IUD correctly positioned in the uterus.**

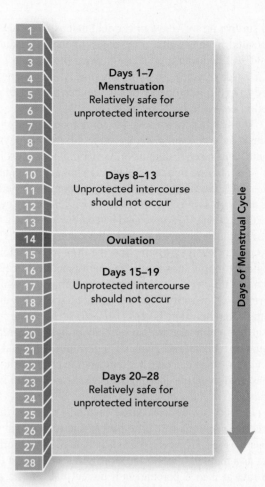

figure 13.6   **The fertility awareness–based method.** This method uses the menstrual cycle to determine when fertilization is likely to occur and when unprotected sexual intercourse should be avoided. If you do not have a 28-day cycle, the variability in your cycle will be in the part of the cycle from menstruation to ovulation.

in the menstrual cycle and abstaining from sex (or using a barrier contraceptive) during the fertile time. Ovulation usually occurs 14 days *before* the menstrual period begins (Figure 13.6). For a woman with a 28-day cycle, ovulation usually occurs on day 14. However, for a woman with a shorter or longer cycle, the time difference is in the first part of the cycle (from menstruation to ovulation), not in the second part of the cycle (from ovulation to menstruation). For example, if a woman has a 21-day cycle, ovulation will usually occur on day 7. If a woman has a 32-day cycle, ovulation will usually occur on day 18.

fertility awareness–based methods
Contraceptive method based on abstinence during the window of time around ovulation when a woman is most likely to conceive.

The ovum is most likely to become fertilized within 24 hours after release from the ovary if it is to happen at all; however, the ovum can remain viable for 4 days. Sperm can survive up to 7 days in cervical mucus. Thus any sperm deposited in the vagina after day 8 of the menstrual cycle could still be around on day 14, when the woman ovulates (in a 28-day cycle). To avoid pregnancy, the couple would need to avoid intercourse or use another method of contraception between day 8 and day 19.

The fertility awareness–based methods require that the woman have a regular cycle (same number of days every month), because abstinence or barrier methods must be used for 7 days before ovulation. Although both regular and irregular cycles are normal, the fertility awareness–based methods are appropriate only for women with a regular cycle.

Ovulation is accompanied by certain signs that a woman can recognize in order to learn her own patterns. Couples also use these signs to pinpoint the time of ovulation when they are trying to conceive. One sign is that cervical mucus becomes thinner and stretchier, resembling egg white, and increases in quantity before ovulation, so the vagina feels wetter. Another sign is that, because of hormone activity, basal body temperature rises by about half a degree when ovulation occurs and remains higher until the end of the cycle. A woman can take her temperature each morning with a basal temperature thermometer to see when this increase occurs.

Fertility awareness–based methods may be the only acceptable options for some people due to personal or religious reasons. However, there is debate over their effectiveness as a method of contraception. Some studies list the failure rate at 3 to 5 percent with perfect use and 25 percent with actual use; other studies conclude that the failure rate is unclear and recommend that couples be informed about the lack of evidence regarding effectiveness and be counseled about other options if possible.[3,5]

WITHDRAWAL

Withdrawal, or *coitus interruptus*, is the removal of the penis from the vagina prior to ejaculation. As a method of contraception, it is controversial. It is not included on the list of recommended contraceptives issued by the American College of Obstetrics and Gynecology or the Planned Parenthood Federation of America. However, while it is significantly less effective than hormonal methods, some studies show levels of effectiveness similar to those of barrier methods (approximately 18–27 percent of women will become pregnant in a year of using withdrawal).[3,6,7]

Withdrawal is highly dependent on the characteristics of the users. Success is dependent on a man's ability to determine when he is about to ejaculate and to have the self-control to withdraw with impending orgasm. Both partners need to be committed to interruption of intercourse at the

withdrawal
A contraceptive method in which the man removes his penis from the vagina before ejaculating.

emergency contraception (EC)
A contraceptive method used after unprotected sex to prevent pregnancy.

sterilization
Surgical procedure that permanently prevents any future pregnancies.

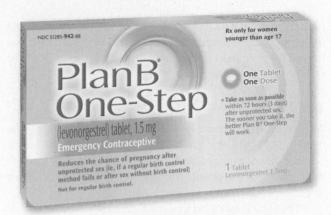

■ Emergency contraception can be taken to prevent pregnancy after unprotected sex or used as a backup when another form of contraception fails, as when a condom breaks.

time of the man's orgasm. Failure rates appear to be higher in unmarried couples. While not generally recommended, withdrawal may be better than no method at all.[2]

EMERGENCY CONTRACEPTION

Also referred to as the *morning-after pill, post-sex contraception*, or *back-up birth control*, **emergency contraception (EC)** can prevent pregnancy after unprotected vaginal intercourse. It is most effective if taken within 48 to 72 hours and must be taken within five days of unprotected intercourse. EC reduces the chance of pregnancy by preventing ovulation and fertilization. It may reduce the likelihood of implantation, but this is not proven. EC will not cause the termination of an existing pregnancy and thus is not an *abortogenic* (abortion-causing) agent.

Emergency contraception is useful when another method fails, such as when a condom breaks or a diaphragm or cervical cap slips out of position. It is also useful in cases of forced sex, including rape and incest. Plan B is an emergency contraceptive now available over the counter for women aged 18 or older. It consists of one pill, containing progesterone only. Other progesterone-only formulations or estrogen-progesterone combinations are available by prescription. The copper IUD may also be used if it is inserted within five days of unprotected sex and has the advantage of providing ongoing contraception.

STERILIZATION

Sterilization is a surgical procedure that is considered a permanent form of contraception. Worldwide, it is the most commonly used form of contraception and is especially popular among couples who do not want to have any more children. Despite counseling prior to sterilization, surgical reversal is sometimes requested due to changing circumstances. The likelihood of pregnancy after a surgical reversal varies widely, with success rates from 10 to 70 percent, and

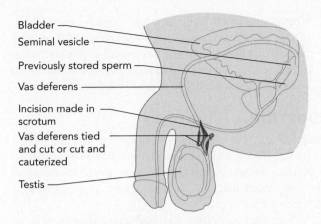

Bladder
Seminal vesicle
Previously stored sperm
Vas deferens
Incision made in scrotum
Vas deferens tied and cut or cut and cauterized
Testis

figure 13.7 **Vasectomy.** With only local anesthesia needed, this surgical procedure offers permanent sterilization.

cannot be guaranteed.[8,9] Besides condoms, sterilization is currently the only form of contraception available to men.

The male sterilization procedure is **vasectomy**. In this procedure, a health care professional makes a small incision or puncture in the scrotum, then ties off and severs the vas deferens, the duct that carries sperm from the testes to the seminal vesicle, where sperm would mix with semen (Figure 13.7). Vasectomy is usually a relatively quick procedure performed with a local anesthetic.

The most common female sterilization procedure is **tubal ligation**. In this procedure, a physician makes an incision in the abdomen, then severs and ties or seals the fallopian tubes, the ducts through which ova pass from the ovaries to the uterus (Figure 13.8). The procedure can be done

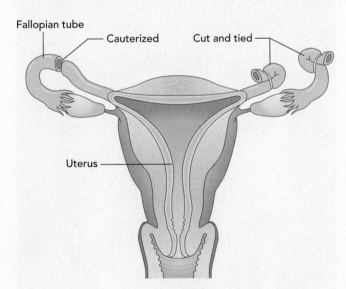

Fallopian tube
Cauterized
Cut and tied
Uterus

figure 13.8 **Tubal ligation.** This surgical procedure is often performed via laparoscopy, which involves creating two small incisions, one for the scope device and the other for the surgical instruments. It usually requires only local anesthesia.

via a surgical method called *laparoscopy*. A laparoscope, a tube that the surgeon can look through with a tiny light on the end, is inserted through a small incision, and the surgical instruments are inserted through another small incision. Recovery usually takes somewhat longer than recovery from a vasectomy. Vasectomies are also associated with less risk of complications than tubal ligation.

Tubal ligation does not alter a woman's menstrual cycle or hormone levels. The ovaries continue to function, but ova are prevented from traveling through the fallopian tubes to the uterus and thus cannot be fertilized. Although in rare cases pregnancy does occur after a vasectomy or tubal ligation, these procedures should be considered permanent.

Another option for permanent sterilization in women, called Essure, involves the placement of a micro-rod in each of the fallopian tubes. Tissue begins to develop around the micro-rods, and after 3 months this tissue barrier prevents sperm from reaching the egg.

Unintended Pregnancy

If you or your partner becomes pregnant unexpectedly, you have to make a monumental decision in a very short period of time. Your options are to (1) carry the pregnancy to term and raise the child, (2) carry the pregnancy to term and place the child in an adoptive family, or (3) terminate the pregnancy.

SIGNS OF PREGNANCY

Some signs of pregnancy are common early on, even before a missed period, as a result of hormonal changes. They can include breast tenderness and swelling, fatigue, nausea and vomiting, and light-headedness or mood swings. Some women have light vaginal bleeding or spotting 10 to 14 days after conception—about the time of a normal period but shorter in duration. If you experience any of these symptoms after unprotected sex or a missed period, you may want to take a pregnancy test.

A rare complication of early pregnancy is **ectopic pregnancy**, a potentially life-threatening condition. The fertilized egg implants or attaches outside of the uterus, usually in the fallopian tube. Signs of ectopic pregnancy are severe lower abdominal pain or cramping on one or both sides, vaginal spotting or bleeding with abdominal pain, or light-headedness, dizziness, or fainting (a possible sign of internal bleeding). If you experience any of these signs, contact your physician or go to the emergency room immediately.

vasectomy
Male sterilization procedure, involving tying off and severing the vas deferens to prevent sperm from reaching the semen.

tubal ligation
Female sterilization procedure involving severing and tying off or sealing the fallopian tubes to prevent ova from reaching the uterus.

ectopic pregnancy
A pregnancy in which a fertilized egg implants or attaches outside of the uterus, usually in a fallopian tube.

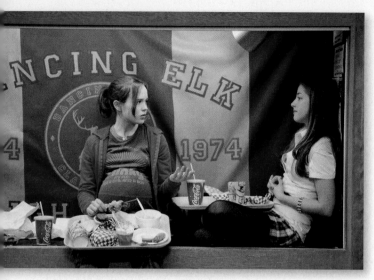

■ In the 2007 movie *Juno*, Ellen Page plays 16-year-old who considers abortion but opts for adoption as the solution to her unintended pregnancy. The movie underplays the hardship experienced by many teenagers who find themselves in this situation.

DECIDING TO BECOME A PARENT

Are you ready to become a parent? Here are some questions to consider:

■ What are your long-term educational, career, and life plans? How would having a child at this time fit in with those plans?

■ What is the status of your relationship with your partner? Is he or she someone you want to commit to and share parenthood with? If you are the mother, the greater part of the pregnancy experience will fall on you, but parenting will involve making decisions with your partner about child rearing (see the box "Supporting Fathers and Families"). Do you have similar goals for a child? Can you communicate well with each other?

■ Do you feel emotionally mature enough to take on the responsibility of raising a child? Parenthood requires patience, sacrifice, and the ability to put aside your own needs to meet the needs of another person.

■ What are your financial resources at this point? Having a child is expensive. In 2008 the total cost of having a child and raising the child through age 18 was estimated at between $160,000 and $367,000.[10] If you are the father, even if you do not want to be emotionally or physically involved, you will probably be legally required to remain financially involved.

■ How large is your social support system? Do you have family members and friends who will help you? Does your community have resources and support services? Social support has been found to be one of the most important factors in helping couples make a successful adjustment to parenthood.

■ What is your health status and age? Do you smoke, drink, or use recreational drugs? Do you have an STD or other medical condition that needs to be treated? Are you under 18 or over 35? Babies born to teenagers and women over 35 have a higher incidence of health problems.

ADOPTION

Adoption can be a positive solution for an unintended pregnancy if you and your partner are not able or willing to become parents at this time in your lives. All forms of adoption require that both biological parents relinquish their parental rights.

In an *open adoption*, the biological parents help to choose the adoptive parents and can maintain a relationship with them and the child. The degree of involvement can range from the exchange of information through a third party to a close and continuous relationship among all parties throughout the child's life. This choice can make it easier for parents to give up a baby, and it allows the child to know his or her biological parents, siblings, and relatives. Many adoption agencies offer this option.

In a *closed adoption*, the more traditional form of adoption, the biological parents do not help choose the adoptive parents, and the adoption records are sealed. This type of adoption provides more privacy and confidentiality than open adoption does. In some states, the child may access the sealed records at the age of 18, and many states are in the process of passing legislation that would open previously sealed records, even for adoptions that occurred decades

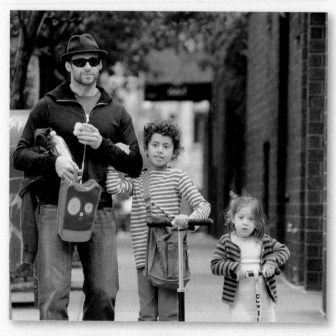

■ Adoption offers the possibility of parenting to people who are not able to conceive a child or who choose not to. Actor Hugh Jackman and his wife, Deborah-Lee Furness, adopted two children after she suffered multiple miscarriages.

Supporting Fathers and Families

No matter the income, education, or cultural background of the father, children do better when their fathers are involved. They learn more, perform better in school, and have healthier behaviors. Children living without the involvement of their fathers are more likely to be poor and less educated, use drugs, be victims of child abuse, engage in criminal behavior, and have more emotional, psychological, and health problems. In 2007, 40 percent of children in the United States were born to unmarried parents. At the time of birth, nearly all unmarried fathers report that they want to be involved in their child's life, and yet by the time a child is 5 years old, 37 percent of fathers have not seen their child for two years. A national survey of dads found that over half feel they can easily be replaced by moms or other men, and half felt unprepared to be fathers.

On Father's Day 2009, Senator Evan Bayh of Indiana introduced the Responsible Fatherhood and Healthy Families Act of 2009 in the U.S. Senate, and Representative Danny Davis of Illinois introduced companion legislation in the House. The act would increase funding for responsible fatherhood programs, adjust the work requirements for temporary government assistance so that two-parent families are not penalized, and change the way states collect and distribute child support. Senator Bayh said, "The government can't pass a law to make men good dads, but we can support local programs that specialize in job training, career counseling, and financial literacy to help those men who embrace their parental responsibility and are trying to earn a livable wage to do right by their kids." Specifically, the bill would

- Fund job training programs and community partnerships to help parents find employment

- Fund financial literacy programs, employment services, and mediation and conflict resolution for low-income parents

- Ensure that child support payments to families do not count as income and result in loss of food stamps

- Prohibit unfair and unequal treatment of two-parent families receiving Temporary Assistance to Needy Families, ensuring the state work participation standard is the same for all families

- Expand the Earned Income Tax Credit to increase the incentive for full-time work and fulfillment of child support obligations

Currently the bill is awaiting a vote in Congress. President Obama has pledged to sign the bill if it is passed. In promoting passage of the bill, Congressman Davis remarked, "Fatherhood is one of life's great privileges, but it is also one of life's great responsibilities." The pending legislation is designed to help fathers fulfill their responsibilities and take a more active role in their children's lives.

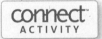

Sources: "Bayh, Davis Introduce Legislation to Promote Healthy Families, Active Fatherhood," retrieved April 27, 2010, from http://bayh.senate.gov/news/press/release/?id=61a8775f-8cb7-4f8b-8025-9073dfe2cc36; "Barack Obama Campaign Promise No. 322: Sign the Responsible Fatherhood and Healthy Families Act," 2009, Politifact, retrieved April 27, 2010, from www.politifact.com/truth-o-meter/promises/promise/322/sign-the-responsible-fatherhood-and-healthy-famili/; Lessons From Responsible Fatherhood Initiatives (Info Sheet 14), 2008, Minnesota Fathers and Families Network; Unmarried Father Involvement (Info Sheet 16), 2008, Minnesota Fathers and Families Network.

ago. One of the reasons for the proposed change is the realization that knowledge about one's biological parents can be important for both psychological and health reasons.

International adoptions have become increasingly common, with children being adopted from countries around the world. A major legislative change now allows children in international adoptions to automatically be granted U.S. citizenship at the time of their adoption.

ELECTIVE ABORTION

Terminating the pregnancy through **elective abortion** is the third option for a woman with an unintended pregnancy. (This type of abortion is called *elective* to distinguish it from **spontaneous abortion**, or miscarriage.) Since 1973 elective abortion has been legal in the United States. In the case of *Roe v. Wade*, the U.S. Supreme Court ruled that the decision to terminate a pregnancy must be left up to the woman, with some restrictions applying as the pregnancy advances through three *trimesters* (divisions of the pregnancy into parts, each about three months long).

Since the passage of *Roe v. Wade*, many attempts have been made at state and national levels to limit access to legal abortion. The debate over abortion between pro-life and pro-choice activists is one of the most highly charged political issues of our time. In 2007 the U.S. Supreme Court upheld the Partial Birth Abortion Ban Act of 2003, the first federal legislature to criminalize a form of abortion.[11] "Partial birth" refers to a rarely performed procedure that aborts a fetus in the third trimester, virtually always for medical reasons. The vast majority of abortions—88 percent—are performed during the first 12 weeks of pregnancy.

International studies show that the legality of abortion does not influence abortion rates. Women around the world seek abortion regardless of the legality of the procedure. In fact, the lowest rates of abortion occur in countries where abortion is legal (Western Europe), and the highest rates of abortion occur in countries where abortion is illegal (Latin America). When

elective abortion
Voluntary termination of a pregnancy.

spontaneous abortion
Involuntary termination of a pregnancy, or miscarriage.

abortion is illegal, it is more likely to be unsafe and to be associated with a higher rate of maternal death.[12]

Unintended pregnancy raises complex emotions. The majority of women who have an abortion report a feeling of relief after the abortion. However, about 20 percent of women experience mild, transient depressive symptoms that pass quickly after an abortion. These are similar to symptoms experienced by 70 percent of women after childbirth. The risk of emotional problems after an abortion is increased if depression is present before an unplanned pregnancy or if the abortion is performed due to fetal abnormalities in a desired pregnancy. Even if women do not regret the decision to terminate a pregnancy, they may still experience feelings of regret and sadness. Expressing such feelings may help the recovery process.[13]

If you are pregnant and considering abortion, seek health care counseling to discuss all your options, the risks associated with the procedure, and the technique to be used. The most common technique currently in use is surgical abortion, but the use of medical abortion is increasing.

increase the risk of infertility or of complications in future pregnancies.

For later stage pregnancies, usually when the mother's life is at risk, a procedure called dilatation and extraction ("partial birth abortion") is sometimes used. Fetal death is caused by a fetal injection; then the cervix is dilated and the contents of the uterus removed by a combination of suction, curette, and forceps.[13]

Medical Abortion   An alternative to surgical abortion is **medical abortion**, in which a pharmaceutical agent is used to induce an abortion. Medical abortions can be performed very early in pregnancy (less than 7 weeks of gestation) or in late pregnancy (after 15 weeks). Between these gestational ages, the surgical techniques are recommended.

The drug mifepristone (RU486) is used during the first 7 weeks of gestation (or 9 weeks of pregnancy, dated from the first day of the last menstrual period). It is taken in a pill and followed 2 or 3 days later by another drug, misoprostol, which induces contractions. Most women have cramp-

International studies show that the legality of abortion does not influence abortion rates. In fact, **the lowest rates of abortion occur in countries where abortion is legal** *(Western Europe), and the highest rates of abortion occur in countries where abortion is illegal (Latin America).*

Surgical Abortion   In **surgical abortion**, the embryo or fetus and other contents of the uterus are removed through a surgical procedure. (Between 2 and 8 weeks of gestation, the term *embryo* is used; after the 8th week, the term *fetus* is used.) The most common method of surgical abortion performed between the 6th and 12th weeks is vacuum aspiration; it is used for about 90 percent of all abortions performed in the United States. A physician performs this procedure in a clinical setting, such as a medical office or hospital. The cervix is numbed with a local anesthetic and opened with an instrument called a dilator. After the cervix has been opened, a catheter, a tubelike instrument, is inserted into the uterus. The catheter is attached to a suction machine, and the contents of the uterus are removed.

The procedure takes about 10 minutes and requires a few hours' recovery before the woman can return home. A follow-up appointment is needed about 2 weeks after the procedure to ensure that the body is healing. When performed in a legal and safe setting, elective abortion does not

surgical abortion
Surgical removal of the contents of the uterus to terminate a pregnancy.

medical abortion
Use of a pharmaceutical agent to terminate a pregnancy.

infertility
Inability to become pregnant after not using any form of contraception during sexual intercourse for 12 months.

ing and bleeding and abort the pregnancy within 2 weeks, although in some cases abortion may occur in a few hours or days. The success rate is nearly 90 percent, and serious complications are rare. After 15 weeks of gestation, different medications are used to induce labor. If abortion does not occur with medication, a surgical abortion is recommended, because the drugs can harm the developing fetus.[13]

Infertility: Causes and Treatment Options

Approximately 10 percent of couples receive specialist care for **infertility**,[14] the inability to become pregnant after not using any form of contraception during sexual intercourse for 12 months. The longer childbearing is delayed, the higher the chances that conception will be difficult and that pregnancy will be complicated.

In about one-third of cases, infertility stems from male factors, such as low sperm count or lack of sperm motility. In another one-third of cases, infertility results from blockage in the woman's fallopian tubes, often scarring that has occurred as a result of pelvic inflammatory disease or another complication of an STD. Blockage can also be caused by an unsterile abortion or by endometriosis, a condition in which uterine tissue grows outside the uterus. In the remaining one-third of cases, the problem is lack of ovulation, abnormalities in the cervical mucus or in anatomy, or unknown causes.

Treatment options for infertility are increasingly being used by couples experiencing difficulty conceiving and by single and lesbian women. Treatments include surgery to open blocked fallopian tubes or correct anatomical problems, fertility (hormonal) drugs to promote ovulation and regulate hormones, and more advanced reproductive techniques. Intrauterine (artificial) insemination is a process whereby sperm are collected and placed directly into a woman's uterus by syringe. This procedure can be helpful if a man has a low sperm count or low sperm mobility. Donor sperm can be used if a man has a genetic abnormality or in the case of a single woman or a lesbian.

In vitro fertilization is a technique by which hormones are used to stimulate egg production in the ovaries, multiple eggs are collected through a surgical procedure, the eggs are fertilized in the clinic, and the fertilized eggs are transferred to the woman's uterus. Other techniques used include gamete intrafallopian transfer and zygote intrafallopian transfer. Both techniques involve induction of multiple eggs with hormones, surgical collection, and manual reintroduction into the fallopian tubes.

Pregnancy and Prenatal Care

Research is now indicating that adverse events and conditions during pregnancy can not only cause **congenital abnormalities** (birth defects) but also influence the individual's development throughout life, affecting cognitive development in childhood and health risks, including mental health risks, in adulthood. The best approach to ensuring good health is to give every child the best possible start in life.

congenital abnormalities
Birth defects.

prepregnancy counseling
Counseling before conception that may include an evaluation of current health behaviors and health status, recommendations for improving health, and treatment of any existing conditions that might increase risk.

PREGNANCY PLANNING

When is the best time to have a child? Although this is a highly personal decision influenced by many factors—educational and career plans, relationship status, health issues, and others—evidence indicates that the least health risk occurs when women have pregnancies between the ages of 18 and 35. Before age 18, a woman's body is still growing and developing. The additional demands of pregnancy and nursing can impair her health, and the baby is more likely to be born early and have a low birth weight.

After age 35, a woman is more likely to have difficulty getting pregnant, because fertility declines as a woman gets older. Women over 35 are also more likely to have medical problems during pregnancy, including miscarriage, and to have a baby who is born prematurely, has low birth weight, or has a genetic abnormality like Down syndrome.

Male fertility also declines with age. After age 35, men are twice as likely to be infertile as men in their early 20s. Men over age 40 have an increased risk of fathering a child with autism, schizophrenia, or Down syndrome.[15]

PREPREGNANCY COUNSELING

Couples who practice family planning can take advantage of **prepregnancy counseling**, which typically includes an evaluation of current health status, health behaviors, and family health history. A woman who smokes, uses drugs, or drinks alcohol will be encouraged to quit *before* trying to become pregnant, as will her partner. Existing health conditions will be treated and medications adjusted to the safest options for pregnancy. This can be especially important if a woman is taking medications for high blood pressure, seizure disorder, or some psychiatric disorders. If obesity is an issue, a woman may be counseled about a weight management program. If a couple appear to be at increased risk for a genetic disease on the basis of their ethnic background or family history, they may be referred at this point for genetic counseling and testing.

NUTRITION AND EXERCISE

Because so many women become pregnant unintentionally, every sexually active woman who might become pregnant should be aware of the importance of healthy lifestyle factors. A balanced, nutritious diet before and during pregnancy helps ensure that mother and child get required nutrients. A baby needs calcium for its growing bones, and this is linked to the mother's calcium intake. Getting folic acid in food or in a folate supplement is also recommended to reduce the risk of neural tube defects (problems in the development of the brain and spinal cord). Women should increase their folic acid intake one month *before* getting pregnant so that they

■ Prenatal care includes regular, moderate physical activity.

have a high level of folic acid in their bodies at the time of conception. It is recommended that all women of child-bearing age who may become pregnant consume at least 400 micrograms of folic acid a day.[16]

Foodborne infections can have more serious effects in pregnant women than in the general population. Pregnant women are advised to avoid unpasteurized foods, soft cheese (for instance, Brie, Camembert, and feta), and raw or smoked seafood. Pregnant women, women who might become pregnant, nursing mothers, and young children are advised to monitor their fish and shellfish intake because of contamination with mercury.[16] For guidelines on safe fish consumption, see Chapter 6.

Weight gain goals during pregnancy vary based on prepregnancy weight status. A woman in the healthy weight range should gain 25 to 35 pounds. An underweight woman should gain 28 to 40 pounds, and an overweight woman 15 to 25 pounds.[16] Note that overweight women should gain *less* weight than women who are underweight or at a healthy weight.

Regular exercise during pregnancy is recommended to help maintain muscle strength, circulation, and general well-being. Women can usually maintain their prepregnancy level of activity. In the second and third trimesters, women should be cautious about exercise that might cause injury or trauma and favor safer forms of exercise like walking and swimming.

MATERNAL IMMUNIZATIONS

Women should be up-to-date on routine vaccinations *before* pregnancy. Especially important are vaccination for rubella (German measles) and hepatitis B. Rubella can cause spontaneous abortion or serious birth defects, including deafness and blindness. Hepatitis B is a highly infectious disease that causes liver damage and can be transmitted from mother to child during pregnancy and delivery (called **vertical transmission**). Pregnant women are also at high risk of complications from influenza and should get a flu shot during the flu season.

MEDICATIONS AND DRUGS

The uterus is a highly protected place, but most substances that the mother ingests or that otherwise enter her bloodstream eventually reach the fetus. These include prescription medications as well as other drugs and toxic substances. Some substances, called **teratogens**, can cause physical damage or defects in the fetus, especially if they are present during the first trimester, when rapid development of body organs is occurring.

Tobacco and alcohol are the most commonly used drugs during pregnancy. Tobacco use is associated with increased risk of spontaneous abortion, low birth weight, early separation of the placenta from the uterine wall, and infant death. Babies living in homes where adults smoke have a higher incidence of respiratory infections and **sudden infant death syndrome (SIDS)**.

Consuming 3 or more ounces of alcohol daily (about six drinks) during pregnancy is associated with **fetal alcohol syndrome (FAS)**. This condition is characterized by abnormal facial appearance, slow growth, mental retardation, and social, emotional, and behavior problems in the child. A safe level of alcohol consumption during pregnancy has not been

vertical transmission
Transmission of an infection or disease from mother to child during pregnancy and delivery.

teratogens
Substances that can cause physical damage or defects in the fetus, especially if they are present during the first trimester, when rapid development of body organs is occurring.

sudden infant death syndrome (SIDS)
Unexpected death of a healthy baby during sleep.

fetal alcohol syndrome (FAS)
Combination of birth defects caused by prenatal exposure to alcohol, characterized by abnormal facial appearance, slow growth, mental retardation, and social, emotional, and behavior problems.

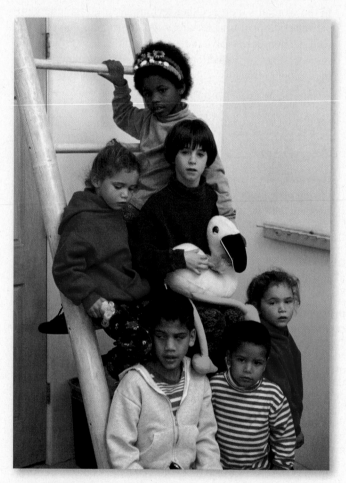

■ Alcohol consumption during pregnancy can cause permanent damage to the fetus, with physical, learning, and behavioral effects. These children with fetal alcohol syndrome exhibit some of the facial characteristics associated with FAS, including a short nose, low nasal bridge, and thin upper lip.

Choosing a Health Care Provider for Labor and Delivery

When you are thinking about prenatal care and delivery, you have a number of options. Factors influencing your choice include your personal preferences, your medical and health history, and the likelihood of complications during your pregnancy. Here is a general description of the kinds of providers who may be available.

Midwives can be certified nurse-midwives or licensed midwives. A certified nurse-midwife has graduated from a school of nursing, passed a nursing certification exam, and received additional training in midwifery. A licensed midwife has completed a training program in midwifery similar to that of a certified nurse-midwife but may or may not have a prior background in nursing. Licensing laws for midwives vary from state to state. Depending on the state, midwives may be allowed to deliver babies at home, in birthing centers, or in hospitals.

Midwives usually take patients who are at low risk for medical or pregnancy complications. If complications develop during prenatal care or delivery, a midwife will refer the case to a family physician or an obstetrician. Midwives tend to view pregnancy and birth as a family event. They are usually trained in support techniques (such as breathing and relaxation techniques) so the woman can have a delivery without anesthetic medications, and they usually stay with the woman throughout labor.

Family physicians have completed 4 years of medical school and 3 years in a residency training program. Some family physicians provide pregnancy-related care only for low-risk pregnancies; others receive extra training so they can manage complicated pregnancies and perform caesarean sections if necessary. Family physicians may deliver babies in birthing centers or hospitals but rarely perform home births. Like midwives, many family physicians view pregnancy and birth as a family event, and some use the same kind of support techniques.

Obstetricians have completed 4 years of medical school and an additional 4 years in a residency training program in obstetrics and gynecology. They are trained to handle all kinds of pregnancies, from low risk to high risk. Obstetricians tend to spend limited time at the bedside of a laboring patient; instead, they monitor labor for signs of problems and are present for delivery. Obstetricians usually have a medical orientation to labor management and delivery.

Perinatologists are obstetricians with additional training in the management of high-risk pregnancy. These specialists consult with and accept referrals from obstetricians. They are usually found at major medical centers. Most women see a perinatologist only if serious complications arise in the pregnancy.

---

established, and even occasional binge drinking may carry significant risk.

Illicit drugs have a variety of effects on a fetus, depending on the chemical action of the drug. Cocaine causes blood vessels to constrict in the placenta and fetus, increasing the risk of early separation of the placenta from the uterine wall, low birth weight, and possible birth defects. Heroin can cause retarded growth or fetal death as well as behavior problems in a child exposed to it in the womb. A baby whose mother used heroin during pregnancy is born addicted and experiences withdrawal symptoms, which can include seizures, irritability, vomiting, and diarrhea. Illicit drugs are also dangerous because they are often contaminated with other agents, such as glass, poisons, and other drugs.[17]

REGULAR HEALTH CARE PROVIDER VISITS

Every pregnant woman should visit her health care provider regularly for *prenatal care* (see the box "Choosing a Health Care Provider for Labor and Delivery"). After the first visit, the health care provider uses the subsequent visits to monitor the fetus for normal growth and development and the woman for complications of pregnancy.

Complications of Pregnancy   Although it is shocking to hear that a woman has died in childbirth in the 21st century, such deaths do occur. Mortality is higher in ethnic and racial minority groups, pointing to the role of socioeconomic factors, such as lack of prenatal care, lack of access to health information, and dietary differences.

Early complications of pregnancy include the diagnosis of an STD, usually treated with antibiotics or antiviral medications, and miscarriage. Approximately 15–50 percent of all pregnancies end in miscarriage, most during the first trimester.

Pregnancy predisposes some women to develop diabetes, called *gestational diabetes*. Most women are screened between 24 and 28 weeks, since the condition occurs midway through pregnancy. Women with gestational diabetes are advised to exercise, control their diet, and monitor glucose levels, but some women need to start taking insulin.

Toward the end of pregnancy, the risk for several conditions increases. An especially dangerous condition is **preeclampsia**, characterized by high blood pressure, fluid retention, possible kidney and liver damage, and potential fetal death. Signs include facial swelling, headaches, blurred vision, nausea, and vomiting. If not treated, the condition can progress to **eclampsia**, a potentially life-threatening disease marked by seizures and coma.

preeclampsia
Dangerous condition that can occur during pregnancy, characterized by high blood pressure, fluid retention, possible kidney and liver damage, and potential fetal death.

eclampsia
Potentially life-threatening disease that can develop during pregnancy, marked by seizures and coma.

Preterm or early labor is another complication of pregnancy. If a woman experiences contractions, cramping, pelvic pressure, or vaginal bleeding before 37 weeks, she should be evaluated to prevent preterm labor.[18]

Complications of Pregnancy for the Child Approximately 1.2 percent of all pregnancies end in infant death. Half of these deaths occur before the fetus is born, and 80 percent occur before the 28th week of pregnancy (**stillbirth**). After birth, the leading causes of infant death are preterm birth, low birth weight, and SIDS.

Rates of both low birth weight and infant mortality are significantly higher for African Americans in the United States than for members of other groups. Reducing such disparities through improved access to health information and prenatal care is a national health goal.[18]

DIAGNOSING PROBLEMS IN A FETUS

About 5 percent of babies born in the United States have a birth defect. Several tests have been developed to detect abnormalities in a fetus before birth. One is the **alpha-fetoprotein (AFP)** triple screen measurement, which can be used to detect problems in brain and spinal cord development, as well as chromosomal abnormalities in the fetus, especially Down syndrome. AFP testing can be done at 16 to 18 weeks of pregnancy.

Ultrasound is the use of high-frequency sound waves to produce a visual image of the fetus in the womb. It is commonly used to determine the size and gestational age of the fetus, its location in the uterus, and any major anatomical abnormalities. It can also reveal the sex of the fetus.

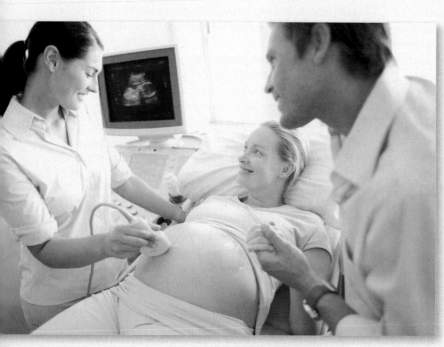

■ Ultrasound is a commonly used prenatal screening tool that can reveal the sex of the fetus, along with other information. Sonograms give expectant parents their first view of their child.

Both **chorionic villus sampling (CVS)** and **amniocentesis** are done to detect chromosomal abnormalities, which cause from 20 to 25 percent of all birth defects. The most common is Down syndrome (see Chapter 2 for more on this syndrome). Chromosomal abnormalities occur with greater frequency as maternal age increases.

In both tests, a needle is passed through the abdomen of the pregnant woman into the uterus. In CVS, a sample is taken from the chorionic villus, part of the placenta (fetal support system) in the uterus. In amniocentesis, a sample of amniotic fluid, the fluid that fills the pouch enclosing the fetus in the uterus, is taken. In both cases, fetal cells from the samples are subjected to chromosomal analysis. CVS can be performed between weeks 10 and 12, and amniocentesis can be performed between weeks 14 and 18.

FETAL DEVELOPMENT

Within 30 minutes of fertilization in the fallopian tube, the single-celled fertilized ovum, called a *zygote*, starts to divide. By the end of 5 days, the cluster of cells has made its way down the tube into the uterus. By the end of a week, it attaches to the uterus and starts to send small rootlike attachments into the uterine wall to draw nourishment. By the end of the 2nd week, it is fully embedded in the lining of the uterus.

The period from week 2 to week 8, called the embryonic period, is a time of rapid growth and differentiation. By 4 weeks, the cluster of cells has divided into cells of different types, forming an embryo, a **placenta**, and an **amniotic sac**. By 8 weeks, all body systems and organs are present in rudimentary form, and some, including the heart, brain, liver, and sex organs, have started to function.

The period from the end of the 8th week after conception to birth is called the fetal period. By 16 weeks, the sex of the fetus can be readily determined, and the mother can feel fetal movements. By 24 weeks, the fetus makes sucking movements with its mouth.

stillbirth
Infant death before or at the time of expected birth.

alpha-fetoprotein (AFP)
Protein produced by the infant and released into the amniotic fluid; AFP measurement is used to screen for some fetal abnormalities.

ultrasound
Technique for producing a visual image of the fetus using high-frequency sound waves.

chorionic villus sampling (CVS)
Technique for testing fetal cells for chromosomal abnormalities by removing cells from the chorionic villus, part of the placenta in the uterus.

amniocentesis
Technique for testing fetal cells for chromosomal abnormalities by removing a sample of amniotic fluid from the amniotic sac.

placenta
Structure that develops in the uterus during pregnancy and links the circulatory system of the fetus with that of the mother.

amniotic sac
Membrane that surrounds the fetus in the uterus and contains amniotic fluid.

Time	Changes/milestones
8 weeks (end of embryonic period)	*By week 8, pregnancy is detectable by physical examination.* Head is nearly as large as body. First brain waves can be detected. Limbs are present. Ossification (bone growth) begins. Cardiovascular system is fully functional. All body systems are present in at least basic form. Crown-to-rump length: 30 mm (1.2 inches) Weight: 2 grams (0.06 ounce)
9–12 weeks (3rd month)	*By week 10, fetus responds to stimulation.* Head is still large, but body is lengthening. Brain is enlarging. Spinal cord shows definition. Facial features begin to appear. Internal organs are developing. Blood cells are first formed in bone marrow. Skin is apparent. Limbs are well molded. Sex can be recognized from genitals. Crown-to-rump length: 90 mm
13–16 weeks (4th month)	*By week 14, skeleton is visible on X-ray.* Cerebellum becomes prominent. Sensory organs are defined. Blinking of eyes and sucking motions of lips occur. Face has human appearance. Head and body come into greater balance. Most bones are distinct. Crown-to-rump length: 140 mm
17–20 weeks (5th month)	*By week 17, mother can feel movement of fetus.* Fatty secretions (vernix caseosa) cover body. Lanugo (silky hair) covers skin. Fetal position is assumed. Limbs are reaching final proportions. Mother feels "quickening" (movement of fetus). Crown-to-rump length: 190 mm
21–30 weeks (6th and 7th months)	*By weeks 25–27, survival outside the womb is possible.* Substantial weight gain occurs. Myelination (formation of sheath around nerve fibers) of spinal cord begins. Eyes are open. Bones of distal limbs ossify. Skin is wrinkled and red. Fingernails and toenails are present. Tooth enamel is forming. Body is lean and well proportioned. Blood cells are formed in bone marrow only. In males, testes reach scrotum at 7th month. Crown-to-rump length: 280 mm
30–40 weeks (8th and 9th months)	*Between weeks 32 and 34, survival outside the womb is probable.* Skin is whitish pink. Fat is present in subcutaneous tissue. Crown-to-rump length: 360–400 mm Weight: 2.7–4.1 kg (6–10 pounds)

figure **13.9**   **Fetal development.**

Sources: Data from Human Anatomy and Physiology, *6th ed., by E.N. Marieb, 2004, San Francisco: Benjamin-Cummings;* Understanding Children and Adolescents, *4th ed., by J.A. Schickedanz et al., 2001, Boston: Allyn & Bacon.*

By week 26, the eyes are open, and by week 30, a layer of fat is forming under the skin. At 36 weeks, the fetus has an excellent chance of survival. A baby is considered to be full term at 38 weeks of gestation, 40 weeks after the mother's last menstrual period. Full-term babies usually weigh about 7½ pounds and are about 20 inches long. An overview of fetal development is shown in Figure 13.9.

Childbirth

By the 9th month, the pregnant woman is usually uncomfortably large and eager to have the baby, despite any apprehension she may harbor about the process of giving birth.

LABOR AND DELIVERY

Labor begins when hormonal changes in both the fetus and the mother cause strong uterine contractions to begin. The pattern of labor and delivery can be different for every woman, but often it begins with irregular uterine contractions.

labor
Physiological process by which the mother's body expels the baby during birth.

cesarean section (C-section)
Surgical delivery of the infant through the abdominal wall.

neonate
Newborn.

When labor begins in earnest, the contractions will become regularly spaced and begin to get stronger and more painful. The contractions cause the cervix to gradually pull back and open (dilate), and they put pressure on the fetus, forcing it down into the mother's pelvis. This first stage of labor can last from a few to many hours.

When the cervix is completely open, the second stage of labor begins. The baby slowly moves into the birth canal, which stretches open to allow passage. The soft bones of the baby's head move together and overlap as it squeezes through the pelvis. When the top of the head appears at the opening of the birth canal, the baby is said to be *crowning*. After the head emerges, the rest of the body usually slips out easily.

The third stage of labor is the delivery of the placenta, which usually takes another 10 to 30 minutes. An overview of the process of labor and delivery is shown in Figure 13.10.

Many techniques have been developed to help women with the discomfort of the labor and delivery process. Childbirth preparation classes help women and their partners learn breathing and relaxation techniques to use during contractions. Several medication options are available in hospitals to further help with the discomfort.

Occasionally the birthing process does not go smoothly. Sometimes the infant is too big to pass through the mother's pelvis or is in the wrong position, either sideways, buttocks first, or face first. Occasionally, the placenta covers the cervix so the baby cannot move into the birth canal. And sometimes the infant just does not tolerate the stress of the process well.

In these situations, the health care provider usually recommends **cesarean section (C-section)**, the surgical delivery of the infant through the abdominal wall. Although many

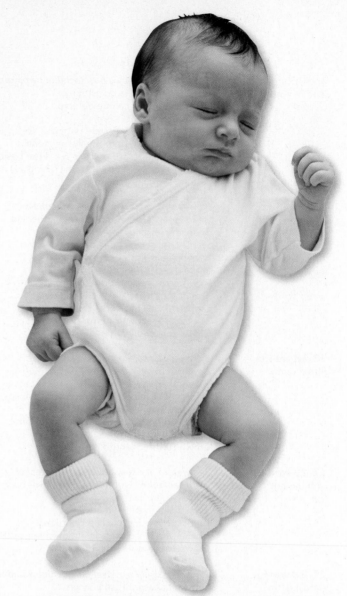

■ The arrival of a newborn signals not just the beginning of a new life but a radical change in how the family will function.

women are not enthusiastic about this option, it has saved many infants' and mothers' lives.

NEWBORN SCREENING

Babies are evaluated at birth to determine whether they require any medical attention or will need developmental support later. The Apgar scale is used as a quick measure of the baby's physical condition: a score of 0 to 2 is given for heart rate, respiratory effort, muscle tone, reflex irritability, and color. The scores are added for a total score of 0 to 10. The baby's neurological condition may also be assessed, and various screening tests may be given, such as tests for hearing and for phenylketonuria (see Chapter 2). Most babies are pronounced healthy and taken home within 24 to 48 hours of birth.

THE POSTPARTUM PERIOD

The first few months of parenthood, known as the postpartum period, are a time of profound adjustment, as parents

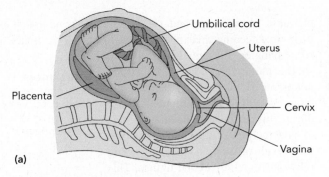

(a)

Early first stage

The cervix thins (*effacement*) and begins to open (*dilation*). Short contractions (30 seconds) occur in 15- to 20-minute cycles. If the mucus plug that blocked the opening of the cervix during pregnancy gives way, light bleeding may occur (*bloody show*). The amniotic sac may also rupture (*water breaking*).

Late first stage

In the transition phase, contractions become stronger and more frequent. These contractions may last from 60 to 90 seconds and occur every 1 to 3 minutes. When the cervix is completely open, with a diameter of about 10 centimeters, it is ready for passage of the baby's head.

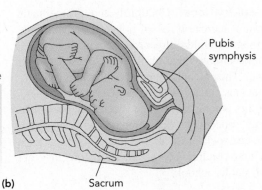

(b)

Second stage

With strong and frequent contractions, the baby moves downward through the pelvic area, past the cervix, and into the vagina. The mother is instructed to "bear down" with the contractions to aid in the baby's passage through the birth canal. The baby's head emerges first, followed by the shoulders and rest of the body.

(c)

Third stage

Contractions of the uterus continue, and the placenta (*afterbirth*) is expelled. If the placenta is not expelled naturally, the health care provider puts pressure on the mother's abdomen to make this happen. The entire placenta must be expelled from the uterus or bleeding and infection may result.

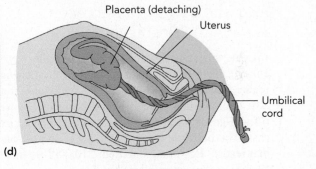

(d)

figure 13.10 **Labor and delivery.** (a) In the first stage of labor, the cervix thins and dilates, ending with the transition phase (b). (c) Delivery of the baby occurs in the second stage. (d) In the third stage, the placenta is expelled.

learn how to care for their newborn (or **neonate**) and the newborn takes his or her place in the family. A few issues that deserve attention are growth and nutrition, illness and vaccinations, and attachment.

Growth and Nutrition Babies have very high calorie requirements. One reason for this is their rapid rate of growth—they triple their birth weight by their first birthday—and another reason is the great relative mass of the infant's organs, especially the brain and liver, compared with muscle. Organs have much higher metabolic and energy requirements than muscle does.

Most organizations agree that breastfeeding is the best way to feed babies. Breast milk is perfectly suited to babies' nutritional needs and digestion; it also contains antibodies that reduce the risk of infections, allergies, asthma, and SIDS. For mothers, breastfeeding enhances bonding with the baby, contributes to weight loss after pregnancy, and may decrease the risk of ovarian cancer and breast cancer after menopause.

Breastfeeding can be more convenient and less expensive than bottle-feeding. New mothers who have difficulty with breastfeeding can get advice and support from a lactation consultant, their health care provider, or support groups like LaLeche League. When a woman is breastfeeding, she may not get her menstrual period for up to 6 months after giving birth; however, ovulation can still occur, so breast-feeding is not a reliable form of birth control.

Because of illness, breast infection, or other reasons, about 10 percent of women are unable to breastfeed, and they bottle-feed their infants instead. Bottle-feeding provides adequate nutrition and enables parents to know how much food the baby is consuming.

Illness and Vaccinations   Childbirth and the neonatal period are times of increased risk of infection for an infant. Starting at 2 months, children receive vaccinations against several childhood diseases that, in the past, caused serious illness and death. They include diphtheria, pertussis (whooping cough), tetanus, measles, rubella (German measles), mumps, and polio, among others. The vaccinations are inexpensive and safe, especially when compared with the physical, emotional, and social costs of childhood diseases. Most states require that children be vaccinated before they are allowed to start public school.

Adjustment and Attachment   Although babies are tiny, they quickly become the center of attention in the household. They spend their time in recurring states of crying, alertness, drowsiness, and sleep. Parents spend much of their time feeding their newborn (at first, every 2 hours or so), changing diapers, and trying to soothe the crying infant. The strong emotional bond between parents and infant known as **attachment** develops during this period, and the infant begins to have feelings of trust and confidence as a result of a comforting, satisfying relationship with parental figures. This sense of trust is crucial for future interpersonal relationships and social and emotional development. Thus a healthy infancy lays the foundation for a healthy life.

attachment
Deep emotional bond that develops between an infant and its primary caregivers.

About 13 percent of women experience depression in the first year after giving birth, referred to as *postpartum depression*. Rapid hormone changes after delivery, broken sleep patterns, self-doubt about one's ability to provide for an infant, a sense of loss of control, and changes in one's support system can all contribute to feelings of sadness, restlessness, loss of interest, guilt, difficulty focusing, and withdrawal. Postpartum depression can have significant effects on a woman's relationships with her partner and baby. Effective treatments exist for depression, and women and their partners should be aware of the signs and symptoms of the condition.

You Make the Call

Egg and Sperm Donation: A Booming Business

Imagine this scenario: You are in your senior year of college, the bills are adding up, and you are starting to realize how big those student loans really are. You're also thinking how nice it would be to take a week off and go on vacation—if only you had some extra cash. You open the campus newspaper and see an ad that reads, "Egg donors needed: $10,000." Is this the answer to all your problems?

The fertility industry has become just that—an industry that addresses people's fertility needs by creating babies. Egg donors (and sperm donors, too) are often recruited on college campuses. College students are among the most coveted donors because they are typically young, healthy, and smart. They usually are also financially limited and thus become an appealing target. But a number of issues arise in association with this practice.

One issue is health risk and safety. A woman who agrees to donate eggs first undergoes personal and family health screening. She is then given a series of hormonal medications, often by injection, to induce the formation of multiple eggs at one time in her ovaries. She then goes to a health care facility to have the eggs collected. During the procedure, for which the woman is sedated, a needle is inserted through the vagina, bladder, or abdominal wall and guided by ultrasound to the ovaries, where the eggs are removed. Potential risks from the medications include nausea, diarrhea, abdominal bloating, shortness of breath, sleeplessness, moodiness, and rarely, ovarian hyperstimulation (a condition in which too many eggs are produced). It is not known how or whether egg donation affects a young woman's own future fertility, but over a woman's reproductive lifespan, she produces many more eggs than she will use for her own pregnancies.

For sperm donations, the man also undergoes personal and family health screening. He has to refrain from intercourse or ejaculation for a few days prior to the donation and then has to ejaculate into a cup. Men produce millions of sperm, so donation does not limit a man's future fertility. The smaller time investment and the lower risk for men translate into less compensation for sperm donation—usually about $150.

Compensation for egg and sperm donations raises another issue. Many countries have banned payments to egg donors, arguing that a child is not a commodity to be bought and sold. When compensation is high, it can induce financially strapped individuals to take actions they might otherwise find morally or ethically repugnant or later think of as coerced.

Perhaps most important, this practice raises questions that must be answered by each prospective donor: What does your DNA mean to you? Is it just a set of genes and chromosomes that you can separate from yourself and your family? Or is a child created with your DNA somehow connected to you? Most egg and sperm donors sign a legal agreement relinquishing all parental rights, and most arrangements are anonymous. Although non-anonymous sperm donation is an option at some sperm banks, it is unlikely that an anonymous donor could ever track down his or her genetic offspring in the future or that the offspring could locate his or her genetic donor. The personal, biological, and ethical implications of these situations are yet to be fully explored.

This rapidly growing area of reproductive technology has been portrayed both as a boon to infertile couples and as a seriously questionable practice. What do you think?

PROS

- Reproductive technology allows many couples and individuals access to pregnancy and childbearing that they would otherwise not have had. It allows them to achieve their dream of parenthood. Often the child is biologically related to one of the parenting adults.

- Men produce millions of sperm, and donation does not limit a man's fertility.

- Women produce more eggs than they use for their own pregnancies and thus can perform a service for an infertile couple without risking their own future childbearing.

- Financial compensation for time spent and medical risks is appropriate.

CONS

- Paying women and men for egg or sperm amounts to buying and selling children.

- Women or men in financial need may be exploited by couples or fertility clinics with the means to pay them.

- A child may suffer psychological harm when told of the donated egg or sperm.

- Donors may struggle with their role (or lack thereof) in the life of a child genetically related to them.

- Egg and sperm donations result in the birth of children who may be related to each other and not know it. As adults, such individuals may meet and become romantically involved, creating the potential for relationships that could be genetically problematic.

connect
ACTIVITY

IN REVIEW

What are the commonly available contraceptive methods?

The most reliable method is abstinence. Other methods include hormonal methods (birth control pills, the transdermal patch, the contraceptive ring, the injectable contraceptive, and the contraceptive implant), barrier methods (male and female condoms, the diaphragm, Lea's shield, the cervical cap, and the contraceptive sponge), the IUD, the fertility awareness–based methods, emergency contraception, and male and female sterilization. Methods vary in their effectiveness, cost, convenience, permanence, safety, protection against STDs, and consistency with personal values.

What are a person's options in the event of unintended pregnancy?

The three options are having and keeping the baby, placing the baby for adoption, and having an abortion. The vast majority of abortions, nearly 90 percent, are performed during the first 12 weeks of pregnancy. Abortion can be performed surgically or medically (with drugs).

What happens when a couple cannot conceive?

Treatments are increasingly available for infertility and include surgery, fertility drugs, intrauterine fertilization, in vitro fertilization, and other advanced technologies.

What are the basics of prenatal care?

Prepregnancy care can include genetic counseling and vaccinations against common infectious diseases, especially rubella and hepatitis B. Once a woman is pregnant, prenatal care includes good nutrition and exercise, avoidance of substances that could harm the fetus, and regularly scheduled health care visits. Problems in the fetus can be diagnosed prenatally by advanced technologies.

What happens during prenatal development?

The fertilized egg (zygote) implants in the uterine wall and begins a period of rapid growth and differentiation. During the first trimester, all the body systems form and start functioning (for example, the heart starts beating), the limbs are molded, and the sex of the fetus can be recognized. During the second trimester, the fetus continues to develop, and the proportion of the body to head becomes more balanced. The third trimester is a period of rapid weight gain. At birth, the typical baby weighs about 7½ pounds and is about 20 inches long.

What happens during labor and delivery?
During the first stage of labor, strong uterine contractions cause the cervix to shorten and open and push the baby down into the mother's pelvis. During the second stage of labor, the baby moves into the birth canal and emerges from the mother's body, usually head first. During the third stage of labor, the placenta is delivered.

What concerns arise during the postpartum period?
Breastfeeding is considered the best way to feed a baby, but bottle-feeding is an acceptable alternative. Newborns are especially vulnerable to infections; they start receiving routine vaccinations at about 2 months. The newborn period is one of profound adjustment for all family members.

Web Resources

American Academy of Family Physicians: This site offers information on many issues for men and women, including contraceptive options, pregnancy and childbirth, reproductive health, and childbirth.
http://familydoctor.org

American Society for Reproductive Medicine: Offering publications on sexual and reproductive health, this organization also provides fact sheets, FAQs, and information booklets.
www.asrm.org

Guttmacher Institute: This organization publishes journals and special reports related to sexual and reproductive health. Online articles address topics such as abortion, pregnancy and childbirth, contraception, and STDs.
www.guttmacher.org

NARAL Pro-Choice America: This pro-choice organization works for better access to effective contraceptive options and to reproductive and other health care services.
www.naral.org

National Adoption Clearinghouse: This organization offers information on adoption, adoption counseling, birth family search, and more, including referrals and links.
www.adoption.org

Planned Parenthood Federation of America: This organization provides health information on birth control, emergency contraception, abortion, adoption, and pregnancy.
www.plannedparenthood.org

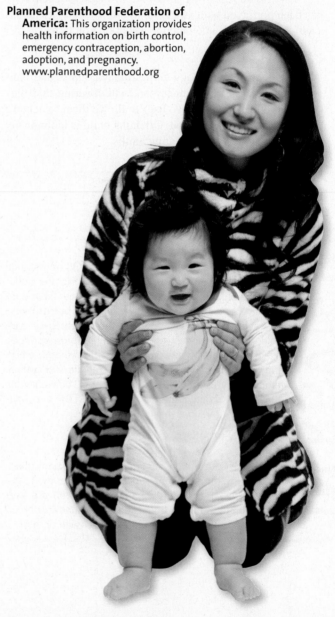

Infectious Diseases

14

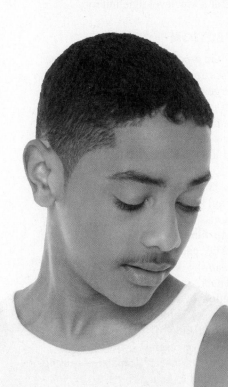

Ever Wonder...

- if there's any risk in getting a tattoo or piercing?

- if you should buy antibacterial soaps and cleaning products?

- which STDs can be cured and which can't?

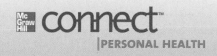

connect™
|PERSONAL HEALTH

http://www.mcgrawhillconnect.com/personalhealth

Prior to 1900 infectious diseases were the leading cause of death in the United States, with 30 percent of

all deaths occurring among young children. Public health measures, vaccinations, and antibiotics are responsible for the reduction in the death rate from infectious diseases in the United States to about 2 percent by the end of the 20th century. Perhaps the greatest reductions in infectious diseases have come from improved sanitation and hygiene practices, especially clean water supplies. In recent years, however, death rates from infectious diseases have started to creep up again, as a result of new diseases such as AIDS and the reemergence of existing diseases once thought vanquished. This chapter provides an overview of infectious diseases, including sexually transmitted diseases, and offers guidelines for protecting yourself from infections.

The Process of Infection

Microorganisms, the tiniest living organisms on earth, do what all living organisms do: eat, reproduce, and die. An **infection** occurs when part of a microorganism's life cycle involves you. An infection is considered an illness or disease if it interferes with your usual lifestyle or shortens your life.

Infections can result in different outcomes. Some infections cause a sudden illness with a high risk of death, such as infection with the Ebola virus. Some stimulate your body's immune response, causing the death of the microorganism, as occurs with the common cold virus. Still others may persist without signs of illness for years and yet be passed on to other people, as is the case with the human immunodeficiency virus (HIV). Finally, some infections are walled off by the immune system, as in the case of tuberculosis, and held at bay for as long as the immune system is healthy.

The process of infection often follows a typical course, with the length of each stage depending on the pathogen (Figure 14.1). Some infections will have a latent phase, when the infectious organism is dormant or walled off in the body prior to causing symptoms. Latent infections may activate at a later point. Other infections are incompletely cleared by the body and continue at a low level indefinitely.

THE CHAIN OF INFECTION

The **chain of infection** is the process by which an infectious agent, or **pathogen**, passes from one organism to another. Pathogens often live in large communities, called *reservoirs*, in soil or water or within organisms. Many pathogens cannot survive in the environment and require a living *host*. To cause infection, pathogens must have a *portal of exit* from the reservoir or host and a *portal of entry* into a new host (Figure 14.2).

A pathogen can exit a host in respiratory secretions (coughing, sneezing); via feces, genital secretions, blood or blood products, or skin; or through an insect or animal bite. The pathogen enters the new host in similar ways: through skin-to-skin contact, genital-to-genital contact, inhalation of respiratory droplets, exposure to blood products, or insect or animal bites. If the transfer from host to host or reservoir to host is carried out by an insect or animal, that organism is said to be a **vector**.

Breaking or altering the chain of infection at any point can either increase or decrease the risk of infection. For example, chlorinating drinking water reduces the number of pathogens and

infection
Disease or condition caused by a microorganism.

chain of infection
Process by which an infectious agent passes from one organism to another.

pathogen
Infectious agent capable of causing disease.

vector
Animal or insect that transmits a pathogen from a reservoir or an infected host to a new host.

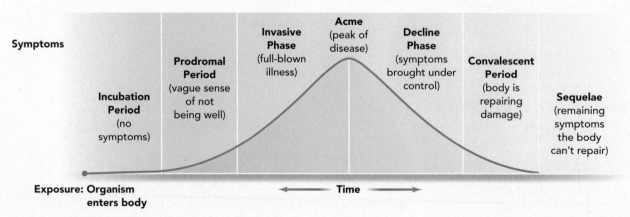

figure **14.1**   **Stages of infection.** At the peak of the disease, either the immune system gains control, medical treatment occurs, or death ensues.

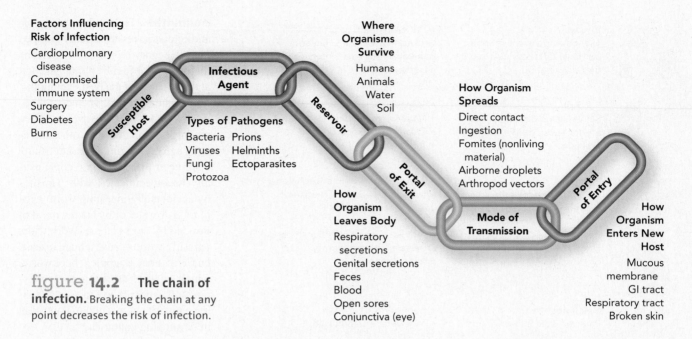

Factors Influencing Risk of Infection
Cardiopulmonary disease
Compromised immune system
Surgery
Diabetes
Burns

Susceptible Host

Infectious Agent

Types of Pathogens
Bacteria   Prions
Viruses   Helminths
Fungi   Ectoparasites
Protozoa

Reservoir

Where Organisms Survive
Humans
Animals
Water
Soil

Portal of Exit

How Organism Leaves Body
Respiratory secretions
Genital secretions
Feces
Blood
Open sores
Conjunctiva (eye)

Mode of Transmission

How Organism Spreads
Direct contact
Ingestion
Fomites (nonliving material)
Airborne droplets
Arthropod vectors

Portal of Entry

How Organism Enters New Host
Mucous membrane
GI tract
Respiratory tract
Broken skin

figure 14.2   The chain of infection. Breaking the chain at any point decreases the risk of infection.

the size of reservoirs for waterborne infections; using condoms disrupts both the portal of exit and the portal of entry for infectious agents that may be present in semen or vaginal secretions; controlling mosquito populations eradicates vectors and disrupts a pathogen's mode of transmission.

The extent or spread of an infection depends on several factors, including the **virulence** (speed and intensity) of the pathogen, the mode of transmission (how an infection spreads from person to person), the ease of transmission, the duration of infectivity (how long a person with infection can spread it to other people), and the number of people an infected person has contact with while he or she is infectious. If an infected person does not transmit the infection to anyone else, that person's disease dies out. If the person transmits it to at least one other person, the infection continues. If the infection is transmitted to many people, an **epidemic** may occur.

PATHOGENS

Millions of different pathogens cause human infections, but they fall into several broad categories (Figure 14.3).

Viruses   Viruses represent some of the smallest pathogens. They are also among the most numerous; it is estimated that there are more different types of viruses than all other living organisms combined.

Viruses consist of a genome (a genetic package of either DNA or RNA), a capsid (protein coat), and in some cases an outer covering or envelope. They are unable to reproduce on their own; they can replicate only inside another organism's cells. Viruses do not survive long outside of humans or other hosts. A virus infects a host cell by binding to its receptors and injecting its genetic material into the cell. Once inside,

the virus can have a number of different effects. It can make many copies of itself, burst the cell, and release the copies to infect more cells. It can persist within the cell, slowly continuing to cause damage or becoming inactive and reactivating at a later time. Some viruses integrate themselves into a cell's DNA and alter the growth pattern of the cells. This process can lead to the development of a tumor or cancer.[1]

Bacteria   Bacteria are single-celled organisms that can be found in almost all environments. They are classified based on shape (spherical, rodlike, spiral), the presence or absence of a cell wall, and growth requirements. Speed of replication varies from 20 minutes to 2 weeks. Some bacteria can enter a dormant or spore state in which they can survive for years.

Many bacteria inhabit a person harmlessly or helpfully and are considered part of the person's **normal flora**. Sometimes, bacteria that are normal in one body location are pathogens in another location, as when *Escherichia coli*, a bacterium that inhabits the large intestine and aids in digestion, enters the bladder, where it causes a bladder or urinary tract infection.

Prions   Prions, the least understood infectious agents, are known to be responsible for the neurodegenerative disease bovine spongiform encephalopathy (BSE), or mad cow disease. The term *prion* was coined as a shortened form of *proteinaceous infectious particle*. Prions are believed to be made

virulence
Speed and intensity with which a pathogen is likely to cause an infection.

epidemic
Widespread outbreak of a disease that affects many people.

normal flora
Bacteria that live in or on a host at a particular location without causing harm and sometimes benefiting the host.

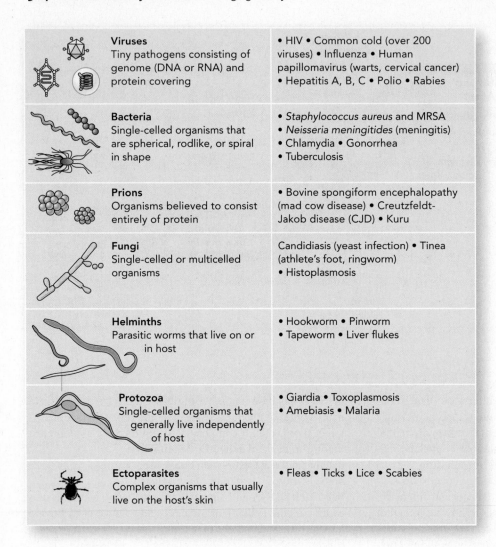

	Viruses Tiny pathogens consisting of genome (DNA or RNA) and protein covering	• HIV • Common cold (over 200 viruses) • Influenza • Human papillomavirus (warts, cervical cancer) • Hepatitis A, B, C • Polio • Rabies
	Bacteria Single-celled organisms that are spherical, rodlike, or spiral in shape	• *Staphylococcus aureus* and MRSA • *Neisseria meningitides* (meningitis) • Chlamydia • Gonorrhea • Tuberculosis
	Prions Organisms believed to consist entirely of protein	• Bovine spongiform encephalopathy (mad cow disease) • Creutzfeldt-Jakob disease (CJD) • Kuru
	Fungi Single-celled or multicelled organisms	Candidiasis (yeast infection) • Tinea (athlete's foot, ringworm) • Histoplasmosis
	Helminths Parasitic worms that live on or in host	• Hookworm • Pinworm • Tapeworm • Liver flukes
	Protozoa Single-celled organisms that generally live independently of host	• Giardia • Toxoplasmosis • Amebiasis • Malaria
	Ectoparasites Complex organisms that usually live on the host's skin	• Fleas • Ticks • Lice • Scabies

figure **14.3** **Main types of pathogens.**

Helminths Helminths, protozoa, and ectoparasites are broadly grouped in the category *parasites*—organisms that live on or in a host and get food at the expense of the host. Helminths, or parasitic worms, include roundworms, flukes, and tapeworms. They are large compared with other infectious agents, ranging in length from 1 centimeter to 10 meters. People usually become infected with parasites by accidentally ingesting worm eggs in food or water or by having the skin invaded by worm larvae. Worldwide, parasitic worms cause a huge disease burden. For example, hookworm, which attaches to the human intestine and causes blood loss, is a leading cause of anemia and malnutrition in developing countries.[1,2]

Protozoa Protozoa are single-celled organisms; most can live independently of host organisms. Protozoal infection is a leading cause of disease and death in Africa, Asia, and Central and South America. Infection may be transmitted by contaminated water, feces, or food, as is the case in protozoal infections such as giardia, toxoplasmosis, and amebiasis; by air, as is the case in *Pneumocystis carinii* pneumonia; or by a vector, such as the mosquito in the case of malaria.[1,2]

entirely of protein. They are found in brain tissue and appear to alter the function or shape of other proteins when they infect a cell, initiating a degeneration of brain function. Prions appear to spread by the ingestion of infected brain or nerve tissue.[1]

Fungi A fungus is a single-celled or multicelled organism. Several kinds of fungi, including yeasts and molds, cause infection in human beings. Fungi reproduce by budding or by making spores; many fungal infections result from exposure to spores in the environment, such as in the soil or on tile floors. Except for tinea (ringworm) in children, fungal infections rarely spread from person to person.

Dermatophytes are a group of fungi that commonly infect the skin, hair, or nails; they are responsible for tinea, athlete's foot, and nail fungus. The yeast *Candida* may be part of a person's normal flora but can overgrow and cause a yeast infection in the vagina or mouth. All of the fungi can become serious infections in a person with a compromised immune system (for example, someone with HIV infection or AIDS, someone undergoing chemotherapy for cancer, or someone taking immunosuppressant drugs following an organ transplant).[1]

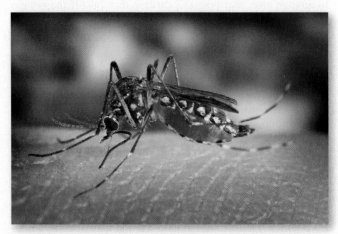

■ Skin is an excellent physical barrier, but the female mosquito is able to penetrate it with her proboscis. Mosquitoes serve as vectors for several diseases caused by bloodborne pathogens, including encephalitis, West Nile virus, and malaria.

Ectoparasites Ectoparasites are complex organisms that usually live on or in the skin, where they feed on the host's tissue or blood. They cause local irritation and are frequently vectors for serious infectious diseases. Examples are fleas, ticks, lice, mosquitoes, and scabies.[1,2]

The Body's Defenses

A single square inch of skin on your arm is home to thousands of bacteria. A sneeze projects hundreds of thousands of viral particles into the air. Bacteria can double in number every 20 minutes, and a virus can replicate thousands of times within a single human cell. Although you are substantially larger than microorganisms, you feel the power of their numbers each time you catch a cold. Considering these facts, our ability to overcome invasion and survive infectious diseases is remarkable.

acids make it difficult for most organisms to survive. The small intestine contains bile and enzymes that break down pathogens. The vagina normally has a slightly acidic environment, which favors the growth of normal flora and discourages the growth of other bacteria. The body protects pores and hair follicles in the skin by excreting fatty acids and lysozyme, an enzyme that breaks down bacteria and reduces the likelihood of infection. The physical and chemical barriers to infection are illustrated in Figure 14.4.

immune system
Complex set of cells, chemicals, and processes that protects the body against pathogens when they succeed in entering the body.

THE IMMUNE SYSTEM

The **immune system** is a complex set of cells, chemicals, and processes that protects the body against pathogens when

A single square inch of skin on your arm is home to thousands of bacteria. Although you are substantially larger than microorganisms, you feel the power of their numbers each time you catch a cold.

EXTERNAL BARRIERS

The skin is the first line of defense against infection. Most organisms cannot get through skin unless it is damaged, such as by a cut, burn, or infection, or if passage is aided by an insect bite or needle stick. Most portals of entry into the body, such as the mouth, lungs, nasal passages, and vagina, are lined with mucous membranes. Although these linings are delicate, mucus traps many organisms and prevents them from entering the body. Nasal passages and ear canals have hair that helps trap particles. The lungs are protected by the cough reflex and by cilia, tiny hairlike structures that rhythmically push foreign particles up and out. Damage to these physical barriers increases risk of infection.

If pathogens get past these barriers, they often encounter chemical defenses. Saliva contains special proteins that break down bacteria, and stomach

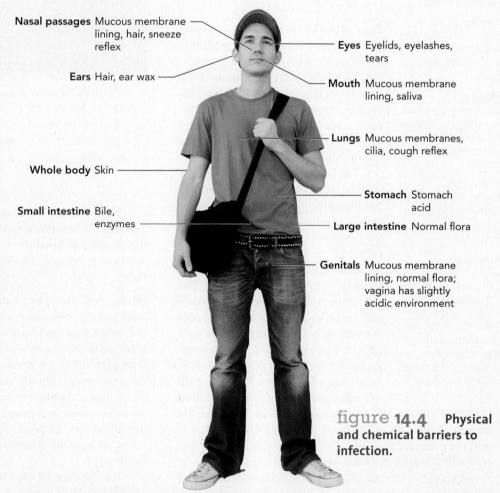

Nasal passages Mucous membrane lining, hair, sneeze reflex

Ears Hair, ear wax

Whole body Skin

Small intestine Bile, enzymes

Eyes Eyelids, eyelashes, tears

Mouth Mucous membrane lining, saliva

Lungs Mucous membranes, cilia, cough reflex

Stomach Stomach acid

Large intestine Normal flora

Genitals Mucous membrane lining, normal flora; vagina has slightly acidic environment

figure **14.4** **Physical and chemical barriers to infection.**

they succeed in entering the body. It has two subdivisions: the **innate immune system**, a rapid response designed to catch and dispose of foreign particles or pathogens in a non-specific manner, and the **acquired immune system**, a highly specialized response that recognizes specific targets.

The Innate Immune System The body's initial reaction to tissue damage, whether it is due to trauma or infection, is an **acute inflammatory response**, a series of changes that increase the flow of blood to the site. A complicated series of molecular and cellular events occurs when the innate immune system is activated. Signs of the inflammatory response are redness, warmth, pain, and swelling.

The cells of the innate immune system are neutrophils, macrophages, and natural killer cells. Neutrophils and macrophages are white blood cells that travel in the bloodstream to areas of infection or tissue damage. These phagocytes ("cell eaters") digest damaged cells, foreign particles, and bacteria. Natural killer cells are white blood cells that recognize and destroy virus-infected cells or cells that have become cancerous.

The Acquired Immune System Your acquired (or adaptive) immunity develops as you are exposed to potential infections and vaccinations. Each time the cells of the acquired immune system are exposed to a pathogen, they form a kind of memory of it and can mount a rapid response the next time they encounter it.

The defining white blood cells of the acquired immune system are **lymphocytes**, which circulate in the bloodstream and lymphatic system. If the lymphocytes encounter an **antigen** (a marker on the surface of a foreign substance), they rapidly duplicate and "turn on" their specific function. The two main types of lymphocytes are *T cells* and *B cells*. T cells monitor events that may be occurring inside the body's cells. If a cell is infected, molecules on its surface are altered that indicate it is now "nonself." *Helper T cells* "read" this message and trigger the production of killer T cells and B cells; helper T cells also enhance the activity of the cells of the innate immune system and of B cells once they are activated. *Killer T cells* attack and kill foreign cells and body cells that have been infected by a virus or have become cancerous. *Suppressor T cells* slow down and halt the immune response when the threat has been handled.

innate immune system
Part of the immune system designed to rapidly dispose of pathogens in a non-specific manner.

acquired immune system
Part of the immune system that recognizes specific targets.

acute inflammatory response
Series of cellular changes that bring blood to the site of an injury or infection.

lymphocytes
White blood cells that circulate in the bloodstream and lymphatic system.

antigen
Marker on the surface of a foreign substance that identifies it to immune cells as "nonself."

antibodies
Proteins that bind to specific antigens and trigger events that destroy them.

immunity
Reduced susceptibility to a disease based on the ability of the immune system to remember, recognize, and mount a rapid defense against a pathogen it has previously encountered.

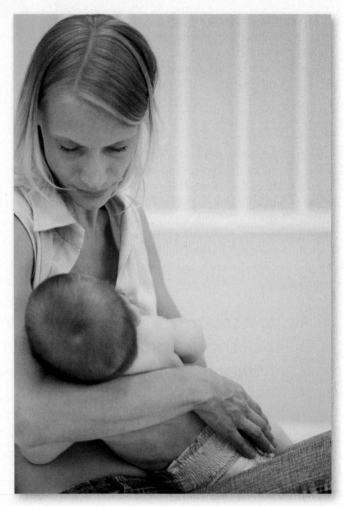

■ Antibodies for some diseases are passed from mothers to babies in breast milk. Breastfeeding has been shown to reduce the incidence of infections, allergies, and diarrhea in infants and even to promote good health later in the child's life.

B cells monitor the blood and tissue fluids. When they encounter a specific antigen, they mature to become cells that produce **antibodies**—proteins that circulate in the blood and bind to specific antigens, triggering events that destroy them.

Immunization Once a person has survived infection by a pathogen, he or she often acquires **immunity** to future infection by the same pathogen. The reason for this is that some B and T cells become *memory cells* when exposed to an infectious agent; if they encounter the same antigen in the future, they can respond rapidly, destroying the invader before it can cause illness. Immunization is based on this principle: The immune system is exposed to part of an infectious agent so that an immune response is triggered. On subsequent exposures, the immune system mounts a rapid response, preventing disease.

The concept of immunization was first introduced in 1796 by English physician Edward Jenner. Jenner realized that people who had been infected with cowpox (a disease that causes mild illness in humans) seldom became ill or died when exposed to smallpox (a related but often fatal disease). Jenner's observation led to the development of **vaccines**, preparations of weakened or killed microorganisms or parts of microorganisms that are administered to confer immunity to various diseases. Since 1900, vaccines have been developed for many infectious diseases, and significant reductions in death rates from these diseases have occurred (see the box "Vaccinations: Not Just for Kids" and Figure 14.5).[3]

Vaccination serves two functions. The first is to protect an individual by stimulating an immune response. The second is to protect society. Widespread vaccination shrinks the reservoir of infectious agents, protecting the community through "herd" immunity. For example, widespread use of the smallpox vaccine has led to the elimination of naturally occurring smallpox worldwide. All future generations benefit from the earlier smallpox vaccination campaigns and no longer require vaccination themselves. Deaths from vaccine-preventable diseases are at an all-time low, but high vaccination levels are necessary to maintain this effect.[4]

RISK FACTORS FOR INFECTION

Your risk for infections depends on numerous factors, some within your control and others beyond your individual control.

Controllable Risk Factors   You can reduce your risk of infection by adopting behaviors that support and improve the health of your immune system. One such behavior is eating a balanced diet; poor nutrition is associated with a higher risk of infectious disease. Other behaviors that support a healthy immune system are exercising, getting enough sleep, and managing stress. Vaccination, when available, can boost your immune system and facilitate a quicker response to pathogens. Good hygiene practices like hand washing reduce the risk of many infections, and protecting your skin from damage keeps many pathogens out of your body. Avoiding tobacco and environmental tobacco smoke improves your defenses against respiratory illness.

Uncontrollable Risk Factors   Age plays a role in vulnerability to infection, with higher risks at both ends of the lifespan. Newborns and young children are at increased risk because they have not been exposed to many infections; pregnancy and breast feeding confer **passive immunity**—a mother's antibodies can pass to the fetus or child to provide temporary immune protection. Older people are at increased risk due to a gradual decline in the immune system that can occur with aging. Other factors that increase vulnerability include undergoing surgery, having a chronic disease such as diabetes or lung disease, and being bedbound.

Genetic predisposition may play a role in susceptibility to infectious disease. It is unclear why certain people develop an overwhelming, life-threatening illness when exposed

vaccines
Preparations of weakened or killed microorganisms or parts of microorganisms that are administered to confer immunity to various diseases.

passive immunity
Temporary immunity provided by antibodies from an external source—such as passed from mother to child in breast milk.

Vaccine ▼ Age Group ▶	19–26 years	27–49 years	50–59 years	60–64 years	≥65 years
Tetanus, diphtheria, pertussis (Td/Tdap)	Substitute 1-time dose of Tdap for Td booster; then boost with Td every 10 years				Td booster every 10 yrs
Human papilloma virus (HPV)	3 doses (females)				
Varicella	2 doses				
Zoster				1 dose	
Measles, mumps, rubella (MMR)	1 or 2 doses		1 dose		
Influenza*	1 dose annually				
Pneumococcal (polysaccharide)	1 or 2 doses				1 dose
Hepatitis A	2 doses				
Hepatitis B	3 doses				
Meningococcal	1 or more doses				

For all persons in this category who meet the age requirements and who lack evidence of immunity (e.g., lack documentation of vaccination or have no evidence of prior infection)

Recommended if some other risk factor is present (e.g., on the basis of medical, occupational, lifestyle, or other indications)

* In July 2010, the CDC recommended that all persons 6 months and older receive the seasonal influenza vaccine for the 2010–2011 season.

figure **14.5**   **Recommended adult immunizations.** Additional information about specific recommendations and vaccines can be found at www.cdc.gov/vaccines.

Source: "Recommended Adult Immunization Schedule—United States, 2010," Centers for Disease Control and Prevention, 2010, Mortality and Morbidity Weekly Report, 59, *(1).*

Public Health in Action

Vaccinations: Not Just for Kids

As a child, you almost certainly received a series of routine vaccinations. As an adult, you need vaccinations, too. It's especially important for college students to be up-to-date on their vaccinations because of crowded living quarters and close social interactions. Check Figure 14.5 and this list to see if your vaccinations are current:

- **Tetanus, diphtheria, and acellular pertussis (Tdap) vaccine.** This vaccine boosts immunity against three diseases; most adults received a similar series in childhood.

- **Human papillomavirus (HPV) vaccine.** The vaccine is recommended for all girls and women aged 9 to 26 years—ideally, prior to the onset of sexual activity. However, women with a history of HPV infection, abnormal Pap tests, or genital warts may still benefit from vaccination, since the vaccine protects against multiple strains of HPV. The vaccine has also been approved for males aged 9 to 26 to reduce risk of genital warts.

- **Varicella (chickenpox) vaccine.** Many adults have immunity to chickenpox from a childhood exposure. If you are not sure whether you had chickenpox, you can have a blood test to assess your immunity.

- **Herpes zoster (shingles) vaccine.** Herpes zoster is a reactivation of the varicella (chickenpox) virus; it increases in frequency with age or in times of stress.

- **Mumps, measles, and rubella (MMR) vaccine.** A single dose is recommended for all adults born during or after 1957; many people receive the vaccine in childhood. A second dose is recommended for college students, international travelers, health care workers, and in outbreaks. Many colleges require proof of two doses prior to enrollment.

- **Influenza vaccine (seasonal).** Vaccination against influenza is recommended for all people aged 6 months and older. The vaccine is available as a shot or a nasal spray and becomes available each fall for that year.

- **Pneumococcal vaccine.** A single dose of the pneumococcal vaccine is recommended routinely for all adults 65 years of age or older and for younger adults if they have risk factors for pneumonia, such as HIV, compromised immune function, diabetes, heart disease, chronic lung disease, alcoholism, liver disease, kidney disease, or sickle cell disease.

- **Hepatitis A vaccine.** Hepatitis A vaccination is recommended for certain persons who have liver disease or are receiving clotting factors; men who have sex with men; people who use intravenous drugs; people in certain occupations, such as food workers; and people who plan to travel where hepatitis is common, such as Mexico, Central America, or South America.

- **Hepatitis B vaccine.** Hepatitis B vaccination is recommended for all sexually active persons not in a long-term, mutually monogamous relationship; men who have sex with men; and injection drug users. It is also recommended for persons with chronic liver disease, kidney disease, HIV infection, or other sexually transmitted diseases, and for those who work in health care or other settings where they could be exposed to blood products.

- **Meningococcal vaccine.** The vaccine protects against a dangerous form of meningitis and is recommended for first-year college students living in the dormitories, military recruits, people in other close living situations, and travelers to areas where infection is common.

- **Other vaccinations.** Other vaccines may be recommended for you (for example, for rabies, yellow fever, and typhoid fever) if you were not immunized in childhood, if you plan to travel to other countries, or if you have other risks based on your occupation or exposures.

connect ACTIVITY

Sources: "Recommended Adult Immunization Schedule, United States, 2010," U.S. Department of Health and Human Services, "CDC's Advisory Committee on Immunization Practices Recommends Universal Influenza Vaccination," February 24, 2010, retrieved from www.cdc.gov/media/ pressrel/2010/r100224.htm; January 15, 2010, Morbidity and Mortality Weekly Report, 59 (1) pp. 1–4; data from Global Alliance for Vaccines and Immunization, retrieved from www.gavialliance.org.

to a pathogen while others develop only a mild fever. Certain sociocultural factors are associated with higher risk for infectious disease; in many situations, these are not controllable risk factors. Overcrowded living environments (including dormitories, fraternities, and sororities) increase the risk for any infectious disease that is spread from person to person, such as influenza, meningitis, and tuberculosis. Poverty is associated with increased risk for many illnesses, probably owing to poor nutrition, stress, and lack of access to health care, among other factors.

DISRUPTION OF IMMUNITY

Because the immune system is so complex, it is occasionally subject to malfunctions. Two such disruptions are autoimmune diseases and allergies.

Autoimmune Diseases   Sometimes, a part of the body is similar enough to an antigen on a foreign agent that the immune system mistakenly identifies it as "nonself." Other times, the immune control system fails to turn off an immune response once an infection is over. In both cases, a process of self-destruction can ensue, causing damage to body cells and tissues. Autoimmune diseases vary in their effects, depending on which part of the body is seen as foreign. Autoimmune diseases include rheumatoid arthritis, psoriasis, multiple sclerosis, scleroderma, and lupus erythematosis. Genetics is known to play a role in some autoimmune diseases.[1] For unknown reasons, most autoimmune diseases are more common in women than in men.

Allergies   Allergic reactions occur when the immune process identifies a harmless foreign substance as an infectious agent and mounts a full-blown immune response. Allergic responses to substances like pollen or animal dander, for example, may include a runny nose, watery eyes, nasal congestion, and an itchy throat. Asthma, a condition characterized by wheezing and shortness of breath, is caused by inflammation of the bronchial tubes and spasm of the muscles around the airways in response to an allergen or other trigger (see the box "Asthma: A Treatable Condition").

Anaphylactic shock is a life-threatening systemic allergic response requiring immediate medical attention.

anaphylactic shock
Hypersensitive reaction in which an antigen causes an immediate and severe reaction that can include itching, rash, swelling, shock, and respiratory distress.

Immunity and Stress   As described in Chapter 3, stress can have a significant impact on the immune system. Short-term stress can actually enhance immune system functioning by activating the body's responses to stressors like puncture

■ The incidence of asthma has increased dramatically in recent years, particularly among ethnic minorities, low-income populations, and children living in inner cities.

Highlight on Health

Asthma: A Treatable Condition

Asthma is a chronic lung condition that affects the airways, or bronchial tubes (the tubes that carry air in and out of the lungs). In asthma, inflammation makes the smooth muscle that lines the airways very sensitive. The muscles go into spasm in response to irritants in the air, making the airways even narrower and reducing the amount of air that can move in and out. Symptoms range from mild to life threatening and include wheezing, coughing, shortness of breath, chest tightness, and difficulty breathing.

Rates of asthma have been increasing over the past 50 years, especially among children and in racial and ethnic minorities. About 20 million Americans have asthma, nearly 9 million of them children. What causes the disorder is unclear, but it does run in families and is more common in people with allergies. Exposure to cigarette smoke and other irritants early in life and some infections may play a role.

An asthma attack—a sudden worsening of symptoms—can be set off by a range of triggers, including exercise, cold air, pet dander, foods, air pollution, tobacco smoke, and viral infections. Although asthma cannot be cured, it can be controlled. Some medications work over the long term to reduce inflammation; others provide quick relief by relaxing the muscles causing the spasm. The National Heart, Blood, and Lung Institute offers the following recommendations:

■ If you think you might have asthma, see your physician to get tested. Medications can significantly improve the quality of your life.

■ Identify your irritants and learn to avoid them.

■ Respond quickly at the onset of an attack to treat it effectively, and seek medical care if your medications are not controlling symptoms.

■ If your asthma is exacerbated by exercise, ask your physician how to use your medications so that you can lead an active life.

■ Get annual flu shots. People with asthma are at increased risk of complications if they get a respiratory infection.

wounds, scrapes, and animal bites. Chronic, long-term stress, however, suppresses immune system functioning; the longer lasting the stress, the greater the negative effect on immune system functioning.[5]

Changing Patterns in Infectious Disease

In 1969 the surgeon general of the United States reportedly declared before Congress that it was time to close the book on infectious diseases. Dramatic declines in the death rate from

FOOD PRODUCTION AND DISTRIBUTION CHANGES THAT AFFECT DISEASE TRANSMISSION

Much of our food is grown in one part of the country or in a foreign country, shipped to a central processing plant, packaged, and then distributed to locations from coast to coast. This widespread distribution of food lowers some costs and makes production more convenient, but it may decrease nutrient value and increase the risk that contaminated food will cause infectious disease in many people.

More than 250 organisms are associated with food-related illnesses. They include viruses, bacteria, prions,

Allergic reactions occur when the immune process identifies a harmless foreign substance—like pollen—as an infectious agent and mounts a **full-blown immune response.**

infectious diseases during the 20th century inspired this bold statement (Figure 14.6). Within a little more than 10 years, however, the first cases of what would soon be identified as human immunodeficiency virus (HIV) infection were causing perplexity and alarm in hospitals in several U.S. cities. Since then, the appearance of other new infections, changes in patterns of infection, and the development of antibiotic resistance in many strains of bacteria have demonstrated that infectious diseases remain an important health concern.

and parasites. As described in Chapter 2, a national network of public health officials monitors reported cases of foodborne illness in the United States and investigates unusual increases in cases involving particular strains of pathogens. For example, in October 2006, an outbreak of salmonella poisoning with cases in 47 states was traced to a single peanut butter processing plant in Georgia.[6] For guidelines on avoiding foodborne illness, see the tips provided in Chapter 6.

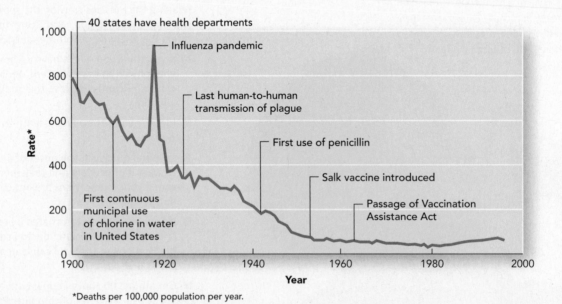

*Deaths per 100,000 population per year.

figure 14.6   **Death rate from infectious diseases, United States, 20th century.**

Sources: Adapted from "Achievements in Public Health, 1990–1999: Control of Infectious Disease" (MMWR serial online), 1999, Morbidity and Mortality Weekly Report, 48 (29), p. 621, www.edc.gov/mmwr; "Trends in Infectious Disease Mortality in the United States During the 20th Century," by G.L. Armstrong, L.A. Conn, and R.W. Pinner, 1999, Journal of the American Medical Association, 281, pp. 61–66; "Water Chlorination Principles and Practices: AWWA Manual M20," American Water Association, 1973, Denver, CO: Author.

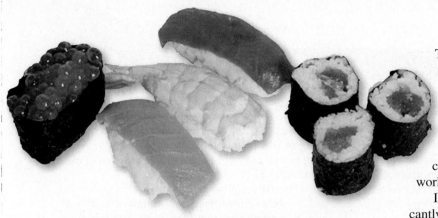

BEHAVIOR-RELATED CHANGES THAT AFFECT DISEASE TRANSMISSION

Disease transmission has also been affected by changes in behavior, including travel, sexual behavior, drug use, and body art.

Travel and Disease Before the advent of modern transportation systems—for example, when it took weeks to cross the ocean on a ship—a passenger who became sick en route could be quarantined (separated from others to prevent transmission of disease). Nowadays, people can travel immense distances in hours, carrying incubating pathogens with them. University students and staff are particularly vulnerable to disease transmission because higher education is an international endeavor, with academics traveling around the world in pursuit of their interests.

The severe acute respiratory syndrome (SARS) outbreak in 2003 is an excellent example of how travel affects the spread of disease and how public health agencies detect and contain disease outbreaks. In March 2003 the World Health Organization activated a Global Outbreak Alert (a system for monitoring outbreaks) concerning an atypical pneumonia that was believed to have originated in southern China at the end of 2002. By February 2003 it had spread to Hong Kong, Vietnam, Singapore, Germany, and Canada. By the time the disease was contained in July 2003, there had been 8,098 probable cases and 774 deaths in 26 countries.

SARS is caused by a previously unknown corona virus and is spread directly from person to person by coughing, sneezing, and skin contact. Air travel was identified as a key reason for its rapid spread. With no vaccine or treatment available, isolation and quarantine of potentially infected people was the key to stopping the spread of infection.

During the outbreak, airlines and travelers were alerted to the early symptoms, which can progress fairly rapidly to a severe form of pneumonia.

Travelers boarding planes that were departing from cities with SARS cases were screened for symptoms and prevented from traveling if symptomatic. If a traveler became ill in flight, health officials boarded the plane upon arrival to examine and possibly quarantine the individual. Travelers were advised to avoid cities with SARS cases, and many locales suffered financially until the advisory ended. Countries around the world remain on alert for a recurrence.

International surveillance and preparedness have significantly improved as a result of this experience.[7] In 2009, when the governments of Mexico and the United States reported to the World Health Organization what appeared to be a rapidly spreading new influenza virus (subsequently identified as 2009 H1N1 or swine flu), the World Health Organization's Global Alert and Response was again activated to launch a coordinated response to the outbreak. Although almost 18,000 people in 214 countries have died thus far from swine flu, the pandemic has not been as severe as once feared (see the box "H1N1: An Influenza Pandemic").[8]

Sexual Behavior and Disease Sexual behavior also affects the transmission of disease. A variety of factors make a difference in how likely it is that a person will be exposed to a sexually transmitted disease (STD). These factors can be categorized as partner variables, susceptible person variables, and sex act variables.

Partner variables that increase the risk of being exposed to an STD include the total number of sex partners a person has, how frequently he or she acquires new sex partners, and the number of concurrent sexual partners. Certain types of partners are associated with an increased risk of infection; the highest risks are associated with commercial sex workers (people who are paid to have sex) and unknown partners (for example, a person someone hooks up with at a party).[9]

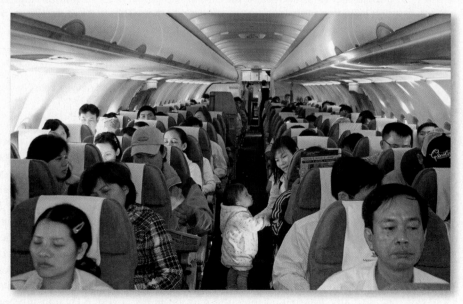

By allowing people to travel immense distances in short time periods, air travel facilitates the global spread of infectious disease.

Highlight on Health

H1N1: An Influenza Pandemic

In 1918–1919, the infamous "Spanish flu" swept the globe, causing an estimated 50 million deaths. The world saw two more influenza pandemics—worldwide epidemics—in the 20th century: the "Asian flu" of 1957 and the "Hong Kong flu" of 1968. In each of these pandemics, serious illness and death were not limited to high-risk groups, such as older adults or infants; in 1918–1919, death rates were highest among healthy young adults. Thus, in April 2009 reports out of Mexico of an influenza-like illness causing deaths among otherwise healthy young adults were met with worldwide concern. Would this become a new influenza pandemic?

The cause of the illness was identified as a new strain of influenza A, eventually termed 2009 H1N1 flu. Two types of influenza virus, influenza A and influenza B, cause "flu" in humans. Influenza A is further divided into subtypes based on antigens on the surface of the virus, called H and N; subtypes are named according to these antigens, such as "H1N1." Like other viruses, the influenza virus is subject to frequent minor genetic changes as well as infrequent, abrupt, major genetic change. When a slight change occurs, many people will have partial immunity from previous infection with a similar strain or vaccination. When a substantial change occurs, however, most people will have little or no immunity to the new strain.

Seasonal influenza can involve subtypes of either influenza A or influenza B, with slightly different strains circulating each year. Between 5 and 20 percent of the U.S. population is infected with seasonal influenza annually, and approximately 36,000 people die from it, most of them 65 or older.

Epidemic influenza usually involves influenza A, since it is more likely to undergo major genetic changes than influenza B. Influenza A can also affect animal species, including birds, pigs, horses, dogs, and others. These infections are usually species-specific, but cross-species

infection does occur when genes from different strains mix. This was the case with H5N1 influenza, or avian (bird) flu, which infected people in several Asian countries beginning in the late 1990s. Although avian flu is very serious in humans, it does not spread easily from person to person and so far has remained localized.

The 2009 H1N1 influenza (initially called swine flu) involved a mix of genes from four different strains of the virus, two from pigs, one from birds, and one from humans. The outbreak was a concern because the strain is easily transmitted from person to person and can spread rapidly. On June 11, 2009, the World Health Organization declared it a worldwide pandemic because it had spread to more than 70 countries.

Most cases of the flu in the United States in the 2009–2010 flu season were caused by 2009 H1N1. Although most people recovered without needing medical treatment, an estimated 12,000 people have died in the United States to date from 2009 H1N1, 87 percent of them younger than 65. Besides young adults, other groups at high risk of serious complications include pregnant women, young children, and people with underlying health conditions. A vaccine released in October 2009 was recommended for these groups.

History suggests this will not be the last influenza pandemic. Recommendations for influenza immunization will change and adapt in response to new viruses and affected populations. In 2010, influenza vaccine became universally recommended for all people aged six months or older. One thing remains clear—basic good health habit recommendations will remain the same. Avoid people who are sick, stay home when you are sick, wash your hands often, avoid touching your face unless you have washed your hands, and take good care of your immune system. For more information on protecting yourself from influenza, visit www.flu.gov.

Sources: "World Now at the Start of 2009 Influenza Pandemic," World Health Organization statement to the press June 11, 2009, retrieved May 3, 2010, from www.who.int/mediacentre/news/statements/2009/h1n1_pandemic_phase6_20090611/en/index.html; "CDC Estimates of 2009 H1N1 Influenza Cases, Hospitalization and Deaths in the United States, April–February 13, 2010," Centers for Disease Control and Prevention, retrieved May 3, 2010, from http://www.cdc.gov/H1N1flu/pdf/Estimates5_Short%20Table.pdf.

Variables associated with increased susceptibility to infection include gender, age at first intercourse, and the general health of the susceptible person. Women are at greater risk than men due to anatomy (the larger mucosal surface of the vagina and the cervix in comparison to the penis). Young women are at particular risk because the cervix is more susceptible to infection in the first few years after the start of menstruation. The overall health of a person is important because it affects the strength of the immune response and the integrity of the mucosal surfaces. For instance, a person with one sexually transmitted infection may be more likely to contract a second infection, as discussed later in this chapter.

The sexual acts performed by a couple also affect disease transmission. Nonpenetrative sex (fondling, mutual masturbation) has the lowest risk, followed in increasing order of risk by oral sex, penile-vaginal intercourse, and penile-anal intercourse. Other factors further increase or decrease the risk of transmission. The risk of exposure increases with the number of sexual acts. The amount of lubrication, either natural from foreplay or applied, affects risk, because abrasions to the mucosa make it easier for the STD to be transmitted. Forced sex or violent sex increases the risk of abrasions and of STD transmission.

The most effective ways to prevent the transmission of STDs are to abstain from intimate sexual activities and to

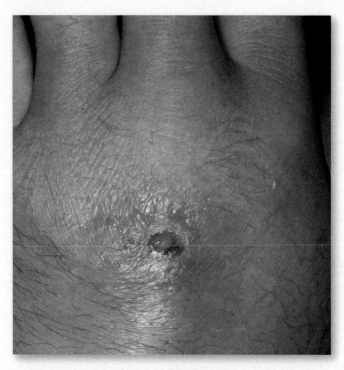

■ A skin infection caused by MRSA is easy to get and hard to treat.

throat, and sinus infection among the top 10 impediments to academic performance.[23] Assess your risk for infectious disease by completing the immunizations table and answering the questions in the Chapter 14 Personal Health Portfolio.

Pertussis (Whooping Cough) *Whooping cough* is the common name for an infection of the respiratory tract caused by the pertussis bacterium. It is highly contagious, transmitted by inhaling respiratory droplets from an infected person's cough or sneeze. Initial infection may seem similar to a common cold, with nasal congestion, runny nose, mild fever, and a dry cough, but after 1 to 2 weeks, the coughing occurs in spells lasting a few minutes and ending in a "whooping" sound as the person gasps for air. The cough can persist for months.

Most infants and young children are vaccinated against pertussis, but immunity begins to wear off after 5 to 10 years, leaving adolescents and young adults susceptible to infection. Studies on college campuses show that among students with a prolonged cough, approximately 30 percent may have pertussis. Pertussis is treated with antibiotics if diagnosed early. Reported cases of pertussis have increased 20-fold in the past 30 years. It is now recommended that all adolescents and adults receive a booster vaccination to enhance their immunity against this infection.[24]

Staphylococcus Aureus Skin Infections *Staphylococcus aureus* (often called "Staph"), a common bacterium carried on the skin or in the noses of healthy people, is one of the most common causes of skin infection. Some strains of Staph are becoming increasingly resistant to antibiotics. Initially seen in hospitals, methicillin-resistant *Staphylococcus aureus* (MRSA) is becoming common in community settings. MRSA is transmitted from person to person by skin-to-skin contact, through the sharing of personal items, or through contact with contaminated surfaces. Outbreaks of infection have been reported among athletes and people in shared living situations (such as on college campuses).

Usually Staph infections are mild, taking the form of a pimple or small boil (sometimes mistaken for a spider bite). Sometimes these infections can spread, creating a large abscess (pocket of infection), which can require incision, drainage, and treatment with antibiotics. Less often, Staph can cause infection of the blood, lungs, or muscle. These cases usually require hospitalization and intravenous antibiotic treatment.

Good hygiene practices can reduce the risk of Staph infection. Keep your hands clean by washing frequently with soap and water, or use an alcohol-based hand sanitizer. Shower after exercising, and avoid sharing personal items such as towels, razors, clothing, and uniforms. Keep cuts and scrapes clean and covered until healed. If you have been diagnosed with a Staph infection, avoid skin-to-skin contact (including contact sports) until the area has healed.[25]

Urinary Tract Infections Urinary tract infections (UTIs) are believed to be the most common bacterial infection. They are more common in women than in men. The vast majority of UTIs are caused by the bacterium *E. coli*, although they can be caused by other bacteria. Symptoms include pain or burning with urination, pain in the lower abdomen, urgency and frequency of urination, and, if the kidneys become involved, pain in the back and fever. Recent sexual activity and history of UTI are risk factors for infection. If a woman is at risk for STDs or has vaginal symptoms, such as discharge or irritation, she should be tested to rule out STDs. Treatment includes fluids and antibiotics, although *E. coli* is becoming increasingly resistant to commonly used antibiotics.[26]

Sexually Transmitted Diseases

Sexually transmitted diseases (STDs) are infections that are spread from one person to another predominantly through sexual contact. Some health experts prefer the term *sexually transmitted infection* (*STI*), because often there are no symptoms, and by definition, a disease is an infection that causes symptoms. However, the CDC continues to use the term *sexually transmitted disease*, and this text follows their usage.

The primary pathogens responsible for STDs are viruses and bacteria. We begin this section with HIV infection, one of the most serious threats to public health worldwide, and

Table 14.1   Infectious Diseases on Campus

Illness	Cause (Pathogen)	Incubation	Symptoms	Home Treatment	When to Seek Medical Care	Prevention
Common cold	Over 200 different viruses, including rhinovirus, adenovirus, coronavirus	1–4 days	Runny nose (often clear initially, then turning thicker, darker), nasal congestion, mild cough, sore throat, low-grade fever (<101° F), sneezing.	Usually resolves on its own; fluids, rest, over-the-counter decongestant, antihistamines, cough suppressant, antipyretic/analgesic; avoid alcohol and tobacco.	Inability to swallow, worsening symptoms after 3rd day, difficulty breathing, stiff neck.	Hand washing, avoid sharing personal items, balanced nutrition, exercise, adequate sleep.
Influenza ("the flu")	Influenza A or B virus	1–5 days	Sudden-onset fever (usually >101° F), headache, tiredness (can be extreme), body aches, cough, sore throat, runny or stuffy nose.	Usually resolves on its own; same as for common cold; in addition, antiviral medications can be used by prescription.	Immediately if in group with high risk for complications, such as pregnant women, those with chronic lung or heart disease, those with asthma. Otherwise, difficulty breathing, severe headache or stiff neck, confusion, fever lasting more than 3 days, new pain localizing to one area (ear, chest, sinuses).	Annual flu shot in October or November, frequent hand washing; avoid close contact with sick people.
Strep throat	*Streptococcus* bacteria	2–5 days	Sudden-onset sore throat and fever (often >101° F); may have mild headache, stomachache, nausea; back of throat red and white pus on tonsils, sore lymph nodes in neck; absence of cough, stuffy nose, or other cold symptoms (as most common cause of sore throat is common cold).	Salt water gargles, analgesics, antipyretics, throat lozenges.	Strep throat is treated with antibiotics to reduce duration of symptoms and reduce risk of complications. If symptoms are consistent with strep, a health provider visit is appropriate.	Same as common cold.
Acute sinus infection	Virus: most common cause; same as common cold Bacteria: *Streptococcus, Haemophilus influenza*; less common, often as complication of common cold or allergies	Varies	Pain or pressure in the face, stuffy or runny nose, upper teeth pain, fever; may have headache, bad breath, yellow or green nasal discharge.	Same as for common cold: decongestants or antihistamines; nasal irrigation; most sinus infections resolve on their own with opening and drainage of the sinuses.	Fever >101° F after 3 days, no improvement in facial pain or pressure after 2 days of home treatment with decongestant, cold symptoms continue beyond 10 days or worsen after 7 days.	Same as common cold. Early treatment of nasal congestion with decongestant or antihistamine.

Illness	Cause (Pathogen)	Incubation	Symptoms	Home Treatment	When to Seek Medical Care	Prevention
Mononucleosis ("mono")	Epstein-Barr virus (EBV)	4–6 weeks	High fever (>101° F), severe sore throat, swollen glands, weakness and fatigue; loss of appetite; nausea, and vomiting can occur.	Usually resolves on its own; rest, fluids; avoid contact sports until symptoms resolve due to risk of spleen rupture.	Fever >101° F after 3 days, unable to maintain fluids; low energy, body aches, swollen glands lasting longer than 7–10 days; severe pain in belly can indicate spleen rupture and is a medical emergency.	Do not kiss or share utensils or foods with someone who has mono; EBV is spread from saliva.
Bronchitis or cough	Virus: same as common cold Bacteria: rare Other lung irritants: tobacco smoke	Varies	Initial dry, hacking cough; after a few days, may be productive of mucus; may have associated low fever and fatigue; often develops 3–4 days into a cold; may last 2–3 weeks.	Rest, fluids, cough drops, and avoidance of lung irritants such as tobacco; over-the-counter cold medications may help.	If you feel short of breath, have history of asthma or chronic lung disease, or develop signs of pneumonia: high fever, shaking chills, shortness of breath; also, if symptoms last more than 4 weeks.	Avoid tobacco smoke; get annual flu shot; good hand washing.
Meningitis	Virus: fairly common, usually not serious Bacteria: less common, must be treated immediately to avoid brain damage and death	Varies	Stiff and painful neck, fever, headache, vomiting, difficulty staying awake, confusion, seizures.	Home treatment is not appropriate if signs of meningitis are present until a health care provider determines if symptoms are due to a virus or bacteria; if viral cause, home treatment to relieve fever and pain symptoms is appropriate.	Immediately if signs of meningitis are present.	Viral: Immunization against some of the pathogens reduces risk; these include measles, mumps, rubella; chicken pox; *Neisseria meningitides* (meningococcal vaccine). Bacterial: Antibiotics when you have come in close contact with someone who is infected; insect repellent; special immunizations for certain areas of the world.
Cellulitis	Bacteria: most common are *Streptococcus* and *Staphylococcus aureus*	Varies	Infected area will be warm, red, swollen, and painful; if infection spreads, may have associated fever, chills, swollen glands.	Warm compresses; keep area clean and dry; topical antibiotics if small area of skin involved.	Cellulitis is usually treated with antibiotics; any symptoms of cellulitis should be evaluated by a health care provider.	Healthy skin protects you from infection; keep cuts, burns, and insect bites clean and dry; treat chronic skin conditions such as eczema, ulcers, psoriasis; avoid intravenous drug use; avoid piercing and tattoos.

then we discuss the other STDs by type of pathogen. See Table 14.2 on page 326 for information relating to the incubation period, symptoms, complications, screening and diagnosis, and treatment of each STD discussed.

HIV/AIDS

Acquired immunodeficiency syndrome (AIDS) is caused by the human immunodeficiency virus (HIV). Since the first case was diagnosed in 1981, more than 20 million people have died from HIV/AIDS. The pandemic is considered the most serious infectious disease challenge in public health today. At the end of 2008, an estimated 33.4 million people worldwide were infected, two-thirds of them in sub-Saharan Africa and another 20 percent in Asia (Figure 14.7). In 2008 2.7 million new infections and 2.0 million deaths occurred. Over 90 percent of infections among children and 70 percent of overall deaths were in sub-Saharan Africa. Furthermore, in sub-Saharan Africa an estimated 14.1 million children have lost one or both parents to AIDS.[27]

Currently, there appear to be two patterns of infection. In sub-Saharan Africa, the epidemic is in the general population, with women representing 61 percent of the people living with HIV, and transmission is predominantly via heterosexual contact. In other parts of the world, HIV remains concentrated in populations of increased risk, such as men who have sex with men, injection drug users, and sex workers and their sexual partners.[27]

An estimated 1.4 million people are living with HIV in North America. In the United States, sexual contact is involved in about 85 percent of newly diagnosed HIV infections (men who have sex with men account for more than half of all infections, and high-risk heterosexual sex accounts for 14 percent), and intravenous drug use is involved in about 10 percent. Racial and ethnic minority populations continue to be affected disproportionately (see the box "Disproportionate Risk for HIV Infections").[28]

HIV most likely originated from a similar virus, the simian immunodeficiency virus found in chimpanzees in Africa. It is believed to have jumped from animal host to human host approximately 50 to 75 years ago. The virus may have entered a human being from the bite of an infected chimpanzee or during the slaughtering of a chimpanzee. Once in a human host, the simian immunodeficiency virus

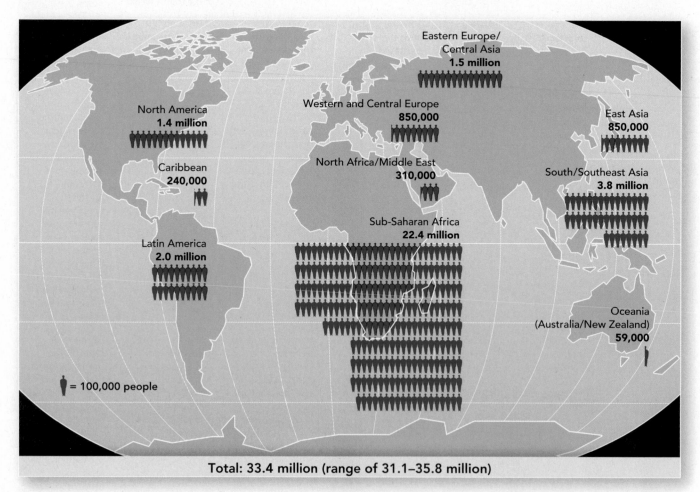

figure 14.7   Adults and children estimated to be living with HIV in 2008.

Source: 2009 AIDS Epidemic Update. Copyright © Joint United Nations Programme on HIV/AIDS (UNAIDS) and World Health Organization (WHO).

Disproportionate Risk for HIV Infections

Who's at Risk?

Certain groups are at disproportionate risk for HIV infections. Here is a profile of new HIV cases in the United States.

By sex

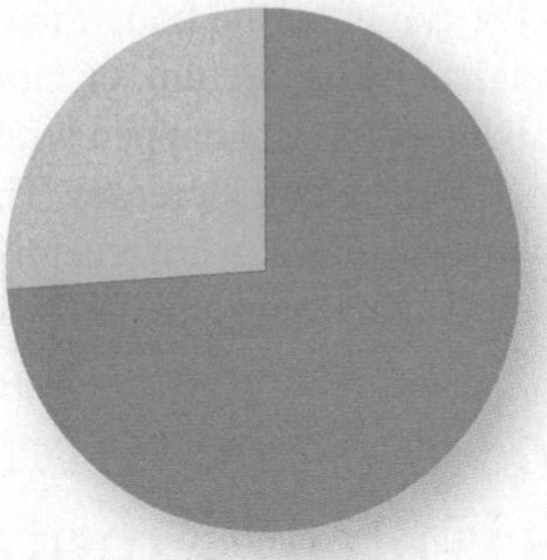

- Male 74%
- Female 26%

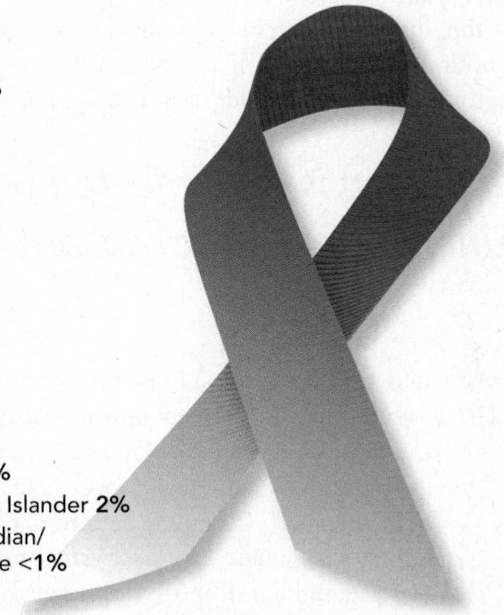

By ethnicity

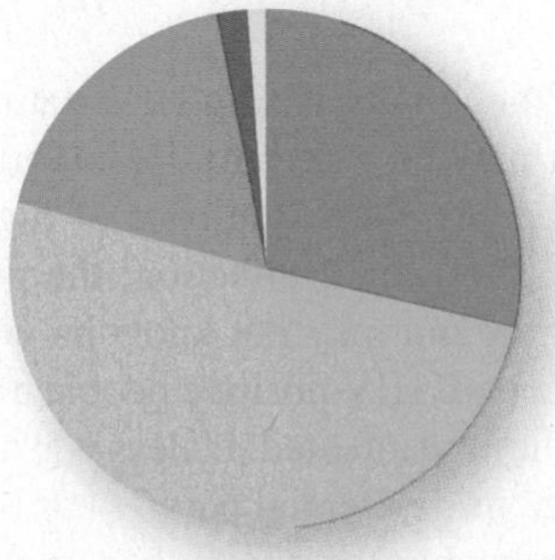

- White 29%
- Black 51%
- Hispanic 18%
- Asian/Pacific Islander 2%
- American Indian/Alaska Native <1%

By risk behavior

Male
- MSM* 71%
- IDU** 10%
- MSM and IDU 4.9%
- High-risk heterosexual contact 14%
- Other <1%

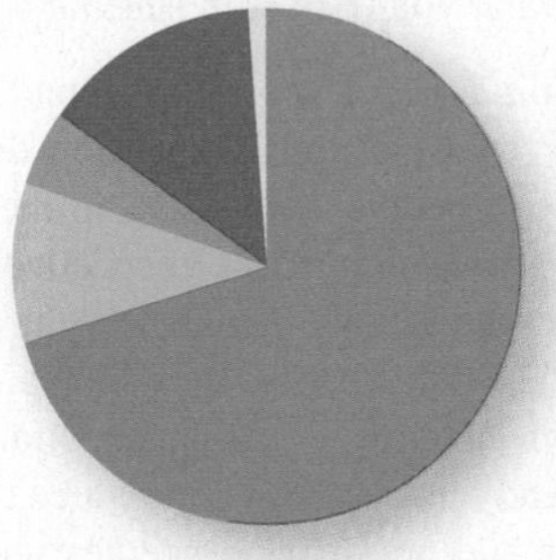

*Men who have sex with men
**Injection drug use

Female
- IDU** 16%
- High-risk heterosexual contact 83%
- Other 1%

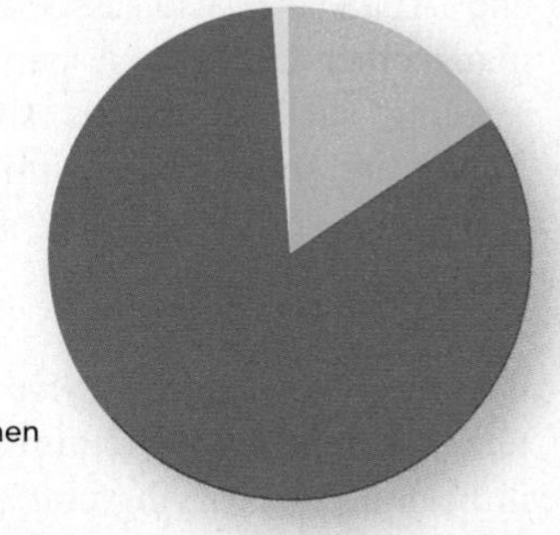

Source: "HIV/AIDS in the United States," Centers for Disease Control and Prevention, 2009, retrieved May 4, 2010, from www.cdc.gov/hiv/resources/factsheets/us.htm.

evolved through mutation into human immunodeficiency virus.[29] There are two main strains of the virus: HIV-1 is the predominant strain in North America and most of the rest of the world; HIV-2 is found primarily in Africa.

Course of the Disease   HIV targets the cells of the immune system, especially macrophages and CD4 cells (a subcategory of helper T cells). Once inside these host cells, the virus uses the cell's DNA to replicate itself and disable the host cell. During the initial infection with HIV, known

as *primary infection*, the virus replicates rapidly. Within 4 to 11 days of exposure, several million viral copies may circulate in the bloodstream. The immune system mounts a rapid response in an attempt to control and remove the virus, but HIV is able to mutate quickly and avoid complete eradication.

Between 40 and 90 percent of people infected with HIV experience an acute infection phase approximately 4 to 6 weeks after exposure, with symptoms such as fever, weight loss, fatigue, sore throat, lymph node swelling, night sweats, muscle aches, rash, and diarrhea. The symptoms may last for a few weeks and are easily mistaken for those of other infections, such as influenza, mononucleosis, or herpes.[30]

After the early phase, the immune system and the virus come to a balance with the establishment of a *viral load set point*, a level of virus that continues to circulate in the blood and body fluids. During this phase, a person is asymptomatic and may remain so for 2 to 20 years. The virus continues to replicate, and the immune system continues to control it without completely removing it.

Eventually the immune system is weakened significantly and can no longer function fully, signaling the onset of AIDS. Symptoms of AIDS include rapid weight loss,

addition, some people may have a higher viral load set point during the equilibrium period. Antiviral treatment (discussed in a later section) lowers the level of circulating virus and may reduce the risk of transmission.

Sexual Conduct   The primary exposure risk for 85 percent of cases of HIV infection in the United States is sexual contact.[28] HIV can enter the body through the mucosa or lining of the vagina, penis, rectum, or mouth. If the mucosa is cut, torn, or irritated (as can happen with intercourse or if there is another STD), the risk increases. The sexual behaviors associated with transmission are receptive anal sex, insertive anal sex, penile-vaginal sex, and oral sex.

When a person is first infected with HIV, the immune system mounts a rapid response, but **the virus is able to mutate quickly** *and avoid complete eradication.*

cough, night sweats, diarrhea, rashes or skin blemishes, and memory loss. These symptoms are due to **opportunistic infections**—infections that occur when the immune system is no longer able to fight them off. Common opportunistic infections include *Pneumocystis carinii* pneumonia, Kaposi's sarcoma (a rare cancer), and tuberculosis.

opportunistic infections
Infections that occur when the immune system is weakened. These infections do not usually occur in a person with a healthy immune system.

A note of caution: The symptoms associated with acute HIV infection and AIDS are also associated with many other illnesses. A person experiencing such symptoms should not automatically assume they are signs of HIV infection or AIDS. However, if the person is at risk, he or she should get tested for HIV infection.

Methods of Transmission   HIV cannot survive long outside of a human host, and thus transmission requires intimate contact. The virus can be found in varying concentrations in an infected person's blood, saliva, semen, genital secretions, and breast milk. It usually enters a new host either at a mucosal surface or by direct inoculation into the blood. HIV is not transmitted through casual contact, such as by shaking hands, hugging, or a casual kiss, nor is it spread by day-to-day contact in the workplace, school, or home setting. Although HIV has been found in saliva and tears, it is present in very low quantities. It has not been found in sweat.

Risk of HIV transmission is influenced by factors associated with the host (the already infected person), the recipient (the currently uninfected person), and the type of interaction that occurs between the host and recipient (behaviors). An important host factor is the level of virus circulating in the blood. High levels of circulating virus, such as during the initial infection stage, increase the risk of transmission. In

Although discussing HIV status with a potential sexual partner may be awkward, its importance cannot be overemphasized. As noted, the time of highest circulating virus is shortly after initial infection; the person may not have any symptoms and may not know he or she is infected. In fact, 25 percent of HIV-positive people in the United States do not know they are infected. Unless you have a conversation about whether your potential partner has been tested for HIV, what risky behaviors he or she has engaged in, and what other sexual partners he or she has been involved with, you do not know what your risk is in starting a sexual relationship.[28]

Injection Drug Use   The second most common method of HIV transmission is injection drug use, reported by 18 percent of people with AIDS in the United States. Another 4 percent and 5 percent, respectively, report both injection drug use and being a man who has sex with other men as combined risk factors. Individuals can reduce their risk of HIV infection by avoiding injection drug use. People who are already using drugs can reduce their risk by using sterile needles and not sharing needles with others. Communities can play a role in decreasing the spread of HIV by implementing needle exchange programs and ensuring adequate access to drug treatment programs.

Contact With Infected Blood or Body Fluids   HIV can be transmitted by direct contact with the blood or body fluids of an infected person. The risk of transmission again varies depending upon how much virus is in the body fluid, how much fluid gets onto another person, and where the fluid contacts the other person. A small amount of infected blood on the intact skin of another person carries essentially no risk. A larger amount of blood on cut or broken skin or mucosal membranes has a greater risk. The accidental injection of infected blood through a needle stick has an even greater risk.

These types of exposure are most likely to occur in health care settings, and to reduce the risk of transmission of HIV, hepatitis B and C, and other bloodborne infections, the **universal precautions** approach has been instituted in these settings.

Universal precautions include the use of gloves, gown, mask, and other protective wear (such as eyewear or face shields) in settings where someone is likely to be exposed to the blood or infected body fluids of another person. These precautions should be taken with every patient.[31]

Perinatal Transmission Perinatal, or vertical, transmission—the transmission of HIV from an infected mother to her child—can occur during pregnancy, during delivery (when the fetus is exposed to the mother's blood in the birth canal), or after delivery (if the baby is exposed to the mother's breast milk). The risk of transmission from mother to child can be reduced through the use of antiretroviral medications during pregnancy and around the time of delivery. Infected mothers also reduce the risk to their babies by electing not to breastfeed.

In the United States, women are routinely offered HIV testing as part of prenatal care. If she tests positive, a woman is offered preventive therapy with antiretroviral medications to reduce her child's risk. In untreated women with HIV, approximately 30 percent of infants are infected; in treated women, less than 2 percent are infected.

HIV Testing The earlier HIV infection is recognized, the sooner treatment can begin, the longer a person is likely to remain symptom free, and the fewer people he or she is likely to expose to the virus. The only way to confirm HIV infection is by laboratory testing.

To increase the number of HIV cases that are diagnosed early, the CDC recommends that everyone between the ages of 13 and 64 be tested for HIV infection at least once during routine medical care. Testing is strongly recommended for anyone who has engaged in any of the following behaviors or has a partner who has done so:

- Injected drugs, including steroids
- Had unprotected vaginal, anal, or oral sex with men who have had sex with men
- Had multiple partners or anonymous partners or has exchanged sex for drugs or money
- Been diagnosed with an STD

Anyone who continues to engage in these risk behaviors should be tested at least annually. All pregnant women should be screened for HIV.[32]

Most HIV tests are designed to detect antibodies to HIV circulating in the bloodstream. After an HIV exposure, it can take 2 to 8 weeks for a sufficient quantity of antibodies to be produced for an HIV test to detect them. This time is referred to as a "window period"—a time when the HIV test may result in a false negative. If the test is done within the first 3 months after a potential exposure, the test should be repeated 3 months later.

Several HIV screening tests are available. The standard test is an enzyme immune assay (EIA) that screens a person's blood for antibodies to HIV. Newer EIA tests use oral fluid or urine instead of blood, and some can deliver results in about 20 minutes. If the result of any of these screening tests is positive, a confirmatory test called a Western blot is performed. The Western blot also detects antibodies to HIV but can distinguish false positives from actual infection. It is also possible to test for recent HIV infection by looking for the actual virus through a viral load test. This test is used if HIV infection is suspected based on acute symptoms, but it is not used routinely because of its greater cost.

An over-the-counter home test called the Home Access HIV-1 Test System is licensed and approved by the FDA. The consumer collects a small amount of blood from a finger prick, places the blood on a card, mails the card to a registered laboratory, and telephones for results using an identification number. All people with a positive result are referred to a health clinic

universal precautions
A set of precautions designed to prevent transmission of bloodborne infections. Blood and certain body fluids of *all* patients are considered potentially infectious for HIV and hepatitis B and C. Protective barriers, such as gloves, aprons, and protective eyewear, are used in health settings.

- Actress Scarlett Johansson has said that she gets tested for HIV twice a year. The CDC recommends that people aged 13 to 64 get tested for HIV at least once during routine medical care.

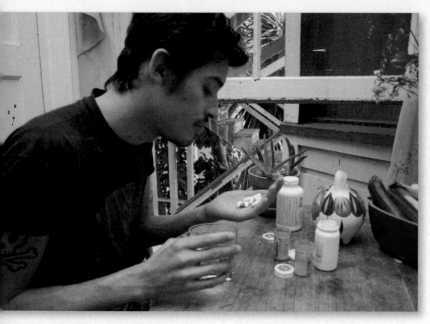

■ People with HIV manage the disease with antiretroviral medications. Multiple drugs are used since the virus can quickly become resistant to individual drugs.

because the positive result must be confirmed by the Western blot test. Consumers are warned to use only FDA-approved test kits, since others may not be as accurate.[33,34]

Management of HIV/AIDS   The development of new medications and improved understanding of the HIV disease process have contributed to prolonged survival by some people infected with HIV. Educating people in low- and middle-income countries and getting them medication has been a major challenge, but international efforts have shown tremendous progress in recent years.[35]

drug cocktails
Complicated drug combinations used to overcome drug resistance in different strains of HIV.

microbicide
Compound or chemical in the form of a cream, gel, or suppository that would kill microorganisms and that could be applied topically to the vagina or rectum before intercourse, reducing the risk of STD transmission.

Antiretroviral Agents   The most important medications in HIV treatment are antiviral drugs—or, more accurately, antiretroviral drugs, since HIV is a type of virus called a retrovirus. Antiretroviral medications do not cure the infection, but they slow the rate at which the virus replicates and destroys the immune system, thus prolonging life and improving the quality of life for people who are HIV-positive.

Drug Cocktails   If a single antiretroviral medication is used, resistant strains develop fairly quickly. To combat resistance, scientists have developed complicated drug combinations, called **drug cocktails**, that usually include a medication from two to four of the drug categories. A viral strain is less likely to develop several mutations allowing it to evade the combination of

drugs than to develop one or a few mutations allowing it to evade a single drug. However, the complexity, cost, and risk of side effects for the person taking the drugs are all increased.

New Prevention Possibilities   Since the identification of the virus, researchers have been attempting to develop safe and effective measures to reduce risk of infection. An HIV vaccine would be ideal but is challenging. The immune system does not seem to be able to clear HIV and produce immunity; instead, the virus produces lifelong infection. Furthermore, the virus is a moving target; it mutates frequently and develops new strains rapidly. That said, multiple vaccine trials are under way.[36]

Another avenue being pursued is the development of a **microbicide**, a compound or chemical in the form of a cream, gel, or suppository that would kill microorganisms and that could be applied topically to the vagina or rectum before intercourse.[36] In addition, adult male circumcision is recognized as an intervention to reduce risk of HIV infection, possibly due to the fact that removing the foreskin results in a toughening of the skin covering the penis.

BACTERIAL STDS

Bacterial STDs are curable infections if identified early. Undiagnosed, they can cause serious consequences, including pelvic inflammatory disease, reduced fertility, ectopic pregnancy, and increased risk for HIV transmission.[37,38]

Chlamydia   The most commonly reported bacterial STD is chlamydia infection. Rates of infection are increasing in the United States, with an estimated 1.1 million cases diagnosed annually. Young women are at greatest risk for chlamydia, with rates three times that of young men. Seven percent of women aged 15 to 24 visiting family planning clinics are infected. Although all racial and ethnic groups are affected, Black women have rates eight times higher than those of White women.[37,38]

All sexually active women under age 26 should be screened regularly for chlamydia, as should women who are at increased risk because they have a new sexual partner or multiple sexual partners or are infected with another STD. There is debate about the cost effectiveness of screening all sexually active men under age 26. Men should be tested if they have symptoms or have a

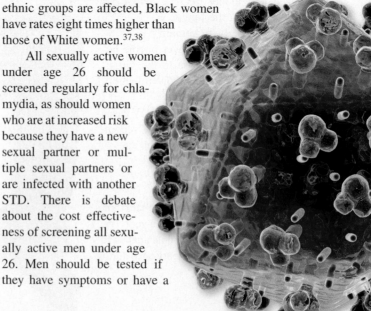

new sexual partner or if their sexual partner has been diagnosed with chlamydia. They also should be aware that rates of chlamydia infection are increasing among men and that they can be infected yet have no symptoms.

Gonorrhea The second most commonly reported bacterial STD is gonorrhea. As with chlamydia, the highest rates occur in young women. Rates of gonorrheal infection have remained stable, with an estimated 356,000 cases diagnosed annually.

Regular screening is recommended for women at high risk of infection—those who are under 25 and have had two or more sex partners in the past year, who exchange sex for money or drugs, or who have a history of repeated episodes of gonorrhea. It is less clear if asymptomatic men should be screened, because most men eventually develop symptoms.

Gonorrhea is treated with antibiotics, but drug resistance is a growing problem. Cephalosporins are the only class of antibiotics now available to treat gonorrhea infection.[37–39]

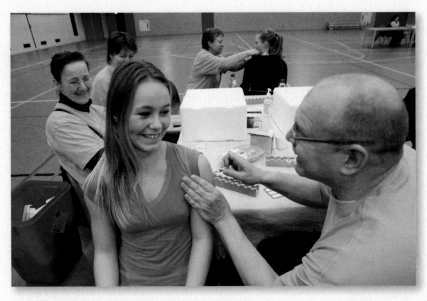

■ The vaccine Gardasil, approved for females 9 to 26 years of age, protects against strains of HPV that cause 70 percent of cervical cancer cases and 90 percent of genital warts cases.

Pelvic Inflammatory Disease Pelvic inflammatory disease (PID) is an infection of the uterus, fallopian tubes, and/or ovaries. The infection occurs when bacteria from the vagina or cervix spread upward into the uterus and fallopian tubes. The bacteria involved are usually from STDs, such as chlamydia or gonorrhea, but they can be bacteria that are normally found in the vagina.

Symptoms of PID include fever, abdominal pain, pelvic pain, and vaginal bleeding or discharge. If PID is suspected, a combination of antibiotics is prescribed to cover gonorrhea, chlamydia, and vaginal bacteria. If symptoms are severe, hospitalization may be required. About 18 percent of women with PID develop chronic abdominal or pelvic pain that lasts more than 6 months.

PID can cause severe consequences and can be life threatening if untreated. Most of the long-term problems arise from scarring in the fallopian tubes, which increases the risk of ectopic pregnancy and infertility.[37,38]

Syphilis Rates of syphilis decreased throughout the 20th century but began to increase in 2001. Since then, rates among men who have sex with men have increased rapidly, such that rates among men are now six times those among women (they were nearly equal 10 years ago). Although rates in women are lower than they are in men, they are increasing. In particular, rates among Black women have increased.[37,38] Syphilis progresses through several stages. If left untreated, it can lead to serious complications, including death (see Table 14.2).

Screening is recommended for all pregnant women at their initial prenatal care visit and for persons at increased risk for syphilis infection. This includes men who have sex with men, commercial sex workers, and anyone who tests positive for another STD, exchanges sex for drugs, or has sex with partners who have syphilis.

Bacterial Vaginosis Bacterial vaginosis (BV) is an alteration of the normal vaginal flora; Lactobacillis, the usually predominant bacteria, is replaced with different bacteria, causing a vaginal discharge and unpleasant odor. It is not clear why women develop bacterial vaginosis. Although it is not considered an STD, women who have never had sex rarely experience the condition. Treatment of male partners does not alter the rate of recurrence for women.

BV is diagnosed by an evaluation of the vaginal flora under a microscope. Treatment is recommended not just because the symptoms are unpleasant but also because BV has been associated with increased risk of PID, complications in pregnancy, and transmission of HIV. The condition is treated with the antibiotic metronidazole, which can be taken orally or vaginally.[38]

VIRAL STDS

Viral STDs cannot be cured, making prevention even more important than in cases of bacterial STDs. Vaccination is an option for some of the viral STDs, and symptoms can be treated.

Human Papillomavirus Human papillomavirus (HPV) is the most common STD in the United States. There are more than 100 types of HPV. Some types are associated with genital warts, others with cancers of the cervix, vulva, penis, anus, and other areas. Strains associated with cancer are called high-risk strains; of these, two strains (HPV 16,

Table 14.2 Common Sexually Transmitted Diseases

Infection	Incubation	Signs and Symptoms	Complications	Screening and Diagnosis	Treatment	Prevention
Bacterial						
Chlamydia (*Chlamydia trachomatis*)	1–3 weeks	No symptoms for 75% of women and 50% of men. **If symptoms:** watery discharge, burning with urination.	Pelvic inflammatory disease (PID), chronic pelvic pain, infertility, and ectopic pregnancy in women; epididymitis (red, swollen testicles) and, rarely, sterility in men. **If untreated in pregnant women:** premature birth and newborn eye and lung infections.	Urine or sample collected from penis, cervix, rectum, or throat.	Antibiotics, sex partners need testing and treatment prior to resuming sexual intercourse.	Condoms.
Gonorrhea (*Neisseria gonorrhoeae*)	2–5 days	No symptoms in most women and some men. **If symptoms:** pain or burning with urination, discharge from penis, itching inside penis in men; pain or burning with urination, vaginal discharge, vaginal bleeding between periods, pain during sex in women. Rectal infection: discharge, soreness, bleeding, or pain. Throat infection: sore throat.	Pelvic inflammatory disease (PID), chronic pelvic pain, infertility, and ectopic pregnancy in women; epididymitis (red, swollen testicles) and infertility in men; can spread to blood and joints. **If untreated in pregnant women:** risk of newborn eye, joint, and blood infection.	Urine or sample collected from cervix, penis, rectum, or throat.	Antibiotics, sex partners need testing and treatment prior to resuming sexual intercourse.	Condoms.
Syphilis (*Treponema pallidum*)	**Primary stage:** 10–90 days **Secondary stage:** 3–6 weeks after primary stage **Late stage:** years after initial untreated infection	No symptoms for most people. **If symptoms:** **Primary stage**—single sore (chancre) at site of exposure; sore is round, firm, and painless sore resolves without treatment after 3–6 weeks. **Secondary stage:** skin rash that includes non-itchy, rough, reddish brown spots on palms and soles of feet; may have fever, swollen lymph nodes, headache, and fatigue; resolves without treatment.	**Late stage:** without treatment, infection remains in body and 15% of people will develop deterioration of the brain, arteries, bones, heart, and other organs; death possible. **If untreated in pregnant women:** risk of fetal death or infant developmental delay, seizures, or other complications.	Blood test for antibodies to syphilis.	Antibiotics will cure if diagnosed within the first year of infection.	Avoidance of high-risk behaviors; condoms.
Viral						
HIV (human immuno-deficiency virus)	4–6 weeks	No symptoms for 10–60% of people. **If symptoms:** fever, fatigue, sore throat, lymph node swelling, muscle aches; may include weight loss, rash, night sweats, and diarrhea; often mistaken for other illnesses.	Acquired immunodeficiency syndrome (AIDS) 2–20 years after initial infection if untreated; symptoms include opportunistic infections, weight loss, rashes, and skin changes. **Pregnant women:** can be transmitted to fetus; reduced risk with treatment of mother.	Blood, saliva, or urine test.	No cure; management of infection is with antiretroviral medications that reduce the rate of viral replication and slow the rate of immune system decline.	Condoms; post-exposure prophylaxis (taking an antiretroviral medication as soon as possible after high-risk sexual encounter or assault can reduce risk of infection).

Infection	Incubation	Signs and Symptoms	Complications	Screening and Diagnosis	Treatment	Prevention
HPV (human papillomavirus, more than 40 strains)	Weeks to months	No symptoms for most people. **If symptoms:** Genital warts: small bumps or clusters of bumps in genital area. Cervical cancer: irregular bleeding.	In 90% of cases, immune system clears infection within 2 years; cancers of cervix, vulva, vagina, anus, and penis. **Pregnant women:** very rarely, newborn can develop throat infection during vaginal birth.	Genital warts: visual identification. Cervical cancer: routine Pap testing starting at age 21 for all women.	Warts: topical medications or cryotherapy (freezing). Cervical cancer: see Chapter 16.	Vaccination for women and men; Pap testing for women reduces risk of cervical cancer; condoms can reduce risk, but virus can infect areas of genitalia not covered by male and female condoms.
Genital herpes (herpes simplex virus type 1 or type 2)	2–7 days	No symptoms for most people. **If symptoms:** one or more blisters on or around the mouth, genitals, or rectum, which break open, leaving a painful sore that resolves after 2–4 weeks (for first infection); may have association with fever and lymph node swelling.	Recurrent outbreaks, usually less severe than initial one and decrease in severity with time. **Pregnant women:** potential life-threatening infection in newborn if infection during pregnancy or outbreak at time of vaginal birth.	Culture of ulcer or blood test.	No cure; antiviral medications can shorten and prevent outbreaks.	Use of antiviral medications can reduce risk of transmission from an infected person to an uninfected partner (transmission can occur even when lesions are not present); condoms can reduce risk but virus can infect areas of genitalia not covered by male and female condoms.
Hepatitis B	6 weeks– 6 months	No symptoms for 30% of people. **If symptoms:** fever, loss of appetite, nausea, vomiting, abdominal pain, dark urine, yellow color of skin or eyes.	Chronic hepatitis B: increased risk of liver failure due to scarring of liver and liver cancer. **Pregnant women:** can transmit infection to newborn.	Blood tests can look for virus and evidence of immune response.	No treatment for acute infection; if chronic infection develops, several medications can be used but are not suitable for all people.	Vaccination recommended routinely for most people; vaccination can be effective if given within 24 hours after exposure; condoms.
Protozoan						
Trichomoniasis (*Trichomonas vaginalis*)	5–28 days	No symptoms in most men. **If symptoms:** slight burning of penis or mild discharge in men; frothy, yellow-green vaginal discharge with strong odor; vaginal soreness or itching in women.	**If untreated in pregnant women:** increased risk of premature delivery.	Identification under a microscope.	Antibiotics; treatment of both partners prior to resuming sexual activity.	Condoms.

Sources: Sexually Transmitted Disease Surveillance, 2007, Centers for Disease Control and Prevention, 2008, Atlanta: Author; "Sexually Transmitted Diseases Treatment Guidelines 2006," Centers for Disease Control and Prevention, (n.d.), retrieved from www.cdc.gov/STD/treatment/default.htm; "Updated Recommended Treatment Regimens for Gonococcal Infections and Associated Conditions—United States, 2007," Centers for Disease Control and Prevention, 2007, retrieved from www.cdc.gov/STD/treatment/2006/updated-regimens.htm.

18) are associated with 70 percent of cervical cancer cases. Strains associated with genital warts are called low-risk strains; of these, two strains (HPV 6, 11) are most commonly associated with genital warts.

Estimates are that 26.8 percent of U. S. women aged 14 to 69 are infected with HPV and that 44.8 percent of women aged 20 to 24 are infected.[40] HPV is transmitted by skin-to-skin contact, usually through penetrative vaginal or anal sex.

The virus is easily transmitted during sexual intercourse. Weeks to months after exposure to low-risk strains of HPV, both men and women can develop genital warts—flat or raised, small or large, pinkish lesions—on the penis, scrotum, vagina, anus, or skin around the genital area. They can be treated with topical medications but this is primarily for cosmetic reasons and may not alter the risk of transmission.

Men are not routinely screened for high-risk HPV infection. Most women with HPV are diagnosed through screening with the Papanicolaou smear (Pap test). The Pap test was implemented as a way to detect cervical cancer or precancerous lesions. After infection with HPV, the cells of the cervix undergo specific changes that can be identified under a microscope. If mild abnormalities in the cervical cells are noted, HPV testing can be performed to determine if a high-risk (cancer-causing) strain of HPV is present. Among women with HPV infection, the majority will clear the infection within two years. A small percentage of women will go on to have persistent infection and increased risk for cervical cancer. Risk appears to be higher in women who smoke and have impaired immune systems. Given the high rates of spontaneous clearance and the very low rates of cervical cancer in young women, the Pap screening recommendations were recently changed and now recommend that screening start at age 21 years of age (rather than the previous age of 18) regardless of the age of onset of sexual activity.[41]

Men and women who have receptive anal intercourse are at high risk for anal HPV infection and anal cancer. A test called an anal pap can be used to collect a sample of cells from the rectum to be evaluated for precancerous changes. Currently, anal pap or HPV testing is not recommended as a routine screening for men, but men at high risk should discuss this test with their health care provider.[42] Consistent and correct use of condoms may reduce the risk of transmission of HPV but may not provide full protection, since HPV can infect skin not covered by the condom.

Two vaccines are available to reduce risk of HPV infection. Gardasil protects against four HPV strains (HPV 6, 11, 16, and 18). Two of these strains—16 and 18—cause 70 percent of cervical cancer cases, and the two others—6 and 11—cause 90 percent of genital warts. The vaccine is approved for females 9 to 26 years of age and males 9 through 26 years of age and should be given ideally before the onset of sexual activity. Cervarix is the second vaccine and protects against two strains of HPV (HPV 16 and 18). It is currently only approved for females 10 through 25 years of age. [43,44]

Genital Herpes Genital herpes is caused by the herpes simplex virus (HSV), which has two strains, called HSV-1 and HSV-2. Both strains can infect the mouth,

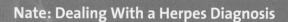

Life Stories

Nate: Dealing With a Herpes Diagnosis

Nate, a second-year student at a community college, had just come home from the student health center after being diagnosed with genital herpes. A week ago he had noticed a sore on his penis and had gone to the doctor to get it checked out even though he felt embarrassed. The doctor did a culture and gave him the results today. He also gave him a prescription for a medication that would help reduce the number of future outbreaks, though Nate would carry the virus with him forever.

Nate was still in shock at the results. He couldn't believe he had an STD. He found himself wondering how he got it—he had been with his current girlfriend, Stacy, for over a year. The doctor had explained that he may have contracted herpes from a previous partner and just not had any symptoms yet. The doctor told him he needed to discuss his diagnosis with his girlfriend. That thought filled Nate with dread and embarrassment. He felt confused as he did not know if he had this virus from previous relationships or if he had contracted it from Stacy. What if Stacy had cheated on him and had given him the infection?

To make matters worse, Stacy had just left for a quarter-long internship in a city three hours away. They had been arguing a lot before she left, and they hadn't talked much since then. He worried about how she was going to react. Would she suspect him of cheating and possibly break up with him? His mind raced forward—if they broke up and he started dating again, he would eventually have to tell other women that he had herpes. He couldn't *not* tell them and have sex with them—he would never do something like that—but what if they didn't want to date him or have sex with him after he told them?

Nate brought his thoughts back to the present situation. He felt stuck and alone. He missed Stacy—she was the one he told everything. Even though they had been fighting, he didn't want to break up. He knew he needed to talk with her to work through their problems and tell her about his diagnosis. He sent her a text asking if they could talk later that day and spent the rest of the afternoon planning what to say.

connect
ACTIVITY

genitals, or skin. HSV-1 is often associated with lesions in and around the mouth (cold sores). This type of herpes is frequently acquired in childhood from nonsexual transmission, although up to 30 percent of genital herpes cases have been associated with HSV-1. The type more frequently associated with genital herpes is HSV-2.[38]

Because there is no cure for HSV infection, prevention is particularly important (see the box "Nate: Dealing With a Herpes Diagnosis"). Condoms partially protect people against infection with HSV, but they are not 100 percent effective. Condoms must be used at all times and not just when a lesion is present since the virus can be spread even without evidence of a sore. Several different vaccines for HSV are currently under study. Antiviral medications are available that shorten the course of outbreaks and reduce their frequency. These medications may also reduce the risk of transmission to sexual partners.

Hepatitis Hepatitis (inflammation of the liver) can be caused by several viruses, but the most common ones are hepatitis A, B, and C. We discussed hepatitis C earlier in the context of injection drug use, the most common route of acquiring the infection. Hepatitis A and B are both easily transmitted through sexual acts. Hepatitis A is transmitted through fecal-oral contact and can be spread through contact with contaminated food or water. The people at greatest risk for sexual transmission of hepatitis A are those who have oral-anal contact or penile-anal intercourse. A safe and effective vaccine is available for hepatitis A and is recommended for men who have sex with men, illicit drug users, people with chronic liver disease, and the general population in areas that have high rates of hepatitis A or before travel to such areas.[38]

Most hepatitis B infections in the United States are sexually transmitted, although the infection can also be spread by exposure to infected blood. Worldwide, hepatitis B is a major cause of liver disease, liver failure, and liver cancer; unlike hepatitis A, it can cause chronic liver disease. The chance of developing chronic disease varies by age at the time of infection, with risk decreasing with age of exposure. Chronic infection carries an increased risk of liver failure and liver cancer.

A safe and effective vaccine for hepatitis B is available, and universal vaccination of all children is recommended. Adolescents and adults who were not vaccinated in childhood and are sexually active should be vaccinated; some colleges encourage hepatitis B vaccinations for all entering students. Vaccinations are currently required for all health care workers, and all pregnant women are screened for the virus.

OTHER STDS

Several other nonbacterial, nonviral infections are transmitted sexually or involve the genital area. Most are treatable infections.

hot tip

If you find out you have an STD, you need to tell your former partners so that they can also be tested. You can do this with an anonymous e-card at www .inspot.org.

Trichomoniasis Trichomoniasis is caused by a protozoan and is transmitted from person to person by sexual activity. Sexual partners of the infected person need to be contacted and treated to prevent the further spread and recurrence of the infection.[38]

Candidiasis Candidiasis is usually caused by the yeast *Candida albicans*. Symptoms of yeast infection include vaginal discharge, itching, soreness, and burning with urination. Yeast infections are not usually acquired through sexual intercourse, but they can be mistaken for an STD because the symptoms are similar. *C. albicans* can be a normal part of the vaginal flora and may overgrow in response to changes in the vaginal environment, such as when a woman takes antibiotics or if she has diabetes.

Candidiasis is treated by antifungal medications available over the counter that can be taken orally as a pill or applied to the vagina with a tablet or as a cream. If a woman is unsure of the diagnosis, has recurrences, or is at risk for STDs, she should have the diagnosis confirmed by a health care provider before she treats herself.[38]

Pubic Lice and Scabies Pubic lice and scabies are ectoparasites that can be sexually transmitted. Pubic lice (or "crabs") infect the skin in the pubic region and cause intense itching. Scabies can infect the skin on any part of the body and, again, cause intense itching. In adults, both pubic lice and scabies are most often sexually transmitted, but in children, scabies is usually acquired through nonsexual contact. Both infections are treated with a medicated cream or shampoo called permethrin or lindane. Bedding and clothing must be decontaminated to prevent reinfection.

Prevention and Treatment of Infectious Diseases

There are many steps that you as an individual can take to protect yourself from infectious diseases. Each of these measures will in turn reduce the risk of spread and the rates of disease in your community.

■ Support your immune system by eating a balanced diet, getting enough exercise and sleep, managing stress, not smoking, and adopting other practices that are part of a healthy lifestyle.

■ Follow government recommendations for vaccinations for both adults and children. If you are in a high-risk group, get a flu shot when it is offered in the fall.

■ If you have been exposed to an infectious disease, minimize the chances that you will pass it on to someone else. For example, if you have a cold or the flu, follow good hygiene practices such as washing your hands frequently; stay home from work; and avoid crowded public places.

Challenges & Choices

Tips for Telling a Partner You Have an STD

Telling a partner you have an STD is not easy. Being candid and honest at the outset of the relationship is highly recommended. Here are some tips:

- If you are currently undergoing treatment for the STD, tell your partner; do not have sex until treatment is complete.

- Be open about how you contracted the STD and share the information you have about the disease. Do not share any medication you are taking. Most antibiotics are effective only if you take the entire course prescribed for you.

- Encourage your partner to be tested if it is possible that he or she has become infected. This might

happen if you realize you have an STD after you and your partner begin a sexual relationship. Symptoms of some STDs don't appear for some time; other STDs don't have any visible symptoms at all.

- If your partner resists getting tested, emphasize that consequences can be very serious if an STD is left untreated.

- You can be reinfected with an STD after you have been treated if your partner isn't treated as well. Some STDs are passed back and forth between partners several times, sometimes becoming more resistant to treatment. Make sure you are both free of infection before you start or resume sexual activity.

If you have been exposed to an STD, take appropriate action (see the box "Tips for Telling a Partner You Have an STD").

- Minimize your use of antibiotics. Don't buy antibacterial soaps, try to avoid meat or poultry from animals that have been fed antibiotics, and don't take antibiotics for viral infections. When prescribed antibiotics for a bacterial infection, take them as directed and complete the full course of treatment.

- Practice the ABCDs of STD prevention and follow recommended screening guidelines. If you have been exposed to an STD or have symptoms, see your physician

for testing and treatment, and tell any sexual partners that they have been exposed so that they can be treated too.

- If you are planning a trip to a new part of the country or a new country, learn what infectious diseases are common in that location and how you can decrease your risk of infection while visiting or living there.

- Reduce the likelihood that new diseases will take hold in your community, such as by getting rid of any standing water in your yard where mosquitoes could breed.

Infectious diseases will always be part of human existence. By being vigilant, we can reduce their negative impact on our lives.

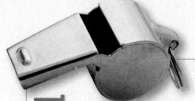

You Make the Call

Should Colleges Tighten Vaccination Requirements?

In November 2007 a student at the University of Southern Maine was diagnosed with mumps. Although mumps is usually mild, it occasionally has serious complications, and it is extremely contagious. At the time, USM students were required by state law to show proof that they had received one dose of measles-mumps-rubella (MMR) vaccine. Following the diagnosis, the requirement was changed to two doses of MMR vaccine. Students who could not show such proof or who did not comply with the requirement were not allowed on campus. The student with mumps was sent home for 9 days to reduce the risk of a widespread outbreak.

This case exemplifies the ethical dilemma frequently faced by society, in which individual freedom is pitted against the collective welfare of the community, or the "common good." College campuses are uniquely vulnerable to these issues. Colleges and universities are small communities of people living in close contact with each other, whether in residence halls, off-campus housing, classrooms, or shared eating facilities. In addition, students, faculty, and staff frequently travel around the world for recreation, academic research, and family opportunities. As such, they have an increased likelihood of exposure to infectious disease. Returning students, faculty, and staff can bring infections back to campus, where they may spread rapidly.

The University of Southern Maine implemented a relatively mild requirement—a second immunization. Some health experts have proposed stricter requirements in such situations, including the following:

- *Immunizations for a range of diseases could be required prior to entry onto campus.* Currently most colleges require one or two doses of MMR and recommend but do not require immunization for such diseases as meningococcal infection, varicella (chickenpox), pertussis (whooping cough), 2009 H1N1 influenza, and other childhood and adult infectious diseases. To increase "herd" immunity and reduce the risk of outbreaks, colleges could require immunization for all these diseases.

- *Travel to high-risk areas by students, faculty, and staff could be restricted.* Currently the CDC and the World Health Organization offer travel warnings, precautions, and news of outbreaks in the states and around the world; occasionally they recommend that travelers avoid certain areas or countries if an outbreak risk is high. Colleges could similarly limit or restrict travel.

- *Travelers returning from certain parts of the world could be prevented from entering campus for a certain period of time.* The CDC recommends that travelers returning from countries with outbreaks of new and emerging diseases monitor themselves for symptoms for 10 days prior to returning home or stay at home for 10 days after returning. Colleges could enforce this restriction on campus.

- *Individuals with infectious diseases could be quarantined.* This course of action has been proposed in the event of a pandemic flu outbreak. Colleges could house students, faculty, or staff in separate facilities for the duration of their illness so that the disease could be contained.

Each of these proposals has its advantages and its drawbacks. Some people think colleges and universities should tighten their restrictions to protect the community and promote the common good. Others see such restrictions as violations of personal freedom, if not civil rights. What do you think?

PROS

- Required vaccination reduces the risk of disease for the entire college community. When vaccination levels are high overall, even the few who aren't vaccinated are protected by herd immunity, because widespread vaccination shrinks the reservoir of infectious agents.

- College campuses are unique, tightly linked communities with a high risk of contagion should an infectious agent be introduced.

- Colleges have a responsibility to protect students and other community members from unnecessary risk. Requiring vaccination and taking other restrictive measures helps ensure health and safety for everyone.

CONS

- Individuals should have freedom of choice about health risks and what they do with their bodies. They should not have to take personal risks, such as those associated with vaccination, for the good of the community.

- Travel advisories by the CDC and the World Health Organization are usually issued as recommendations. Colleges do not have the right to enforce a different standard.

- Isolation and quarantine are difficult to enforce, and the threat of such treatment may discourage people from

seeking appropriate medical care. Thus, these measures could actually increase the risk of infectious disease outbreaks.

connect ACTIVITY

Source: "Mumps Confirmed on USM Campus," News Releases 2007–2008, University of Southern Maine, November 29, 2007; "Recommendations for Institutional Prematriculation Immunization," American College Health Association, 2009, retrieved May 4, 2010, from www.acha.org/topics/vaccine.cfm.

IN REVIEW

What causes infection, and how does the body protect itself from infectious diseases?

Several different types of pathogens cause infection and illness in humans, categorized as viruses, bacteria, prions, fungi, helminths, protozoa, and ectoparasites. Infection occurs when one of these microorganisms gains entry to the body and reproduces, sometimes causing symptoms of illness. The body has external barriers to keep pathogens out and a complex immune system to destroy them when they get in.

What changing patterns in infectious diseases are occurring?

Technological advances, like blood banks, organ transplants, and centralized food distribution, have created new opportunities for widespread disease transmission, as have global travel, changes in sexual behavior, injection drug use, and tattooing and piercing. Overuse of antibiotics has led to the appearance of resistant strains of many bacteria.

What are the most common infectious diseases?

Currently the top four infectious diseases worldwide are pneumonia, diarrhea, tuberculosis, and malaria. On college campuses in the United States, the top four are pertussis (whooping cough), mumps, *Staphylococcus aureus* skin infections, and urinary tract infections.

What are the most serious and most common sexually transmitted diseases?

HIV/AIDS is the most serious STD because it is fatal, although it is now possible, with medications, to live with HIV infection as a chronic condition for many years. The virus attacks and eventually overwhelms the immune system, leaving the body vulnerable to opportunistic infections like tuberculosis. The bacterial STDs, which include chlamydia, gonorrhea, pelvic inflammatory disease, syphilis, and bacterial vaginosis, can be treated with antibiotics. The viral STDs, which include human papillomavirus, genital herpes, and hepatitis A and B, can be controlled but not cured. Other STDs include trichomoniasis, candidiasis, and pubic lice and scabies.

How can infectious diseases be prevented?

The best defense is being in good health, so a healthy lifestyle is important. Getting all recommended vaccinations also helps, as do avoiding exposure, practicing safer sex, and minimizing unnecessary use of antibiotics.

Web Resources

CDC National Center for Infectious Diseases Traveler's Health: This comprehensive Web site offers information on safe food and water, tips on traveling with children, travelers with special needs, illness and injury abroad, cruises, and air travel. Its Travel Notices section is updated regularly for health warnings and precautions.
www.cdc.gov/travel

CDC National Prevention Information Network: This site focuses on prevention of HIV/AIDS, STDs, and tuberculosis.
www.cdcnpin.org

HIV InSite: Gateway to AIDS Knowledge: This organization looks at AIDS from a global perspective, offering research and news information about advances in knowledge about this disease, treatment approaches, and trends in the spread of the disease.
http://hivinsite.ucsf.edu

National Foundation for Infectious Diseases: Publications offered by NFID include immunization guides, clinical updates, reports on special populations, and a newsletter.
www.nfid.org

National Institute of Allergy and Infectious Diseases: This organization provides publications on AIDS, allergies, asthma, hepatitis, Lyme disease, SARS, and West Nile virus.
www.niaid.nih.gov

World Health Organization: Infectious Diseases: This site offers a comprehensive list of health topics that provide in-depth information on infectious diseases worldwide, including STDs.
www.who.int/health-topics/idindex.htm

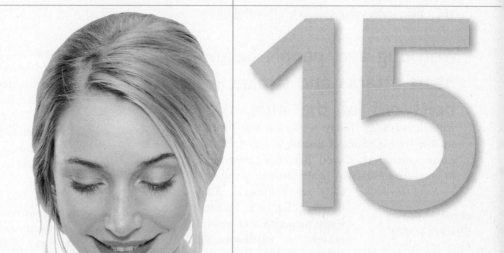

15

Cardiovascular Health

Ever Wonder...

- how anger and stress affect your heart?

- why it's bad to have high blood pressure?

- how to know if someone is having a heart attack—and what to do?

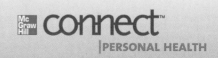

http://www.mcgrawhillconnect.com/personalhealth

Not long ago, people believed that heart attacks and strokes were like bolts out of the blue, happening without warning. Today we know that heart attacks and strokes are the result of disease processes that begin much earlier, often in childhood. Behavior patterns that contribute to good cardiovascular health include maintaining a physically active lifestyle, eating a heart-healthy diet, and avoiding tobacco. Early detection and treatment of precursors to **cardiovascular disease (CVD)**, such as high blood pressure, diabetes, and elevated cholesterol levels, can help people of all ages reduce the risk of developing this disease. This chapter presents an overview of CVD, along with guidelines for living a heart-healthy life.

cardiovascular disease (CVD)
Any disease involving the heart and/or blood vessels.

The Cardiovascular System

Basic knowledge of the **cardiovascular system** is necessary to understand the various forms of cardiovascular disease.

The cardiovascular system consists of a network of blood vessels (arteries, veins, and capillaries) and a pump (the heart) that circulate blood throughout the body. The heart is a fist-sized muscle with four chambers, the right and left atria and the right and left ventricles, separated from one another by valves.

The right side of the heart is involved in **pulmonary circulation**—pumping oxygen-poor blood to the lungs and oxygen-rich blood back to the heart. The left side of the heart is involved in **systemic circulation**—pumping oxygen-rich blood to the rest of the body and returning oxygen-poor blood to the heart (Figure 15.1).

In pulmonary circulation, oxygen-poor (or deoxygenated) blood returning from the body to the heart enters the right atrium via large veins called the inferior and superior **vena cava**. After the right atrium fills, it contracts and moves the blood into the right ventricle. The

cardiovascular system
The heart and blood vessels that circulate blood throughout the body.

pulmonary circulation
Pumping of oxygen-poor blood to the lungs and oxygen-rich blood back to the heart by the right side of the heart.

systemic circulation
Pumping of oxygen-rich blood to the body and oxygen-poor blood back to the heart by the left side of the heart.

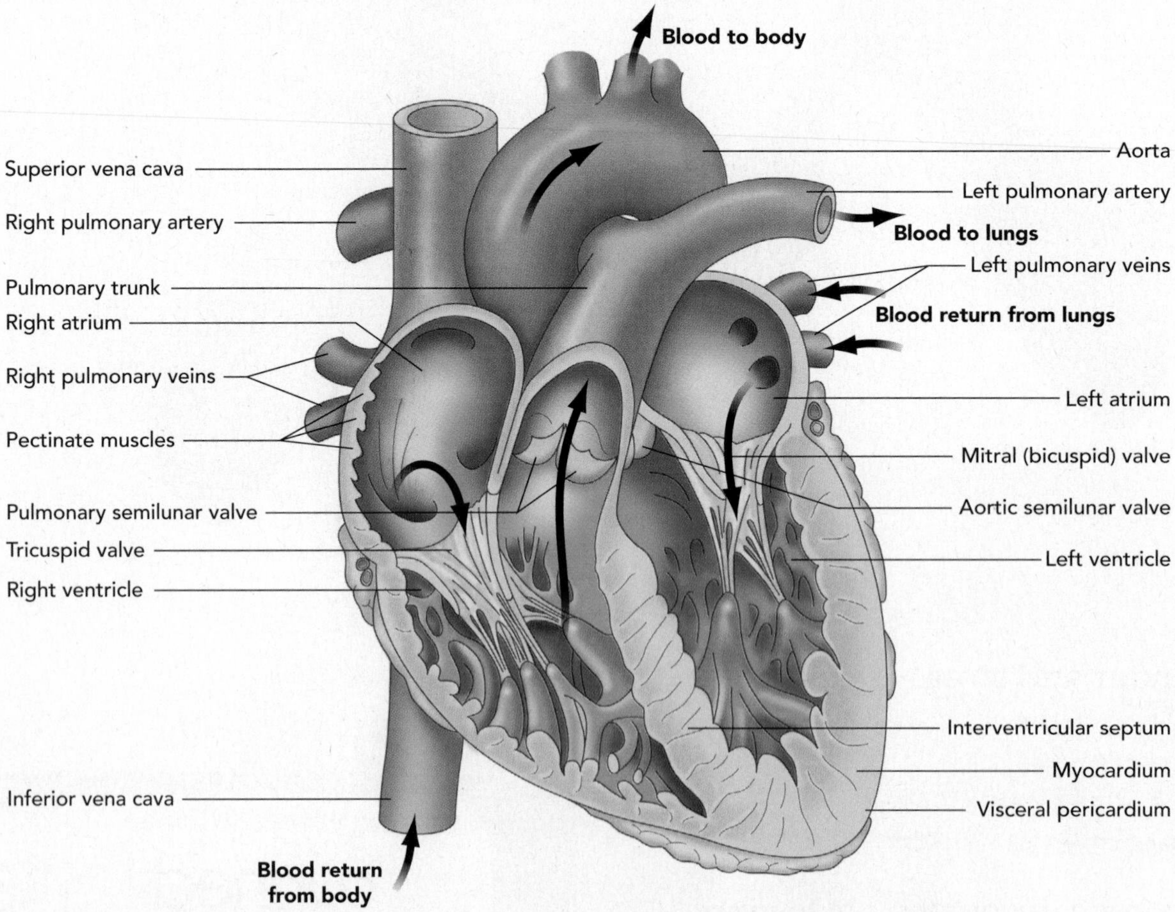

figure **15.1**   **The heart, showing interior chambers, valves, and major arteries and veins.**

vena cava
Largest veins in the body; they carry oxygen-poor blood from the body back to the heart.

aorta
Largest artery in the body; it leaves the heart and branches into smaller arteries, arterioles, and capillaries carrying oxygen-rich blood to body tissues.

coronary arteries
Medium-sized arteries that supply blood to the heart muscle.

right ventricle fills and contracts, moving the blood into the lungs via the right and left pulmonary arteries. The pulmonary artery branches into a network of smaller arteries and arterioles that eventually become the pulmonary capillaries. Capillaries are the smallest blood vessels; some capillary walls are only one cell thick, readily allowing the exchange of gases and molecules. In the interweaving network of capillaries, the red blood cells in the blood pick up oxygen and discard carbon dioxide, a waste product from the cells. The capillaries then unite and form venules, and venules join to become pulmonary veins. The pulmonary veins return oxygen-rich blood from the lungs to the left atrium of the heart.

In systemic circulation, the left atrium fills and contracts to move oxygen-rich blood into the left ventricle. The left ventricle fills, contracts, and moves oxygen-rich blood into the body via the **aorta**, the largest artery in the body. The aorta branches into smaller and smaller arteries, and

eventually, oxygen-rich, nutrient-rich blood enters the capillaries located throughout the body. At these sites, red blood cells release oxygen and nutrients to the tissues and pick up carbon dioxide to be carried back to the lungs. The capillaries unite to form veins and eventually connect to the inferior and superior vena cava, which returns the oxygen-poor blood to the heart. The cycle then repeats.

Like other muscles of the body, the heart needs oxygen and nutrients provided by blood; the blood being pumped through the heart does not provide nourishment for the heart muscle itself. Two medium-sized arteries, called **coronary arteries**, supply blood to the heart muscle. The main vessels are the right coronary artery and the left coronary artery, each distributing blood to different parts of the heart (Figure 15.2). Blood flow is important, because when a vessel is narrowed, the muscle that it supplies does not get enough blood.

The four chambers of the heart contract to pump blood in a coordinated fashion. The contraction occurs in response to an electrical signal that starts in a group of cells called the **sinus node** or **sinoatrial (SA) node** in the right atrium. The signal

sinus node or **sinoatrial (SA) node**
Group of cells in the right atrium where the electrical signal is generated that establishes the heartbeat.

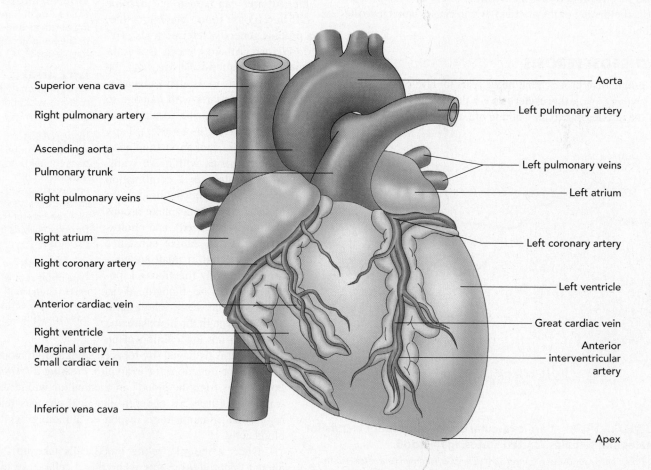

Superior vena cava — Aorta

Right pulmonary artery — Left pulmonary artery

Ascending aorta — Left pulmonary veins

Pulmonary trunk — Left atrium

Right pulmonary veins —

Right atrium — Left coronary artery

Right coronary artery — Left ventricle

Anterior cardiac vein — Great cardiac vein

Right ventricle — Anterior interventricular artery
Marginal artery —
Small cardiac vein —

Inferior vena cava —

Apex

figure **15.2** **Blood supply to the heart.** The heart muscle is supplied with oxygen and nutrients via the coronary arteries.

spreads through a defined course leading first to contraction of the right and left atria, then to contraction of the right and left ventricles. The contraction and relaxation of the ventricles are what we feel and hear as the heartbeat. The contraction phase is called *systole* and the relaxation phase is called *diastole*.

Cardiovascular Disease

The leading cause of death for men and women in the United States, cardiovascular disease (CVD) accounts for 34.3 percent of all deaths. Approximately 831,000 Americans die each year from various forms of this disease. Some good news can be seen in the fact that the death rate from CVD for men has decreased over the past 30 years and more recently for women (Figure 15.3). The drop in the death rate is believed to be the result of lifestyle changes, improved recognition and treatment of risk factors, and improved treatment of disease. The drop in death rate has been slower for women than for men, and some reasons for this are discussed later in the chapter.[1]

Cardiovascular disease is a general term that includes heart attack, stroke, peripheral artery disease, congestive heart failure, and other conditions (Figure 15.4). The disease process underlying many forms of CVD is atherosclerosis (hardening of the arteries), which causes damage to the blood vessels.

ATHEROSCLEROSIS

A progressive process that takes years to develop and starts at a young age, **atherosclerosis** is a thickening or hardening of the arteries due to the buildup of fats, cholesterol, cellular

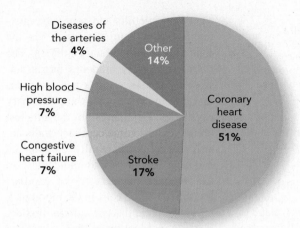

figure 15.4   **Percentage of deaths from types of CVD, United States, 2010.**

Source: "Heart Disease and Stroke Statistics—2010 Update," American Heart Association, 2010, Dallas: Author.

waste products, calcium, and other substances in artery walls. Autopsies of people aged 15 to 35 who died from unrelated trauma show that some young people already have the beginnings of significant atherosclerosis.[2]

Healthy arteries are strong and flexible. Arteries can harden and become stiff in response to too much pressure, a process generally referred to as *arteriosclerosis*. Atherosclerosis is a common form of arteriosclerosis, and the terms are often used interchangeably. Atherosclerosis starts with damage to the inner lining and the formation of a **fatty streak** in an artery. Fatty streaks consist of an accumulation of lipoproteins within the walls. A **lipoprotein** is a combination of proteins, phospholipids (fat molecules with phosphate groups chemically attached), and **cholesterol** (a waxy, fatlike substance that is essential in small amounts for certain body functions). Lipoproteins can be thought of as packages that carry cholesterol and fats through the bloodstream.

When the inner lining of an artery wall is damaged (by tobacco smoke, high blood pressure, or infection, for example), creating a *lesion*, lipoproteins from the blood can accumulate within the wall. Here, they can undergo chemical changes that trigger an inflammatory response, attracting white blood cells.

Once at the site, white blood cells take up the altered lipoproteins. Some white blood cells leave the site, cleaning lipids from the artery wall, but if blood

atherosclerosis
Thickening or hardening of the arteries due to the buildup of lipid (fat) deposits.

fatty streak
Accumulation of lipoproteins within the walls of an artery.

lipoprotein
Package of proteins, phospholipids (fat molecules with phosphate groups chemically attached), and cholesterol that transports lipids in the blood.

cholesterol
Type of fat that is essential in small amounts for certain body functions.

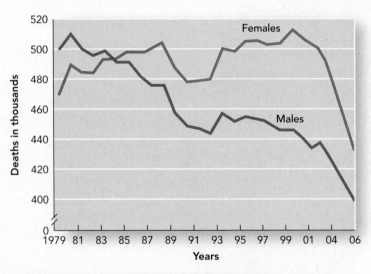

figure 15.3   **Cardiovascular disease mortality trends for males and females, United States, 1979–2006.**

Sources: Centers for Disease Control and Prevention/National Center for Health Statistics, www.cdc.gov/nchs; "Heart Disease and Stroke Statistics—2010 Update," American Heart Association, 2010, Dallas: Author.

lipoprotein levels are high, more lipoproteins continue to accumulate. Many of the white blood cells die within the lesion, forming a core of lipid-rich material—a fatty streak.

The process may stop at this point, leaving a dynamic lesion that can still undergo repair, or may develop further in the artery wall. Together with the white blood cells, smooth muscle cells release collagen and other proteins to form a **plaque**, an accumulation of debris that undergoes continuing damage, bleeding, and calcification. Plaques cause the artery wall to enlarge and bulge into the *lumen*, the channel through which the blood flows, slowing blood flow and reducing the amount of blood that can reach the tissue supplied by the artery. Plaques can also break off and completely block the artery, preventing any blood from flowing through (Figure 15.5).

Heart attacks, strokes, and peripheral vascular disease are all consequences of the narrowing of arteries caused by atherosclerosis. A diagnosis of one of these diseases suggests risk for the others. Atherosclerosis may also weaken an artery wall, causing a stretching of the artery known as an **aneurysm**. Aneurysms can rupture, tear, and bleed, causing sudden death.

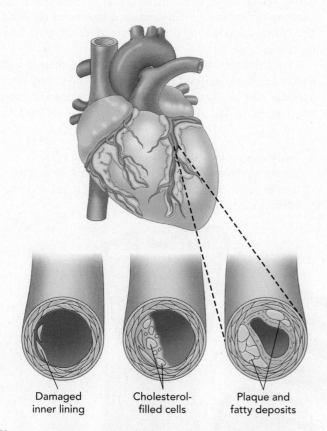

figure 15.5 **The process of atherosclerosis.** The process begins with damage to the lining of an artery and progresses to narrowing or blockage of the artery by fatty deposits and plaques.

Damaged inner lining

Cholesterol-filled cells

Plaque and fatty deposits

CORONARY HEART DISEASE

When atherosclerosis involves a coronary artery, the result is **coronary heart disease (CHD)** and, often, a heart attack. Coronary heart disease (also called coronary artery disease) is the leading form of CVD. An estimated 17.6 million Americans are living with CHD. Those who survive a heart attack are often left with damaged hearts and significantly altered lives.

Heart Attack and Angina   When a coronary artery becomes narrowed or blocked, the heart muscle does not get enough oxygen-rich blood, a condition called **ischemia**. If the artery is completely blocked, the person has a heart attack, or **myocardial infarction (MI)**. The blockage may be caused by an atherosclerotic plaque that has broken loose or a blood clot (a *thrombus*) that has formed in a narrowed or damaged artery. The latter condition is called a **coronary thrombosis** and may cause sudden death. During a heart attack, the area of muscle supplied by the blocked coronary artery is completely deprived of oxygen. If blood flow is not quickly restored, that part of the heart muscle will die.

The severity of a heart attack is determined by the location and duration of the blockage. If the blockage occurs close to the aorta where the coronary arteries are just starting to branch, a large area of heart muscle is deprived of oxygen. If the blockage is farther out in a smaller coronary artery, the area of muscle supplied is smaller. The duration of the blockage is usually determined by the time between onset of symptoms and initiation of medical or surgical treatment to reopen the artery. Duration is directly dependent on how quickly a person recognizes the symptoms of a myocardial infarction and gets help.

A heart attack may occur when extra work is demanded of the heart, such as during exercise or emotional stress, or it may occur during light activity or even rest. A classic symptom of a heart attack is chest pain, often described as a sensation of pressure, fullness, or squeezing in the midportion of the chest. However, symptoms vary, and 37 percent of women and 27 percent of men typically do not have chest pain or discomfort during a heart attack. The American Heart Association does not list different symptoms of presentation for men and women—both can have a range of symptoms, including pain radiating to the jaw, back, shoulders, or arms (see the box "Signs of a Heart Attack"). However, women

plaque
Accumulation of debris in an artery wall, consisting of lipoproteins, white blood cells, collagen, and other substances.

aneurysm
Weak or stretched spot in an artery wall that can tear or rupture, causing sudden death.

coronary heart disease (CHD)
Atherosclerosis of the coronary arteries.

ischemia
Insufficient supply of oxygen and nutrients to tissue, caused by narrowed or blocked arteries.

myocardial infarction (MI)
Lack of blood to the heart muscle with resulting death of heart tissue; often called a heart attack.

coronary thrombosis
Blockage of a coronary artery by a blood clot that may cause sudden death.

Highlight on Health

Signs of a Heart Attack

Recognizing the signs of a heart attack and getting treatment quickly are critical to survival. Although symptoms may vary, the following signs may indicate that a heart attack is occurring:

■ *Chest discomfort.* Most heart attacks involve discomfort in the center of the chest that lasts more than a few minutes, or that goes away and comes back. It can feel like uncomfortable pressure, squeezing, fullness, or pain.

■ *Discomfort in other areas of the upper body.* Symptoms can include pain or discomfort in one or both arms, the back, neck, jaw, or stomach.

■ *Shortness of breath.* May occur with or without chest discomfort.

■ *Other signs.* These may include breaking out in a cold sweat, nausea, light-headedness, weakness, or faintness.

Note: For both men and women, chest pain or discomfort is the most common symptom of heart attack. However, women are more likely than men to experience middle or upper back pain, neck pain, jaw pain, shortness of breath, nausea or vomiting, weakness or fatigue, insomnia, or loss of appetite as their presenting symptoms. Women are less likely than men to believe they are having a heart attack and more likely to delay seeking treatment.

If you or someone you are with experiences one or more of these signs, seek emergency medical treatment by calling 911 immediately.

Sources: American Heart Association, www.americanheart .org; "Symptom Presentation in Women with Acute Coronary Syndromes: Myth vs. Reality," by J.G. Canto, R.J. Goldberg, M.M. Hand, et al., 2007, Archives of Internal Medicine, 167 (22), pp. 2405–2413.

attacks are preceded by angina. The difference between a heart attack and angina is that the pain of angina resolves, whereas the pain of a heart attack continues. Angina can be controlled with medical treatment.

Many physical conditions can cause pain in the chest, including irritated esophagus, arthritis of the neck or ribs, gas in the colon, stomach ulcers, and gallbladder disease. Chest pain can also be caused by weight lifting or other heavy lifting or vigorous activity. If you are used to chest pain from any of these causes, you may be inclined to ignore angina or chest pain from a heart attack. Don't let complaisance or confusion delay your efforts to seek help if you experience the signs of a heart attack.

angina
Intermittent pain, pressure, heaviness, or tightness in the center of the chest caused by a narrowed coronary artery.

arrhythmia
Irregular or disorganized heartbeat.

Arrhythmias   The pumping of the heart is usually a well-coordinated event, controlled by an electrical signal emanating from the sinus node in the right atrium, as described earlier. The sinus node establishes a rate of 60 to 100 beats per minute for a normal adult heart. The rate increases in response to increased demand on the heart, such as during exercise, and slows in response to reduced demand, such as during relaxation or sleep. If the signal is disrupted, it can cause an **arrhythmia**, or disorganized beating of the heart. The disorganized beating is usually not as effective at pumping blood.

An arrhythmia is any type of irregular heartbeat. It may be an occasional skipped beat, a rapid or slow rate, or an irregular pattern. Not all arrhythmias are serious or cause for concern. In fact, most people have occasional irregular

■ Automated external defibrillators can be used by the general public and thus decrease the time that it takes to provide defibrillation to someone in cardiac arrest. A variety of models are shown here.

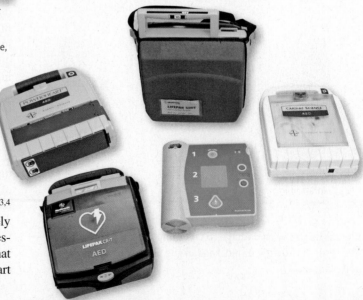

may be less likely to have classic symptoms of a heart attack. They may also be less aware that heart disease is a major health concern and thus less likely to seek help for their symptoms. Although awareness has increased over the past decade, only 54 percent of women are aware that heart disease is the leading cause of death for women, and only 53 percent of women say they would call an ambulance if they were having heart attack symptoms.[1,3,4]

When coronary arteries are narrowed but not completely blocked, the person may experience **angina**—pain, pressure, heaviness, or tightness in the center of the chest that may radiate to the neck, arms, or shoulders. Half of all heart heartbeats every day; some people do not even notice them. However, arrhythmia may cause noticeable symptoms, including palpitations, a sensation of fluttering in the chest, chest pain, light-headedness, shortness of breath, and fatigue.

Arrhythmias occur for a variety of reasons, including damage to the sinus node, chemical imbalances, or the use of caffeine, alcohol, tobacco, cocaine, or medications.

Sudden Cardiac Death **Ventricular fibrillation** is a particular type of arrhythmia in which the ventricles contract rapidly and erratically, causing the heart to quiver or "tremor" rather than beat. Blood cannot be pumped by the heart when the ventricles fibrillate. The result is **sudden cardiac death**—an abrupt loss of heart function. An estimated 7,000 to 14,000 infants and children die each year from sudden cardiac death, and sudden cardiac death is the leading cause of death in high school and college athletes, with an estimated incidence at 1 in 200,000 athletes (see Chapter 2 for a discussion of the genetic contributing factors). Vigorous exercise can be a trigger for lethal arrhythmia when an underlying heart abnormality is present. Under age 35, sudden cardiac death is usually due to congenital cardiac abnormalities. Over age 35, the cause is usually coronary artery disease.

Ventricular fibrillation can be reversed with an electrical shock from a defibrillator, which can restart the heart's normal rhythm. Automated external defibrillators (AEDs) are beginning to show up in public places like gyms and airports. AEDs are designed for use by the general public,

ideally by people who have received training at a CPR, first-aid, or first-responder class. Every minute counts, however: The chances of survival are reduced by 8–10 percent for every minute following cardiac arrest. About 310,000 Americans die each year from sudden cardiac death in emergency rooms or prior to reaching the hospital. Response to sudden cardiac death provides an example of how communities must work together to improve health.

STROKE

When blood flow to the brain or part of the brain is blocked, the result is a **stroke**, or **cerebrovascular accident (CVA)**. Stroke is the third-leading cause of death in the United States, after heart disease and cancer, and is a leading cause of severe, long-term disability.

Ischemic strokes account for 87 percent of all strokes and occur when an artery in the brain becomes blocked, in the same way that a heart attack occurs when a coronary artery is blocked, and prevents the brain from receiving blood flow (Figure 15.6). The blockage

ventricular fibrillation
Type of arrhythmia in which the ventricles contract rapidly and erratically, causing the heart to quiver or "tremor" rather than beat.

sudden cardiac death
Abrupt loss of heart function caused by an irregular or ineffective heartbeat.

stroke, or **cerebrovascular accident (CVA)**
Lack of blood flow to the brain with resulting death of brain tissue.

ischemic strokes
Strokes caused by blockage in a blood vessel in the brain.

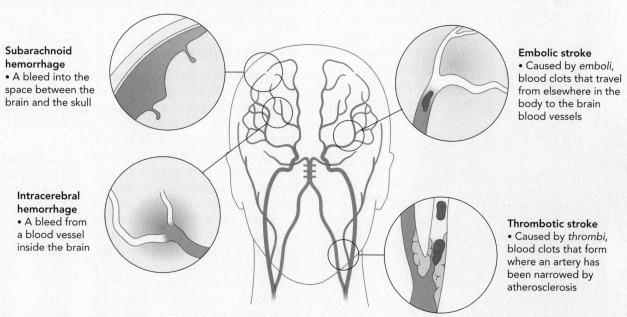

Hemorrhagic stroke
• Caused by ruptured blood vessels followed by blood leaking into tissue; more serious than ischemic stroke

Ischemic stroke
• Caused by blockage in brain blood vessels; potentially treatable with clot-busting drugs

Subarachnoid hemorrhage
• A bleed into the space between the brain and the skull

Embolic stroke
• Caused by *emboli,* blood clots that travel from elsewhere in the body to the brain blood vessels

Intracerebral hemorrhage
• A bleed from a blood vessel inside the brain

Thrombotic stroke
• Caused by *thrombi,* blood clots that form where an artery has been narrowed by atherosclerosis

figure **15.6** **Types of stroke.**

Source: Reprinted with permission from the Harvard Health Letter, April 2000. Copyright © Harvard University. For more information visit www.health .harvard.edu. Harvard Health Publications does not endorse any products or medical procedures.

thrombus
Blood clot that forms in a narrowed or damaged artery.

embolism
Blood clot that travels from elsewhere in the body.

hemorrhagic strokes
Strokes caused by rupture of a blood vessel in the brain, with bleeding into brain tissue.

can be due to a **thrombus** (a blood clot that develops in a narrowed artery) or an **embolism** (a clot that develops elsewhere, often in the heart, travels to the brain, and lodges in an artery).

Hemorrhagic strokes make up 13 percent of strokes and occur when a brain artery ruptures, bleeds into the surrounding area, and compresses brain tissue. There are two types of hemorrhagic stroke. *Intracerebral hemorrhagic* strokes account for 10 percent and occur when the ruptured artery is within brain tissue. *Subarachnoid hemorrhagic* strokes account for 3 percent and occur when the ruptured artery is on the brain's surface and blood accumulates between the brain and the skull. Hemorrhagic strokes may be due to a head injury or a ruptured aneurysm.[1]

As with the heart, different arteries supply different areas of the brain. Strokes may have a variety of symptoms, depending on the area of the brain involved. However, symptoms usually involve the sudden onset of neurological problems, such as headaches, numbness, weakness, or speech problems (see the box "Signs of a Stroke").

Table 15.1   Blood Pressure Guidelines

Category	Systolic	Diastolic
Normal	Less than 120 *and*	Less than 80
Prehypertension	120–139 *or*	80–89
Hypertension Stage 1 Stage 2	 140–159 *or* 160 and above *or*	 90–99 100 and above

Source: "The Seventh Report of the Joint National Committee on Prevention, Detection, Evaluation and Treatment of High Blood Pressure" (NIH Publication No. 03-5233), 2003, Bethesda, MD: National Heart, Lung, and Blood Institute, National Institutes of Health.

A small percentage of people have **transient ischemic attacks (TIAs)** before having a stroke. Sometimes called "ministrokes," TIAs are periods of ischemia that produce the same symptoms as a stroke, but in this case the symptoms resolve within 24 hours with little or no tissue death. A TIA should be viewed as a warning sign of stroke. After a TIA, 3–17 percent of people will have a stroke within the next 90 days. Early recognition and rapid treatment are as important for TIA and stroke as they are for heart disease. Treatment

Untreated high blood pressure can weaken and scar the arteries and makes the heart work harder, weakening it as well.

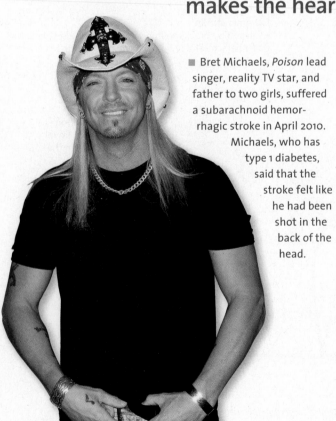

■ Bret Michaels, *Poison* lead singer, reality TV star, and father to two girls, suffered a subarachnoid hemorrhagic stroke in April 2010. Michaels, who has type 1 diabetes, said that the stroke felt like he had been shot in the back of the head.

can improve survival and reduce complications but must be given quickly.

HYPERTENSION

Blood pressure is the pressure exerted by blood against the walls of arteries, and high blood pressure, or **hypertension**, occurs when the pressure is great enough to damage artery walls. Untreated high blood pressure can weaken and scar the arteries and makes the heart work harder, weakening it as well. Hypertension can cause heart attacks, strokes, kidney disease, peripheral artery disease, and blindness.[1,5]

Blood pressure is determined by two forces—the pressure produced by the heart as it pumps the blood and the resistance of the arteries as they contain blood flow. When arteries are hardened by atherosclerosis, they are more resistant. Blood pressure is measured in millimeters of mercury and stated in two numbers, such as 120/80 mm Hg. The upper number represents

transient ischemic attacks (TIA)
Periods of ischemia that temporarily produce the same symptoms as a stroke.

blood pressure
Force exerted by the blood against artery walls.

hypertension
Blood pressure that is forceful enough to damage artery walls.

Signs of a Stroke

Neurological problems that have a sudden onset and are unremitting, especially if they involve only one side of the body, may be signs that a stroke is occurring or has occurred. Although some of the following symptoms may occur with other illnesses, such as migraine headache, the more symptoms there are, and the more severe they are, the more likely they are to be the result of a stroke.

- Sudden numbness or weakness of the face, arm, or leg, especially on one side of the body.
- Sudden confusion, trouble speaking or understanding.
- Sudden trouble seeing in one or both eyes.
- Sudden trouble walking, dizziness, loss of balance or coordination.
- Sudden, severe headache with no known cause.

If you or someone you are with experiences one or more of these symptoms, seek emergency medical treatment by calling 911 immediately. Remember the acronym FAST:

- Facial numbness or weakness
- Arm numbness or weakness
- Slurred speech
- Time to call 911

Source: Adapted from American Stroke Association, www.stroke.org.

systolic pressure, the pressure produced when the heart contracts; the lower number represents **diastolic pressure**, the pressure in the arteries when the heart is relaxed, between contractions. There is no definite line dividing normal blood pressure from high blood pressure, but categories have been established as guidelines on the basis of increased risk for CVD; see Table 15.1.

Prehypertension is a category of blood pressure measurement higher than recommended but not meeting criteria for hypertension; the category has been identified to target people at high risk of developing hypertension. An estimated 28 percent of the U.S. population aged 18 and older have prehypertension. Blood pressure in this range should prompt aggressive lifestyle change and increased monitoring to reduce future risk.

Hypertension is often referred to as the "silent killer," because it usually causes no symptoms. More than 74 million people in the United States (nearly one in three adults) and more than 1 billion people worldwide are estimated to have high blood pressure. Although people are becoming more aware of this condition, 22 percent of people with high blood pressure do not know they have it.[1,5]

In approximately 95 percent of cases, the cause of hypertension is unknown. In Western societies, aging seems to be a factor, but this is not the case in other cultures. Genetics plays a role in some cases. Racial differences exist, with Blacks having the highest rates. Other factors that contribute to elevated blood pressure include high salt consumption, use of alcohol, low potassium levels, physical inactivity, and obesity (see the box "Reducing Sodium: Beyond Individual Action"). Less frequently, medical conditions can cause hypertension. Women can develop hypertension during pregnancy or while taking oral contraceptive pills. Among children and adolescents rates of hypertension are increasing. The trend appears to be following the rising rates of obesity within these age groups.[1]

systolic pressure Pressure in the arteries when the heart contracts, represented by the upper number in a blood pressure measurement.

diastolic pressure Pressure in the arteries when the heart relaxes between contractions, represented by the lower number in a blood pressure measurement.

congestive heart failure Condition in which the heart is not pumping the blood as well as it should, allowing blood and fluids to back up in the lungs.

CONGESTIVE HEART FAILURE

When the heart is not pumping the blood as well as it should, a condition known as **congestive heart failure** occurs. It can develop after a heart attack or as a result of hypertension, heart valve abnormality, or disease of the heart muscle. When the heart cannot keep up its regular pumping force or rate, blood backs up into the lungs, and fluid from the backed-up blood in the pulmonary veins leaks into the lungs. A person with congestive heart failure experiences difficulty breathing, shortness of breath, and coughing, especially when lying down. Blood returning to the heart from the body also gets backed up, causing swelling of the lower legs. When blood fails to reach the brain efficiently, fatigue and confusion can result.

Approximately 5.3 million Americans live with congestive heart failure.[1] Symptoms can be treated with medications that help draw off extra fluid, decrease blood pressure, and improve the heart's ability to pump. Other factors that contribute to the development of congestive heart failure include cigarette smoking, high cholesterol, and diabetes. Lifestyle changes such as weight loss, exercise, and smoking cessation can reduce symptoms and the risk of disease progression.

OTHER CARDIOVASCULAR DISEASES

Other conditions can affect the structure of the heart and blood vessels and their ability to function. Some of these

Reducing Sodium: Beyond Individual Action

Consuming too much sodium can lead to cardiovascular problems like hypertension, heart disease, and stroke. Yet salt shows up in our foods more than we realize, and sometimes in ways we can't control. Even sodium-savvy consumers who try to limit their sodium intake when eating out are often thwarted by menus where almost all the food has high levels of sodium. At Olive Garden, for example, only one of its 16 dinner pastas has fewer than 1,000 milligrams of sodium. Even a serving of Garden Fresh Salad without salad dressing has 550 milligrams of sodium. (The 2010 Dietary Guidelines Advisory Committee Report and the American Heart Association recommend no more than 1,500 mg—about half a teaspoon—per day for everyone.)

Another problem is that we have become accustomed to salty foods—we prefer them over foods with less sodium. While individuals should monitor and seek to limit their own sodium intake, the U.S. Congress, along with a number of public health organizations, has recognized that the challenge of lowering sodium consumption goes beyond individual behavior.

Thus, in 2008 Congress asked the Institute of Medicine (IOM) to develop strategies for reducing Americans' sodium intakes. Projections are that lowering population-wide consumption of sodium would prevent 100,000 deaths a year. In 2010, the IOM returned to Congress with a report that outlined measures that would gradually reduce the levels of sodium in our food, allowing people's tastes to become accustomed to lower levels of sodium without their realizing it or feeling "deprived."

The report called on the FDA to set mandatory standards for sodium content in processed and restaurant/food service foods. In the past, companies have not taken these measures on their own out of fear that customers would switch to other brands that had the high levels of sodium they preferred. With the FDA setting the standards and implementing them across the board, no manufacturer would be at a disadvantage for lowering sodium content. Following the release of the 2010 Dietary Guidelines Advisory Committee Report, which lowered the 2005 sodium recommendation from 2,300 mg to 1,500 mg for the general population, some food manufacturers announced that they would begin to reduce the sodium content in their foods.

The ultimate goal of the IOM's report is for Americans to consume healthy levels of sodium and for their preferences to gradually change to less salty foods. Reflecting on the current status of sodium consumption in the United States, the IOM's conclusion was that in light of the health risks posed by excessive sodium consumption, "the current level of sodium in the food supply [. . .] is too high to be 'safe.' Without major change, hypertension and cardiovascular disease rates will continue to rise, and consumers, who have little choice, will pay the price for inaction."

connect ACTIVITY

Sources: "Strategies to Reduce Sodium Intake in the United States," Institute of Medicine, 2010, Washington, DC: The National Academies Press; "Nutrition Information," Darden Restaurants, Inc., www.olivegarden.com.

conditions are congenital (present from birth), and others occur as progressive diseases.

Heart Valve Disorders Four valves in the heart keep blood flowing in the correct direction through the heart (see Figure 15.1). A normally functioning valve opens easily to allow blood to flow forward and closes tightly to prevent blood from flowing backward. Sometimes a valve does not open well, preventing the smooth flow of blood, and sometimes a valve does not close tightly, allowing blood to leak backward.

These problems can be caused by congenital abnormalities, rheumatic heart disease, or an aging-related degeneration process. When valves are not functioning normally, the flow of blood is altered and the risks of blood clots and infection increase. Often, the person experiences no symptoms; if symptoms do occur, they can include shortness of breath, dizziness, fatigue, and chest pain.

mitral valve prolapse
Heart valve disorder in which the mitral valve, which separates the left ventricle from the left atrium, does not close fully, allowing blood to leak backward into the atrium.

The most common heart valve defect is **mitral valve prolapse** (the mitral valve separates the left atrium from the left ventricle). In this condition, the mitral valve billows backward and the edges do not fully close when the left ventricle contracts to move blood into the aorta, allowing blood to leak backward into the atrium (Figure 15.7). Mitral valve prolapse is common, affecting 5–10 percent of the population. With certain types of mitral valve prolapse, individuals should take antibiotics before dental surgery and other procedures to reduce the risk of infection from bacteria introduced into the bloodstream by the procedure.

Rheumatic Heart Disease A common cause of heart valve disorders and other heart damage is **rheumatic fever**, leading to **rheumatic heart disease**. In this

hot tip
Many grocery stores and drugstores have do-it-yourself machines that check your blood pressure. Get your blood pressure checked the next time you see one.

rheumatic fever
Acute disease that can occur as a complication of an untreated strep throat infection.

rheumatic heart disease
Disease in which the heart is scarred following strep throat infection and rheumatic fever.

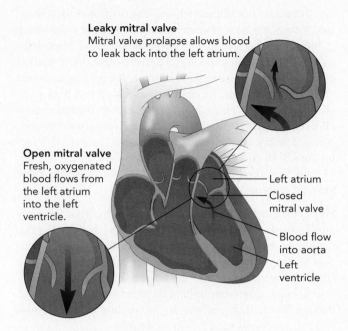

Leaky mitral valve
Mitral valve prolapse allows blood to leak back into the left atrium.

Open mitral valve
Fresh, oxygenated blood flows from the left atrium into the left ventricle.

Left atrium
Closed mitral valve
Blood flow into aorta
Left ventricle

figure **15.7** **Mitral valve prolapse.**

disease, the heart is scarred following an infection with a strain of streptococcus bacteria (usually as strep throat). Symptoms of rheumatic fever include fever, joint pain, fatigue, and rash; when the heart is affected, there can be congestive heart failure, valve dysfunction, or arrhythmia. Acute rheumatic fever can occur 2 to 3 weeks after a strep throat infection (although almost one in three people do not have a sore throat) and last weeks to months.

The condition is prevented by treating strep throat infections with antibiotics. Rheumatic fever often occurs in children, and worldwide it is a major cause of heart disorders. The incidence of rheumatic heart disease has declined significantly in developed countries, partly as a result of aggressive diagnosis and treatment of strep throat.

Congenital Heart Disease   A variety of structural defects that are present at birth can involve the heart valves, major arteries and veins in or near the heart, or the heart muscle. An abnormality can cause the blood to slow down, flow in the wrong direction, or not move from one chamber to the next. Undetected cardiac abnormalities are the leading cause of death in competitive athletes.

More than 35 types of heart defects have been described. One of the more common defects is a **septal defect**, in which an extra hole in the heart allows blood to flow from one atrium to the other or from one ventricle to the other. When a septal defect is present, poorly oxygenated blood from the body mixes with oxygenated blood from the lungs, resulting in lower oxygen supply to the body.[6]

Peripheral Vascular Disease   The result of atherosclerosis in the arteries of the arms or legs (more commonly, the legs), **peripheral vascular disease (PVD)** causes pain,

aches, or cramping in the muscles supplied by a narrowed blood vessel. Although it is usually not fatal, PVD causes a significant amount of disability, limiting the activity level of many older people because of pain with walking. If circulation is severely limited by the ischemia, the affected leg or arm may have to be amputated.

It is a clue to advanced atherosclerosis and indicates the need for lifestyle change or medical treatment in order to reduce the risk of heart attack or stroke. High levels of daily physical activity are associated with better survival and lower risk of death. Anyone who experiences unexplained pain in the legs or arms, especially if it is associated with exercise, should see a health care provider.[1]

Cardiomyopathy   Deaths from **cardiomyopathy**—disease of the heart muscle—account for 1 percent of heart disease deaths in the United States, with the highest rates occurring among men and Blacks. The most common form of cardiomyopathy is *dilated cardiomyopathy*, an enlargement of the heart in response to weakening of the muscle. The cause is often unknown, although a virus is suspected in some cases. Other factors that can weaken the heart muscle are toxins (alcohol, tobacco, heavy metals, and some medications), drugs, pregnancy, hypertension, and coronary artery disease.

Another form is **hypertrophic cardiomyopathy**, an abnormal thickening of one part of the heart, frequently the left ventricle. The thickened wall makes the heart abnormally stiff, so the heart doesn't fill well. Although most people with hypertrophic cardiomyopathy have no symptoms, the condition can cause heart failure, arrhythmia, and sudden death. In fact, 36 percent of cases of sudden death in young competitive athletes are due to hypertrophic cardiomyopathy. The cause of the condition is unknown in about 50 percent of cases, but in the rest, there is a genetic link.[7]

septal defect
Congenital heart defect in which an extra hole allows blood to flow from one atrium to the other or from one ventricle to the other.

peripheral vascular disease (PVD)
Atherosclerosis in the blood vessels of the arms or legs.

cardiomyopathy
Disease of the heart muscle.

hypertrophic cardiomyopathy
Abnormal thickening of one part of the heart, frequently the left ventricle.

Risk Factors for CVD

As discussed in Chapter 2, cardiovascular disease is a multifactorial disease, the result of genetic, environmental, and lifestyle factors interacting over time. Some factors are controllable, while others are not. Worldwide, nine risk factors account for more than 90 percent of the risk for initial heart attack: cigarette smoking, abnormal lipid levels, hypertension, diabetes, abdominal obesity, lack of physical activity, low daily fruit and vegetable intake, excessive alcohol intake, and psychosocial stress. This holds true for men and women and for different ethnic groups.[8,9]

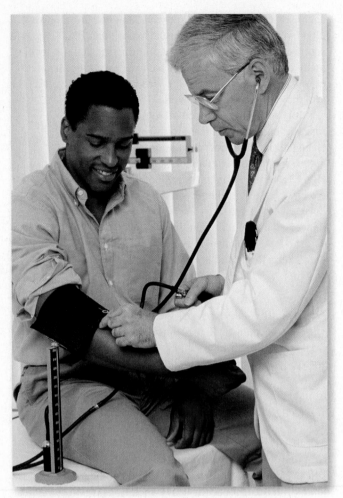

■ African Americans have higher rates of hypertension than the rest of the population, probably due to a combination of genetic, sociocultural, and behavioral factors. Regular screening can help keep blood pressure under control.

MAJOR CONTROLLABLE RISK FACTORS IN CVD

Controllable risk factors are factors associated with CVD that can be altered through individual behavior or community intervention. Given that cardiovascular disease develops gradually, you are never too young to start paying attention to these factors. The American Heart Association lists six major controllable risk factors: tobacco use, hypertension, unhealthy blood cholesterol levels, physical inactivity, overweight and obesity, and diabetes. Ninety percent of persons with heart disease will have at least one of these risk factors.[1]

Tobacco Use   Tobacco use is the leading risk factor for all forms of CVD. Cigarette smokers develop coronary artery disease at two to four times the rate of nonsmokers and have twice the risk of sudden cardiac death as nonsmokers. Cigar and pipe smoking are also associated with an increased risk of coronary artery disease and perhaps an increased risk of stroke, although not as great an increase as with cigarettes.

Tobacco smoke functions in a variety of ways to increase risk. Components of tobacco smoke damage the inner lining of blood vessels, speeding up the development of atherosclerosis. Toxins in tobacco smoke can stimulate the formation of blood clots in the coronary arteries and trigger spasms that close off the vessels. Smoking raises blood levels of LDL cholesterol ("bad" cholesterol) and decreases blood levels of HDL cholesterol ("good" cholesterol). Exposure to environmental tobacco smoke (secondhand smoke) is also a risk factor for CVD; risk appears to be proportional to the amount of daily exposure. The risk for CVD decreases within a few years of quitting smoking.[10]

Hypertension   Hypertension increases the risk for heart attack, stroke, congestive heart failure, and kidney disease; the higher the blood pressure, the greater the risk. Hypertension makes the heart work harder to circulate the blood. The increased work may cause the heart to enlarge, which may lead to congestive heart failure. Hypertension can also cause damage to the lining of arteries, promoting atherosclerosis and causing blood vessel walls to weaken.

There are significant differences in the prevalence of high blood pressure across different minority populations. In Blacks, hypertension not only is more common, but also appears to follow a different course than it does in other groups. It develops earlier, is more severe, and is associated with more complications, such as heart attacks, stroke, and kidney failure. Blacks tend to excrete sodium (salt) at a slower rate than Whites do, possibly making them more sensitive to dietary salt. This difference may contribute to the higher rate of stroke among Blacks. To date, there has not been a clear genetic explanation for the ethnic differences. Socioeconomic and behavioral factors may be involved as well, as discussed later in the chapter.[11]

Unhealthy Cholesterol Levels   Cholesterol is a waxy, fat-like substance essential to the body; it is used in cell membranes, in some hormones, in brain and nerve tissue, and in bile acids that help digest fats. The amount of cholesterol in your body is affected by what you eat and by how fast your body makes and gets rid of cholesterol. Because it is fat-like, cholesterol cannot circulate in the blood in a free-floating state; instead, it is combined with proteins and other molecules in packages called *lipoproteins*.

Lipoproteins are spherical and smaller than red blood cells; they are categorized into five main classes according to density, with each class playing a different role in the body. The categories that have received the most study are total cholesterol and the LDL and HDL subcategories. Levels of total cholesterol are directly related to frequency of coronary heart disease; that is, as cholesterol levels rise, so does the incidence of heart disease (Table 15.2). Nearly half of the adult U.S. population have total cholesterol greater than 200 mg/dl. Among youth aged 12 to 17 years, one in five has at least one abnormal cholesterol level. Rates in overweight or obese youth are even higher.[12]

Table 15.2 Cholesterol Guidelines

Total cholesterol (mg/dl)	
Less than 200	Desirable
200–239	Borderline high
240 or greater	High
LDL cholesterol (mg/dl)	
Less than 100*	Optimal
100–129	Near or above optimal
130–159	Borderline high
160–189	High
190 or greater	Very high
HDL cholesterol (mg/dl)	
Less than 40	Low (undesirable)
60 or greater	High (desirable)
Triglycerides (mg/dl)	
Less than 150	Normal
150–199	Borderline high
200–499	High
500 or greater	Very high

*Achieving a goal of less than 70 is an option if there is a high risk for heart disease.

Source: "Executive Summary of the Third Report of the National Cholesterol Education Program Expert Panel on Detection, Evaluation, and Treatment of High Blood Cholesterol in Adults," 2001, by Journal of the American Medical Association, 285 (19), pp. 2486–2497.

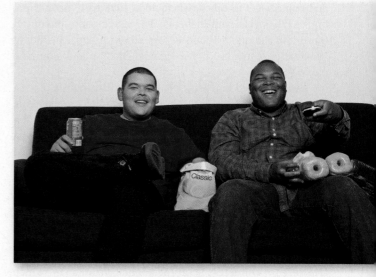

■ Physical inactivity and obesity are two of the major controllable risk factors for cardiovascular disease.

Low-density lipoproteins (LDLs)—"bad" cholesterol—are clearly associated with atherosclerosis. The higher the level of LDLs, the higher the risk of atherosclerosis. Lowering LDL cholesterol through dietary change, exercise, and medication reduces risk. Goals for LDL levels (in mg/dl) are influenced by the number of other risk factors for coronary artery disease a person has (for example, tobacco use, hypertension, older age):[13,14]

■ No risk factors or one other risk factor: <160

■ Two risk factors: <130

■ Already have heart disease or diabetes: <100

■ Very high risk (for example, recent heart attack): <70

High-density lipoproteins (HDLs)—"good" cholesterol—consist mainly of protein and are the smallest of the lipoprotein particles. HDLs help clear cholesterol from cells and atherosclerotic deposits and transport it back to the liver for recycling. High HDL levels provide protection from CVD.

HDL levels are determined mainly by genetics, but they are influenced by exercise, alcohol, and estrogen. They are higher among Blacks and among women, especially before menopause, and they change little with age. The protective effect of HDL is significant: A 1 percent decrease in HDL level is associated with a 3–4 percent increase in heart disease.[13]

Physical Inactivity   A sedentary lifestyle is another major risk factor for CVD, and regular physical activity reduces the risk of CVD and many cardiovascular risk factors, including high blood pressure, diabetes, and obesity. Physical activity conditions the heart, reduces high blood pressure, improves HDL cholesterol levels, helps maintain a healthy weight, and helps control diabetes.

Many adults in the United States are not active at levels that can promote health. About 60 percent of women and 69 percent of men report achieving the minimum recommendation of 150 minutes per week of moderate-intensity activity or 75 minutes per week of vigorous-intensity activity. Prevalence of physical activity differs by racial/ethnic group, with 56 percent of Blacks and 67 percent of Whites meeting the recommendation. College students have the highest reported prevalence—70 percent—of meeting the goal.[15] Exercise is especially important for children, because it is associated with lower blood pressure and weight control and because active children tend to become active adults.

low-density lipoproteins (LDLs) "Bad" cholesterol; lipoproteins that accumulate in plaque and contribute to atherosclerosis.

high-density lipoproteins (HDLs) "Good" cholesterol; lipoproteins that help clear cholesterol from cells and atherosclerotic deposits and transport it back to the liver for recycling.

Excess weight *puts a strain on the heart.*

Overweight and Obesity   Overweight and obesity are associated with increased risk for CVD and greater seriousness of the disease. Excess weight puts a strain on the heart and contributes to other risk factors, such as hypertension, high LDL levels, and diabetes. The association among all these risk factors is found across ethnic groups, including Mexican Americans, non-Hispanic Blacks, and non-Hispanic Whites.

As discussed in Chapter 8, body fat distribution plays a role in CVD risk. Waist-to-hip ratio may play a greater role than absolute body mass index. People with central fat distribution—those who are apple-shaped, as suggested by an abdominal circumference of greater than 40 inches for men and greater than 35 inches for women—have a higher risk for diabetes, high blood pressure, and CVD. Weight loss of 10–15 percent for an overweight individual, if maintained, is associated with an improved cardiovascular risk profile. Diet and exercise are recommended ways to reduce overweight and obesity.[1,8]

Diabetes   **Diabetes** is a metabolic disorder in which the production or use of insulin is disrupted, as described in Chapter 8. Elevated levels of glucose circulating in the bloodstream cause changes throughout the body, including damage to artery walls, changes in some blood components, and damage to peripheral nerves and organs. People with diabetes are two to four times more likely than people without diabetes to develop cardiovascular disease. Their arteries are particularly susceptible to atherosclerosis, and it occurs at an earlier age and is more extensive. The incidence of Type-2 diabetes has doubled in the past 30 years and is expected to double again by 2050. Currently, 9.6 percent of the U.S. adult population has been diagnosed with diabetes. An estimated 30 percent of people with diabetes have not been diagnosed.[1]

Another concern for people with diabetes is that their symptoms of heart attack may be different from the norm. They are more likely to have a "silent" heart attack. Their only symptoms may be nausea, vomiting, sweating, or dizziness, any of which could be easily mistaken for another illness. Control of diabetes reduces risk, and it is especially important for people with diabetes to control other risk factors.[1]

diabetes
Metabolic disorder in which the production or use of insulin is disrupted, so that body cells cannot take up glucose and use it for energy, and high levels of glucose circulate in the blood.

triglycerides
Blood fats similar to cholesterol.

CONTRIBUTING RISK FACTORS IN CVD

Besides the six major controllable risk factors for CVD, other risk factors that can be controlled have been identified. These factors contribute to risk, but their role either is slightly less than that of the major risk factors or has not been as clearly delineated yet.

High Triglyceride Levels   **Triglycerides** are another form in which fat exists in the body. Body triglycerides are derived from fats eaten or produced by the body from other energy sources, such as excess carbohydrates. High blood levels of triglycerides are a risk factor for CVD, although they are not linked to CVD as strongly as are cholesterol levels. A triglyceride level of less than 150 is desirable (see Table 15.2).

High triglyceride levels are associated with excess body fat, diets high in saturated fat and cholesterol, alcohol use, and some medical conditions, such as poorly controlled diabetes. The main treatment for high triglycerides is lifestyle modification, but medications can also be used.

High Alcohol Intake   The relationship between alcohol and CVD is complicated because different levels of alcohol consumption have different effects. Heavy drinking, defined as more than three drinks per day, can damage the heart, increasing the risk of cardiomyopathy, some arrhythmias, and neurological complications. Light to moderate alcohol intake, defined as fewer than two drinks per day, appears to have a protective effect against heart disease and stroke, increasing HDL levels.

The benefit associated with light to moderate alcohol use is seen regardless of the beverage, which suggests that the protective factor is alcohol itself, rather than another substance in some beverages, such as the tannins in red wine. The disadvantages of alcohol consumption are that it may contribute to weight gain, higher blood pressure, and elevated triglycerides, as well as alcoholism in vulnerable individuals. The possible cardiovascular benefits have to be weighed against the disadvantages and potential harm associated with drinking.[1]

Psychosocial Factors   As described in Chapter 3, traits and behavior patterns associated with the so-called Type A

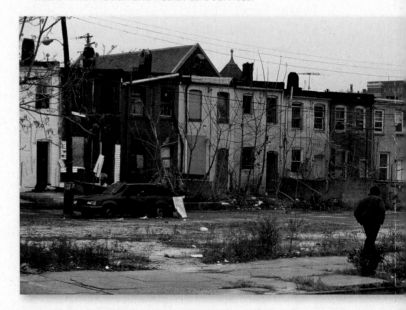

■ Low socioeconomic status is associated with greater risk for cardiovascular disease. Contributing factors may be the stress of poverty and discrimination and lack of access to health information and health care services.

personality—specifically, anger and hostility—have been shown to contribute to CVD risk. These feelings cause the release of stress hormones. When anger, hostility, and stress in general are persistent and pervasive, the continuous circulation of stress hormones in the blood increases blood pressure and heart rate and triggers the release of cholesterol and triglycerides into the blood. All these changes may promote the development of atherosclerosis and, for those with atherosclerosis, increase vulnerability to heart attack or stroke.[16,17]

Low socioeconomic status and low levels of educational attainment are associated with an increased risk for heart attack, stroke, congestive heart failure, and hypertension. Income inequality in a country—the gap between the rich and the poor—is directly related to national rates of death from CVD, coronary artery disease, and stroke. Numerous factors may help explain the link between poverty and poor health. For example, poverty limits people's ability to obtain

discussed so far. Researchers are constantly trying to identify additional risk factors; in this section we consider a few promising areas of ongoing research.

Vitamin D Deficiency Vitamin D has long been known to play an important role in calcium absorption and bone health; however, it is becoming increasingly clear that low levels of vitamin D are associated with heart disease, diabetes, hypertension, and obesity. Vitamin D is believed to affect blood clotting, inflammation, and the cells in the walls of arteries. An estimated 30 to 50 percent of the population has low levels of vitamin D. Although there is currently no guideline for vitamin D screening, vitamin D deficiency may become an important risk factor in the future given that it is relatively easy to treat with sunshine exposure or vitamin supplementation.[21]

lipoprotein(a)
Subgroup of LDL cholesterol that is thought to increase blood clotting.

The strength of a person's relationships and the nature of his or her **basic attitudes toward life** *play important roles in maintaining health and protecting against disease.*

---

the basic requisites for health, such as food and shelter, as well as their ability to participate in society, which creates psychological stress. Poverty also limits access to health-related information, health care, medications, behavior change options, and physical activity. In addition, racism, prejudice, and discrimination can act as psychosocial stressors and lead to increased risk of CVD.[1,9,18,19]

Depression has a bidirectional relationship with CVD; that is, depression increases risk of CVD, and CVD increases risk of depression. Depression can play a role in all stages in the development of CVD. People who are depressed have a more difficult time choosing healthy lifestyle options, making lifestyle changes, initiating access to health care, and adhering to medication regimens. Early diagnosis and treatment of depression may help reduce risk of CVD in vulnerable individuals.[1,9]

People who lack social support or live in social isolation are at increased risk for many health conditions, including CVD. Strong social networks have been shown to decrease the risk of CVD, and social support, altruism, faith, and optimism are all associated with a reduced risk of CVD. Thus, it appears that the strength of a person's relationships and the nature of his or her basic attitudes toward life play important roles in maintaining health and protecting against disease, as discussed in Chapter 4.[20]

POSSIBLE RISK FACTORS IN CVD

Factors that contribute to CVD are not fully understood, and some people with heart disease have none of the risk factors

Lipoprotein(a) A subgroup of LDL cholesterol, **lipoprotein(a)** is similar to LDL but has an additional protein attached. This particular subtype of LDL may increase blood clotting and atherosclerosis. Higher levels of lipoprotein(a) are associated with an increased risk of coronary artery disease. Screening for lipoprotein(a) is possible but not currently recommended.

■ The National Heart, Lung, and Blood Institute, along with a number of corporate sponsors, presents the Red Dress Fashion show during Fashion Week in New York to remind women of the need to protect their cardiovascular health. Fashion industry models and celebrities like Elisabeth Hasselbeck, shown here, walk the runway in red dresses, some of which are later auctioned off to provide financial support for awareness and research efforts.

Steps that decrease LDL levels, such as dietary modifications and medications, also decrease levels of lipoprotein(a).[22,23]

homocysteine
Amino acid that circulates in the blood and may damage the lining of blood vessels.

metabolic syndrome
Condition characterized by a combination of obesity, especially central obesity; elevated blood pressure; dyslipidemia (high triglycerides and low HDL cholesterol); and glucose intolerance, a pre-diabetes condition.

C-reactive protein
Blood marker for inflammation that may indicate an increased risk for coronary heart disease.

Homocysteine High blood levels of **homocysteine**, an amino acid, have been associated with increased risks of CVD. Homocysteine may damage the lining of blood vessels, leading to inflammation and atherosclerosis. Both genetics and diet appear to play a role in setting homocysteine levels. Blood levels of homocysteine are higher in people with diets high in animal protein and low in vitamin B_6, vitamin B_{12}, and folic acid (commonly found in fruits, vegetables, and enriched grains). At this time, there is no recommendation for measuring homocysteine levels in the general population, nor is there evidence to show that reducing homocysteine levels can reduce risk of CVD.[22]

Metabolic Syndrome A condition associated with a significantly increased risk of CVD and the development of Type-2 diabetes, **metabolic syndrome** is characterized by a combination of risk factors. Although several criteria have been identified, the condition is commonly diagnosed when three of the following five risk factors are present:

- Fasting glucose level ≥100
- HDL cholesterol <40 in men or <50 in women
- Triglycerides ≥150
- Waist circumference ≥102 cm for men or ≥88 cm for women
- Systolic blood pressure ≥130 and diastolic blood pressure ≥85

An estimated 34 percent of adult Americans meet the criteria for diagnosis, but prevalence varies by ethnic and racial group. For men, prevalence is 25.3 percent in Blacks, 35.2 percent in Mexican Americans, and 37.2 percent in Whites. For women, prevalence is 38.8 percent in Blacks, 40.6 percent in Mexican Americans, and 31.5 percent in Whites.[1] The causes are believed to be a combination of genetics and central obesity. Recommendations for metabolic syndrome include increasing physical activity, losing weight, and making dietary changes.

Inflammatory Response and C-Reactive Protein
Inflammation is well established as a factor in all stages of atherosclerosis. Several blood test markers can be used to identify and measure an ongoing inflammatory response, and elevated levels of **C-reactive protein**, fibrinogen, and white blood cell count have been associated with an increased risk of CVD. High levels of C-reactive protein are associated with increased risk for coronary heart disease in both men and women and have also been associated with more rapid progression of CVD. Routine screening of all populations for C-reactive protein is not recommended at this time.[22]

Infectious Agents Hard as it may be to believe, increasing evidence suggests that infections play a role in CVD. Infections appear to promote atherosclerosis and may cause atherosclerotic plaques to break free and block arteries. *Chlamydia pneumoniae*, a strain of *Chlamydia* that causes lung infections (not the strain that causes the sexually transmitted disease), was the first organism to be shown to have a potential role. The organism was found in 59 percent of arteries containing atherosclerotic plaques and only 3 percent of arteries without atherosclerotic plaques. Other studies have shown an association between heart attack and stroke in the month of a respiratory infection and pneumonia. Risk appears to be greatest in the few days to a week after infection. Lung infections may stress the heart by causing an increase in oxygen demand. There still is no conclusive evidence to support the use of antibiotics to reduce risk of infection-associated CVD, though flu shots may reduce risk.[24,25]

Fetal Origins Research has shown a relationship between birth weight and risk of CVD, with lower birth weight associated with higher risk. This represents what is called a *programming phenomenon*. Tissues (in this case the heart muscle and blood vessels) may be damaged during a sensitive stage of fetal development in a way that programs them to develop problems later in life. Poor fetal growth has been associated with increased risk of other common adult health problems as well, such as hypertension, stroke, diabetes, and obesity.[26]

NONCONTROLLABLE RISK FACTORS IN CVD

Age, gender, family history, ethnicity and race, and postmenopausal status are the noncontrollable risk factors for cardiovascular disease (see the box "Risk for CVD by Age, Gender, Race/Ethnicity, and Geographical Location"). Individuals with noncontrollable risk factors, especially, should choose healthy behaviors that do not promote CVD.

Age Age is probably the most important noncontrollable risk factor. There is a significant rise in deaths due to heart disease and stroke after age 65. Age alone does not cause CVD, however; there is great variation in CVD among older people of the same age.[1]

Gender Although heart disease is often thought of as a man's disease, CVD is the leading cause of death for both men and women. There are some differences between the sexes, however. A 40-year-old man without evidence of heart disease has a 1 in 2 chance of developing CVD in his lifetime, whereas a 40-year-old woman has a 1 in 3 chance. Women tend to develop heart disease about 10 years later than men, perhaps because of the protective effect of estrogen before menopause. After age 50 (the average age of

Who's at Risk?

Risk for CVD by Age, Gender, Race/Ethnicity, and Geographical Location

Race/ethnicity is a noncontrollable risk factor for CVD. Risk for CVD also varies by the state in which a person lives. Why do you think geographical location makes a difference in risk for CVD?

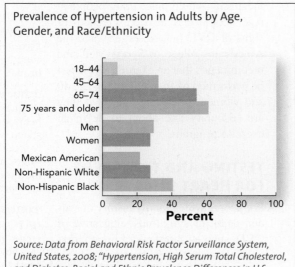

Prevalence of Hypertension in Adults by Age, Gender, and Race/Ethnicity

- 18–44
- 45–64
- 65–74
- 75 years and older

- Men
- Women

- Mexican American
- Non-Hispanic White
- Non-Hispanic Black

Percent (0, 20, 40, 60, 80, 100)

Source: Data from Behavioral Risk Factor Surveillance System, United States, 2008; "Hypertension, High Serum Total Cholesterol, and Diabetes: Racial and Ethnic Prevalence Differences in U.S. Adults, 1999–2006," by C. D. Fryar, M. Hirsch, M. S. Eberhardt, et al., 2010, National Center for Health Statistics Data Brief No. 36.

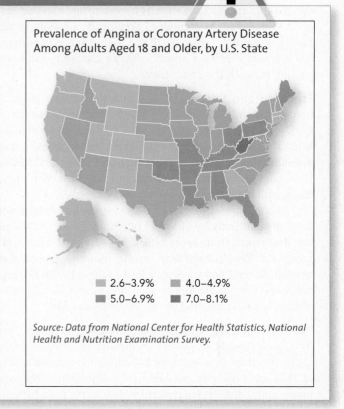

Prevalence of Angina or Coronary Artery Disease Among Adults Aged 18 and Older, by U.S. State

- 2.6–3.9%
- 4.0–4.9%
- 5.0–6.9%
- 7.0–8.1%

Source: Data from National Center for Health Statistics, National Health and Nutrition Examination Survey.

menopause), the difference in risk between men and women starts to decrease.

The death rates for CVD are higher in women, both Black women and White women; this is true of heart attack, stroke, hypertension, and congestive heart failure. One reason for this is that women tend to be older and frailer when they develop heart disease and so are less likely to survive. Another reason is that women are more likely to have either no symptoms before a heart attack or symptoms that make the diagnosis of heart disease more confusing, such as stomach complaints. One study showed that women delay seeking treatment as much as 3.5 hours longer than men do. Because treatment is more effective the sooner it is started, this delay means that more damage occurs. A third reason is that health care providers may also delay treatment because they do not recognize the symptoms or are less likely to think about heart disease in women.[1]

Genetics and Family History   Individuals who have a relative with a history of CVD have a higher risk of CVD themselves. The risk for heart attack appears to be greatest if a male relative had a heart attack before age 55 or a female relative had a heart attack before age 65. The risk for stroke is increased if a relative has had a stroke, regardless of age.

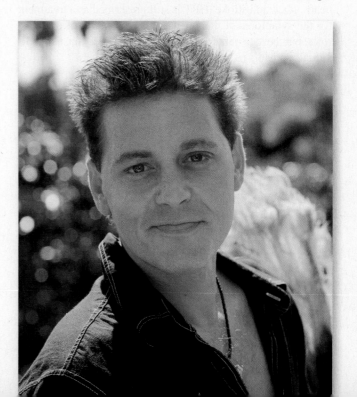

■ Corey Haim, '80s teen heartthrob and co-star of A&E reality TV show *The Two Coreys*, died in March 2010. Although Haim's death was initially thought to have been due to a drug overdose given his past struggles with drug addiction and the over 550 prescription pills he obtained in the month previous to his death, an autopsy revealed that he died from complications related to pneumonia, an inherited heart defect, and hardening of the coronary arteries.

High rates of CVD in a family may be related to genetics or lifestyle patterns or both. A large part of the family risk is due to other risk factors, such as hypertension, elevated lipids, and diabetes. As mentioned previously, a history in the family of sudden cardiac death at a young age is important, since it may signify a genetic risk for cardiomyopathy or another congenital cardiac disease.[7,9]

Ethnicity and Race   Minority and low-income populations in the United States carry a disproportionate burden of CVD. Blacks have a higher risk of CVD and stroke than do Whites, as well as higher rates of hypertension, obesity, and diabetes. Mexican Americans, American Indians, and Native Hawaiians also have a higher risk of CVD than do Whites, along with higher rates of obesity and diabetes.

Recent improvements in cardiovascular health have not been shared evenly by all racial or ethnic groups. Although the death rate from heart attack has declined across all groups, it has declined less among minority groups and women. Several pathways may lead to these health disparities, including differences in such risk factors as hypertension, genetics, stress, and psychosocial factors.[18,27]

Postmenopausal Status   The hormone estrogen has long been thought to protect premenopausal women from CVD. When levels of estrogen fall during menopause, levels of HDL also decline, and body fat distribution shifts to a more central distribution pattern, similar to the male pattern.

For many years, medical practitioners prescribed hormone replacement therapy (HRT) for postmenopausal women to relieve the symptoms of menopause, lower the risk of osteoporosis (bone thinning), and reduce the risk of CVD. The belief in the benefits of estrogen was so strong that at one point, nearly one in three postmenopausal women was on HRT. As described in Chapter 12, research has now shown that HRT actually increases rather than decreases the risk of heart attack and stroke. HRT is still prescribed as a treatment for the symptoms of menopause and prevention of osteoporosis, but these benefits must now be weighed against an individual woman's risk for CVD.[28]

Testing and Treatment

People with no symptoms of CVD are usually not tested for evidence of disease; instead the focus is on screening for risk factors (hypertension, cholesterol levels, family health history, and so on). An exception is people in certain occupations, such as airline pilots or truck drivers, whose sudden incapacity would place other people at risk. People may also be screened for signs of CVD before surgery, and the American College of Sports Medicine recommends that an exercise stress test be performed on men older than age 40 and women older than age 50 if they are sedentary and about to begin an exercise program.

TESTING AND TREATMENT FOR HEART DISEASE

For people with a family history of sudden death or symptoms suggestive of CVD, such as shortness of breath, dizziness, or exertional chest pain, physical examination and diagnostic tests can determine the presence of disease and the extent of the problem. If disease is present, a variety of steps can be taken, from lifestyle changes, to medication, to surgery.

Diagnostic Testing for Heart Disease   Several tests are available to evaluate heart function and determine if underlying disease is present. An **electrocardiogram** (ECG or EKG), a record of the electrical activity of the heart as it beats, can detect abnormal rhythms, inadequate blood flow (possibly due to ischemia or heart attack), and heart enlargement. An **echocardiogram** (or echo), an ultrasound test that uses sound waves to visualize the heart structure and motion, can detect structural abnormalities (changes in the underlying structure of the valves, arteries, or heart chambers), thickness of the muscle walls, and how well the heart pumps. An **exercise stress test** evaluates how well the heart functions with exercise.

Blood tests can be performed to detect certain proteins in the blood that are released by a damaged heart muscle. A variety of other procedures produce images of the heart, heart valves, and any blocked or narrowed coronary arteries; they include **coronary angiogram** (injection of a dye with multiple X-rays), computerized tomography (CT) scans, and magnetic resonance imaging (MRI).

electrocardiogram
Record of the heart's electrical activity as it beats.

echocardiogram
Diagnostic test for a heart attack in which sound waves are used to visualize heart valves, heart wall movement, and overall heart function.

exercise stress test
Procedure that evaluates how well the heart functions with exercise.

coronary angiogram
Diagnostic test for a heart attack in which a dye is injected into a fine catheter that is passed into the heart and X-rays are taken as the dye moves through the heart, showing any blocked or narrowed coronary arteries.

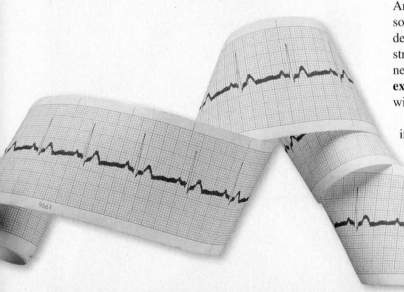

Medical Management of Heart Disease Multiple categories of medications can be used in the treatment of heart disease, depending on the underlying problem. There are medications that help control heart rhythm (anti-arrhythmics), dilate the coronary arteries and reduce angina (anti-anginals), decrease blood clotting (anti-coagulants), and dissolve blood clots during a heart attack (thrombolytics).

When a heart attack occurs, emergency treatment is critical. The effectiveness of treatment depends on the time elapsed from first symptoms until the reestablishment of blood flow to the heart muscle. Thrombolytics are most effective when given within the first hour after a heart attack. Other medications are used to control risk factors and reduce the chance of developing heart disease or a recurrence of heart disease. These include anti-hypertensives, cholesterol-lowering medications, and antiplatelet medications.

Surgical Management of Heart Disease Every day thousands of people have heart surgery; there are many different types of surgery, depending on the underlying problem. For structural abnormalities, surgeons can repair or replace heart valves, close septal defects (holes) that allow blood to flow abnormally, reposition arteries and veins that are attached incorrectly, and repair aneurysms in the aorta. If the problem is related to abnormal electrical conduction through the heart, a cardiologist can destroy a small amount of heart tissue in an area that is disturbing the flow of electricity or can implant a defibrillator into the chest that will automatically shock the heart if a life-threatening arrhythmia develops. Also, often as a last resort, a surgeon can replace a damaged heart completely with a heart from a donor.

If the underlying abnormality is related to coronary artery disease, a few surgical options exist. One is **angioplasty**, in which a balloon catheter (a thin plastic tube) is threaded into a blocked or narrowed artery and inflated to stretch the vessel open again. A *coronary stent*, a springy framework that supports the vessel walls and keeps the vessel open, is often permanently placed in the artery to prevent it from closing again. Another surgical option is **coronary artery bypass grafting**, usually just called *bypass*. A healthy blood vessel is taken from another part of the body, usually the leg, and grafted to the coronary arteries to allow a bypass of blood flow around a narrowed vessel.

angioplasty
Procedure to reopen a blocked coronary artery, in which a balloon catheter (a thin plastic tube) is threaded into the narrowed area and inflated to stretch the vessel open again.

coronary artery bypass grafting
Surgical procedure in which a healthy blood vessel is taken from another part of the body and grafted to the coronary arteries to allow a bypass of blood flow around a narrowed vessel.

TESTING AND TREATMENT FOR STROKE

Before the 1990s, little could be done to alter the natural course of a stroke. Today we know that the same thrombolytic (clot-dissolving) medications used in heart attacks can decrease the damage incurred by a stroke. These medications can be administered only within the first 3 hours of the onset of symptoms. Thus, it is critical that a person experiencing symptoms of a stroke receive medical care immediately.

Diagnostic Testing for Stroke At the hospital, a CT scan or an MRI can be used to generate images of the brain and blood flow and to determine whether a stroke has occurred. These tests can also show whether a stroke has been caused by a blockage or by a hemorrhage. Further testing may be done to find the source of the blockage. The carotid arteries, the large arteries on the sides of the neck that supply blood to the brain, are examined to see if they are blocked with atherosclerotic plaques. If so, part of the plaque may have broken off and become the source of an embolism blocking a blood vessel in the brain.

Management of Stroke If a stroke is found to be thrombotic (caused by a blockage) and there is no evidence of bleeding in the brain, thrombolytic medications can be administered to dissolve the clot and restore blood flow to the brain. Thrombolytic medications must not be given if the stroke is hemorrhagic, because they can cause increased

■ About two-thirds of individuals who suffer a stroke survive and require rehabilitation. When a stroke has caused muscle weakness or paralysis, therapy focuses on regaining use of impaired limbs, improving coordination and balance, and developing strategies for bypassing deficits.

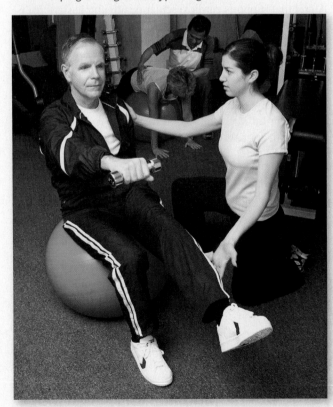

bleeding. Aspirin and other anticlotting medications can be used after a thrombotic stroke to reduce the risk of another stroke. Control of blood pressure and other risk factors is important for all people who have a stroke, whether thrombotic or hemorrhagic.

Rehabilitation is a component of treatment for stroke. If an area of the brain is damaged or destroyed, the functions that were controlled by that part of the brain will be impaired. Rehabilitation consists of physical therapy (to strengthen muscles and coordination), speech therapy (to improve communication and eating), and occupational therapy (to improve activities of daily living and job retraining if appropriate). Progress and return of functions vary by individual. Some people recover fully within a few days to weeks, while others are left with long-term impairment.

Promoting Cardiovascular Health

As scientists learn more about the progressive nature of cardiovascular disease, the significance of early prevention becomes clearer. Adopting healthy lifestyle habits now, regardless of your age or current health status, is the best way to reduce your risk of developing CVD in the future.[29] Complete the Personal Health Portfolio for this chapter to assess your cardiovascular health.

EATING FOR HEART HEALTH

A diet that supports cardiovascular health emphasizes fruits, vegetables, whole grains, low-fat dairy products, fish, and lean meat and poultry. The American Heart Association Dietary Guidelines are summarized in the box "Choosing a Heart-Healthy Diet."

Micronutrients appear to play a role in cardiovascular health. Many micronutrients, especially antioxidants, are more plentiful in a plant-based diet than in a diet based on foods from animal sources. Foods high in important antioxidants are brightly colored fruits and vegetables and nuts and seeds (see Chapter 6). Experts recommend that micronutrients be consumed in foods rather than in supplements.

Specific foods have been shown to alter cholesterol levels. Soy products and legumes, such as lentils and chickpeas, have both been shown to decrease LDL. Garlic appears to have a similar effect on total cholesterol, although fresh garlic (one to two cloves per day) is recommended over synthesized garlic capsules. Foods rich in fiber also help reduce cholesterol levels; they include fruits, vegetables, oats, and barley.

Challenges & Choices

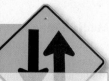

Choosing a Heart-Healthy Diet

The American Heart Association encourages all Americans, young and old, to adopt a heart-healthy diet. AHA guidelines include the following recommendations:

- Balance your calories in to calories out. Don't eat more calories than you use each day. Aim for at least 30 minutes of moderate physical exercise on most days of the week.

- Eat a variety of nutritious foods from all the food groups. Eat plenty of nutrient-rich foods such as fruits, vegetables, and whole-grain products. These are high in vitamins, minerals, and fiber and are low in calories.

- Aim to eat fish twice a week; omega-3 fatty acids may reduce risk of CVD.

- Eat less of the foods that are low in nutrients and high in calories:
  - Choose lean meats and poultry without skin, and prepare them without added saturated fats and trans fat.
  - Choose fat-free or 1 percent fat dairy products.
  - Avoid consumption of trans fatty acids, found in foods containing partially hydrogenated vegetable oils, such as fried foods, margarines, and commercial baked goods.
  - Aim to limit dietary cholesterol to no more than 300 mg per day.
  - Cut back on drinks and foods with added sugar.
  - Aim to eat less than 1,500 mg of salt per day.
  - If you drink alcohol, drink in moderation—for women, no more than one drink per day, and for men, no more than two drinks per day.

Source: Data from the American Heart Association, www.americanheart.org.

EXERCISING REGULARLY

Exercise has an effect on many CVD risk factors. It has a direct conditioning effect on the heart, improving the health of the heart muscle and enhancing its ability to pump blood efficiently. Exercise helps in weight loss and weight-maintenance programs by increasing energy output. It also has more subtle effects, such as improving HDL levels and increasing the number of insulin receptors, which enhances the ability of people with diabetes to use insulin.

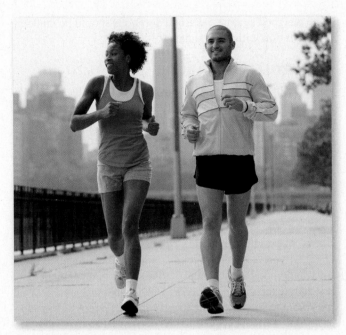

Cardiorespiratory endurance exercise is one of the best antidotes to heart disease. The current recommendation for most adults is 30 minutes of moderate-intensity physical activity on most days of the week or 20 minutes of vigorous activity on three days of the week.

Even low-intensity activities, such as walking, gardening, or climbing stairs, can be helpful (see the box "Studying Doesn't Have to Be Sedentary").

AVOIDING TOBACCO USE

Smoking poses both an immediate hazard for heart attack and a long-term hazard for atherosclerosis. Because nicotine is so addictive, the best prevention is never to start smoking. If you do smoke, quitting now can significantly reduce your risk of developing CVD.

CONTROLLING BLOOD PRESSURE

Regular screening for hypertension is recommended for individuals over age 15.[1] For anyone in the prehypertension or hypertension category, lifestyle changes are recommended, including weight reduction, dietary changes, low salt intake, physical activity, and moderate alcohol intake.[5] If lifestyle changes alone do not reduce blood pressure, medications are recommended. Hypertension can be controlled in most cases, but sometimes it takes lifestyle change plus two or more medications.

The DASH diet was developed to reduce elevated blood pressure (see Chapter 6). The 2005 *Dietary Guidelines for Americans* recommends a limit of 1,500 mg of sodium per day for individuals with hypertension, middle-aged and older adults, and Blacks.

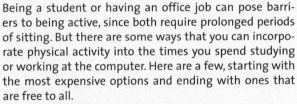

Consumer Clipboard

Studying Doesn't Have to Be Sedentary

Being a student or having an office job can pose barriers to being active, since both require prolonged periods of sitting. But there are some ways that you can incorporate physical activity into the times you spend studying or working at the computer. Here are a few, starting with the most expensive options and ending with ones that are free to all.

Treadmill desks allow people to work on the computer or do office work while walking on a treadmill. The accompanying desk is elevated to the height of the treadmill and the pace is set very low—1 to 2 miles an hour. For a 150-pound person, walking 1 mile per hour burns more than 100 calories an hour. Even just standing burns an extra 20 calories an hour over sitting. Treadmill desks are designed to fit around a treadmill, so if you already own a treadmill, you can buy a desk for about $500. Models that include a treadmill and a desk can cost upward of $4,500.

Another option to keep you moving is to use an exercise-ball chair instead of a conventional chair. This type of chair has an exercise ball for the seat and a frame around it with support for the back and roller-ball feet. The advantage of using an exercise-ball chair is that the unstable nature if the seat makes the body constantly readjust and stabilize itself, primarily with the core muscles. However, these types of chairs may not be best for people who type a lot and are thus at risk for carpal tunnel syndrome or tendinitis. Exercise ball chairs cost about $100.

Low and no-cost ways to get exercise while in front of a computer or a book include buying lightweight dumbbells or an exercise band (so that you can do arm exercises while reading or waiting for files to download) or doing simple exercises (such as standing up and sitting back down 10 times) every half hour or so. Another strategy is to drink water while you study or work so that you will need to get up frequently for bathroom trips.

Low-intensity exercise like the activities described here is not meant to replace moderate- or vigorous-intensity exercise that you should be getting during the week, but it can help you to stay active and prevent unwanted weight gain—both of which are important in avoiding cardiovascular disease.

Sources: "Walking While You Work," *Good Morning America,* 2007, retrieved May 10, 2010, from http://abcnews.go.com/GMA/WaterCooler/story?id=3771802&page=1; "How to Exercise While Sitting at Your Computer," Wikihow, retrieved May 10, 2010, from www.wikihow.com/Exercise-While-Sitting-at-Your-Computer.

MANAGING CHOLESTEROL LEVELS

The National Cholesterol Education Program recommends that all adults over age 20 have their cholesterol checked at least once every 5 years. If you find that your LDL cholesterol levels, in combination with other risk factors, put you at risk for CVD, your physician will work with you to develop an LDL goal and a plan for reaching it. Exercising, maintaining a healthy weight, and dietary changes, including reducing total and saturated fat intake and increasing dietary fiber, are first-line actions. However, as with high blood pressure, these changes may not be enough for some people and medication may be required.[13]

USING ASPIRIN THERAPY

Nearly 36 percent of American adults—more than 50 million people—take aspirin regularly to reduce their risk of CVD. Aspirin inhibits the clotting function of platelets and thus reduces the risk of blood clots. However, aspirin also increases the risk of bleeding, and the higher the aspirin dose, the greater the risk of bleeding. Aspirin is generally recommended for anyone who has a history of heart attack, unstable angina, ischemic stroke, or transient ischemic attack if the person has no contra-indications (such as allergy to aspirin or a history of bleeding ulcer). In others, both men and women, benefits have to be weighed against risks, and decisions should be made in collaboration with a physician.[30]

CONTROLLING DIABETES

People with diabetes must control their blood glucose levels to reduce their risk of cardiovascular complications. People with diabetes also have to control their other CVD risk factors, such as high cholesterol levels, high triglyceride levels, and high blood pressure, all of which are more likely to occur in association with this disorder.[1]

MANAGING STRESS AND IMPROVING MENTAL HEALTH

Stress, anger, hostility, and depression can all contribute to CVD. If you frequently feel overwhelmed by negative feelings and moods, try some of the stress management and relaxation techniques described in Chapters 3 and 4. You may want to increase your social support system by expanding your connections to family, friends, community, or church. You may want to simplify your schedule and slow down. Meditating can lower blood pressure and blood cholesterol levels, thereby slowing the process of atherosclerosis. Biofeedback may help reduce blood pressure. Hypnosis may be useful to help control hypertension and other chronic health problems. Whatever approach you choose to manage stress and enhance your mental health, try to incorporate a daily practice into your life.

You Make the Call

Screening for Cardiovascular Disease in Athletes: How Much Is Enough?

Did you play sports in high school? Are you on a college team or participating in intramural activities? Do you exercise vigorously on your own? If so, you should be aware that sudden cardiac arrest is the most common cause of death in young athletes (those younger than age 35). Vigorous exercise is a trigger for lethal arrhythmias in athletes with unrecognized heart disease, typically congenital disease. On average, only 11 percent of athletes will survive a sudden cardiac arrest—a worse outcome than might be expected, given their age, fitness level, and the fact that many of these events are witnessed. The low survival rates may be due to the underlying congenital disease, the exertion at the time of arrest, or slow recognition by bystanders of what has happened. These low survival rates highlight the critical importance of early recognition of underlying disease.

If you played sports in high school, you may or may not have participated in a screening physical prior to sports participation. This is because there is no national mandate regarding screening standards for high school athletes. On the college level, there are no requirements for intramural sports teams or other school-affiliated teams, such as ultimate Frisbee teams. However, the National College Athletic Association (NCAA) has recently mandated a pre-participation evaluation for all Division I, II, and III athletes. The traditional evaluation involves a visit to a health care provider for screening questions concerning an athlete's personal and family history and a physical exam, with findings suggestive of heart disease prompting further evaluation. This screening has limitations because 60–80 percent of athletes have no symptoms, many have no family history of CVD or don't know their family history, and results of physical exams are normal in many people with congenital heart problems.

In 1979 a national program that added ECG screening to the traditional screening was started in Italy. The addition of ECG identified many asymptomatic athletes whose conditions would have gone unrecognized by traditional screening. Since adding ECG screening, the incidence of sudden cardiac death among athletes in Italy has been reduced by 90 percent. The European Society of Cardiology (ESC) and the International Olympic Committee (IOC) recently adopted similar recommendations.

Some health experts think the United States should add ECG screening as a national preparticipation requirement for high school and college athletes, pointing to the healthy young people whose lives would be saved. The prohibiting factor is cost: If national screening were adopted, an estimated 10 million athletes would require screening at a theoretical cost of $2 billion dollars a year or approximately $330,000 for each athlete detected with cardiac disease. Another problem is the number of false-positive results that would occur—abnormal ECG findings in athletes who do not have underlying cardiac disease. An estimated 10 percent of results could be false positives. These athletes would have to go through the stress of an additional workup and temporary disqualification from their sport.

In a 2009 review the American Heart Association (AHA) did not recommend the addition of ECG screening for American athletes. The AHA concluded that a national screening program would not be practical given the financial resources, staffing, and logistics that would be required. However, the AHA did recognize that at present we do not have full knowledge of how many young athletes die per year of sudden cardiac arrest and thus called for a national mandatory reporting system for sudden cardiac deaths in young competitive athletes.

Proponents of the additional ECG screening argue that any measures that save the lives of otherwise healthy young adults are worth the time and money invested. Opponents respond that such measures are unrealistic and impractical at this time. What do you think?

PROS

- Because survival rates from sudden cardiac arrest are very low, prevention is critical.

- Although it may be expensive and result in some false positives, the ECG is a straightforward, noninvasive test, and further evaluation is done with another noninvasive test, the echocardiogram.

- Italy demonstrated the will to save lives by adding ECG screening to its other athletic screening requirements. If a small country like Italy can institute such screening, a large, wealthy country like the Untied States should be able to do so, too.

- Cost should not be a factor when the lives of otherwise healthy young adults are at stake.

CONS

- The high rate of false positives from ECGs means that many athletes would be unnecessarily sidelined from their sports while awaiting further evaluation.

- Because of its larger population and geographical size, the United States cannot do ECG screening with the same ease as Italy or other European countries. The United States does not have the infrastructure (staffing, finances) to support a national program adding ECG screening.

- There isn't even a national requirement for the traditional screening (personal history, family history, and physical exam) in the United States right now. Thus, it is unrealistic to talk about adding an ECG requirement.

connect
ACTIVITY

Source: "Sudden Deaths in Young Competitive Athletes: Analysis of 1866 Deaths in the United States, 1980–2006," by B. J. Maron, J. J. Doerer, T. S. Hess, et al., 2009, Circulation, 119 (8), pp. 1085–1092.

IN REVIEW

What is the cardiovascular system, and how does it work?

The heart, a four-chambered, fist-sized muscle, pumps blood throughout the body (systemic circulation) and to and from the lungs (pulmonary circulation) via the blood vessels—arteries, veins, and capillaries. Arteries carry oxygen-rich blood to the body's cells, and veins carry deoxygenated blood back to the heart and from there to the lungs, where oxygen is replenished. The only exceptions are the pulmonary arteries, which carry oxygen-poor blood to the lungs, and the pulmonary veins, which carry oxygen-rich blood back to the heart.

What is cardiovascular disease?

The disease process underlying most forms of CVD is atherosclerosis, a condition in which the arteries become clogged and blood flow is restricted, causing heart attack, stroke, or peripheral vascular disease. A disturbance in the electrical signals controlling the heartbeat can cause an arrhythmia (disorganized beating) and sudden cardiac arrest. Other forms of CVD are hypertension (high blood pressure), congestive heart failure, heart valve disorders, rheumatic heart disease, congenital heart disease, and cardiomyopathy (disease of the heart muscle). A stroke occurs either when a blood vessel serving the brain is blocked or when a blood vessel in the brain ruptures.

What are the risk factors for CVD?

The six major controllable risk factors are tobacco use, hypertension, unhealthy blood cholesterol levels, physical inactivity, overweight and obesity, and diabetes. The four major noncontrollable risk factors are older age, a genetic predisposition, Black or other minority racial/ethnic status, and postmenopausal status. Numerous other contributing and possible risk factors have been identified, including psychosocial factors such as a hostility-prone personality, chronic stress, low socioeconomic status and education, depression, and social isolation.

How is CVD diagnosed and treated?

If warranted by family history or symptoms, diagnostic tests can be performed to determine if CVD is present; tests include electrocardiogram, echocardiogram, exercise stress test, blood tests, and a variety of procedures that produce images of the heart and blood vessels. CVD can be managed medically (with drugs) and surgically. Stroke is diagnosed by procedures that produce images of the brain. Some strokes can be treated with drugs, but many cause brain damage requiring rehabilitation.

What are the best ways to promote cardiovascular health?

Eating a heart-healthy diet from a young age is important, as are getting regular exercise, avoiding tobacco use, knowing and managing blood pressure and cholesterol levels, controlling diabetes, and managing stress.

Web Resources

Cancer

16

LYMPHOMA:08

MARATHON:09

Ever Wonder...

- if it's safer to tan at a tanning salon than in the sun?

- what cancer screening tests you or your parents should be getting?

- if someone who gets cancer can ever be fully cured?

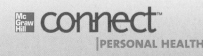

http://www.mcgrawhillconnect.com/personalhealth

Cancer is the second leading cause of death in the United States. In the past, people with cancer often hid their diagnosis; the word *cancer* was not used even in obituaries. Today, with greater understanding of this complex condition, cancer patients are diagnosed earlier and have higher survival rates, better prospects for a cure, and more social support. Although there is still much to learn, there is cause for optimism.

The American Cancer Society projects an estimated 1.53 million new cancer cases in 2010 and more than 569,000 deaths from cancer, about 1,500 per day. Cancer causes about 23 percent of all deaths in the United States, with lung cancer the leading killer among both men and women. The four most common cancers—lung, colon, breast, and prostate—combined account for nearly half of all cancer deaths[1] (Figure 16.1). In this chapter we provide an overview of the many forms cancer takes and the steps you can follow to reduce your risk of developing this disease.

What Is Cancer?

Cancer is a condition characterized by the uncontrolled growth of cells. It develops from a single cell that goes awry, but a combination of events must occur before the cell turns into a **tumor**. The process by which this occurs is called *clonal growth*, the replication of a single cell such that it produces thousands of copies of itself in an uncontrolled manner. With 30 billion cells in a healthy person, the fact that one out of three people develops cancer is not surprising; what is surprising is that two out of three people do not.

cancer
Condition characterized by the uncontrolled growth of cells.

tumor
Mass of extra tissue.

HEALTHY CELL GROWTH

Healthy cells have a complicated system of checks and balances that control cell growth and division. From the start, beginning with the single-celled fertilized egg, cells develop in contact with other cells, sending and receiving messages about how much space is available for growth. Healthy cells in solid tissues (all tissues except the blood) require the presence of neighboring cells. This tendency to stick together serves as a safety mechanism, discouraging cells from drifting off and starting to grow independently.

Healthy cells divide when needed to replace cells that have died or been sloughed off. Each time a cell divides, there is a possibility that a mutation, an error in DNA replication, will occur. Mutations are always occurring randomly, but the risk of mutations is increased by exposure to certain substances, such as tobacco smoke, radiation, and toxic chemicals. Certain mutations may start the cell on a path

Estimated New Cases*		Estimated Deaths	
Male	**Female**	**Male**	**Female**
Prostate 217,730 (28%)	Breast 207,090 (28%)	Lung and bronchus 86,220 (29%)	Lung and bronchus 71,080 (26%)
Lung and bronchus 116,750 (15%)	Lung and bronchus 105,770 (14%)	Prostate 32,050 (11%)	Breast 39,840 (15%)
Colon and rectum 72,090 (9%)	Colon and rectum 70,480 (10%)	Colon and rectum 26,580 (9%)	Colon and rectum 24,790 (9%)
Urinary bladder 52,760 (7%)	Uterine corpus 43,470 (6%)	Pancreas 18,770 (6%)	Pancreas 18,030 (7%)
Melanoma of the skin 38,870 (5%)	Thyroid 33,930 (5%)	Liver and intrahepatic bile duct 12,720 (4%)	Ovary 13,850 (5%)
Non-Hodgkin's lymphoma 35,380 (4%)	Non-Hodgkin's lymphoma 30,160 (4%)	Leukemia 12,660 (4%)	Non-Hodgkin's lymphoma 9,500 (4%)
Kidney and renal pelvis 35,370 (4%)	Melanoma of the skin 29,260 (4%)	Esophagus 11,650 (4%)	Leukemia 9,180 (3%)
Oral cavity and pharynx 25,420 (3%)	Kidney and renal pelvis 22,870 (3%)	Non-Hodgkin's lymphoma 10,710 (4%)	Uterine corpus 7,950 (3%)
Leukemia 24,690 (3%)	Ovary 21,880 (3%)	Urinary bladder 10,410 (3%)	Liver and intrahepatic bile duct 6,190 (2%)
Pancreas 21,370 (3%)	Pancreas 21,770 (3%)	Kidney and renal pelvis 8,210 (3%)	Brain and other nervous system 5,720 (2%)
All sites 789,620 (100%)	All sites 739,940 (100%)	All sites 299,200 (100%)	All sites 270,290 (100%)

*Excludes basal and squamous cell skin cancers and in situ carcinoma except urinary bladder.

figure **16.1**   Leading sites of new cancer cases and deaths, 2010 estimates.

Source: American Cancer Society, Facts and Figures 2010. *Atlanta: American Cancer Society, Inc. Reprinted with permission.*

toward cancer. Specific mechanisms are designed to correct genetic mutations and destroy cells with mutations.

As one mechanism, enzymes within the nucleus of each cell scan the DNA as it replicates, looking for errors. If an error is detected, the enzyme repairs it, or the cell destroys

or the bloodstream, and travel to nearby lymph nodes or to distant sites in the body. At a new site, the cancerous cell can grow and become a secondary tumor, or **metastasis**. When a cancer spreads from one part of the body to another, it is said to have *metastasized*.

In the past, people with cancer often hid their diagnosis; the word *cancer* was not even used in obituaries.

itself. As another safety mechanism, cells are programmed to divide a certain number of times, and then they become incapable of further division. The immune system also helps watch for cells that are not growing normally and destroys them.

A special protective mechanism exists for certain cells called **stem cells**. These are cells that did not differentiate into specific cell types (for example, nerve cells, skin cells, bone cells) during prenatal development. Instead, they retain the ability to become different cell types, and they are capable of unlimited division. A small number of stem cells are present within most tissue types, where they are needed to replace lost or damaged cell lines.

Because stem cells do not have a predetermined number of cell divisions, they pose a risk for cancer. As a safety mechanism, they are located deep within tissues, where they are protected from factors that increase the risk of genetic mutations, such as exposure to the sun, chemicals, and irritation.

CANCER CELL GROWTH

Cancer starts from a single cell that undergoes a critical mutation, either as a result of an error in duplication or in response to a **carcinogen** or radiation. This *initiating event* allows a cell to evade one of the restraints placed upon healthy cells. To become a cancer, however, it must escape all the control mechanisms. Usually this process requires a series of 5 to 10 critical mutations within the cell's genetic material. It may take many years for these changes to progress to cancer, or they may never do so.

In time, perhaps a period of years, another mutation, such as one in an **oncogene** (a gene that drives cell growth regardless of signals from surrounding cells), may allow the cell line to divide forever rather than follow its preprogrammed number of divisions. A condition of cell overgrowth, called *hyperplasia*, develops at the site, and some cells may become abnormal, a condition called *dysplasia*. Eventually, a mass of extra tissue—a tumor—may develop.

A **benign tumor** grows slowly and is unlikely to spread. Benign tumors are dangerous if they grow in locations where they interfere with normal functioning and cannot be completely removed without destroying healthy tissue, as in the brain. A **malignant tumor** is capable of invading surrounding tissue and spreading. Malignant cells do not stick together as much as normal cells, and as the tumor grows, some cancer cells may break off, enter the lymphatic system

CLASSIFYING CANCERS

Cancers are classified according to the tissue in which they originate, called the *primary site*. If a cancer originates in the cells lining the colon, for example, it is considered colon cancer, even when it metastasizes to other, secondary sites. The most common sites of metastases are the brain, liver, and bone marrow. When a cancer is still at its primary site, it is said to be *localized*. When it has metastasized, it is referred to as *invasive*. The greater the extent of metastasis, the poorer the *prognosis* (likely outcome).

Cancers are staged at time of diagnosis—a process that helps guide treatment choices and predict prognosis. The stage of disease is a description of how far the cancer has spread. One common staging system uses five categories (stages 0–IV). Stage 0 is also called cancer *in situ*, an early cancer that is present only in the layer of cells where it began. Stage I cancers are generally small and localized. Stages II and III are locally advanced and may or may not involve local lymph nodes. Stage IV cancers have metastasized to distant sites.

TYPES OF CANCER

Different tissues of the body have different risks for cancer, due in part to their different rates of cell division. Four broad types of cancer are distinguished, based on the type of tissue in which they originate. **Carcinomas** arise from epithelial tissue, which includes the skin, the lining of the intestines and body cavities, the surface of body organs, and the outer portions of the glands. Epithelial tissue is frequently shed and replaced. From 80 to 90 percent of all cancers originate in epithelial tissues. **Sarcomas** originate in connective tissue, such as bone, tendon, cartilage, muscle, or

stem cells
Undifferentiated cells capable of unlimited division that can give rise to specialized cells.

carcinogen
Cancer-causing substance or agent in the environment.

oncogene
Gene that drives a cell to grow and divide regardless of signals from surrounding cells.

benign tumor
Tumor that grows slowly and is unlikely to spread.

malignant tumor
Tumor that is capable of invading surrounding tissue and spreading.

metastasis
Cancer that has spread from one part of the body to another.

carcinomas
Cancers that arise from epithelial tissue.

sarcomas
Cancers that originate in connective tissue.

fat tissues. **Leukemias** are cancers of the blood and originate in the bone marrow or the lymphatic system. **Lymphomas** originate in the lymph nodes or glands.

Risk Factors for Cancer

Because some cancers occur as a result of random genetic mutations, there is an element of chance in the development of the disease. Other cancers are associated with inherited genetic mutations. Still others occur as a result of exposure to carcinogens. Some such exposures can be limited by lifestyle behaviors, such as using sunscreen and avoiding tobacco, but others are beyond individual control and require the involvement of local authorities, the larger society, or even the international community, as in the case of air pollution (see the box "Cancer Mortality and Risk Factor Disparities").

Risk factors are associated with a higher incidence of a disease but do not determine that the disease will occur. For example, if you smoke, you are 20 times more likely to develop lung cancer than a nonsmoker. Smoking does not guarantee you will get lung cancer, but your risk, relative to that of a nonsmoker, is greater. Conversely, if you do not smoke, you still may get lung cancer, but your risk is much lower than that of a smoker. The most significant risk factor for most cancers is age. Advancing age increases the risk for cancer; 77 percent of cancers occur in people aged 55 or older.[1]

leukemias
Cancers of the blood, originating in the bone marrow or the lymphatic system.

lymphomas
Cancers that originate in the lymph nodes or glands.

FAMILY HISTORY

A family history of cancer increases an individual's risk. Examining your family health tree can help you understand whether you have an increased risk for any cancers. Family history does alter some cancer screening recommendations, such as when to start screening, how frequently to have screenings repeated, and what types of tests to have performed. However, genes are not the entire story. Genes interact with environmental exposures and lifestyle behaviors to alter risk. The social determinants of health—including socioeconomic and cultural factors—are also influential (see the box "Addressing Cancer Disparities").

LIFESTYLE FACTORS

Some environmental agents (carcinogens) have a direct impact on a cell, causing an initial genetic alteration that can lead to cancer. Other

---

Who's at Risk?

Cancer Mortality and Risk Factor Disparities

Cancer affects people of all races and ethnicities, but disparities in incidence (number of new cases) and mortality (number of deaths) between population groups are striking. Consider the following:

■ Black men have the highest incidence of prostate cancer and are more than twice as likely as White men to die from it.

■ White women have the highest incidence of breast cancer but Black women are more likely to die from it.

■ Hispanic women have the highest incidence of cervical cancer, followed by Black women, and then White women. Black women are more than twice as likely as White women and Asian American women to die from cervical cancer and somewhat more likely than Hispanic women.

■ Prior to 1980, Blacks and Whites had similar mortality rates for colon cancer, but since 1980, mortality rates have steadily increased for Blacks. Blacks are less likely than Whites to receive recommended surgery, chemotherapy, or radiation treatment for colon cancer.

Multiple factors contribute to cancer mortality disparities, but most are believed to be attributable to socioeconomic barriers to early cancer detection and treatment. Consider the following:

■ Inadequate health insurance: 1 in 5 Blacks, 1 in 3 Hispanics, and 1 in 10 Whites were uninsured in 2008. Blacks with private health insurance have a 30 percent higher survival rate from colon cancer than those without insurance.

■ Low income: 1 in 4 Blacks and Hispanics, and 1 in 10 Whites lived below the poverty line in 2008. Poverty is associated with increased tobacco use, obesity, inactivity, and lack of access to health care—all risk factors for disease.

■ Dietary and physical activity differences: reduced access to fresh fruits, vegetables, and safe exercise environments are a bigger problem in lower income communities.

■ Cultural practices: women in cultures that promote earlier marriage may have reduced risk of breast cancer due to earlier childbearing.

Recognizing health disparities is important because interventions can be designed to target underlying factors. Cancer risk factor and mortality disparities need not be with us forever.

Source: "Cancer Facts and Figures 2010," American Cancer Society, 2010, retrieved July 1, 2010, from www.cancer.org/Research/CancerFactsFigures/index.

and the type of cigarettes smoked, with higher tar content being more dangerous.[1]

Nutrition and Physical Activity Nutrition and physical activity are the second most important contributors to cancer risk for the general population. Diets rich in fruits, vegetables, and whole grains appear to decrease the risk for many cancers, including lung, colon, rectal, breast, stomach, and ovarian cancers. Diets high in fiber appear to decrease the risk of colon cancer and possibly the risk of breast, rectal, pharyngeal, and stomach cancers.

Only 5 percent of college students report eating the recommended 5 or more servings of fruits and vegetables per day.[2] Fruits and vegetables are rich in antioxidants, chemicals that protect against damage to tissues. Although fruits and vegetables can have trace amounts of pesticides and herbicides, which can be toxic in high amounts, there is no evidence currently that the amounts in foods outweigh the proven benefits of consuming fruits and vegetables. To date, there is no clear evidence that taking supplements produces the same benefits in cancer-risk reduction that eating the whole foods provides. In addition, high-dose supplements of beta-carotene (an antioxidant) have actually been shown to increase risk of developing some cancers. Consuming organic foods over conventionally grown food does not appear to provide any additional cancer risk reduction. To help encourage people to eat fruits and vegetables, the National Cancer Institute has partnered up with other government agencies in the "Fruits and Veggies—More Matters" public health initiative (www.fruitsandveggiesmatter.gov).[3]

Cooking meats at high temperatures, such as when grilling, frying, or broiling, may produce chemicals that increase risk for colon cancer. Processed meats, which are high in nitrites, also appear to increase risk. Studies have not shown an increase in cancer risk associated with coffee, saccharin, aspartame, or food irradiation.

Exercise is directly linked to a reduction in risk of breast and colon cancers, though its effect on other cancers is less clear. The benefits of exercise on cancer risk are independent of exercise's impact on weight. Exercise alters body functions in a positive way; for example, it increases the rate at which food travels through the intestines, thus reducing the exposure of the bowel lining to potential carcinogens. Appropriate exercise after a cancer diagnosis and during treatment can also help people feel better, eat better, and recover faster.[1,4–7]

Overweight and Obesity Overweight and obesity increase the risk of developing many types of cancer as well as the risk of dying from cancer once it occurs. Overweight and obesity not only make it harder to detect cancers at an early stage but also delay diagnosis and may make treatment more difficult.

Although it is not clear how fat cells contribute to an increased risk of cancer, several pathways are possible. Fat cells produce hormones, some of which (such as estrogen)

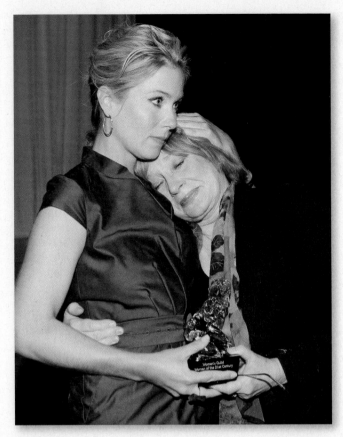

■ A family history of cancer can indicate that a person may have a genetic predisposition to the disease, especially if the cancer occurred in a first-degree relative (like a parent) at an early age. Christina Applegate, whose mother is a repeat breast cancer survivor, was diagnosed with breast cancer in 2008. Testing revealed that she had inherited a mutation of the BRCA1 gene, which is linked to breast cancer.

agents, called *cancer promoters*, have a less direct effect, enhancing the possibility that a cancer will develop if an initiating event has already occurred in a cell.

Tobacco Use Tobacco use is the leading preventable cause of cancer in the United States. It is responsible for 30 percent of all cancer deaths and 87 percent of all lung cancer deaths. Smokers are more likely than nonsmokers to die from their lung cancer—23 times more likely if they are men and 13 times more likely if they are women.[1]

Tobacco use increases the risk of cancers of the mouth, throat, lung, and esophagus by directly exposing them to the chemicals in tobacco smoke. It increases the risk of other cancers, including bladder, pancreas, stomach, liver, kidney, and bone-marrow cancers, because other chemicals from tobacco are absorbed into the bloodstream and travel to distant sites. Individual risk from tobacco use depends on the age at which the person starts smoking, the number of years the person smokes, the number of cigarettes smoked per day,

Public Health in Action

Addressing Cancer Disparities

Do you live in rural America? Do you earn less money than the average American? Are you uninsured? Your answers to these questions are indicators of whether or not you are likely to develop cancer someday and how likely you are to die from it.

Although the number of new cases of cancer and the number of deaths from cancer are reported by race and ethnicity, factors such as income, education, geographical location, housing, and cultural beliefs are believed to be stronger indicators of risk. These factors influence risk behaviors (such as tobacco use), access to health care, and quality of health care.

As an example, let's consider cancer screening tests. Getting the recommended tests in a timely way increases the likelihood that a cancer will be detected or diagnosed at an earlier, more treatable stage. However, in our current health system screening tests are not free. Many people receive screening tests through a health plan covered by health insurance, but lower paying jobs are less likely to offer health insurance than higher paying jobs. In addition, the cost of health insurance can be prohibitive for many poor people with or without jobs, so they go without health insurance, and uninsured people are significantly less likely to receive cancer screening tests. Rural Americans are less likely than urban Americans to receive cancer screening, in part because fewer physicians practice in rural communities. Rural residents are also less likely than urban residents to have health insurance. If

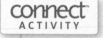

uninsured people do develop cancer, it is diagnosed at a later, less treatable stage, and their chances of survival are reduced.

In an attempt to reduce barriers to screening for breast and cervical cancer, the Centers for Disease Control and Prevention (CDC) implemented the National Breast and Cervical Cancer Early Detection Program in 1990. The program provides low-income, uninsured, and underserved women access to breast and cervical cancer screening, including clinical breast exams, Pap tests, mammograms, and further diagnostic testing or treatment as necessary. Since 1991 the program has served 3.6 million women throughout all 50 states, the District of Columbia, 5 U.S. territories, and 12 American Indian/Alaskan Native tribes or tribal organizations.

The CDC recently launched the Colorectal Cancer Control Program in an attempt to reduce disparity in rates of colorectal cancer screening. The program targets low-income, under- or uninsured men and women aged 50 to 64 and will operate similarly to the National Breast and Cervical Cancer Detection Program. At present, an estimated 40 percent of individuals who should be screened for colorectal cancer have not been screened. The lowest screening rates are among racial and ethnic minorities and the uninsured. Addressing the economic factors influencing access to cancer screening is just one way to reduce cancer disparities.

Sources: National Healthcare Disparities Report, 2006, *Centers for Disease Control and Prevention, Agency for Healthcare Research and Quality, U.S. Department of Health and Human Services;* "National Breast and Cervical Cancer Early Detection Program," *Centers for Disease Control and Prevention, retrieved May 13, 2010, from www.cdc.gov/cancer/nbccedp/index.htm;* "Colorectal Cancer Control Program," *Centers for Disease Control and Prevention, retrieved May 13, 2010, from www.cdc.gov/cancer/crccp/.*

---

are linked to cancer. Fat cells may trigger an inflammatory reaction, alter insulin production, or release proteins that trigger cell growth, all of which may contribute to the development of cancer. Fat cells may also accumulate more environmental toxins. Maintaining a healthy BMI throughout your lifespan is another way to reduce your cancer risk.[1,6]

Alcohol Consumption and Cancer Risk   Alcohol consumption of more than one drink a day for women and two drinks a day for men increases the risk for cancers of the

alone. Red wine does not appear to offer a protective effect against cancer; wine, beer, and hard liquor all increase risk.[1,8]

ENVIRONMENTAL FACTORS

Some cancers are caused by exposure to carcinogens in the environment, but some exposures are more controllable than others.

Sunlight and Other Sources of Ultraviolet Radiation
Ultraviolet (UV) radiation, the rays of energy that come

Overweight and obesity *not only make it harder to detect cancers at an early stage but also delay diagnosis and may make treatment more difficult.*

mouth, throat, esophagus, liver, and breast. Regular intake of a few drinks per week may increase risk of breast cancer. Alcohol and tobacco used together amplify the risk for cancer and are associated with a greater risk than is either one

from the sun (or sun lamps and tanning beds), can damage DNA and cause skin cancer. The sun's ultraviolet radiation has two types of rays: ultraviolet B (UVB) and ultraviolet A (UVA). UVB rays are more likely to cause sunburns and

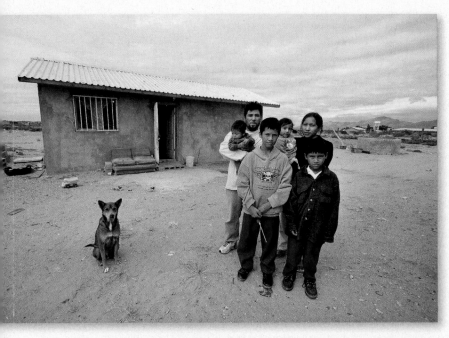

■ Being poor and living in a rural locale are risk factors for cancer. This low-income family living in the desert has less access to well-paying jobs, health insurance, health information, and health care services, including cancer screening tests, than a more affluent family living in an urban environment.

have long been associated with skin cancers. UVA rays tend to pass deeper into the skin and are now believed to cause skin cancer and premature aging of the skin.

The risk for the two milder forms of skin cancer, basal cell and squamous cell carcinomas, is cumulative; the more UV exposure over the years, the higher the risk. The risk for melanoma, the most dangerous form of skin cancer, appears to be related more to the timing and number of sunburns. Sunburns that occur during childhood seem to be the most dangerous, and the more sunburns, the greater the risk.

People who live in certain regions of the world have a higher risk of developing skin cancers because of their location close to the equator or in areas affected by the hole in the ozone layer of the atmosphere. The ozone layer, which protects the earth from the sun's damaging UV rays, is being disrupted by chemical pollution and is thinning over Antarctica and southern portions of the globe. Australia has one of the highest rates of skin cancer in the world, presumably because of this environmental condition.[9,10]

Other Forms of Radiation Ionizing radiation, radiation with enough energy to displace electrons from atoms, can also cause cancer. An estimated 82 percent of ionizing

radiation comes from natural sources, such as radon (a naturally occurring radioactive gas in the ground in certain regions of the world). The other 18 percent is from human-made sources, such as medical X-rays, nuclear medicine, and consumer products (such as tobacco, building materials, and television and computer screens).[11]

Residents in many parts of North America are exposed to low levels of radon in their homes, particularly homes with basements. In regions known to have high levels of radon in the ground, testing of homes is recommended, followed by the installation of a ventilation system if levels are found to be elevated.

Nuclear fallout is an environmental source of radiation. Survivors of nuclear bomb explosions and tests have high levels of cancer, particularly cancers of the bone marrow and thyroid. The nuclear reactors used in power plants have not been shown to emit enough ionizing radiation to place surrounding communities at risk. However, accidental releases of radioactive gases have occurred, and accidents at power plants, such as the one at Chernobyl in 1986, have contaminated land for miles around and caused an untold number of cancers in those exposed to radiation and radioactive debris.

Radiation in medical settings is used in the treatment of cancers or diagnostic imaging. High-dose radiation for cancer treatment has been shown to increase the risk for leukemia and thyroid and breast cancers years later. Lower levels of radiation are used in diagnostic X-rays and CT scans. The amount of radiation per procedure is low, but exposures can accumulate if someone needs many tests. To reduce risk, the number of medical procedures should be minimized as much as possible, especially in children.[11,12]

There is ongoing debate over the risk associated with non-ionizing radiation, such as radiofrequency from cell phones and cordless phones. Some studies have shown an increased risk of brain cancer and greater risk with greater number of hours of use. Other studies have shown no

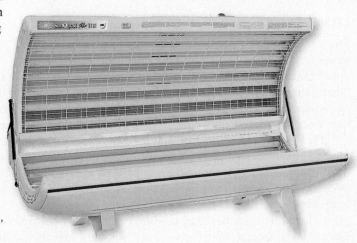

■ Although the risks of sun exposure are well known and include not only skin cancer but premature aging of the skin, tanning is still popular in the United States.

increased risk. Given the pervasive use of cell phones, this remains an important area of study.[13]

Chemical and Physical Carcinogens Many other substances in the environment have been associated with different forms of cancer. Environmental carcinogens include metals (such as arsenic, mercury, and lead), natural fibers (such as asbestos and silica), combustion by-products (including motor vehicle exhaust, diesel exhaust, and soot), solvents (benzene, toluene), polychlorinated biphenyls, and pesticides. Your exposure to environmental carcinogens varies depending on where you live, where you work, what your hobbies and recreational activities are, and what you eat, among other factors. Exposures are higher and rates of cancer are higher in cities, farming states, and industrial areas and near hazardous waste sites.[13–15]

Infectious Agents Some viruses are known to cause cancer. Human papillomavirus (HPV) is linked to cancers of the cervix, anus, vagina, penis, and mouth. The hepatitis B and C viruses are associated with liver cancer. Certain strains of Epstein-Barr virus, which causes mononucleosis, are associated with Hodgkin's lymphoma, non-Hodgkin's lymphoma, and some stomach cancers. Human immunodeficiency virus (HIV) suppresses the immune system and allows several types of cancer to develop. The only bacterium linked to cancer thus far is *Helicobacter pylori*, which causes a chronic irritation of the stomach lining and is associated with stomach ulcers and an increased risk of stomach cancer.[16–19]

Common Cancers

Since 1930 changes have occurred in the rates of different cancers in the United States (Figure 16.2). The most dramatic change in overall rates can be seen for lung cancer. The increase in lung cancer for both sexes is believed to be the result of higher rates of smoking. Rates of smoking increased among women about 20 to 30 years after they increased in men, and there has been a corresponding increase in lung cancer among women.

LUNG CANCER

The leading cause of cancer death for both men and women in the United States and the second most commonly diagnosed cancer is lung cancer. In 1987 lung cancer overtook breast cancer as the leading cause of cancer death for American women. The incidence rates are declining for men and have reached a plateau for women.[1]

The leading risk factor for lung cancer is the use of tobacco products in any form. A genetic link has been identified that makes people more likely to become addicted to tobacco, makes it harder to quit, and increases the risk of lung cancer.[20,21] Other risk factors are exposures to carcinogenic chemicals, arsenic, radon, asbestos, radiation, air pollution, and environmental tobacco smoke. Recently, experts

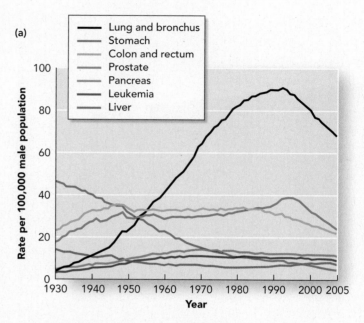

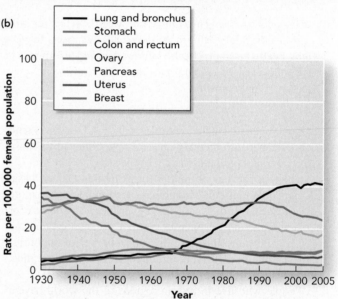

figure 16.2 **Cancer death rates by site, 1930–2005; (a) death rates for men; (b) death rates for women.**
Source: From "U.S. Mortality Data 1960–2005," U.S. Mortality Volumes 1930 to 1959, National Center for Health Statistics, Centers for Disease Control and Prevention, 2009.

determined that dietary supplements containing beta-carotene, a form of vitamin A, further increase the risk for lung cancer in people who smoke. Reducing risk factors, especially exposure to tobacco smoke and environmental tobacco smoke, is the first line of defense against this disease.

Signs and symptoms of lung cancer include coughing, blood-streaked sputum, chest pain, difficulty breathing, and recurrent lung infections. Unfortunately, symptoms do not appear in most people until the disease is advanced, a factor that frequently delays detection of the disease. There is currently no routine screening test for lung cancer. Chest X-rays, examination of sputum, and a form of computerized tomography called *spiral CT* can detect early-stage lung cancer, but there is no evidence that utilizing these tests increases survival from lung cancer. A large study called the National Lung Screening Trial is under way to determine whether screening high-risk, heavy smokers by these methods can improve survival.[22]

If symptoms suggest lung cancer and an abnormality is found on an X-ray or CT scan, the diagnosis is confirmed by a biopsy, performed either by surgery or by **bronchoscopy**. People with small tumors that can be removed surgically have the best prognosis. For more advanced cancers or

COLON AND RECTAL CANCER

The third leading cause of cancer death and the third most commonly diagnosed cancer is colon and rectal cancer. During the 1990s, the incidence of colon and rectal cancer declined in the United States along with the number of deaths from the disease. The decrease may be due to improved screening and treatment, and early detection and removal of **colon polyps**.[1–3]

bronchoscopy
Procedure in which a fiber-optic device is inserted into the lungs to allow the health care provider to examine lung tissue for signs of cancer.

colon polyps
Growths in the colon that may progress to colon cancer.

A genetic link has been identified that makes people more likely to become addicted to tobacco, makes it harder to quit, and increases the risk of lung cancer.

for people who are unable to tolerate surgery, radiation or a combination of radiation and chemotherapy is used. If the cancer has spread to distant sites, radiation and chemotherapy can be used for *palliative care* (care provided to give temporary relief of symptoms but not to cure the cancer). The 1-year survival rate for lung cancer is 42 percent, and the 5-year survival rate is 16 percent.[1]

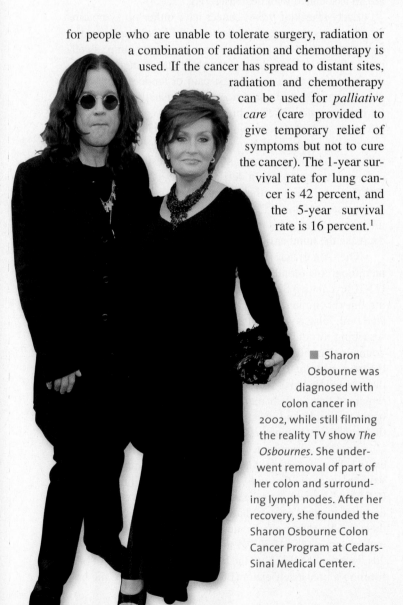

■ Sharon Osbourne was diagnosed with colon cancer in 2002, while still filming the reality TV show *The Osbournes*. She underwent removal of part of her colon and surrounding lymph nodes. After her recovery, she founded the Sharon Osbourne Colon Cancer Program at Cedars-Sinai Medical Center.

The most important risk factor for colorectal cancer is age. More than 90 percent of colorectal cancers are diagnosed in people over age 50. A personal or family history of colon polyps or inflammatory bowel disease also increases risk, as does a family history of colorectal cancer, especially in a first-degree relative. Other factors associated with an increased risk for colon and rectal cancer include smoking, alcohol use, obesity, physical inactivity, a diet high in fat or red or processed meat, and inadequate amounts of fruits and vegetables. Aspirin and hormone replacement therapy may reduce the risk for colon and rectal cancer.[1,2,3]

Warning signs of colorectal cancer include a change in bowel movements, change in stool size or shape, pain in the abdomen, and blood in the stool. The signs do not usually occur until the disease is fairly advanced. Screening tests are available that can enhance early detection of polyps or cancer.

Four techniques can be used to "visualize" the colon. In a **flexible sigmoidoscopy**, a thin, flexible fiber-optic tube is inserted into the rectum and moved through the lower third of the colon. In a **colonoscopy**, a longer scope is used and the entire colon is viewed (Figure 16.3). If a polyp is found, it can be biopsied during the procedure. In a **double-contrast barium enema** the colon is partially filled with a contrast material and then

flexible sigmoidoscopy
Procedure in which a fiber-optic device is inserted in the colon to allow the health care provider to examine the lower third of the colon for polyps or cancer.

colonoscopy
Procedure in which a fiber-optic device is inserted in the colon to allow the health care provider to examine the entire colon for polyps or cancer.

double-contrast barium enema
Test for colon polyps or cancer in which contrast material is inserted into the colon and X-rays are taken of the abdomen, revealing alterations in the lining of the colon if polyps or cancer is present.

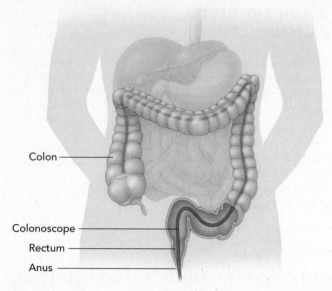

Colon

Colonoscope

Rectum

Anus

figure **16.3** **Colonoscopy.** A colonoscopy allows the entire colon to be examined and facilitates the removal of growths, such as polyps, that may become cancerous.

Source: From Fit & Well: Core Concepts and Labs in Physical Fitness and Wellness, 8th ed. Copyright © 2009 The McGraw-Hill Companies. Used with permission of The McGraw-Hill Companies.

X-rays are taken. A colon cancer or polyp will alter the lining of the colon and can be seen. In **CT colonography** (or virtual colonoscopy), a CT scanner is used to take multiple pictures of the colon and can detect polyps or cancer.

Several other tests can be used that primarily screen for colon cancer but are not as good at detecting polyps. These include the fecal occult blood test, the stool immunochemical test, and the stool DNA test. The first two screen for trace amounts of blood, which can signal a cancer or a bleeding polyp. The DNA test looks for changes in DNA known to be related to colon cancer.[23]

CT colonography
Screen for colon polyps or cancer using a CT scanner.

The American Cancer Society recommends that people of average risk start colorectal cancer screening at age 50. For people with higher than average risk (for example, someone who has a close family member with colon cancer or polyps), earlier and more frequent screening may be recommended.

Surgery is the most common treatment for colon and rectal cancer; it can cure the cancer if it has not spread. Chemotherapy and/or radiation is added if the cancer is large or has spread to other areas. The 1-year survival rate for all stages of colorectal cancer is 83 percent; the 5-year survival rate is 65 percent.

BREAST CANCER

The second leading cause of cancer death in women and the most commonly diagnosed non-skin cancer in women is breast cancer. Breast cancer occurs in men as well as women, but it is less common. There are an estimated 207,090 cases

expected in women and 1,970 cases expected in men in the United States in 2010.[1]

There are both controllable and noncontrollable risk factors for breast cancer. Among the noncontrollable factors are early onset of menarche (first menstruation), late onset of menopause, family history of breast cancer in a first-degree relative, older age, and higher socioeconomic class. As discussed in Chapter 2, a mutation in the BRCA1 or BRCA2 gene is associated with an increased risk of breast cancer. Although inherited susceptibility accounts for only 5 percent of all breast cancer cases, having these genes confers a lifetime risk of developing the disease ranging from 35 to 85 percent.

Controllable risk factors for breast cancer that increase risk include never having children or having a first child after age 30, being obese after menopause, taking hormone replacement therapy, and drinking more than two alcoholic beverages a day. Breastfeeding, engaging in moderate or vigorous exercise, and maintaining a healthy body weight are all associated with decreased risk.

Early stages of breast cancer have either no symptoms or symptoms that may be detected only by a mammogram. Symptoms of later stages include a persistent lump; swelling, redness, or bumpiness of the skin; and change in nipple appearance or discharge. Breast pain or tenderness is common in women without cancer and is usually not a cause for concern; more likely explanations are hormonal changes, infection, or breast cysts, which are rarely cancerous.

Breast cancer can be detected at an early stage by a mammogram, a low-dose X-ray of the breast. The effectiveness of mammography in detecting cancer depends on several factors, including the size of the cancer, the density of the breasts, and the skills of the radiologist. Although mammograms cannot detect all cancers, they have been shown to decrease the number of women who die from breast cancer.

The American Cancer Society recommends annual mammograms for all women aged 40 and older. In 2009, the U.S. Preventative Services Task Force recommended reversing this recommendation, citing the anxiety and cost associated with false positives. It recommended that women begin screening through mammograms at age 50 and that women younger than 50 talk with their doctors about their risk for breast cancer and the value of mammography based on their individual risk factors. Institutions like the ACS have remained firm in their recommendations that mammograms begin at age 40 and insurance companies continue to cover the procedure for women 40 and older.[24]

Another screening technique for breast cancer is breast exam. The American Cancer Society recommends that women in their 20s and 30s have a clinical breast exam (CBE) performed by a health care provider every 3 years and that women over 40 have a breast exam performed by their health care provider annually near the time of their mammogram. The ACS also suggests that, beginning in their 20s, women be told about the benefits and limitations of performing a breast self-exam (BSE) every month (see the box

"Breast Self-Exam"). The ACS considers it acceptable for women to choose not to do self-exams or to do them only occasionally. The Preventative Services Task Force recommended in 2009 that women not perform breast self-exams but instead be on the lookout for any changes in their breasts during the course of daily activities.

Any suspicious lumps, changes, or mammogram findings that are suggestive of cancer are typically followed by a biopsy so that cells or tissues can be evaluated under the microscope, the only way to make a definitive diagnosis. There are several noncancerous causes of lumps in the breast; in younger women, a lump is much more likely to be caused by a cyst or a benign tumor called a fibroadenoma.

Other screening tools, including ultrasound and magnetic resonance imaging (MRI), are sometimes used to help determine whether a lump or abnormality is cancerous.

Surgery is usually the first line of treatment for breast cancer, either a lumpectomy (removal of a section of the breast around the cancer) or a mastectomy (removal of the entire breast). Lymph nodes under the arm on the affected side are often tested to determine whether the cancer has spread from the breast. Radiation, chemotherapy, and hormonal therapy are frequently used in the treatment of breast cancer.

The 5-year survival rate for all stages of breast cancer is 90 percent. For cancer that is localized (no lymph node

Highlight on Health

Breast Self-Exam

Performing a monthly breast self-exam (BSE) can help you learn how your breasts normally feel so you can identify any changes that occur. Almost all women have some lumps and bumps in their breast tissue that change throughout the month. The best time to do your exam is a few days after your period when the breast tissue is least tender. If you no longer menstruate or have very irregular periods, do the exam on the same day every month.

If you choose to do a BSE, follow these steps:

- Lie down and put a pillow under your right shoulder. Place your right arm behind your head.

- Use the finger pads of your three middle fingers on your left hand to feel for lumps or thickening in your right breast. Use overlapping dime-sized circular motions of the finger pads to feel the breast tissue.

- Use three different levels of pressure—light, medium, and firm—to feel all the breast tissue. Use each pressure level to feel the breast tissue before moving on to the next spot. If you're not sure how hard to press, talk with your health care provider. A firm ridge in the lower curve of each breast is normal.

- Move around the breast in an up-and-down pattern starting at an imaginary line drawn straight down your side from the underarm and move across the breast to the middle of the chest (breast bone).

- Repeat the exam on your left breast, using the finger pads of the right hand and moving the pillow under your left shoulder.

- While standing in front of a mirror with your hands pressing firmly down on your hips, look at your breasts for any changes of size, shape, contour, or dimpling. (Pressing down on your hips contracts the chest wall muscles and enhances any breast changes.)

- Examine each underarm while sitting up or standing and with your arm only slightly raised so you can easily feel in the area.

If you notice any change—such as the development of a lump or swelling, skin irritation or dimpling, nipple pain or retraction, redness or scaliness of the nipple or skin, or a discharge other than breast milk—see your health care provider right away for an evaluation. Most of the time, these changes are not cancer.

These BSE guidelines represent a change in previous recommendations, based on an extensive review of the medical literature and input from an expert advisory group.

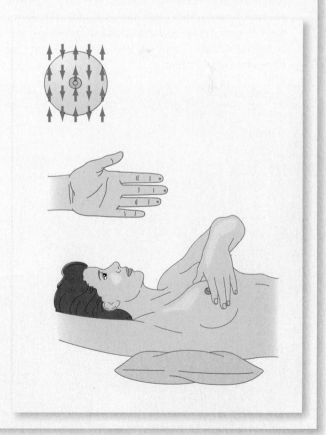

involvement), it is 98 percent; for cancer that has spread regionally (only local lymph node involvement), it is 84 percent; and for cancer that has distant metastases, it is 23 percent.[1]

PROSTATE CANCER

The second most common cause of cancer death in men and the most commonly diagnosed cancer in men is prostate cancer. The incidence of prostate cancer is significantly higher among Black men than White men, as is the death rate. The number of diagnosed cases of prostate cancer increased in the early 1990s, probably as a result of better screening, and has leveled off since 1995. Death rates declined during the same period, although death rates for Black men remain twice as high as those for White men.[1]

The most important risk factor for prostate cancer is age. More than 60 percent of prostate cancer cases are diagnosed in men aged 65 and older. Other risk factors include a family history of prostate cancer, being Black, and possibly having a high animal-fat diet. The risk of dying from prostate cancer appears to increase with increasing body weight. Lycopene, an antioxidant food in red and pink fruits and vegetables may reduce risk.

In its early stages, prostate cancer usually has no signs or symptoms. Advanced prostate cancer can be associated with

■ Prostate cancer has a high rate of survival. Former president of South Africa Nelson Mandela was diagnosed with prostate cancer in 2001 when he was 83 years old. His treatment consisted of seven weeks of radiation therapy, and all reports indicate that he has been cancer-free since the completion of treatment.

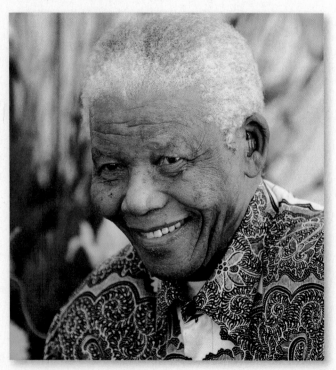

difficulty urinating, pain in the pelvic region, pain with urination, or blood in the urine. These symptoms can also be caused by more common, noncancerous conditions, such as benign enlargement of the prostate gland and bladder infections.

Two screening tests are available to detect prostate cancer. One is a *digital rectal exam*, in which a health care provider inserts a gloved finger into the rectum and palpates the prostate gland. The other is the *prostate-specific antigen (PSA) test*, a blood test that detects levels of a substance made by the prostate (prostate-specific antigen) that are elevated when certain conditions are present, including benign prostate enlargement, infection, and prostate cancer. If PSA levels are elevated, a rectal ultrasound and prostate biopsy can be performed to assess and diagnose the cause.

At present, it is unclear whether the benefits of screening tests for prostate cancer—earlier detection of cancer when it is most treatable—outweigh the negatives. As with mammography, screening tests for prostate cancer can produce false positives, requiring further invasive follow-up tests. Sometimes, fast-growing prostate cancers do not elevate PSA levels, causing a false negative result from a PSA test. To further complicate the situation, some prostate cancers grow very slowly and would not actually lead to an earlier death. The treatment of these cancers can sometimes cause more harm and side effects than if they were left untreated. The American Cancer Society recommends that all men discuss with their health care providers whether they should have a digital rectal exam and PSA screening annually starting at age 50; the ACS also recommends that Black men and men with a family history of prostate cancer begin having screening done at age 45.[1]

Treatment for prostate cancer depends on the stage of the cancer and the man's age and other health conditions. In its early stages and in a younger man, prostate cancer is usually treated with surgery (removal of the prostate gland) and radiation, sometimes in combination with chemotherapy, and hormonal medication, which blocks the effects of testosterone and can cause tumors to shrink. Later stages are treated with chemotherapy, radiation, and hormonal medication. Radiation is sometimes administered by the implantation of radioactive seeds, which destroy cancer tissue and leave normal prostate tissue intact.

The 5-year survival rate for all stages of prostate cancer is 99 percent. For cancers detected at local or regional stages, the 5-year survival rate is close to 100 percent. In studies that follow prostate cancer for more than 5 years, the survival rate decreases to 93 percent at 10 years and to 79 percent at 15 years.[1]

CANCERS OF THE FEMALE REPRODUCTIVE SYSTEM

Cancer can develop throughout the female reproductive system but occurs more frequently in the cervix, uterus, and ovaries.

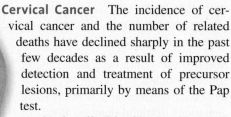

Cervical Cancer The incidence of cervical cancer and the number of related deaths have declined sharply in the past few decades as a result of improved detection and treatment of precursor lesions, primarily by means of the Pap test.

As described in Chapter 14, cervical cancer is closely related to infection with certain strains of the human papillomavirus (HPV). However, HPV infection is common in women, and the majority of women never develop cervical cancer. Persistent infection and progression to cancer are influenced by other factors, such as tobacco use, immunosuppression, multiple births, early sexual activity, multiple sex partners, socioeconomic status, and nutritional status. Currently two vaccines are available and reduce the risk of HPV infection, as described in Chapter 14.

In its early stages, cervical cancer usually does not cause any symptoms. Warning signs of more advanced cancer include abnormal vaginal discharge or abnormal vaginal bleeding. Pain in the pelvic region can be a late sign of cervical cancer. Early detection through the Pap test has significantly reduced the rates of cervical cancer and mortality. The Pap test, recommended for all women, is performed as part of a pelvic exam. A small sample of cells is collected from the cervix with a swab or brush, placed on a slide or into a liquid suspension, processed, and then examined under the microscope to detect cells that may be abnormal. Pap tests are good but not perfect, occasionally giving either a false negative or a false positive. HPV tests can be used with liquid Pap suspensions to identify HPV strains and are particularly helpful if the Pap results are unclear.

Treatment for cervical cancer involves removing or destroying precursor cells. Invasive cervical cancer is treated with a combination of surgery, local radiation, and chemotherapy.

Uterine Cancer Also called *endometrial cancer*, uterine cancer usually develops in the endometrium, the lining of the uterus. Uterine cancer is diagnosed more often in White women than in Black women, but the death rate among Black women is nearly twice the rate among White women. Black women tend to have more advanced cancer when they are diagnosed, perhaps as a result of having less access to health care.

The risk for uterine cancer is related to a woman's exposure to estrogen, so factors that increase estrogen—such as obesity and estrogen replacement therapy without progesterone—increase risk. Other factors associated with increased risk include young age at menarche, late-onset menopause, irregular ovulation, and infrequent periods. Pregnancy and oral contraceptives reduce the risk of uterine cancer. Warning signs of uterine cancer include abnormal uterine bleeding (spotting between periods or spotting after menopause), pelvic pain, and low back pain. Pain is usually a late sign of uterine cancer.

Uterine cancer is frequently detected at an early stage in postmenopausal women because of vaginal bleeding. If uterine cancer is diagnosed, a hysterectomy—surgical removal of the uterus—is usually performed. Depending on the stage of cancer, other treatment methods may also be used, including radiation, chemotherapy, and hormonal therapy.[1]

Ovarian Cancer The leading gynecological cause of cancer death and the fifth overall cause of cancer death in women is ovarian cancer. Ovarian cancer has a low rate of survival because most cases are not diagnosed until they have spread beyond the ovaries. If ovarian cancer is diagnosed early, survival is as high as 94 percent. Between 90 and 95 percent of women with ovarian cancer have no risk factors.

The strongest risk factor is a family history of ovarian cancer in a first-degree relative, especially if the BRCA1 or BRCA2 gene is involved. Women with either of these genetic mutations have a 20–60 percent chance of developing ovarian cancer. Risk is also increased in women with a personal history of breast, colon, or endometrial cancer. Factors that reduce risk include use of oral contraceptive pills, pregnancy, and breastfeeding. Avoidance of postmenopausal hormone replacement therapy may also reduce risk. Women with the BRCA1 or BRCA2 gene mutation may consider more aggressive measures to reduce risk, including removal of the ovaries and fallopian tubes.

The early stages of ovarian cancer have few signs or symptoms. At later stages, a woman may notice swelling of the abdomen, bloating, or a vague pain in the lower abdomen. A screen to increase early detection would be beneficial, given the improved survival with early diagnosis. However, to date, no such screen has proved successful.[25,26] Most women, as part of their annual checkup with a Pap test, undergo a "bimanual exam," in which a health care provider feels the uterus and ovaries with two gloved fingers in the vagina and a hand on the lower abdomen. The exam occasionally detects ovarian cancer but usually only when the disease is advanced.

Several blood tests have been evaluated for use as a screening tool and another potential screening tool is a pelvic ultrasound, in which sound waves are used to visualize the ovaries and show whether they are enlarged or contain a mass. At present, there is no generally recommended screen.

Treatment for ovarian cancer depends on the stage at diagnosis. Typically, all or part of the ovaries, uterus, and fallopian tubes are surgically removed and the lymph nodes are biopsied to determine whether the cancer has spread. Chemotherapy and radiation may then be recommended.

Treatment options currently under investigation include vaccinations, targeted drugs, and immunotherapy.[26]

SKIN CANCER

The three forms of skin cancer are basal cell cancer, squamous cell cancer, and melanoma. More than 2 million cases of basal cell and squamous cell cancers occur each year in the United States. Most of these are curable, although both can be disfiguring and, if ignored, fatal. Melanoma is a less common but more serious form of skin cancer. Skin cancers occur in all racial and ethnic groups, but they are more common in people with lighter skin colors.

All forms of skin cancers are linked directly to ultraviolet light exposure—both UVA and UVB.[27] The most effective way to reduce risk for skin cancer is to limit UV exposure, whether from the sun or from the UV lights in tanning salons. Recommended ways of achieving this goal, in order of importance, are staying out of the sun during midday (10:00 a.m. to 4:00 p.m.), wearing protective clothing (including a hat to shade the face and neck, long sleeves, and long pants), using a broad-spectrum sunscreen with a **sun protective factor (SPF)** of 15 or higher, and wearing sunglasses that offer UV protection (see the box "Sunscreen and Other Sun Protection Products"). Tanning beds and sun lamps should also be avoided. Parents should be particularly vigilant about protecting their children.

Melanoma   Because it is capable of spreading quickly to almost any part of the body, melanoma is a particularly dangerous form of cancer. Rates of melanoma have increased over the past 30 years, especially in young White women and older White men.

The risk of melanoma is greatest for people with a personal history of melanoma, a large number of moles (especially those that are large or unusual in shape or color), or a family member with melanoma. The risk is greater in people with fair skin and sun sensitivity (burning easily). Rates in Whites are 10 times greater than rates in Blacks, but the disease does occur in Blacks. Melanoma can occur on any part of the body, but it is directly related to sun exposure, especially intermittent, acute UV light exposure, as from exposure to sunlight (sunburns) or to UV light in tanning salons. Exposure during childhood or adolescence may be particularly dangerous.

> **sun protective factor (SPF)**
> Measure of the degree to which a sunscreen protects the skin from damaging UV radiation from the sun.

All forms of skin cancers *are directly linked to ultraviolet light exposure.* *The most effective way to reduce risk for skin cancer is to* **limit UV exposure,** *whether from the sun or from the UV lights* *in* **tanning salons.**

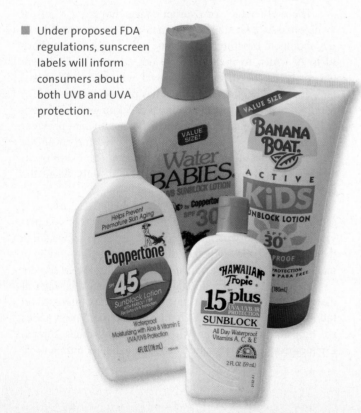

■ Under proposed FDA regulations, sunscreen labels will inform consumers about both UVB and UVA protection.

Melanomas usually develop in pigmented, or dark, areas on the skin. Signs suggestive of melanoma are changes in a mole: a sudden darkening or change in color, spread of color outward into previously normal skin, an irregular border, pain, itchiness, bleeding, or crusting. You can monitor your skin for these signs by using the "ABCD" test for melanoma (Figure 16.4).

Early detection of skin cancer usually occurs as a result of individuals' monitoring their own skin and visiting a health care provider for evaluation of any changes or progressive growth. The ACS recommends that people have a skin exam (visual inspection of the skin all over the body) as part of a regular physical examination every 3 years between ages 20 and 40 and annually after age 40.

Treatment for melanoma begins with surgically excising (cutting out) and doing a biopsy of any suspicious lesions. If melanoma is confirmed, a larger area of surrounding skin is removed, which improves the chance of survival. Chemotherapy and immunotherapy can be added for advanced stages. The overall 5-year survival rate for melanoma is 91 percent; if the melanoma is diagnosed at an early stage, the 5-year survival rate is 98 percent.[1]

Consumer Clipboard

Sunscreen and Other Sun Protection Products

Sun exposure is the most preventable risk factor for skin cancers. Sunscreens, if used properly, can reduce the damaging effects of UV radiation. Historically, sunscreens protected primarily against UVB exposure, long been known to cause sunburns and skin damage and to be associated with skin cancer. Data now indicate that UVA exposure also causes skin cancer, in addition to aging (wrinkling and sagging) and other skin damage. UVA penetrates the skin more deeply than UVB and is responsible for tanning. The FDA has proposed new sunscreen labeling regulations designed to provide consumers with information they need about UVA and UVB radiation.

Currently, sunscreen labels display the SPF (sun protective factor) of the product. (SPF may stand for *sunburn protective factor* on the new labels.) SPF indicates the amount of time you can stay in the sun without burning compared to how long you could stay if you weren't wearing the sunscreen. An SPF of 15 means that a person can stay out in the sun 15 times longer than he or she could without sunscreen before a sunburn would occur. SPF refers to UVB protection only. An SPF of 15 or more is recommended.

Some FDA-approved sunscreens protect against both UVB and UVA by including ingredients that block UVA radiation, such as titanium dioxide and zinc oxide. A sunscreen containing the ingredient Mexoryl or Helioplex also blocks UVA. The new FDA proposals call for products to indicate the amount of UVA protection they provide using a ranking system of one to four stars. Labels will also have to state clearly if the product provides no UVA protection. In addition, labels will have to carry the following message:

> Warning: UV exposure from the sun increases the risk of skin cancer, premature skin aging, and other skin damage. It is important to decrease UV exposure by limiting time in the sun, wearing protective clothing, and using a sunscreen.

Sunscreen should be applied liberally to all sun-exposed areas. Most people do not apply enough. An average-sized adult in a swimsuit needs about 4 ounces of sunscreen for one application. It should be applied at least 20 to 30 minutes before going outside—it takes that long for sunscreen to be absorbed. It should also be reapplied frequently, at least every 2 hours and/or after swimming or sweating.

Combination products, such as sunscreen and insect repellent, result in a reduction in the effect of SPF by up to one-third. When using a combination product, use one with a higher SPF and reapply it more frequently. The protectiveness of clothing can vary. Hats typically offer an SPF between 3 and 6; summer-weight clothing has an SPF of about 6.5; newer sun-protective clothing can have an SPF of up to 30+.

The UV index is a rating system developed by the National Weather Service and the Environmental Protection Agency to predict UV levels in the next few days on a scale of 1 to 10+. If UV levels are going to be unusually high, a UV alert may be issued. You can check the UV index at www.epa.gov/sunwise/uvindex.html.

Sources: "2007 Sunscreen Proposed Rule," U.S. Food and Drug Administration, retrieved from www.fda.gov/cder/drug/infopage/sunscreen/default .htm; "EPA Sunwise," U.S. Environmental Protection Agency, retrieved from www.epa.gov/sunwise/uvindex.html; "Rulemaking History for OTC Sunscreen Drug Products," U.S. Food and Drug Administration, retrieved May 18, 2010, from www.fda.gov/Drugs/DevelopmentApprovalProcess/ DevelopmentResources/Over-the-CounterOTCDrugs/StatusofOTCRulemakings/ucm072134.htm.

A—Asymmetry: Is one half unlike the other?

B—Border irregularity: Does it have an uneven, scalloped edge rather than a clearly defined border?

C—Color variation: Is the color uniform, or does it vary from one area to another, from tan to brown to black, or from white to red to blue?

D—Diameter larger than ¼ inch: At its widest point, is the growth as large as, or larger than, a pencil eraser?

figure **16.4** The ABCD evaluation of moles for melanoma.

Basal Cell and Squamous Cell Carcinomas Sun-exposed areas of the body are susceptible to basal cell and squamous cell cancers. People at high risk include those with fair skin; blonde, red, or light brown hair; blue, green, or hazel eyes; and freckles and moles. Other risk factors are cumulative sun exposure and age, with rates increasing after age 50. However, both types are increasing among younger people.

The signs of a basal cell cancer include new skin growth; a raised, domelike lesion with a pearl-like edge or border; or a sore that bleeds and scabs but never completely heals. The signs of a squamous cell cancer include a red, scaly area that does not go away; a sore that bleeds and does not heal; or a raised, crusty sore. Squamous cell cancers often develop from a precancerous spot called an actinic keratosis, a red, rough spot that develops in a sun-exposed area.

Early detection of basal and squamous cell cancers involves monitoring the skin and having any persistent changes evaluated. The ACS recommends the same skin exams for these cancers as for melanoma. Treatment usually involves local removal and destruction of the cancer by surgery, heat, or freezing, with radiation therapy sometimes an option.[1]

TESTICULAR CANCER

Although testicular cancer accounts for only 1 percent of all cancers in men, it is the most common malignancy in men 20 to 35 years of age. The incidence of testicular cancer has nearly doubled worldwide over the past 40 years. It is not clear why this increase is occurring, but some researchers speculate that it could be due to fetal exposure to higher levels of estrogen during prenatal development as a result of environmental toxins. Because of improved treatment methods, however, the survival rate has increased. In the United States, testicular cancer occurs nearly 4.5 times more often in White men than in Black men. Rates for men of Hispanic, Asian, and Native American backgrounds fall between those for White and Black men.[28,29]

The risk for testicular cancer is 3 to 17 times higher in men with a history of an undescended testicle (one of the testes fails to descend into the scrotum and is retained in the abdomen or inguinal canal). However, only 7–10 percent of men diagnosed with testicular cancer have a history of this condition. Other risk factors include a family history of testicular cancer, a personal history of testicular cancer in the other testicle, abnormal development of the testes, and infertility or abnormal sperm.[28,29]

Warning signs of testicular cancer include a painless lump on the testicle and swelling or discomfort in the scrotum. Testicular cancer is usually detected by an individual, often during a testicular self-exam. Back pain and difficulty breathing can develop in the later stages after cancer metastasizes.

Men can perform a self-exam, although there are no specific recommendations for how often it should be performed (see the box "Testicle Self-Exam"). If a lump is detected, an ultrasound is performed, and if the ultrasound suggests cancer, a biopsy is performed to confirm the diagnosis.

Testicular cancer is treated with surgery to remove the testicle; depending on the stage of disease, radiation or chemotherapy may be needed as well. Testicular cancer is highly treatable, with 95 percent of cases at all stages being cured. The cure rate is 99 percent if the cancer is diagnosed at an early stage. Even in a man with a late-stage diagnosis and extensive metastases, testicular cancer can be cured. International cycling champion Lance Armstrong, after being diagnosed at age 25 with advanced-stage testicular cancer with metastases to the brain and lungs, was successfully treated and went on to win the world's most prestigious cycling events.[28,29]

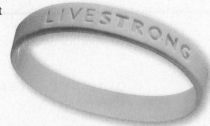

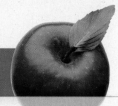

Highlight on Health

Testicle Self-Exam

The testicle self-exam has not been studied enough to show whether it reduces the death rate from testicular cancer. For this reason, the ACS has not set a recommendation for this self-exam for the general population. Testicular cancer is often first detected by a man noticing a change in his own testicles, so some health providers do teach and recommend it.

To perform a self-exam:

■ Stand in front of a mirror. Look for any changes or swelling on the skin of the scrotum.

■ Examine each testicle with both hands. Place your index and middle fingers under the testicle with the thumbs placed on top. Roll the testicle gently between the thumbs and fingers. It's normal for one testicle to be slightly larger than the other.

■ Find the epididymis, the soft, tubelike structure behind the testicle that collects and carries sperm. If you are familiar with this structure, you won't mistake it for a suspicious lump. Cancerous lumps usually are found on the sides of the testicle but also can appear on the front.

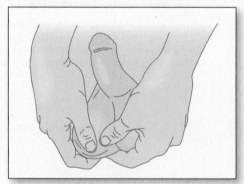

If you find a lump, see your doctor right away. Testicular cancer is highly curable, especially when it's detected and treated early. In almost all cases, testicular cancer occurs in only one testicle, and men can maintain full sexual and reproductive function with the other testicle.

Sources: Testicular Cancer Resource Center, 2004, "How to Do a Testicular Self-Examination"; National Cancer Institute, 2005, "Questions and Answers About Testicular Cancer."

ORAL CANCER

Cancers that develop in the mouth or the pharynx (the back of the throat), which can involve the lips, tongue, gums, or throat, are classified as oral cancers. The rate of new cases has been declining since the 1980s, and death rates have remained stable since 2000. Oral cancers are more common in men than in women.[1]

The major risk factor for oral cancers is tobacco use (smoking cigarettes, cigars, or a pipe or using smokeless tobacco); high levels of alcohol consumption also increase the risk. Early signs of oral cancer include a sore in the mouth that does not heal or bleeds easily; a lump or bump that does not go away or that increases in size; or a patch of redness or whiteness along the gums or skin lining the inside of the cheeks. Late signs of oral cancer can include pain or difficulty swallowing or chewing.

Oral cancers are usually detected by a doctor or dentist, or the individual may report a sore that does not heal. A biopsy is necessary to confirm the diagnosis. Treatment usually starts with surgery to remove as much as possible of the cancer, along with local radiation. If the cancer is advanced, chemotherapy can be added. The 5-year survival rate for all stages of oral cancer is 61 percent.

LEUKEMIA

Leukemia is a group of cancers that originate in the bone marrow or other parts of the body where white blood cells form. Leukemia is the overproduction of one type of white blood cell, which prevents the normal growth and function of other blood cells and can lead to increased risk of infection, anemia, and bleeding. The ACS projected an estimated 43,050 new cases of leukemia in 2010 and an estimated 21,840 deaths.

Risk factors include cigarette smoking and exposure to certain chemicals, particularly benzene, a chemical found in gasoline products and in cigarette smoke. Ionizing radiation can increase the risk for several types of leukemia; people who survive other cancers are at risk for developing leukemia as a result of radiation treatment. Infection with a virus, human T-cell leukemia/lymphoma virus (HTLV-1), can increase the risk of leukemia and lymphoma, another cancer of the white blood cells.

Symptoms of leukemia often occur because healthy white blood cells, red blood cells, and platelets are unable to perform their functions. These symptoms include fatigue, increased incidence of infection, and easy bleeding and bruising. Symptoms can appear suddenly in acute leukemia, but in chronic leukemia, they may appear gradually.

Because the symptoms are fairly nonspecific, early detection of leukemia can be challenging. There is no recommended screening test, but a health care provider can diagnose leukemia with a blood test or bone marrow biopsy if symptoms are present. The most effective treatment is chemotherapy. Therapy can also include blood transfusion, antibiotics, drugs to boost the function of healthy blood cells, and drugs to reduce the side effects of chemotherapy. Bone marrow transplantation can be effective for certain types of leukemia.

LYMPHOMA

Cancers that originate in the lymph system, part of the body's immune system, are called lymphomas. There are two main types: Hodgkin's lymphoma (about 11 percent of all lymphoma) and non-Hodgkin's lymphoma (about 89 percent). Lymphomas can start almost anywhere, since the lymph system exists throughout the body (Figure 16.5). In the past 30 years, rates of lymphoma have nearly doubled. About 95 percent of lymphomas occur in adults, with an average age at diagnosis in the 60s. However, a childhood form of lymphoma exists.[1]

Factors that increase risk for lymphoma include infections, medications, or genetic changes that weaken the immune system. HIV infection explains some of the increase in lymphoma rates. Radiation, herbicides, insecticides, and some chemical exposures also increase risk. However, the majority of people with lymphoma do not have clearly identified risk factors.

Symptoms of lymphoma depend on where it originates. A swollen lymph node is a common presentation, but the majority of swollen lymph nodes are not due to lymphoma. If the lymphoma originates in the thymus, it can cause a cough or shortness of breath; in the abdomen, it can cause swelling or pain. Other general symptoms associated with lymphoma include weight loss, fever, drenching night sweats, and severe itchiness.

■ Michael C. Hall of the TV show *Dexter* announced in January 2010 that he had been undergoing treatment for Hodgkin's lymphoma. Later that year he was reported to have fully recovered. The five-year survival rate for Hodgkin's lymphoma is 85 percent.

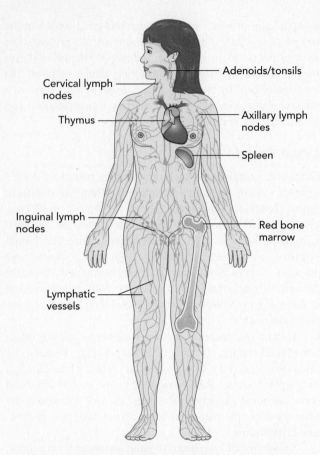

figure 16.5   The lymph system. Structures include the lymph nodes and lymph vessels, the adenoids/tonsils, the thymus gland, the spleen, and the bone marrow. Clusters of lymph nodes can occur anywhere along the lymphatic vessels. Prominent areas include the neck (cervical lymph nodes), armpits (axillary lymph nodes), and groin (inguinal lymph nodes).

Labels in figure:
- Adenoids/tonsils
- Cervical lymph nodes
- Thymus
- Axillary lymph nodes
- Spleen
- Inguinal lymph nodes
- Red bone marrow
- Lymphatic vessels

Diagnosis is made by a biopsy of the swollen lymph node or other tissue. Imaging studies, such as chest X-ray, CT scans, and MRIs, are important to determine if and how far the lymphoma has spread. Treatment often includes a combination of surgery, chemotherapy, and radiation. Treatment can sometimes involve immunotherapy or bone marrow transplant. The 5-year survival rate for Hodgkin's and non-Hodgkin's lymphoma is 85 and 67 percent, respectively.[1]

screening test
Test given to a large group of people to identify a smaller group of people who are at higher risk for a specific disease or condition.

Cancer Screening

Early detection is the key to successful treatment of cancer, and **screening tests** are the key to early detection. Cancer screening involves trying to identify risk factors, precancerous lesions, or undetected cancers in an asymptomatic person. An ideal screening test would always detect precursors or cancer at an early, treatable stage and never produce a false negative or false positive result.

Unfortunately, no screening test meets the ideal. Screening recommendations for breast, colon, prostate, uterine, testicular, and cervical cancers are summarized in the box "Cancer Detection Guidelines." No screening recommendations exist for some cancers, including lung and ovarian cancers, because to date, no test has been shown to improve detection without increasing harm.

Genetic screening can also be done to assess cancer risk. At this time, it is being reserved for members of high-risk families, that is, families with multiple members with cancer. Complete the Personal Health Portfolio for this chapter to assess your personal risk and protective factors.

Cancer Treatments

Surgery is the oldest treatment for cancer; newer options include chemotherapy, radiation, biological therapies, bone marrow transplantation, and gene therapy.

SURGERY

Surgery remains a mainstay in the diagnosis and treatment of cancer. When a cancer is detected early and is small and localized, surgery can cure it, as when an *in situ* cancer of the breast is removed via a lumpectomy. Sometimes an organ affected by cancer can be removed surgically without threatening life, as in the case of prostate or testicular cancer. Certain cancers are unlikely to spread widely, such as a basal cell carcinoma, and surgery often cures these cancers as well. If a cancer has spread, surgery may still be performed as part of the treatment.

CHEMOTHERAPY

Chemotherapy is a drug treatment administered to the entire body to kill any cancer cells that may have escaped from the local site to the blood, lymph system, or another part of the body. More than 50 chemotherapy medicines have been developed; different combinations are used for different cancers. All chemotherapeutic drugs operate by a similar mechanism—they interfere with rapid cell division. Because cancer cells divide more rapidly than normal cells, they are more vulnerable than healthy cells to destruction by chemotherapy.

Other normal tissues that divide rapidly are also harmed by chemotherapy, including the hair, stomach lining, and white blood cells. The timing and dosage must be carefully adjusted so the drugs kill cancer cells but do not damage normal cells beyond repair.

RADIATION

Radiation causes damage to cells by altering their DNA; it can be used to destroy cancer cells with minimal damage to surrounding tissues. Radiation is a local treatment that can be used before or after surgery or in conjunction with chemotherapy. It can also be used to control pain in patients with cancer that cannot be cured.

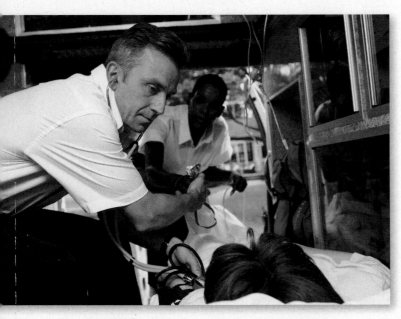

The Heimlich Maneuver

The Heimlich maneuver is used to dislodge an object blocking the airway of a person who is choking. To perform this maneuver (also referred to as abdominal thrusts), follow these four steps:

1. Stand behind the person and put your arms around his or her waist.
2. Make a fist with one hand and place the thumb side of your fist against the victim's upper abdomen, just below the rib cage and above the navel.
3. Grasp your fist with your other hand and thrust upward. Do not squeeze the rib cage. Confine the force of your thrust to your hands.
4. Repeat the upward thrusts until the object is expelled.

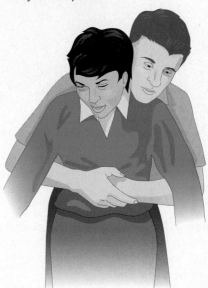

The Heimlich Institute provides special instructions for rescuing infants and children, people the rescuer cannot reach around, people with asthma, and people who are unconscious. For details, visit its Web site at www.heimlichinstitute.org.

■ According to the CDC, more than 50 people die from unintentional drug overdoses every day in the U.S. The rate of lethal overdoses has increased dramatically in the last 10 years, making poisoning the second leading cause of unintentional death.

Choking Death rates for choking are highest in children under 4 years of age and adults over 65 years of age. Rates soar in adults over 75 years of age. Most choking emergencies occur when a piece of food or a swallowed object becomes lodged in the throat, blocking the tracheal opening and cutting the oxygen supply to the lungs. Muscles in the trachea may spasm and wrap tightly around the object.[1]

A person whose airway is obstructed may gasp for breath, make choking sounds, clutch the throat, or look flushed and strained. If a person's airway is only partially blocked, he or she may cough forcefully. Do not slap someone on the back if he or she is coughing; usually the coughing will clear the obstruction. If the person continues to have difficulty breathing, coughing is shallow, the person is not coughing, or the person cannot talk or breathe, a rescue technique like the **Heimlich maneuver** is needed (see the box "The Heimlich Maneuver").

Heimlich maneuver
Technique used to help a person who is choking.

Temperature-Related Injuries Each year scores of people die from excessive heat, particularly older adults and people with weak hearts. The danger is highest for people 75 years of age and older. High temperatures can be exacerbated by high humidity, which prevents the evaporation of perspiration from the skin and makes it difficult for the body to control its core temperature.

On average, 36 children die of hyperthermia in vehicles each year.[26] These children may be forgotten or unintentionally left in the vehicle by an adult, or they may have been playing in an unattended vehicle. Temperatures inside vehicles can quickly reach dangerous levels. Vehicle child hyperthermia deaths can occur when the ambient temperature outside is as low as 70° F. Children's thermoregulatory systems are not as efficient as those of adults, so their core body temperature can rise three to five times faster than an adult's. Children should never be left in a vehicle, even if the windows are down, or allowed to play in an unattended vehicle, and adults should establish a "look before you leave" policy any time they vacate a vehicle.

Excessive cold is dangerous as well and can lead to hypothermia, a condition in which body temperature drops

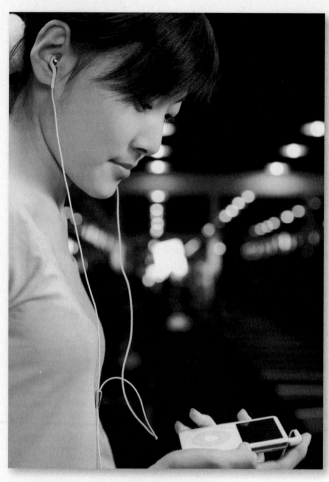

■ Many audio devices now include a package insert warning about the dangers of hearing loss from listening at high volumes.

to dangerously low levels. See Chapter 7 for more information on hypothermia and guidelines on how to avoid it. If you are with someone who is experiencing hypothermia, seek medical treatment immediately.

Excessive Noise Exposure to loud noise can damage hearing and lead to permanent hearing loss. Some **noise-induced hearing loss (NIHL)** is inevitable and irreversible as we age, so people should protect their hearing from additional, avoidable damage.[27]

Common sources of environmental noise include machinery, power tools, traffic, airplanes, and construction. Loud music is also a hazard. When you listen to loud music for a prolonged period, you experience a "temporary threshold shift" that makes you less sensitive to high volumes. In effect, the ears adapt to the environment by anesthetizing themselves (see the box "MP3 Players and Hearing Loss").

Providing Emergency Aid You can help provide care to other people who have been injured or are in life-threatening situations if you learn first aid and emergency rescue techniques. **Cardiopulmonary resuscitation (CPR)** is used when someone is not breathing and a pulse cannot be found. It consists of mouth-to-mouth resuscitation to

restore breathing, accompanied by chest compressions to restore heartbeat. Unfortunately, bystanders provide CPR only 20 to 30 percent of the time when needed, largely out of apprehension of placing their mouth on someone else's mouth. In 2008 the American Heart Association (AHA) announced that hands-only CPR—with chest compressions only—is just as effective for sudden cardiac arrest as standard CPR with mouth-to-mouth breathing. Mouth-to-mouth resuscitation should still be used for children. It should also be used for adults who suffer from a lack of oxygen caused by near-drowning, carbon monoxide poisoning, or drug overdose.[28] Check the AHA's Web site (www.americanheart .org) for the latest guidelines.

Training is required to perform CPR; many organizations offer classes, including the American Heart Association and the American Red Cross. Check the yellow pages or your community or campus resource center for information on where to take a class in first aid or rescue techniques.

noise-induced hearing loss (NIHL)
Damage to the inner ear, causing gradual hearing loss, as a result of exposure to noise over a period of years.

cardiopulmonary resuscitation (CPR)
Technique used when a person is not breathing and a pulse cannot be found; differs from pulmonary resuscitation by including chest compressions to restore heartbeat.

WORK SAFETY

Safety in the workplace improved steadily throughout the 20th century as a result of occupational laws and advances in safety technology. The part of the body most frequently injured is the back, accounting for 24 percent of total injuries.

Improper lifting of heavy objects is a major cause of back injury. When you are lifting an object, bend your knees and hips and lower your body toward the ground, keeping your back as upright as you can. Keep your feet about shoulder-width apart. Grasp the object and lift it gradually with straight arms, using your leg muscles to stand up. Put the object down by reversing these steps (Figure 17.3).

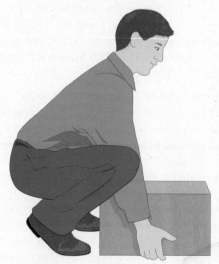

figure **17.3**   **Proper lifting technique.**

Consumer Clipboard

MP3 Players and Hearing Loss

Some MP3 and iPod users who listen to music at high volumes have been found to have hearing loss comparable to that found in aging adults. Noise levels from these portable media players can reach 115 to 125 decibels. Exposure to 125 decibels for an hour can cause permanent hearing loss, as can exposure to 115 decibels for half a minute per day. If you have listened to music at the highest volume for even a few seconds, or if you have felt pain in your ears from loud music, you may already have experienced some hearing damage.

Loud noise destroys hair cells at the nerve endings in the inner ear. These tiny hair cells translate sound vibrations into electrical currents that go to the brain. Noise-induced hearing loss is usually a gradual process that can take 10 to 20 years. Early symptoms of hearing loss include ringing or buzzing in the ears; difficulty understanding speech, especially in noisy settings; and a slight muffling of sounds. More serious symptoms include dizziness, discomfort, and pain in the ears. People who listen to loud music should have their hearing tested periodically, because hearing loss can be unnoticeable until damage is extensive.

Consumer complaints have led iPod and MP3 manufacturers to develop solutions to noise-induced hearing problems. In 2006, in response to a lawsuit charging that iPod use caused hearing damage, Apple announced a free download of software for the iPod Nano that allows listeners to set a volume limit. Manufacturers have also developed different kinds of headphones to address hearing loss issues. "Isolator" earphones sit deeper in the ear canal and block out external sound, so that volume does not have to be cranked up so high. "Supra-aural" headphones sit on top of the ears and deliver sound at lower decibel levels.

However, researchers have found that it is not so much the type of earphone that makes a difference in hearing loss as it is the volume level. Listeners are advised to protect their hearing by avoiding prolonged exposure to sounds above 85 decibels. Another recommendation is the 60 percent/60 minute rule—using MP3 players at volume levels no more than 60 percent of maximum and no more than 1 hour a day. Sound is too loud if it prevents normal conversation, if you have to shout to be heard, if it causes ringing in your ears, if you have trouble hearing for a few hours after exposure, or if the person next to you can hear the music from your headphones. Since most people experience a gradual loss of hearing as they grow older, it is important to use safe listening strategies to protect your hearing while you are young.

Sources: "Researchers Recommend Safe Listening Levels for iPod," Hearing Loss Web, 2006, retrieved May 26, 2008, from www.hearinglossweb .com/Medical/Causes/nihl/mus/safe.htm; "Prevent Tech-Related Hearing Loss," by G. Hughes, 2006, retrieved May 26, 2008, from http://tech .yahoo.com/blog/hughes/35.

Although not necessarily related to work, another common source of back pain is carrying a heavy backpack. Backpacks should weigh no more than 10–20 percent of a person's body weight. If you use a backpack, buy one with wide, padded shoulder straps, a waist strap, and a padded back to distribute weight and enhance comfort. Carry heavier items in the center of your backpack.

Extensive computer use can cause strain on the neck, back, arms, hands, and eyes. If your body is not properly aligned while you are using your computer, you may end up with irritated or pinched nerves, inflamed tendons, or headaches. Research on computer workstations has provided information on how to minimize this strain on the body (Figure 17.4).

When motions and tasks are repeatedly performed in ergonomically incorrect ways, injuries to the soft tissues, known as **repetitive strain injuries**, can occur. A common repetitive strain injury is **carpal tunnel syndrome (CTS)**, the compression

repetitive strain injuries
Injuries to soft tissues that can occur when motions and tasks are repeatedly performed in ergonomically incorrect ways.

carpal tunnel syndrome (CTS)
Compression of the median nerve in the wrist caused by certain repetitive uses of the hands.

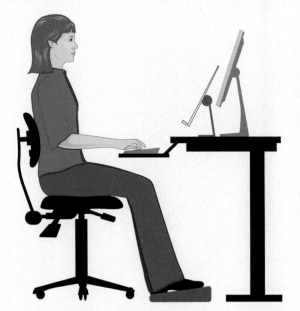

figure **17.4**   **Proper workstation setup.** Your hips should be slightly higher than your knees, and your feet should be flat on the floor or on a footrest slightly in front of your knees. Your monitor should be an arm's length away from you, and your eyes should be level with the top of the screen. When you type, your wrists should be in a neutral position, tilted neither up nor down.

of the median nerve in the wrist caused by certain repetitive uses of the hands, including working at the computer, playing video games, and text messaging. The median nerve is located inside a "tunnel" created by the carpals (wrist bones) and tendons in the hand (Figure 17.5). When the tendons become inflamed through overuse or incorrect use, they compress the median nerve. The symptoms of CTS are numbness, tingling, pain, and weakness in the hand, especially in the thumb and first three fingers. Symptoms are often worse at night, when pain can radiate up into the shoulder.

The first steps in addressing this condition are correcting ergonomic problems in the workstation, taking frequent breaks from repetitive tasks, and doing exercises that stretch and flex the wrists and hands. If symptoms persist, a physician should be consulted.

NATURAL DISASTERS

A sudden event resulting in loss of life, severe injury, or property damage is typically defined as a *disaster*.[19] Disasters can be caused by humans, as in the case of terrorist attacks, or by natural forces. Tornadoes, hurricanes, floods, wildfires, and earthquakes are among the most devastating natural disasters that occur in the United States and around the world. In 2005 Hurricane Katrina devastated New Orleans and the U.S. Gulf Coast, causing loss of life and billions of dollars of damage. In 2008 a cyclone (the name for a hurricane in the Indian Ocean) hit Myanmar (Burma),

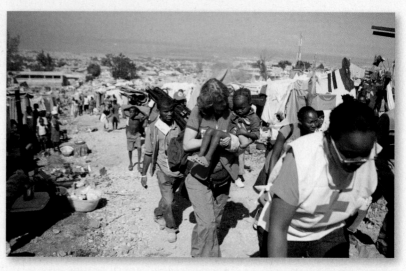

■ Major disasters, like the earthquake that struck Haiti in March 2010, require the coordinated responses of governments and international organizations. The Red Cross and Red Crescent were among the aid agencies that contributed money to support relief and recovery efforts after the Haiti earthquake.

flooding the low-lying coastal delta that was home to millions of people. In January 2010 a magnitude 7.0 earthquake struck Haiti, killing an estimated 200,000 people and leaving 1 million people homeless.

When natural disasters occur on this scale, governments and international aid organizations have to provide the assistance and relief that people need to recover. Individuals can help themselves by preparing as much as they can for the types of disasters that are likely to occur where they live (for example, tornadoes in the Midwest, hurricanes on the East Coast). The National Center for Environmental Health (part of the CDC) provides detailed information on preparedness for all types of events, including natural disasters and severe weather emergencies. Visit their Web site at www.cdc.gov/nceh.

Violence: Working Toward Prevention

More than many of the other health topics discussed in this text, violence is a societal issue. Although violent acts are committed by individuals, the causes of violence are rooted in social and cultural conditions. This does not mean that people who commit violent crimes are not held accountable for their actions—they are. In fact, the United States incarcerates a larger proportion of its population than does any other nation.[29]

It does mean that taking action individually to reduce violence is difficult for people, unlike deciding to improve their diet or get more exercise. What you as an individual can do about violence falls into two categories: knowing how to reduce your own risk of encountering violence and working to create safer communities and to prevent violence in society. To assess how well you protect yourself from

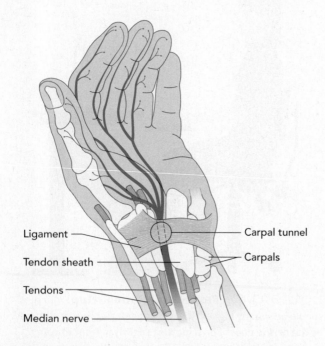

Ligament

Tendon sheath

Tendons

Median nerve

Carpal tunnel

Carpals

figure 17.5 **Carpal tunnel syndrome (CTS).**

Source: Core Concepts in Health, 10th ed. Copyright © 2006 by The McGraw-Hill Companies. Used with permission of the McGraw-Hill Companies.

encountering violence, answer the questions in Chapter 17's Personal Health Portfolio.

VIOLENCE IN THE UNITED STATES

Violence is defined as the use of force or the threat of force to inflict intentional injury, physical or psychological, on oneself or another person. Murder, robbery, and **assault** are all violent crimes, but violence also occurs in association with child abuse, sexual harassment, suicide, and several other kinds of conduct.

violence
Use of force or the threat of force to inflict intentional injury, physical or psychological, on oneself or another person.

assault
Attack by one person on another using force or the threat of force to intentionally inflict injury. *Aggravated assault* is an attack that causes bodily injury, usually with a weapon or other means capable of producing grave bodily harm or death. *Simple assault* is an attack without a weapon that causes less serious physical harm.

Crime Rates and Violence Facts

Rates of violent crime in the United States are lower than those in many other developed countries, except in one area—homicide, especially homicide committed with a firearm. The number of firearm homicides is higher in the United States than in any other country; it is almost 15 times higher than in Canada.[30] Most experts attribute this difference to the ready availability of firearms in the United States.[30]

The U.S. Federal Bureau of Investigation (FBI) and the Department of Justice count cases of homicide, assault, robbery, and rape as violent crimes. *Aggravated assault* accounts for about two-thirds of violent crime and robbery for less than one-third; rape accounts for about 7 percent and homicide about 1 percent. Firearms are involved in about a third of all violent crimes and in about 70 percent of homicides. Among women killed in the United States, about a third are killed by their husbands or boyfriends. About one in five child homicide victims is killed by a family member.[30]

What Accounts for Violence?

Age and sex are among the most reliable risk factors for violence.[31] The typical offender is a young male between the ages of 14 and 24. Forty-four percent of those arrested for violent crimes are under 25 years of age. Men are much more likely to commit a violent act than women are; 82 percent of those arrested for violent crimes are men.[32] Women do commit violent acts, but it is often in self-defense.

Being a member of a minority group is a significant risk factor for violence. Although Blacks make up 12 percent of the population, they make up nearly half (47 percent) of all

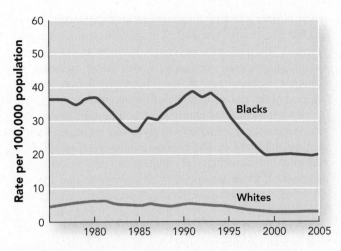

figure 17.6 Homicide rates by race of victim, United States, 1976–2006
Source: Bureau of Justice Statistics, www.ojp.usdoj.gov/bjs.

homicide victims (Figure 17.6).[33] Similarly, Blacks account for 52 percent of homicide offenders. Thirty-seven percent of those arrested for violent crimes are Black, 60.5 percent are White, and the remainder are Native American, Asian, or Pacific Islander. (People of Hispanic ethnic origin are included in the racial categories "Black" and "White" in these statistics.)

Like risk factors for mental illness, risk factors for violence occur at many levels. Risk factors at the societal and cultural levels—social determinants of health—include

■ The availability of firearms in the United States is linked with higher rates of firearm-related homicide than in other developed countries, and states with the highest rates of gun ownership have higher rates of suicide than states with lower rates of gun ownership. Firearms safety training is essential for anyone who owns a gun.

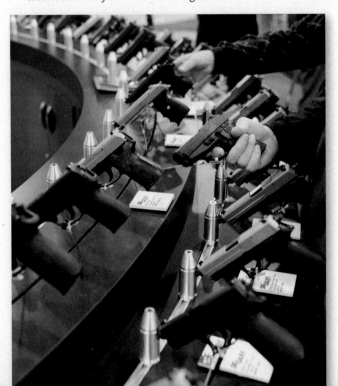

The **United States incarcerates a larger proportion** *of its population than does any other nation.*

poverty, poor schools, disorganized neighborhoods, use of alcohol and drugs, availability of guns, exposure to media violence, and lack of economic, educational, and employment opportunities. Violence is also more common on college campuses than in the general population, perhaps because of the transient nature of the community.

Risk factors at the family level include child abuse, substance abuse or criminal activity by family members, lack of positive role models, and chaotic family organization. Risk factors at the individual level include such biological factors as genetics, brain structure, brain chemistry, and medical disorders; low intelligence; certain personality traits, such as aggressiveness and poor impulse control; and a history of previous criminal or antisocial behavior.[31] Other individual risk factors include attention deficit disorder and hyperactivity in children; deficits in cognitive and social cognitive functioning; poor behavior control; and early antisocial and aggressive behaviors.

Conversely, protective factors, which buffer young people from the effects of risk factors, include high IQ, a positive social orientation, and involvement in school activities.[34] No single factor is sufficient to explain why violence occurs or why levels of violent crime rise or decline in different time periods.

Trends in Violent Crime   Rates of violent crime in the United States declined precipitously from the early 1990s to 2004. In 2005 and 2006, rates of all violent crimes except forcible rape increased, but they may have decreased again in recent years. The estimated rate of violent crime in 2008 was 454.5 per 100,000 inhabitants according to FBI statistics.[33] Experts have proposed a variety of explanations for violent crime trends:[34]

- *Demographics.* Rates of violence fall when the segment of the population responsible for most occurrences of violent crime—young men aged 14 to 24—decreases in size. This commonly offered argument is inadequate to explain the decline in crime in the 1990s, however, because the size of this group changed very little between 1994 and 2003.
- *Crack cocaine.* The boom in crack cocaine in the 1980s, accompanied by drug wars and gun violence, was followed by a steep decline in demand for crack in the early 1990s. Marijuana replaced crack as the drug of choice among younger drug users; the marijuana trade is associated with less violence than is the trade in crack.
- *Economic expansion.* The economy improved in the 1990s, creating more opportunities for people to earn a living in legitimate ways.
- *Law enforcement and incarceration.* Mandatory sentencing policies, as exemplified by "three strikes" laws (automatic maximum sentences for people convicted of a third felony, even a nonviolent one), and the sharp increase in incarceration rates in the 1980s and 1990s removed many criminals from the streets. The prison population in the United States quadrupled between 1980 and 2000.

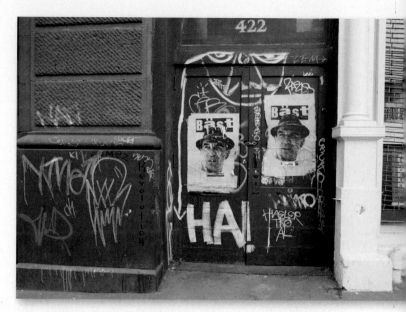

■ Although some graffiti rises to the status of art, most is simple vandalism. When graffiti is not promptly removed, it sends a message of neglect, hurting neighborhoods and communities and lowering quality of life.

- *Expansion of resources for victims.* Resources for those affected by domestic violence increased in the 1980s and 1990s, including hotlines, shelters, legal advocates, and increased availability of judicial protections (such as restraining orders).

None of these explanations is sufficient by itself to explain the fluctuations in the crime rate over the past two decades. Some combination of these factors and others is probably responsible for the overall trends.

YOUTH VIOLENCE

Among people aged 10 to 24, homicide is the second leading cause of death in the United States (unintentional injuries are the first).[35]

Although mass killings in schools like those that occurred at Columbine High School in 1999 and Virginia Tech in 2007 are rare, they are shocking and traumatizing, and their effects are long lasting.

Schools have responded to violence primarily by tightening security and strengthening punitive measures. Congress has mandated a **zero-tolerance policy** that calls for expelling any student who brings weapons or drugs to school.

Youth gangs are associations of adolescents and young adults aged 12 to 24 organized to control a territory, usually in an inner city, and to conduct illegal activities like drug trafficking.

zero-tolerance policy
Policy stating that any student who brings weapons or drugs to school will be expelled.

youth gangs
Associations of adolescents and young adults aged 12 to 24 organized to control a territory and conduct illegal activities.

Who's at Risk?

Violence and College Students

A 2005 survey revealed the following facts about violence on college campuses.

■ For every 1,000 women on a college campus, there are about 35 incidents of rape. Approximately 15–20 percent of college students experienced forced intercourse during their college years. About 15–20 percent of college men acknowledged forced intercourse. Only 5 percent of attempted and completed rapes were reported to law enforcement.

■ Non-Hispanic Whites are more likely than students of other races to be victims of overall violence. Black students are somewhat more likely than White students to experience a simple assault.

■ Male students are twice as likely as female students to be victims of overall violence. Out of every 14 college men, 1 had been physically assaulted or raped by an intimate partner.

■ More than one-third of lesbian, gay, bisexual, and transgender undergraduate students experienced harassment. Some 20 percent of faculty, staff, and students feared for their physical safety because of their sexual orientation or gender identity.

■ Between 25 and 30 percent of college women and between 11 and 17 percent of college men were stalked. Most of the victims knew their stalker. Stalking is more prevalent among college students than in the general population. About 10 percent of stalking incidents resulted in forced or attempted sexual contact.

■ Some 15 percent of college women and 9.2 percent of college men were in emotionally abusive relationships; 2.4 percent of women and 1.3 percent of men were in a physically abusive relationship; and 1.7 percent of women and 1.0 percent of men were in a sexually abusive relationship.

■ Alcohol and other drugs were implicated in 55–74 percent of sexual assaults on college campuses.

■ About 93 percent of crimes against students occurred off campus. Strangers committed 58 percent of all violent crimes against students. Only 35 percent of violent crimes against students were reported to law enforcement.

Source: Campus Violence White Paper, *by J. Carr, February 5, 2005, Baltimore, MD: American College Health Association.*

Many gang members derive a sense of belonging, purpose, and self-esteem not otherwise available in their lives, as well as security, protection, and a source of income, from gang membership.[36]

Efforts to reduce gang violence focus on preventing adolescents from joining gangs by keeping them in school and providing opportunities for legitimate success, such as meaningful employment opportunities. Community social controls can be increased by strengthening social institutions, such as schools and churches, and encouraging parents and community leaders to play a role in supervising adolescents' activities.

Programs are needed in prisons, such as job training and drug treatment programs, that prevent the recycling of adult gang members back into the community crime scene. Finally, efforts to remove guns from the streets need to be enhanced.[36]

VIOLENCE ON THE COLLEGE CAMPUS

Although colleges are often viewed as safe havens, violence is more prevalent on the college campus than in the general population (see the box "Violence and College Students").[37] According to the U.S. Department of Education, thousands of violent crimes occur every year on U.S. college and university campuses, including murder, assault, and rape.

Most colleges have responded to campus violence by raising the visibility of campus security officers, tightening security controls, and implementing stringent discipline programs. Two federal laws regulate how campus crime is treated. The Jeanne Clery Disclosure of Campus Security Policy and Campus Crime Statistics Act (originally known as the Campus Security Act) requires colleges and universities receiving federal funding to disclose information about crime on and around their campuses. The first of these laws was named after Jeanne Clery, a 19-year-old student at Lehigh University, who was raped and murdered in her residence hall in 1986. The law was amended in 2000 to require colleges to inform the community about where they can obtain information about convicted, registered sex offenders enrolled as students or working or volunteering on campus.

The Campus Sexual Assault Victims' Bill of Rights Act requires college administrators to provide justice, medical treatment, and psychological counseling for crime victims and survivors. Amendments to this law require colleges to promote educational awareness programs on sexual assault, facilitate the reporting of sexual assault, and help survivors who want to change their academic and living situations, among other requirements. Schools that fail to comply may lose federal funds, including student loan funding.

The deadliest incident of campus violence in U.S. history, in which 32 people died, occurred at Virginia Polytechnic Institute and State University (Virginia Tech) in 2007. A nonprofit victims' rights organization called Security on Campus (SOC) requested a federal investigation of the school's response to the shootings, which consisted of two

Advances in Emergency Alert Systems

In the light of natural disasters like Hurricane Katrina in 2005 and school shootings like the one at Virginia Tech in 2007, both the federal government and campus administrations have been implementing new and innovative ways to disseminate information in times of crisis.

The Federal Emergency Management Agency (FEMA), which is responsible for distributing information at the federal, state, local, and tribal level before, during, and after a disaster, is upgrading its emergency alert system, which formerly only broadcast messages via radio and television. During working hours, only 40 percent of people are reachable by radio or television, and in the middle of the night over 92 percent of people are neither watching TV nor listening to the radio. The upgraded system will allow FEMA to send messages to people by cellular and residential phone and e-mail. It will also be able to provide translations of messages for non-English-speaking communities. People with disabilities, a group that was formerly difficult to reach in times of emergencies, will have increased ways to receive information. Hearing-impaired individuals will be able to receive e-mails or be texted with links to information posted on the Internet. The system is still under development and testing. FEMA also provides a booklet, *Are You Ready? An In-Depth Guide to Citizen Preparedness*, to help individuals prepare for any kind of disaster. The booklet can be downloaded for free at www.fema.gov.

College campuses have also expanded the ways in which they can communicate with students and faculty during an emergency. Multiple means of contact by e-mail, phone messages, text messages, and siren and/or verbal warnings from communication towers have been implemented. At some campuses, part of freshman orientation includes signing up for campus alerts. Students can opt to receive e-mail and/or phone alerts to multiple e-mail addresses and phone numbers. Some schools have started using social networking sites like Facebook and Twitter to distribute safety alerts. All of these measures speed up the distribution of information and the likelihood that students will receive it. What methods does your campus have in place for distributing emergency alerts?

connect ACTIVITY

Sources: "Integrated Public Alert and Warning System (IPAWS)," U.S. Department of Homeland Security, Federal Emergency Management Agency, 2009, retrieved May 21, 2010, from www.fema.gov/emergency/ipaws/; "FSU ALERT Emergency Notification System," Florida State University, retrieved May 21, 2010, from www.safety.fsu.edu/EmergencyManagement/fsualert.html.

---

attacks separated by about 2 hours. SOC claimed that the school violated the Jeanne Clery Act by failing to issue warnings in a timely way. In 2010, the Department of Education issued a report that found the school had indeed violated the act.

In response to the Virginia Tech incident, colleges and universities across the country have revamped their security plans (see the box "Advances in Emergency Alert Systems"). The U.S. Department of Education provides data on the safety of college campuses. To find out about your campus, visit www.ope.ed.gov/security.

Hazing Hazing is "any action taken or situation created intentionally, whether on or off fraternity premises, to produce mental or physical discomfort, embarrassment, or ridicule."[38] Hazing is typically imposed as an initiation rite or a requirement for joining an organization, usually a fraternity, sorority, or athletic team. Hazing activities have included kidnapping, alcohol chugging, forced swallowing of food and nonfood items, sleep deprivation, beatings, and calisthenics to the point of exhaustion. Deaths have occurred as a result of hazing, most often fraternity hazing. A common cause is alcohol poisoning.

Hazing is illegal in many states and may be either a misdemeanor or a felony, depending on the state and the severity of the offense. Parents whose children have died in these senseless incidents have filed wrongful death suits against both colleges and fraternities.

Free Speech vs. Hate Speech Hate speech—defined as verbal, written, or symbolic acts that convey a grossly negative view of particular persons or groups based on their gender, ethnicity, race, religion, sexual orientation, or disability[39]—is a particularly troublesome phenomenon on many college campuses. Its intent is to humiliate or harm rather than to convey ideas or information, and it has the potential to incite violence. Epithets, slurs, taunts, insults, and intimidation are common modes of hate speech; posters, flyers, letters, phone calls, e-mail, Web sites, and even T-shirts are media by which the message is distributed.

hazing
Actions taken to cause mental or physical discomfort, embarrassment, or ridicule in individuals seeking to join an organization.

hate speech
Verbal, written, or symbolic acts that convey a grossly negative view of particular persons or groups based on their gender, ethnicity, race, religion, sexual orientation, or disability.

The U.S. Supreme Court has made it clear that **colleges and universities cannot suppress speech** *simply because it is offensive.*

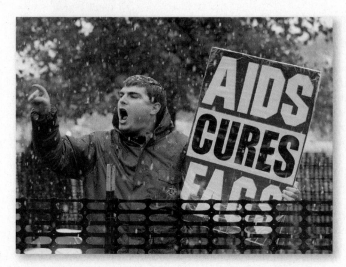

■ No matter how offensive, hate speech is protected by the First Amendment. Some experts recommend increasing conversation, debate, and diversity on campus as a way to expose and combat bigotry.

Some schools have adopted speech codes that require civility in discourse for all campus community members.[39] Some of these codes have been struck down by the courts as a violation of First Amendment rights. According to the rulings, hate speech must be proven to inflict real, not trivial, harm before it can be regulated. The U.S. Supreme Court has made it clear that colleges and universities cannot suppress speech simply because it is offensive. For this reason, many colleges and universities have adopted conduct codes that regulate certain actions associated with hate speech but not the speech itself.[39]

SEXUAL VIOLENCE

Sexual violence includes not just rape but also sexual harassment, stalking, and other forms of forcible or coercive sexual activity.

Sexual Assault **Sexual assault** is any sexual behavior that is forced on someone without his or her consent. At the least, the victim is made to feel uncomfortable and intimidated; at the worst, he or she is physically and emotionally harmed.[40,41] Sexual assault includes forced sexual intercourse (rape), forced sodomy (oral or anal sexual acts), child molestation, incest, fondling, and attempts to commit any of these acts. Another category of victimization is called **sexual coercion**, defined as imposing sexual activity on someone through the threat of nonphysical punishment, promise of reward, or verbal pressure rather than through force or threat of force.

According to different studies, 25–60 percent of men (15–25 percent of college men) have engaged in sexual assault and coercive sexual behavior.[42] The causes of this behavior are complex and probably include personality traits in the perpetrator as well as situational factors, including time and place of assault, use of alcohol and other drugs, and the relationship between victim and perpetrator. Rape prevention efforts need to include a focus on changing the environment that promotes violence against women.

Rape A study called the Sexual Victimization of College Women Survey found that about 35 women per 1,000 female students were victims of completed or attempted rape in any given academic year. These researchers estimated that 20–25 percent of college women experience completed or attempted rape during their college years. First-year college women are at highest risk for sexual assault during the first few weeks of their first semester (see the box "The Red Zone").

In the general population, more than half of rape and sexual assault victims are under the age of 18, and one in five are under the age of 12.[43] When a victim is younger than the "age of consent," usually 18, the perpetrator can be charged with **statutory rape** whether there was consent or not. Only 25–50 percent of all rapes are reported to the police, for a variety of reasons.[42] Victims may be embarrassed or traumatized, may not be sure that what happened to them qualifies as rape, may think they won't be believed, may blame themselves or feel guilty, or may not want to identify someone they know as a rapist (see the box "Heather: A Case of Sexual Assault").

Relatively few rapes are *stranger rapes*, that is, rapes committed by someone unknown to the victim. In about 60 percent of rapes and sexual assaults, the victim knows the perpetrator.[44] In 40 percent of cases, the perpetrator is a friend or an acquaintance; *acquaintance rape* can be committed by a classmate, coworker, or someone else casually known to the victim. *Date rape*, sexual assault by a boyfriend or someone with whom the victim has a dating relationship, is a type of acquaintance rape. In about 18 percent of rapes and sexual assaults, the perpetrator is the victim's intimate partner or husband.[44] Many states now allow rape charges to be brought by a woman against her husband.

Acquaintance rape survivors are more likely to have consumed alcohol or drugs before the assault, possibly reducing their awareness of signs of aggression in the rapist or their ability to respond to violence.[40]

Sexual predators also use so-called date rape drugs, including rohypnol, gamma hydroxybutyrate (GHB), ketamine, and Ecstasy, to incapacitate their victims. To avoid this risk, drink bottled beverages, watch bartenders mix your drink, and do not ever leave drinks unattended.

sexual assault
Any sexual behavior that is forced on someone without his or her consent.

sexual coercion
The imposition of sexual activity on someone through the threat of nonphysical punishment, promise of reward, or verbal pressure rather than through force or threat of force.

statutory rape
Sexual intercourse with someone under the "age of consent," usually 18, whether consent is given or not.

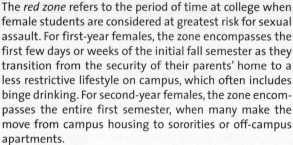

Highlight on Health

The Red Zone

The *red zone* refers to the period of time at college when female students are considered at greatest risk for sexual assault. For first-year females, the zone encompasses the first few days or weeks of the initial fall semester as they transition from the security of their parents' home to a less restrictive lifestyle on campus, which often includes binge drinking. For second-year females, the zone encompasses the entire first semester, when many make the move from campus housing to sororities or off-campus apartments.

Counseling centers, student affairs offices, and public safety centers at colleges and universities use Web-based and print media to warn female students about the red zone. Although sexual assault is a serious health problem on many college campuses, college students sometimes prefer to call these assaults "unwanted sex" and not sexual assaults. The reluctance to view these events as assaults is likely due to an acquaintance relationship between the victim and her assailant.

These safety tips for college students from the Rape, Abuse, and Incest National Network (RAINN) are particularly important for the red zone time period.

1. Trust your instincts. If you feel unsafe in any situation, go with your gut. If you see something suspicious, contact your resident assistant or campus police immediately.

2. Avoid being alone or isolated with someone you don't know well. Let a trusted friend know where you are and whom you are with.

3. Get to know your surroundings and learn a well-lit route back to your dorm or place of residence. If you are new to the campus, familiarize yourself with the campus map and know where the emergency phones are.

4. Be careful when leaving online away messages. Leaving information about your whereabouts or activities reveals details of your location that are accessible to everyone. Avoid putting your dorm room, campus address, or phone number on your personal profile where everyone can see it.

5. Form a buddy system when you go out. Arrive with your friends, check in with each other throughout the night, and leave together. Don't go off alone. Make a secret signal with your friends for when they should intervene if you're in an uncomfortable situation.

6. Never loan your room key to anyone, and always lock your door. Don't let strangers into your room.

7. Practice safe drinking. Don't accept drinks from people you don't know or trust and never leave your drink unattended—if you've left your drink, just get a new one. Always watch while your drink is being prepared. At parties, don't drink from punch bowls or other large, common-use containers.

8. Watch out for your friends. If a friend seems out of it, is too intoxicated for the amount of alcohol he or she has had (which signals that he or she may have been drugged), or is acting out of character, get him or her to a safe place immediately. If you suspect that you or a friend has been drugged, call 911, and be explicit with doctors about symptoms.

9. Don't let your guard down. The college campus environment can foster a false sense of security. Don't assume people you've just met will look out for your best interests; remember that they are essentially strangers.

10. Try not to go out alone at night. Walk with roommates or someone you trust. If you'll be walking home alone, ask a trusted friend to accompany you. At night, avoid going to the ATM or exercising alone.

It is important to remember that sexual assault is a crime of motive and opportunity. If you or a friend has been affected by sexual violence, contact the National Sexual Hotlines at 1-800-656-HOPE, or online at www.rainn.org.

Sources: "'The Red Zone': Temporal Risk for Unwanted Sex Among College Students," by W.F. Flack, M.L. Caron, S.J. Leinen, et al., 2008, Journal of Interpersonal Violence, 23 (9), pp. 1177–1196; "RAINN's 2009 Back-to-School Tips for Students," by the Rape Abuse & Incest National Network, 2009, retrieved May 21, 2010, from www.rainn.org/news-room/sexual-assault-news/2009-back-to-school-tips%20. National Sexual Assault Hotlines (1-800-656-HOPE) and online at http://rainn.org. Used with permission.

Male Rape   In about 5 percent of completed and attempted rapes in the United States, the victim is male. About 1 in 33 men report being a victim of a completed or attempted rape in his lifetime.[45] Like women, men are reluctant to report that they have been raped. They may feel embarrassed or ashamed, or they may not want to believe they have been raped.

Law enforcement personnel, medical personnel, and social service agencies may be less supportive of male rape victims than of female rape victims because of similar misperceptions and misinformation.[45] The law is clear, however, on defining forced penetration as rape or sodomy. Male rape victims require the same level of medical treatment, counseling, and support as female victims.

Effects of Rape   Rape is a crime about dominance, power, and control. For many victims, the effects of rape can be profoundly traumatic and long lasting. Physical injuries usually heal quickly, but psychological pain can endure.

Victims often experience fear, anxiety, phobias, guilt, nightmares, depression, substance abuse, sleep disorders, sexual dysfunctions, and social withdrawal. They may develop rape-related post-traumatic stress disorder, experiencing flashbacks and impaired functioning. Between 4 and

Life Stories

Heather: A Case of Sexual Assault

Heather was a freshman in her first semester at a large university a few hundred miles from the midsize city where she grew up. During Welcome Week, her R.A. put up some flyers around her dorm floor about sexual assault, but Heather didn't stop to read them. One night during the second week of classes, Heather and her roommates attended an off-campus party where there were several kegs. She got very drunk and left her friends to hang out with a cute and funny junior, Tom, and continued to drink for the next hour until she started to feel like she was going to be sick. She thought Tom was being helpful when he showed her to a bedroom at the house where he said she could rest until she felt better. But once they were in the room alone, Tom started kissing her. She tried to turn away, but she was too drunk to resist him or say anything. He then sexually forced himself on her.

When she realized what had happened the next day, she tried to forget about it. But over the next week she found herself unable to concentrate on her classes. She was worried she might be pregnant or have gotten an STD. She cycled through feeling guilty for getting so drunk, angry at Tom, and embarrassed. She went back and forth about whether she had really been raped that night. Did it matter that she had been as drunk as she was? Did she say no or try to resist? What would happen if she reported the incident—would her parents find out? Would anyone believe her?

Heather didn't have many people to talk to since it was only the second week

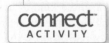

of school, but one of her high school friends who was a year ahead of her was a sophomore at the same school. Heather texted her and they met up at Keisha's apartment. Heather was nervous about sharing something so personal, but Keisha quickly jumped in and said that something similar had happened to her during freshman year. Heather told her how she felt embarrassed, angry, and confused about whether she had been raped. Keisha reminded her that Tom should have stopped when she turned away from him and didn't return his advances. If she didn't report the incident, she asked, how many other girls would Tom do this to? Keisha also explained that because Heather was 18, her parents would not find out unless she told them herself.

Keisha encouraged Heather to report the incident, but she also warned her about the school administration, which she felt had not handled her own report well. She had been made to sign a gag order that threatened the possibility of suspension if she violated it—and technically she was violating it by telling her story to Heather. Keisha advised Heather to contact the Rape Victim Advocacy Program, which Keisha had done only after her bad experience with the campus administration. Heather did so, and RVAP listened to her story and advised her about what to do next, which included filing sexual assault charges against Tom, making an appointment with an off-campus counselor, and getting pregnancy and STD tests at the campus clinic.

---

30 percent of victims contract an STD from the rape, and many worry that they may have been infected with HIV.[40] Some state laws now mandate HIV testing of an alleged rapist if the victim requests it.

Many victims blame themselves for the rape, and our society tends to foster self-blame. Myths about rape include the false beliefs that women or men who are raped did something to provoke it, put themselves in dangerous situations and so deserved it, or could have fought off their attacker. The fact is that no matter what a person does, nobody ever has the right to rape.

What to Do If You Are Raped There is no one way to respond to rape that works in all cases, and authorities recommend that you do whatever you need to do and can do to survive. No matter how you respond, remember that your attacker is violating your rights and committing a crime; rape is not your fault.

After the rape, seek help as soon as you can. If you choose to call the police, there is a better chance that the perpetrator will be brought to justice and will be prevented from raping others. The police will probably take you to the hospital, where you will be given a rape exam and treated for your injuries. You should also contact your local Rape Victim Advocacy Program (RVAP) or the Rape, Abuse, Incest

National Network (RAINN). RVAP or RAINN will inform you of your rights under the Campus Sexual Assault Victims' Bill of Rights Act (CSAVBRA) and provide advocate support during campus and local law enforcement investigations.

Rape counseling is critical to your recovery from the attack. Talking about the rape, either one-on-one with a rape counselor or in a rape survivors' support group, can help you come to terms with your reactions and feelings. Rape crisis hotlines are available when you need immediate help, although research suggests an increasing reluctance among young people to use the phone to discuss sexual assault. One such hotline is the RAINN hotline at (800) 656-HOPE. It takes time to recover from rape, so be patient and take care of yourself.

Culture of Secrecy An investigative report by the Center for Public Integrity (CPI) suggests that colleges and universities are underreporting sexual assaults as required under the Jeanne Clery Disclosure of Campus Security Policy and Campus Crime Statistics Act. This gap in reporting is largely caused by loopholes in the systematic collection of sexual assault data. Crime statistics under the Clery Act are polled from diverse campus programs and centers and local law enforcement agencies. Licensed mental health counselors and pastoral counselors are exempt under confidentiality provisions by the Family Education Reporting Protection

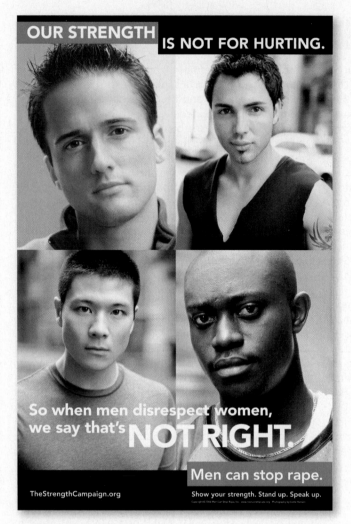

OUR STRENGTH IS NOT FOR HURTING.

So when men disrespect women, we say that's NOT RIGHT.

Men can stop rape.

TheStrengthCampaign.org

Show your strength. Stand up. Speak up.

■ The organization Men Can Stop Rape takes a nontraditional approach to sexual violence prevention, emphasizing healthy masculinity and redefining male strength.

Act. Many of these counselors are housed in rape victim advocacy programs, student health centers, and hospitals. When victims seek help from these types of counselors and not the police, their assaults are not reported.[46,47]

More troublesome are controversial policies used by some colleges and universities to investigate sexual assault reports.[48] Some rely on mediation procedures whereby the alleged perpetrator and alleged victim meet with a college administrator who serves as a mediator to resolve the situation. Both the Department of Justice and the Department of Education explicitly discourage the use of mediation to resolve sexual assault complaints. Mediation processes that do not provide both the alleged victim and alleged perpetrator legal representation and/or advocates may violate the legal rights specified under CSAVBRA. Moreover, sexual assault charges are potentially felony counts that should not be subjected to informal investigations. Gag orders that prevent the alleged victim and alleged perpetrator from disclosing the outcome of a sexual assault complaint have also

come under question. According to the CPI, college female victims who come forward with a sexual assault complaint often feel betrayed by mediation and gag policies.[49] It is recommended that in addition to the police, victims of sexual assault contact an advocacy group like RVAP or RAINN, which can ensure that their rights are being upheld.

Child Sexual Abuse Any interaction between a child and an adult or an older child for the sexual gratification of the perpetrator is defined as **child sexual abuse**. This definition includes intercourse, fondling, and viewing or taking pornographic pictures. Rates of child sexual abuse are difficult to verify because many cases go unreported.

The most frequently abused children are aged 9 to 11.[50] Girls are sexually abused three times as often as boys.[32] The abuse is usually committed by a family member or other person known to the family. **Incest**, sexual activity between family members, is a particularly traumatic form of child sexual abuse because of the profound betrayal of trust involved.

child sexual abuse
Any interaction between a child and an adult or an older child for the sexual gratification of the perpetrator.

incest
Sexual activity between family members.

Victims of sexual abuse usually suffer long-term effects, including anxiety, depression, post-traumatic stress disorder, and sexual dysfunctions. The seriousness of these problems is influenced by the frequency of abuse, the kind of sexual abuse, the child's age when the abuse began, the child's relationship with the abuser, the number of perpetrators, the victim's sex, and the perpetrator's sex.

Child sexual abusers may or may not be pedophiles. A pedophile is a person who is sexually attracted to children. Individuals who are not pedophiles and abuse or molest children are more likely to be opportunists with psychological problems and poor impulse control.

Convicted sex offenders are required to register with the Division of Criminal Justice Services in the state in which they reside. These agencies are authorized to disclose the location of sex offenders if it is considered necessary to protect the public. The Adam Walsh Child Safety and Protection Act of 2007 enhanced penalties for child sexual abuse, tightened registration requirements for sex offenders, and contained measures to combat Internet predators.

Pedophiles and other sex offenders have found a community on the Internet, where they exchange stories and buy and sell child pornography. Sexual predators have also accessed social networking sites like Facebook and MySpace. State justice department officials are pushing for state and federal laws that will require these sites to protect users under age 18 through age identity verification and parental consent.[51] Some opponents to these controls argue that there is no simple way to screen for sexual predators, identify underage users masquerading as adults, or ensure that underage users have parental permission.

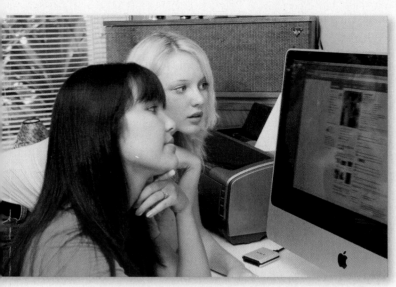

■ Many teens interact safely with strangers online every day. What puts them at risk is giving out their names and other personal information and meeting strangers in person.

The sites themselves, however, are pursuing technologies that can effectively protect users from potential abuses. MySpace, for example, contracted with a national database of convicted sex offenders to detect offenders who were using their site. In one week, MySpace deleted 29,000 convicted sex offenders from its site. In the future, social networking sites will likely face fraud charges if they misrepresent the security of their sites and, possibly, lawsuits if users fall prey to sex offenders and other abusers.

Sexual Harassment **Sexual harassment** includes two broad types of behavior or situations: (1) A person in a position of authority, such as an employer or a teacher, offers benefits for sexual favors or threatens retaliation for the withholding of sex; (2) suggestive language or intimidating conduct creates a hostile atmosphere that interferes with a person's work or academic performance.

Of all sexual harassment claims, 95 percent result from actions that create a hostile environment.[52,53] A hostile environment can be created by visual images (for example, sexually explicit photos), language (for example, jokes, derogatory comments, obscene e-mails), or behavior (for example, inappropriate touching).

Under federal regulations, colleges and universities are liable for sexual harassment perpetrated by their faculty or staff, regardless of whether the advance is accepted or rejected. About 60 percent of college women and men report being sexually harassed. Only about 10 percent report this harassment to university officials.

If you have experienced sexual harassment, keep a written record of all incidents of harassment, including the date, time, place, people involved, words or actions, and any witnesses. If you can, speak up and tell your harasser that the behavior is unacceptable to you. If you do not feel comfortable confronting the harasser in person, consider doing so by letter.

If confrontation does not change the harasser's behavior, complain to a manager or supervisor. If that person does not respond properly to your complaint, consider using your organization's internal grievance procedures. Legal remedies are also available to you through your state Human Rights Commission and the federal Equal Employment Opportunity Commission.

Stalking and Cyberstalking Another form of potentially dangerous conduct is **stalking**, in which a person repeatedly and maliciously follows, harasses, or threatens another person. Women are four times as likely as men to be victims of stalking; it is estimated that 1 in 12 women and 1 in 8 college women have been stalked.[54]

The harassment typically includes surveillance at work, school, or home; frequent disturbing telephone calls; vandalism of the target's property; physical encounters; and attempts to get the victim's family and friends to aid the stalker. Targets of stalkers live in constant fear.

Many states have passed laws to protect individuals who are being stalked, but in some cases it is difficult to arrest and prosecute stalkers without violating their rights, such as the right to be present in a public place. If you plan to report a stalker to the police, keep a written record of all stalking incidents. Include dates, times, locations, witnesses, and types of incidents (personal encounters, telephone calls, e-mails).

A variation on stalking is **cyberstalking**, the use of electronic media to pursue, harass, or contact another person who has not solicited the contact.[55] Online stalkers may send threatening, harassing, sexually provocative, or other unwanted e-mails to the target,

sexual harassment
Behavior in which a person in authority offers benefits for sexual favors or threatens retaliation if sexual favors are withheld, or sexually oriented behavior that creates an intimidating or hostile environment that interferes with a person's work or academic performance.

stalking
Malicious following, harassing, or threatening of one person by another.

cyberstalking
Use of electronic media to pursue, harass, or contact another person who has not solicited the contact.

NEIGHBORHOOD CRIME WATCH

We immediately report all SUSPICIOUS PERSONS and activities to our Police Dept.

or attack or impersonate the person on bulletin boards or in chat rooms. Laws against cyberstalking are in place in some states, but prosecution is hampered by Internet protocols that preserve anonymity as well as by constitutional protection of free speech rights. If you are experiencing this kind of harassment, you can contact the stalker's Internet service provider (ISP) and complain about their client; they will often take action to try to stop the conduct.

FAMILY AND INTIMATE PARTNER VIOLENCE

Violence in families can be directed at any family member, but women, children, and older adults are the most vulnerable. Violence between intimate partners is called **intimate partner violence** or **domestic violence**.

Family Violence Family violence is a broad term that includes several forms of violence and abuse, including child abuse and elder abuse.

Maltreatment of a child, or **child abuse**, includes physical abuse, sexual abuse, emotional abuse, and neglect. It occurs in all cultural, ethnic, and socioeconomic groups, with the highest rates of abuse occurring among the poorest children and among those who are disabled.[56,57] The highest number of victims are among newborns and infants, who are the most fragile, followed by teenagers.

Abusive parents often lack the emotional resources to cope with the stress of childrearing; they may not be knowledgeable about normal child development and have unrealistic expectations of their children. Some may have been abused themselves as children. Social determinants like unemployment, poverty, isolation, as well as alcohol or drug abuse, can be contributing factors. When a case of child abuse comes to light, the abusive parent or guardian is usually removed from the home to keep the child safe. Therapy typically focuses on the abuser but includes all family members.[58]

Maltreatment of an older adult, or **elder abuse**, can include physical abuse (slapping, bruising); sexual abuse; emotional abuse (humiliating, threatening, intimidating); financial abuse (illegal or improper exploitation of funds); and neglect (abandonment, denial of food or health-related services). The abuser is usually a family member, often an adult child, who is taking care of an aging parent or other elderly relative. Interventions for elder abuse include counseling and support groups for caregivers; battered women's services tailored to the needs of older women; family

---

intimate partner violence or **domestic violence**
Violence between two partners in an intimate relationship.

child abuse
Maltreatment of a child; can be physical, sexual, or emotional abuse or neglect.

elder abuse
Maltreatment of an older adult; can be physical, sexual, emotional, or financial abuse or neglect.

battered woman syndrome
Cycle of abuse in an intimate relationship, characterized by escalating tension, a violent episode, and a period of lowered tension and nonviolence.

---

counseling that attempts to improve relationships within the family; and community services such as Meals on Wheels, home health programs, and elder day care.

Intimate Partner Violence Intimate partner violence, or domestic violence, is defined as abuse by a person against his or her partner in an intimate relationship. This definition includes the intentional use of fear and humiliation to control another person. The vast majority of domestic violence victims—95–98 percent—are women.[59] The American Medical Association has stated that the home is more dangerous for women than city streets.[60]

Cycle of Abuse Domestic violence is usually characterized by a cycle of abuse, a recurring pattern of escalating violence. If the couple is heterosexual, the pattern is sometimes referred to as **battered woman syndrome**, but it can occur in any relationship, including gay and lesbian partnerships.

Typically, tension builds up in the relationship until there is a violent outburst, followed by a "honeymoon" period in which the abuser is contrite, ashamed, apologetic, and non-violent.[50] Often he begs his partner to forgive him and promises it will never happen again. Unless the abuser gets help, however, the violence does recur and the cycle repeats itself, almost always becoming more severe (Figure 17.7).

Research indicates that men who batter are more likely to abuse drugs and alcohol, suffer from mental illness, and have financial problems. Most women who are battered eventually leave their abusive relationships, but they may make several attempts before they succeed. Battered women's shelters provide a safe haven where the woman and her children cannot be found by the abuser. They provide housing, food, and resources to help the woman start a new life. When shelters aren't available, private homes are sometimes available as safe houses, and churches, community centers, and YWCAs may also offer temporary facilities.[50]

Dating Violence Dating violence is widespread. Researchers estimate that one in five college students have been physically abused in dating relationships.[61] Studies show that individuals at risk for dating violence are more likely than others to have been sexually assaulted, to have peers who have been sexually victimized, and to accept dating violence. Perpetrators are more likely than others to abuse alcohol or drugs, to have adversarial attitudes toward others, to have sexually aggressive peers, and to accept dating violence.[61,62]

Resources for Survivors of Intimate Partner Violence If you are concerned that someone you know may be in an abusive relationship, try talking to the person about the nature of the relationship and giving him or her information about resources available in your community. Encourage the person to maintain contact with friends and family members while getting support to leave the relationship and begin building a new life.[50] Help is available from social service agencies, educational programs, hotlines, shelters, advocacy

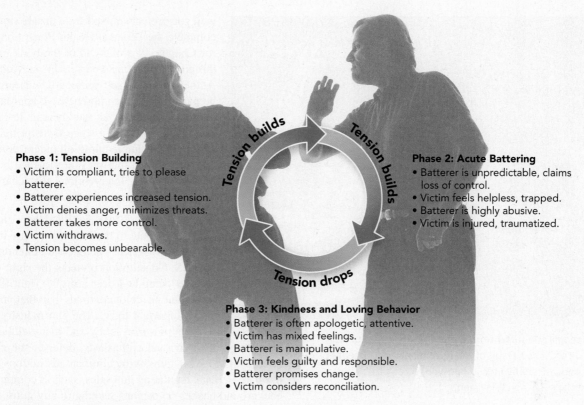

Phase 1: Tension Building
- Victim is compliant, tries to please batterer.
- Batterer experiences increased tension.
- Victim denies anger, minimizes threats.
- Batterer takes more control.
- Victim withdraws.
- Tension becomes unbearable.

Phase 2: Acute Battering
- Batterer is unpredictable, claims loss of control.
- Victim feels helpless, trapped.
- Batterer is highly abusive.
- Victim is injured, traumatized.

Phase 3: Kindness and Loving Behavior
- Batterer is often apologetic, attentive.
- Victim has mixed feelings.
- Batterer is manipulative.
- Victim feels guilty and responsible.
- Batterer promises change.
- Victim considers reconciliation.

figure 17.7 **Cycle of domestic violence.**

Source: Adapted from Understanding Abuse, Gay Partner Abuse Project, www.gaypartnerabuseproject.org.

organizations, and informational books and packets provided by national, state, and local organizations.

WORKPLACE VIOLENCE, HATE CRIMES, AND TERRORISM

Violence can occur where there are high levels of stress, where there is bias, and where there is perceived injustice. In most cases, however, multiple risk factors are present; very often, the perpetrator of violence is psychologically disturbed.

Violence in the Workplace Workplace violence is defined as violent acts, including physical assault and threats of assault, directed toward persons at work or on duty. It can include threatening or aggressive behavior, verbal abuse, intimidation, or harassment. Employers can take measures to lower the risk of workplace violence, such as careful pre-employment screening, appropriate security measures in the workplace, the establishment of procedures for resolving disputes, awareness training for employees and management, and employee assistance programs that provide counseling for employees experiencing psychological problems or high levels of stress.

Hate Crimes A **hate crime** is defined as a crime motivated by bias against the victim's ethnicity, race, religion, sexual orientation, or disability. Hate crimes tend to be excessively brutal, are frequently inflicted at random on people the perpetrators do not know, and are often committed by multiple perpetrators.[63]

Most states have hate crime laws in place, as does the federal government. Many colleges and universities have policies prohibiting hate crimes and harassment of individuals in targeted groups, as well as programs that promote cultural knowledge and diversity.[64] Because hate crimes against lesbian, gay, bisexual, and transgender (LGBT) persons have increased on campuses in recent years,[40] many colleges and universities have specific policies forbidding violence directed toward LGBT students.[65]

hate crime
Crime motivated by bias against the victim's ethnicity, race, religion, sexual orientation, or disability.

terrorism
Violence directed against persons or property, including civilian populations, for the purpose of instilling fear and engendering a sense of helplessness.

Terrorism **Terrorism** is a form of violence directed against persons or property, including civilian populations, for the purpose of instilling fear and engendering a sense of helplessness. Often, terrorist acts are committed in supposed furtherance of political or social aims. For many, the September 11, 2001, attacks on the World Trade Center in New York City and the Pentagon in Washington, D.C., remain the most traumatizing events of the 21st century.

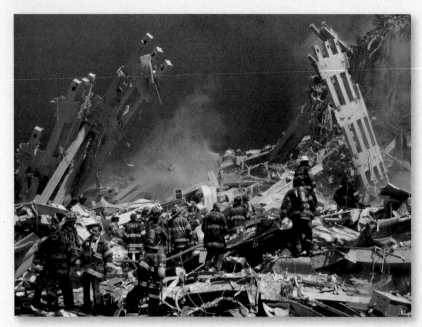

■ Some people still suffer from symptoms of post-traumatic stress disorder as a result of the terrorist attacks of September 11, 2001, including individuals who weren't there but viewed the events on television.

In response to the September 11 attacks, the U.S. government created the Department of Homeland Security to prevent and guard against future attacks and the Homeland Security Advisory System, a color-coded warning system, to alert citizens of the likelihood of attack. In 2005 Congress passed a counterterrorism measure called the Real ID Act, establishing minimum standards for driver's licenses and state-issued ID cards, and in 2007 Congress passed the John Doe provision as part of the renewal of the Homeland Security bill, protecting people who report suspicious activity from being sued by those they report.

The December 25, 2009, attempted bombing of a jetliner over Detroit by a would-be terrorist who was hiding plastic explosives in his underwear led the Transportation Safety Administration (TSA) to accelerate plans for deploying more than 450 full-body scanners at U.S. airports. Full-body scanners are designed to uncover what may not be found by a pat-down search or metal detectors. Opponents to full-body scanners claim they are a violation of privacy rights. Moreover, scanners cannot detect items hidden in body cavities, a common ploy used by drug smugglers and one that terrorist organizations may also try to exploit. Opponents of body scanners recommend the use of more aggressive behavioral profiling, bomb-sniffing dogs, machines that detect the scent of explosives, and heat sensors to increase airline security.

PREVENTING VIOLENCE

Although protecting yourself from terrorism is difficult, there are ways you can limit your risks in life; to assess how

well you protect yourself from unsafe situations, complete the Personal Health Portfolio activity for Chapter 17 at the end of the book (and see the box "Protecting Yourself From Violence"). At the same time, self-protection measures must be part of a more comprehensive approach that addresses violence at the societal level. Current efforts to curb violence focus primarily on arresting and imprisoning offenders. Strategies are also needed that prevent violence before it occurs—that is, interventions that change the social conditions underlying violence.

The Role of Guns: Facilitating Violence
Guns contribute to the lethality of any incident involving violence. The Second Amendment to the U.S. Constitution protects the right of citizens to "keep and bear arms," a right that was important in colonial times but that may not be as important today. The gun industry, along with its powerful lobby and many clubs, organizations, and individual enthusiasts, defends the right of Americans to own guns with minimal restrictions. Some laws are in place regulating gun sales, such as computerized background checks on persons seeking to buy guns, though the U.S. Supreme Court has deemed unconstitutional more severe restrictions, as when in 2009 it overturned Washington, D.C.'s, ban on handguns.

■ The X-rays that are used in backscatter scanners can "see" through clothing. They can detect weapons, dangerous substances, and explosives that might be missed by a metal detector or pat-down search.

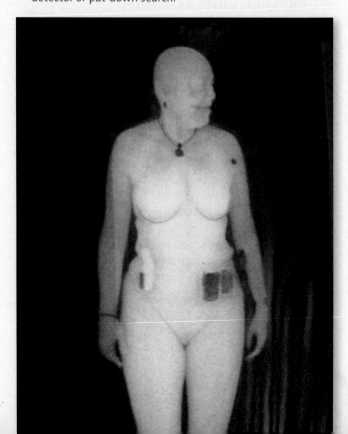

In Your House or Apartment

- Keep doors and windows locked, even when you are at home.

- Before you open your door, make sure the caller is legitimate. If you are expecting a repairperson, insist on proper identification.

- If you have children, tell them not to open the door to strangers.

- If you live alone, use only your initials on your mailbox and in telephone directories.

- If you live in an apartment building, avoid being alone in the laundry room or garage, especially late at night.

On Campus and in Public Places

- Be aware of your surroundings; avoid walking through secluded areas and high-crime neighborhoods.

- Avoid listening to music on headphones; it reduces your attention to warning signs that may be occurring around you.

- Stay with others when possible; groups of three or more are rarely attacked.

- Act and walk in a confident manner. Most assaults occur because the assailant perceives an opportunity to attack someone who appears vulnerable.

- Have your keys ready when getting into your car or opening the door to your residence.

- When carrying packages or luggage, try to keep one arm free.

- Hold your purse firmly under your arm with the strap over your opposite shoulder. Avoid carrying a wallet in a hip pocket, or transfer money and credit cards to a front pocket.

- When you are in any public place, do not display large amounts of cash. Be alert when using an ATM.

- Rely on your instincts. If you think you are being followed, walk quickly to a lighted area. If you feel that you are in immediate danger, scream and run.

- Encourage older and disabled persons to use community transportation services.

- If you jog, do so with a partner. Vary your route and the time you run; and if you run at night, be sure the area is well lighted. Don't wear headphones while jogging.

- Consider taking a class in self-defense.

Source: Adapted from Safety: A Personal Focus *(pp. 178–180), by D. L. Bever, 1996, New York: McGraw-Hill.*

Proponents of gun control support these and other measures, including waiting periods for gun purchases, licensing of guns, and restrictions on access to guns by young people.[66] Proponents of gun control also support the design of safer guns, such as guns with trigger locks, but gun manufacturers point out that gun owners frequently do not use the locks, and the U.S. Congress has concluded that locks are effective only with children younger than age 6.[67]

The gun industry has come under fire in recent years for its marketing practices, which include targeting women, children, and minorities. The marketing campaign aimed at women focuses on empowerment, protection, and participation in shooting sports.[68] These campaigns encourage women to buy guns despite statistics showing that guns in the home are much more likely to kill a family member than a stranger.[68]

The gun industry has also used a variety of strategies to cultivate children as gun enthusiasts, including advertising in youth magazines, financing shooting ranges, providing gun training programs for schools, and manufacturing smaller firearms for children. The huge number of video games that involve shooting also stimulate children's interest in guns.

The gun industry can be expected to increase its marketing to ethnic minorities as well. Rates of gun ownership by Blacks and Hispanics are considerably lower than that for Whites, even though death rates from firearms are higher.[68] The complex issues surrounding the manufacture, sale, and ownership of guns are likely to be part of our national debate for some time to come.

desensitization
Raised threshold of reaction to violence and a loss of compassion.

THE ROLE OF MEDIA AND ENTERTAINMENT: GLORIFYING VIOLENCE

Violent acts occur much more frequently in movies and television shows than they do in real life.[69] Repeated exposure to violence may also lead to habituation and **desensitization**, a raised threshold for reaction to violence and a loss of compassion. Repeated exposure to graphic images of violence also feeds the appetite for more intense violence.[70]

The American Academy of Pediatrics and five other prominent medical groups concluded in 2000 that there is a connection between violence in mass media and increases in both acceptance of aggressive attitudes and aggressive behavior in children. The entertainment industry maintains that these studies demonstrate only possible associations between media violence and aggression. Media defenders warn that attempts at regulation would border on censorship.

In response to this information, communities have organized boycotts of products of companies that sponsor violent and sexually explicit programs. Parents can use blocking technologies to keep their children from seeing selected television programs and Internet sites. The entertainment industry has started to regulate itself, primarily to avoid government regulation.[69] The National Association of Theater Owners, for example, has promised to enforce the movie ratings system vigorously.

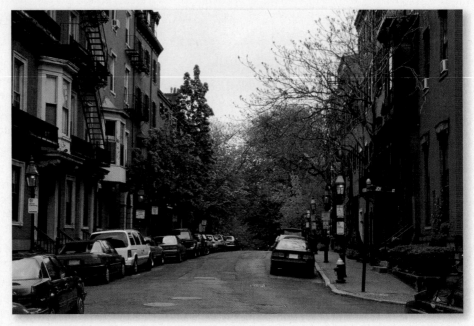

■ Safe neighborhoods and communities provide a setting in which individuals have the opportunity to pursue wellness.

SUPPORTING FAMILIES AND COMMUNITIES

Families play a vital role in reducing violence by teaching children self-control along with constructive ways to deal with anger, frustration, and destructive impulses. Positive family interventions emphasize consistent parenting, clear rules and appropriate consequences, supervision of children's activities, and constructive management of family conflicts.

awareness programs to broad community-based strategies that target the underlying issues surrounding sexual violence.[73] The organization Men Can Stop Rape sponsors a Campus Strength Program that helps students develop and support healthy masculinity and consider the ways men can be allies of women. The Mentors in Violence Prevention Program takes a "bystander" approach to violence

Repeated exposure to violence may lead to a raised threshold for reaction to violence *and* a loss of compassion.

Communities also play a role. Common sense suggests that safe physical environments are less conducive to criminal activity than are run-down environments. Communities where neighbors look out for one another, as with neighborhood watch programs, are less inviting to criminals. Communities also have to support social changes that enhance economic and social stability.[71] To bring about change, communities have used strategies such as cleaning up trash and graffiti and fixing broken windows, providing organized leisure activities and mentoring programs for youth, encouraging parent involvement in school activities, supporting low-income housing to curb an exodus of middle-income residents of all races, and increasing police presence in high-risk areas.[72]

College campuses have an important role to play in the prevention of violence, especially sexual violence. Prevention efforts in this area are undergoing major changes on many college campuses, which are moving away from

prevention in communities and schools. In this model, men are not viewed as potential perpetrators and women are not viewed as potential victims; the focus is on both as bystanders who can confront abusive peers and support abused peers. The American College Health Association has developed a sexual assault prevention toolkit that promotes gender equality, healthy relationships, healthy sexuality, and civility on campus.

Individuals who want to take action against violence have a variety of options, from volunteering at women's shelters to supporting public policies that address the root causes of violence in our society. Keeping a sense of perspective about violence is important, however. Some observers have suggested that Americans live in a media-driven "culture of fear," frightened by overblown accounts of crime, drugs, and violence.[74] The key is to take media portrayals of violence with a grain of salt while using your common sense to keep yourself safe.

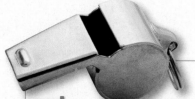

You Make the Call

Should Concealed Weapons Be Allowed on the College Campus?

On August 1, 1966, 25-year-old former marine Charles Joseph Whitman climbed to the top of the bell tower on the University of Texas campus and unleashed a hail of sniper fire, killing and injuring students, faculty, and staff. The Austin police department did not have a SWAT team, and officers were armed only with service revolvers and shotguns, which were not effective in battling Whitman. Some students retreated to their dorm rooms or fraternity rooms, armed themselves with hunting rifles, and began firing at the sniper. This return fire placed Whitman in a position where he could no longer lean over the edge of the tower to effectively take his shots. Most of the sniper damage occurred during the period before the students returned fire, and Whitman was eventually killed by police who gained access to the tower via an underground tunnel.

Almost 40 years later, campus shootings by psychologically deranged men still occur, such as those on the campuses of Virginia Tech and the University of Northern Illinois. But in both of these shooting sprees, there were no armed citizens to confront the assailant. Instead, students, faculty, and staff were forced to hide under desks or to barricade door entrances to classrooms, dorm rooms, or offices as they waited for law enforcement rescue. Recent campus shootings have led colleges and universities to enact several measures, including arming campus security, implementing alert systems, and training students how to survive a classroom shooting.

Students for Concealed Carry on Campus (SCCC) is advocating a more aggressive prevention measure: Change federal and state laws and college and university policies to allow gun-licensed college students to carry concealed handguns on campus. The organization emphasizes that concealed handguns are legal in most states virtually everywhere else—movie theaters, offices, shopping malls, and so on. SCCC proponents hope that educating the public about the discrepancy of gun-free zones on the college campus will motivate citizens to encourage state legislators and campus administrators to amend existing concealed-handgun laws and policies. They argue that while people may *feel* safer knowing that guns are not allowed on campus, they will actually *be* safer if students are allowed to carry guns on campus. Armed students would be able to take immediate action during a campus shooting and potentially save lives, they argue. And in addition, if potential shooters knew that students might be armed, they would be less likely to plan a shooting spree at all. In response to the fear that guns on campus would increase violence, SCCC points out that concealed-weapons permit holders are five times less likely to commit violent crimes than armed individuals without a license.

Opponents of concealed weapons on campus claim that their presence would result in a "Wild West" environment. They maintain that more guns on campus will mean more violence via gun accidents, gun theft, and gun owners who might themselves be mentally unstable. They also argue that guns on campus detract from a healthy learning environment, that strict gun-control measures make cities safer, and that the complicated subject of public safety should not be dictated by public opinion.

Currently, 12 colleges and universities allow people with concealed handgun permits to carry on campus. Opponents do not see these measures as making campuses safer or improving the learning environment. What do you think?

PROS

- Campus shooters would be stopped more quickly if students were allowed to carry concealed weapons.
- Campus concealed-weapons bans are unfair, since concealed weapons are allowed almost everywhere else.
- Concealed-weapons permit holders are five times less likely to commit violent crimes than armed individuals without a license.

CONS

- Guns on campus would lead to more violence on campus.
- Many students and faculty would feel uncomfortable about not knowing whether their instructors and fellow students were armed.
- Studies of students with concealed weapons in simulated shootings have shown that they panic rather than taking effective self-defense actions.

connect
ACTIVITY

Sources: "Students for Concealed Carry on Campus," http://concealedcampus.org/; Gun Facts, www.GunFacts.info.

IN REVIEW

How does injury affect personal health?
Unintentional injuries are the fifth leading cause of death in the United States and the leading cause of death for children and adults aged 1 to 39. Public health experts believe that injuries are preventable if people adopt behaviors that promote safety and if society takes steps to reduce environmental hazards.

What are the leading causes of injury-related death?
The top cause for all age groups is motor vehicle crashes, followed by falls, poisoning, choking, and drowning. Common causes vary by age and race/ethnicity, but males are more likely than females to die from unintentional injuries across all groups until age 80.

How does violence affect personal health?
Many people are the victims of violence and of violent crimes, which include homicide, assault, robbery, and rape. Compared with other developed countries, the United States has higher rates of homicide, especially homicide committed with a firearm.

What forms does violence take in our society?
Teens and young adults commit violent acts in schools and as members of youth gangs. Crimes on college campuses include assaults, rapes, and very rare but high-profile mass shootings. Sexual violence includes sexual assault, child sexual abuse, sexual harassment, and stalking and cyberstalking. Family violence includes child and elder abuse, intimate partner violence, and dating violence. Violence can also occur in the workplace or take the form of a hate crime. Terrorism is violence intended to create fear and helplessness.

Web Resources

American Red Cross: Highlighting news, safety tips, and disaster updates, this Web site features information on a wide range of emergencies.
www.redcross.org

National Center for Injury Prevention and Control: This organization's Web site includes information on various injury-related topics as well as injury care information.
www.cdc.gov/ncipc

National Center for Victims of Crime: This Web site offers information on the cycle of abuse, child abuse, rape, domestic violence, stalking, dating violence, and violence against women.
www.ncvc.org

National Highway Traffic Safety Administration: For information about traffic safety, news, vehicles and equipment, research, and laws and regulations, this organization is an authoritative resource.
www.nhtsa.dot.gov

National Safety Council: This council publishes Injury Facts, an annual compilation of statistics on injuries. Its Web site features information on driving, ergonomics, first aid, and preparedness, among other topics.
www.nsc.org

National Sexual Violence Resource Center: This site operates as a collection and distribution center for information, statistics, and resources on sexual violence.
www.nsvrc.org

Rape, Abuse, and Incest National Network (RAINN): This site provides information about what to do if you or a friend is sexually assaulted, how to reduce your risk of sexual assault, and how to protect your child from sexual abuse.
www.rainn.org

Security on Campus, Inc.: This nonprofit organization organizes the Safe on Campus Peer Education Program, which equips college students to go to high schools and discuss the issues of sexual assault, alcohol, hazing, and crime in college.
www.securityoncampus.org

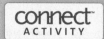
Are you wondering how you are doing in regard to your overall health and well-being? This is the first of a series of self-assessment activities that are included in this book. Your Personal Health Portfolio, the final product of all activities, will be a collection of documents that explore your strengths and challenges. It will represent a snapshot of your health and self-reflections throughout the course.

This first portfolio activity is centered on an adaptation of a well-studied assessment tool (the Rand Corporation's Short Form 36) that will help you take a general look at components of your physical and mental health.

Read each question carefully and circle the point value corresponding to your answer.

PHYSICAL FUNCTIONING

The following items are about activities you might do during a typical day. Does your health now limit you in these activities? If so, how much?

	Yes, limited a lot	Yes, limited a little	No, not limited at all
1. Vigorous activities, such as running, lifting heavy objects, participating in strenuous sports	0	50	100
2. Moderate activities, such as moving a table, pushing a vacuum cleaner, bowling, or playing golf	0	50	100
3. Lifting or carrying groceries	0	50	100
4. Climbing several flights of stairs	0	50	100
5. Climbing one flight of stairs	0	50	100
6. Bending, kneeling, or stooping	0	50	100
7. Walking more than a mile	0	50	100
8. Walking several blocks	0	50	100
9. Walking one block	0	50	100

LIMITATIONS DUE TO PHYSICAL HEALTH

During the past month, have you had any of the following problems with your work or other regular daily activities as a result of your physical health?

	Yes	No
1. Cut down the amount of time you spent on work or other activities	0	100
2. Accomplished less than you would like	0	100
3. Were limited in the kind of work or other activities you did	0	100
4. Had difficulty performing work or other activities (for example, it took extra effort)	0	100

LIMITATIONS DUE TO EMOTIONAL PROBLEMS

During the past month, have you had any of the following problems with your work or other regular daily activities as a result of any emotional problems (such as feeling depressed or anxious)?

	Yes	No
1. Cut down the amount of time you spent on work or other activities	0	100
2. Accomplished less than you would like	0	100
3. Didn't do work or other activities as carefully as usual	0	100

ENERGY/FATIGUE

These questions are about how you feel and how things have been going for you during the past month. For each question, give the one answer that comes closest to the way you have been feeling. How much of the time during the past month . . .

	All of the time	Most of the time	A good bit of the time	Some of the time	A little of the time	None of the time
1. Did you feel full of pep?	100	80	60	40	20	0
2. Did you have a lot of energy?	100	80	60	40	20	0
3. Did you feel worn out?	0	20	40	60	80	100
4. Did you feel tired?	0	20	40	60	80	100

EMOTIONAL WELL-BEING

These questions are about how you feel and how things have been going for you during the past month. For each question, give the one answer that comes closest to the way you have been feeling. How much of the time during the past month . . .

	All of the time	Most of the time	A good bit of the time	Some of the time	A little of the time	None of the time
1. Have you been a very nervous person?	0	20	40	60	80	100
2. Have you felt so down in the dumps that nothing could cheer you up?	0	20	40	60	80	100
3. Have you felt calm and peaceful?	100	80	60	40	20	0
4. Have you felt downhearted and blue?	0	20	40	60	80	100
5. Have you been a happy person?	100	80	60	40	20	0

SOCIAL FUNCTIONING

1. During the past month, to what extent have your physical health or emotional problems interfered with your normal social activities with family, friends, neighbors, or groups? (Circle one number.)

Not at all   100

Slightly   75

Moderately   50

Quite a bit   25

Extremely   0

2. During the past month, how much of the time has your physical health or emotional problems interfered with your social activities (like visiting with friends, relatives, etc.)? (Circle one number.)

All of the time   0

Most of the time   25

Some of the time   50

A little of the time   75

None of the time   100

PAIN

1. How much bodily pain have you had during the past month? (Circle one number.)

None   100

Very mild   80

Mild   60

Moderate   40

Severe   20

Very severe   0

2. During the past month, how much did pain interfere with your normal work (including both work outside the home and housework)? (Circle one number.)

Not at all   100

A little bit   75

Moderately   50

Quite a bit   25

Extremely   0

GENERAL HEALTH

1. In general, you would say your health is

Excellent   100

Very good   75

Good   50

Fair   25

Poor   0

How TRUE or FALSE is *each* of the following statements for you?

	Definitely true	Mostly true	Don't know	Mostly false	Definitely false
2. I seem to get sick a little easier than other people.	0	25	50	75	100
3. I am as healthy as anybody I know.	100	75	50	25	0
4. I expect my health to get worse.	0	25	50	75	100
5. My health is excellent.	100	75	50	25	0

Scoring

Add up your scores from each section and divide by the number of questions in the section to obtain an average score. The highest possible score in each section is 100.

PHYSICAL FUNCTIONING

$$\underline{\qquad}_{1} + \underline{\qquad}_{2} + \underline{\qquad}_{3} + \underline{\qquad}_{4} + \underline{\qquad}_{5} + \underline{\qquad}_{6} + \underline{\qquad}_{7} + \underline{\qquad}_{8} + \underline{\qquad}_{9} = \underline{\qquad}_{\text{raw score}} \div 9 = \underline{\qquad}_{\text{average}}$$

LIMITATIONS DUE TO PHYSICAL HEALTH

$$\underline{\qquad}_{1} + \underline{\qquad}_{2} + \underline{\qquad}_{3} + \underline{\qquad}_{4} = \underline{\qquad}_{\text{raw score}} \div 4 = \underline{\qquad}_{\text{average}}$$

LIMITATIONS DUE TO EMOTIONAL PROBLEMS

$$\underline{\qquad}_{1} + \underline{\qquad}_{2} + \underline{\qquad}_{3} = \underline{\qquad}_{\text{raw score}} \div 3 = \underline{\qquad}_{\text{average}}$$

ENERGY/FATIGUE

$$\underline{\qquad}_{1} + \underline{\qquad}_{2} + \underline{\qquad}_{3} + \underline{\qquad}_{4} = \underline{\qquad}_{\text{raw score}} \div 4 = \underline{\qquad}_{\text{average}}$$

EMOTIONAL WELL-BEING

$$\underline{\qquad}_{1} + \underline{\qquad}_{2} + \underline{\qquad}_{3} + \underline{\qquad}_{4} + \underline{\qquad}_{5} = \underline{\qquad}_{\text{raw score}} \div 5 = \underline{\qquad}_{\text{average}}$$

SOCIAL FUNCTIONING

$$\underline{\qquad}_{1} + \underline{\qquad}_{2} = \underline{\qquad}_{\text{raw score}} \div 2 = \underline{\qquad}_{\text{average}}$$

PAIN

$$\underline{\qquad}_{1} + \underline{\qquad}_{2} = \underline{\qquad}_{\text{raw score}} \div 2 = \underline{\qquad}_{\text{average}}$$

GENERAL HEALTH

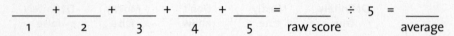

_____ + _____ + _____ + _____ + _____ = _____ ÷ 5 = _____
  1   2   3   4   5   raw score   average

Your scores can be interpreted in the following manner. Mark an X where your score falls on the continuum for each section. Recognize that the behaviors exist on a continuum with low scores indicating areas of concern and higher scores indicating healthier behaviors/feelings.

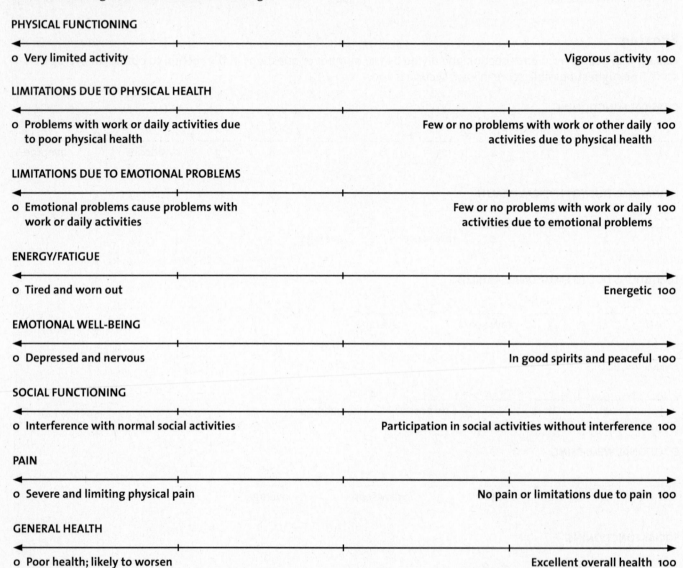

PHYSICAL FUNCTIONING

o Very limited activity — Vigorous activity 100

LIMITATIONS DUE TO PHYSICAL HEALTH

o Problems with work or daily activities due to poor physical health — Few or no problems with work or other daily activities due to physical health 100

LIMITATIONS DUE TO EMOTIONAL PROBLEMS

o Emotional problems cause problems with work or daily activities — Few or no problems with work or daily activities due to emotional problems 100

ENERGY/FATIGUE

o Tired and worn out — Energetic 100

EMOTIONAL WELL-BEING

o Depressed and nervous — In good spirits and peaceful 100

SOCIAL FUNCTIONING

o Interference with normal social activities — Participation in social activities without interference 100

PAIN

o Severe and limiting physical pain — No pain or limitations due to pain 100

GENERAL HEALTH

o Poor health; likely to worsen — Excellent overall health 100

Source: Adapted from the 36-Item Short Form Health Survey developed from the Medical Outcomes Study. Copyright © the RAND Corporation. RAND's permission to reproduce the survey is not an endorsement of the products, services, or other uses in which the survey appears or is applied.

CRITICAL THINKING QUESTIONS

1. Look over your total scores. In what areas do you have high scores—reflecting healthier behaviors and feeling? In what areas do you have lower scores—reflecting possible areas of concern?

2. In areas of higher scores, what helps you maintain healthy behaviors? Consider your personal knowledge about what it means to be healthy and your attitudes and beliefs. Then consider factors in your environment that support healthy patterns—consider how you are supported by friends and family, your school community and living situation, institutions to which you belong, and local or national policies.

3. In areas of lower scores, what are some of the barriers that make improvement difficult for you? As with your strengths, consider each level in the ecological model of health.

4. Finally, consider if there are areas in which you would like to make changes. What would these changes look like? How ready are you to make changes? What steps would you take to start the change process? If you are ready, complete a behavior change contract (see next activity).

This general quality of life assessment is a starting point for exploring your health. In areas where your scores are at the lower or higher end of the continuum, you may already have a sense of what factors contribute to your concerns or strengths. As you continue through each chapter of the book, you will be asked to complete portfolio activities that will help you explore in greater detail factors that influence your general health and well-being. Keep this portfolio activity in mind. Come back and revisit it throughout the term. See if you think differently about various factors in your life as you learn more.

Personal Health Portfolio

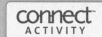

Behavior I want to change: _____

My goal: _____

_____

Remember that your goal should be SMART: specific, measurable, attainable, realistic, and timely.

I will achieve my goal by _____ .
                                        date

Along the way, I will create a series of smaller, incremental goals to help me reach my overall goal:

Incremental goal 1: _____ Target date: _____

Incremental goal 2: _____ Target date: _____

Incremental goal 3: _____ Target date: _____

Benefits associated with this behavior change:

- _____
- _____
- _____

Barriers I expect to encounter:

- _____
- _____
- _____

Strategies for overcoming these barriers:

- _____
- _____
- _____

Signature: _____ Date: _____

Witness signature: _____ Date: _____

A family health tree is a diagram of your family's health history over several generations. As such, it can provide important clues to the genes you have inherited from your parents, grandparents, and ancestors. Constructing a family health tree has three broad steps: (1) mapping the family structure, (2) recording family information, and (3) finding family relationships. Refer to the model provided in Figure 2.1 as you construct your own family health tree. You can use the template provided on the next page, or create one online at www.hhs.gov/familyhistory (which can be printed).

1. Begin with yourself and your immediate family. Then add your cousins, your aunts and uncles, your grandparents, and as many other relatives as you can. The more generations and individuals you include, the more useful your tree will be.

2. When placing children beneath their parents, begin with the oldest on the left. Connect adopted or foster children to their parents with a dotted line to indicate that no biological relationship exists.

3. If a person is deceased, draw an X in the square and write his or her date of death (or age at death) and the cause of death. If a woman has had a miscarriage or stillbirth, indicate that with an X in the square of the deceased child. Because some genetic conditions are more common in certain ethnic groups, include the ethnicity of each person in the oldest generation you include.

4. Now add as much health-related information as you know for each person. Include major diseases or health conditions, such as diabetes, osteoporosis, cancer, heart disease, and so on, and the person's age when diagnosed. Also include surgeries, allergies, mental health problems, and any genetic or chromosomal disorders, such as Down syndrome.

5. Once you have gathered all the information, analyze your family health tree by completing the Critical Thinking Questions. You may want to take your family health tree to your physician or a genetic counselor for a professional opinion on your health risks. He or she may recommend that you modify certain lifestyle behaviors (such as diet or exercise) or have particular screening tests (such as an early test for cancer). You may want to have your physician keep a copy of your family health tree in your medical file for future reference. You may also want to share what you have found out, as well as your physician's recommendations, with your siblings and other family members.

CRITICAL THINKING QUESTIONS

1. What are your family's strengths? Consider such things as longevity, fitness, mental well-being, etc.

2. What are the patterns of disease or illness in your family? Are there certain diseases that appear frequently? Does the pattern suggest a possible genetic link?

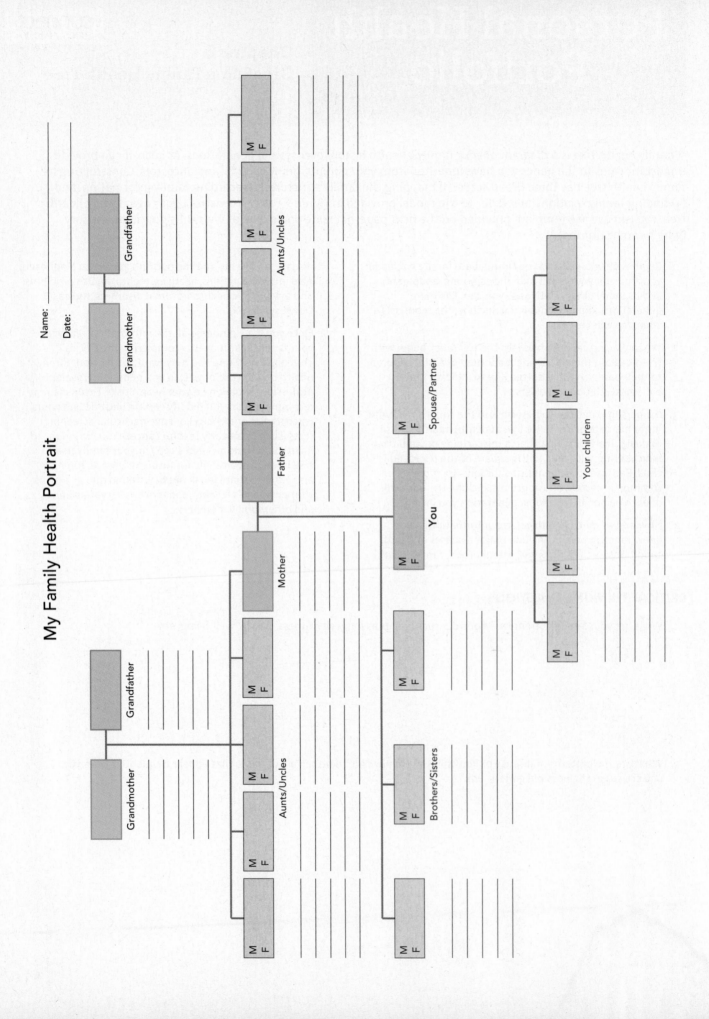

My Family Health Portrait

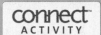
Resilience is described as the ability to regain equilibrium or recover when faced with adversity. Individuals who are resilient are often more self-confident, recognizing their strengths and abilities. For those people whose resilience is low, failures and setbacks are a drain on their energy and motivation, and they are more prone to depression and other mental disorders. Resilience is also important in dealing with stress. Resilient people have the perseverance to deal with stressors in positive ways and rebound more quickly after stressful events.

Take some time and complete the Resilience Scale to gain a better understanding of your ability to respond during times of adversity. Circle the number to the right of each statement that best reflects your feelings. If you are neutral or undecided on a particular item, select 4.

		Strongly disagree					Strongly agree	
1.	When I make plans, I follow through with them.	1	2	3	4	5	6	7
2.	I usually manage one way or another.	1	2	3	4	5	6	7
3.	I am able to depend on myself more than anyone else.	1	2	3	4	5	6	7
4.	Keeping interested in things is important to me.	1	2	3	4	5	6	7
5.	I can be on my own if I have to.	1	2	3	4	5	6	7
6.	I feel proud that I have accomplished things in life.	1	2	3	4	5	6	7
7.	I usually take things in stride.	1	2	3	4	5	6	7
8.	I am friends with myself.	1	2	3	4	5	6	7
9.	I feel that I can handle many things at a time.	1	2	3	4	5	6	7
10.	I am determined.	1	2	3	4	5	6	7
11.	I seldom wonder what the point of it all is.	1	2	3	4	5	6	7
12.	I take things one day at a time.	1	2	3	4	5	6	7
13.	I can get through difficult times because I've experienced difficulty before.	1	2	3	4	5	6	7
14.	I have self-discipline.	1	2	3	4	5	6	7
15.	I keep interested in things.	1	2	3	4	5	6	7
16.	I can usually find something to laugh about.							
17.	My belief in myself gets me through hard times.	1	2	3	4	5	6	7
18.	In an emergency, I'm someone people can generally rely on.	1	2	3	4	5	6	7
19.	I can usually look at a situation in a number of ways.	1	2	3	4	5	6	7
20.	Sometimes I make myself do things whether I want to or not.	1	2	3	4	5	6	7
21.	My life has meaning.	1	2	3	4	5	6	7
22.	I do not dwell on things that I can't do anything about.	1	2	3	4	5	6	7
23.	When I'm in a difficult situation, I can usually find my way out of it.	1	2	3	4	5	6	7
24.	I have enough energy to do what I have to do.	1	2	3	4	5	6	7
25.	It's okay if there are people who don't like me.	1	2	3	4	5	6	7

Scoring

Add up your numbers for each question. Your score will be between 25 and 175.

Score: _____

146 or more: Your score indicates moderately high/high levels of resilience. You are optimistic and see your life as having purpose. Although you have had your share of rough times, you are confident that you can handle future obstacles.

126–145: Your score indicates moderately low/moderate resilience. You have many characteristics of resilience, but you may not be satisfied with all areas of your life. You can move forward with your life, but without enthusiasm. Work to strengthen your resilience and you will have an easier time dealing with the ups and downs of life.

125 or below: Your score indicates low resilience. You may be going through some hard times right now and lack confidence about your ability to get through them. Although your score is on the low end, that doesn't mean you don't have any resilience. If you work to strengthen it, you will make a positive change in your life.

The first critical step in taking the scale is self-awareness. You can then assess how you might want to build on strengths and work on areas of weakness.

Source: The Resilience Scale, by Gail Wagnild and Heather M. Young. © 2009. Used by permission. Scoring adapted from The Resilience Scale User's Guide, by Gail M. Wagnild and Heather M. Young. 2009. The Resilience Center, P.O. Box 313, Worden, Montana 59088.

CRITICAL THINKING QUESTIONS

1. Analyze your score. Was it higher or lower than you expected? What areas of strength or weakness do you see?

2. It has been suggested that when you face adversity and find a way to recover you actually gain confidence for the next time you face a very difficult situation. Think back to your own adolescence. Was it easy? Or did you face issues related to building friendships, becoming comfortable with your body, or participating in sexual activity? How have your past experiences contributed to your resilience today?

3. What people or circumstances have influenced your resilience? Consider your parents, other family members, and friends and the community in which you were raised.

Personal Health Portfolio

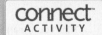
One important aspect of well-being is your perceived meaning in life. Do you believe you have a meaningful life? Are you interested in personal growth and developing your own values?

Researchers believe that there is a relationship between finding meaning in life and a person's well-being. As you search to uncover the meaning in your life, the first step in the process is increasing your self-awareness about your sense of meaning and purpose.

There are two subscales in the questionnaire. The first, Presence of Meaning, measures how meaningful people perceive their life to be. The second, Search for Meaning, measures how actively people are seeking to discover or augment the level of meaningfulness they experience in life.

PRESENCE OF MEANING

	Absolutely untrue			Can't say true or false			Absolutely true	
1. I understand my life's meaning.	1	2	3	4	5	6	7
2. My life has a clear sense of purpose.	1	2	3	4	5	6	7
3. I have a good sense of what makes my life meaningful.	1	2	3	4	5	6	7
4. I have discovered a satisfying life purpose.	1	2	3	4	5	6	7
5. My life has no clear purpose.	7	6	5	4	3	2	1

SEARCH FOR MEANING

	Absolutely untrue			Can't say true or false			Absolutely true	
1. I am looking for something that makes my life feel meaningful.	1	2	3	4	5	6	7
2. I am always looking to find my life's purpose.	1	2	3	4	5	6	7
3. I am always searching for something that makes my life feel significant.	1	2	3	4	5	6	7
4. I am seeking a purpose or mission for my life.	1	2	3	4	5	6	7
5. I am searching for meaning in my life.	1	2	3	4	5	6	7

Scoring

Add up your numbers for each section. Scores will range from 5 to 35.

Presence of Meaning score: _____

Search for Meaning score: _____

If you scored **above** 24 on Presence and also **above** 24 on Search, you feel your life has a valued meaning and purpose, yet you are still openly exploring that meaning or purpose. You likely are satisfied with your life, are somewhat optimistic, experience feelings of love frequently, and rarely feel depressed. You are probably somewhat active in spiritual activities, and you tend not to value pursuing sensory stimulation as much as others. You are generally certain of, and occasionally forceful regarding, your views and supportive of having an overall structure in society and life. People who know you would probably describe you as conscientious, thoughtful, easy to get along with, somewhat open to new experiences, and generally easygoing and emotionally stable.

If you scored **above** 24 on Presence and **below** 24 on Search, you feel your life has a valued meaning and purpose, and you are not actively exploring that meaning or seeking meaning in your life. One might say that you are satisfied that you've grasped what makes your life meaningful, why you're here, and what you want to do with your life. You probably are satisfied with your life, are optimistic, and have healthy self-esteem. You frequently experience feelings of love and joy and rarely feel afraid, angry, ashamed, or sad. You probably hold traditional values. You are usually certain of, and often forceful regarding, your views and likely support structure and rules for society and living. You are probably active in and committed to spiritual pursuits. People who know you would probably describe you as conscientious, organized, friendly, easy to get along with, and socially outgoing.

If you scored **below** 24 on Presence and **above** 24 on Search, you probably do not feel your life has a valued meaning and purpose, and you are actively searching for something or someone that will give your life meaning or purpose. You are probably not always satisfied with your life. You may not experience emotions like love and joy that often. You may occasionally, or even often, feel anxious, nervous, or sad and depressed. You are probably questioning the role of spirituality in your life, and you may be working hard to figure out whether there is a God, what life on Earth is really about, and which, if any, religion is right for you. People who know you would probably describe you as liking to play things by ear or "go with the flow" when it comes to plans, occasionally worried, and not particularly socially active.

If you scored **below** 24 on Presence and also **below** 24 on Search, you probably do not feel your life has a valued meaning and purpose and are not actively exploring that meaning or seeking meaning in your life. You may not always be satisfied with your life, or yourself, and you might not be particularly optimistic about the future. You may not experience emotions like love and joy that often. You may occasionally, or even often, feel anxious, nervous, or sad and depressed. You probably do not hold traditional values and may be more likely to value stimulating, exciting experiences, although you are not necessarily open-minded about everything. People who know you would probably describe you as sometimes disorganized, occasionally nervous or tense, and not particularly socially active or especially warm toward everyone.

Sources: Adapted from "The Meaning in Life Questionnaire: Assessing the presence of and search for meaning in life," by M. F. Steger, P. Frazier, S. Oishi, and M. Kaler, 2006, Journal of Counseling Psychology, 53, pp. 80–93; "Understanding the search for meaning," by Michael F. Steger, Todd B. Kashdan, Brandon A. Sullivan, and Danielle Lorentz, April 2008, Journal of Personality, 76, pp. 197–227.

CRITICAL THINKING QUESTIONS

1. Analyze your scores for each scale. Were they higher or lower than you expected? What areas of strength do you see? Where is there room for growth?

2. Think about the environmental factors in your life, like your friends, family, school, and community. How do they affect your pursuit of meaning in life?

3. After having taken this assessment and considered the results, do you want to be able to find more meaning in your life? If so, what are some actions you can take to begin this process? (You may want to refer to the "Enhancing Your Spirituality" sections in Chapter 4.)

Part 1   Sleep Diary

A sleep diary can help identify habits that interfere with quality sleep. The diary can also be a source of valuable information if you need to consult a medical professional about sleep. Use the sleep diary on the following page to track your sleep for seven days. You may want to keep it close to your bed so that you will remember to fill it out before you go to sleep and when you awake.

Part 2   Do You Have Symptoms of a Sleep Disorder?

Ask yourself the following questions:

- Do you have trouble falling asleep three nights a week or more?
- Do you wake up frequently during the night?
- Do you wake up too early and find it difficult to get back to sleep?
- Do you wake up unrefreshed?
- Do you snore loudly?
- Are you aware of gasping for breath or not breathing while you are sleeping, or has anyone ever told you that you do this?
- Do you feel sleepy during the day or doze off watching TV, reading, driving, or engaging in daily activities, even though you get eight hours of sleep a night?
- Do you have nightmares?
- Do you feel unpleasant, tingling, creeping sensations in your legs while trying to sleep?

If you answer yes to any of these questions, it is possible that you are suffering from a sleep disorder. The first step to take is to make sure you have good sleep habits and practices, as described in Chapter 5. If you are doing everything you can to ensure a good night's sleep, consult your physician. He or she may refer you to a sleep disorder specialist.

Sources: Part 1: "Weekly Sleep Diary," Helpguide, www.helpguide.com. Part 2: Adapted from National Sleep Foundation, 2004, www.sleepfoundation.org.

CRITICAL THINKING QUESTIONS

1. Analyze your sleep over the week. What was the average number of hours you slept for the five weekday nights? What was the average number of hours you slept on the weekend? Discuss the factors (individual and environmental) that affected the duration or quality of your sleep. For example, perhaps you slept worse on the days you drank Pepsi after dinner, or perhaps you slept worse on the weekend because your neighbors had a noisy party. Conversely, perhaps you slept well because you didn't play video games before going to sleep or because your partner goes to sleep and wakes up at the same time you do.

2. In Part 2, did you answer yes to any of the questions? If so, do you think you need to see your doctor about your sleep quality?

3. Overall, do you think you are meeting your sleep needs? Why or why not? If you are not meeting your sleep needs, what are some things you can do to change this?

SLEEP DIARY

	Day 1 Date:	Day 2 Date:	Day 3 Date:	Day 4 Date:	Day 5 Date:	Day 6 Date:	Day 7 Date:
Daytime Activities & Pre-Sleep Ritual (Fill in each night before going to bed)							
Exercise What did you do? When? Total time?							
Naps When? Where? How long?							
Alcohol & Caffeine Types, amount and when							
Feelings Happiness, sadness, stress, anxiety; major cause							
Food & Drink (Dinner/snacks) What and when?							
Medications or **Sleep Aids** Types, amount and when							
Bedtime Routine Meditation / Relaxation? How long?							
Bed Time							
Sleeping & Getting Back to Sleep (Fill in each morning)							
Wake-up Time							
Sleep Breaks Did you get up during the night? If so, what did you do?							
Quality of Sleep & **Other Comments**							
Total Sleep Hours							

Source: "Weekly Sleep Diary." Helpguide, www.helpguide.org

Personal Health Portfolio

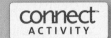

Chapter 6
Assessing Your Diet

For this activity, you will need to use the USDA's online MyPyramid Tracker, located at www.mypyramidtracker .gov. You will need to complete the free registration in order to use the site. The nutrition tracker provides an online assessment tool that will help you evaluate the quality of your diet.

Part 1

Complete the food log below, recording all the food you eat and drink in one full day. Make sure to include everything you drink—water, soft drinks (even diet), coffee, alcohol, and so on. List the foods you eat and drink and the serving size (1/2 apple, 2 cups of pasta, 24 oz. Diet Mountain Dew, etc.).

Day/Date: _____

Food/Drink item	Serving size/Amount

Part 2

Now enter the information from your food log in the "Assess Your Food Intake" section of MyPyramid Tracker (go to www.mypyramidtracker.gov, complete the free registration, and click on the Assess Your Food Intake link). Enter the foods you recorded in your journal, select serving sizes and quantities for each, and then click the Save & Analyze button, which will take you to the "Analyze Your Food Intake" section. Review all the reports you see listed and pay special attention to the "Nutrient Intakes From Foods" and your "MyPyramid Stats" sections.

CRITICAL THINKING QUESTIONS

1. Analyze how well your food intake for the day matches up to your MyPyramid recommendations. (To view how your food intake compares with your MyPyramid recommendations, click the Calculate MyPyramid Stats link in the "Analyze Your Food Intake" section.) Did you meet your recommendations for milk, meat and beans, vegetables, fruits, and grains?

2. Now analyze your food intake in terms of calories, fat, fiber, sugar, sodium, and cholesterol (click the Calculate Nutrient Intakes from Foods link in the "Analyze Your Food Intake" section). How did you do in these areas? How many calories did you consume?

3. Based on your analysis in the first two questions, do you think you need to make any dietary changes? Why or why not? If you do need to make changes, what specific dietary modifications do you need to make and how can you realistically achieve them? Consider both behavioral and environmental strategies.

You may want to analyze your diet for a few more days—or even longer—to get a better idea of how well your diet is meeting your nutritional needs. Make a note of your login for MyPyramid Tracker as you will be using the site again for the Personal Health Portfolio activity in Chapter 7.

Personal Health Portfolio

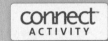

For this activity, you will need to use the USDA's online MyPyramid Tracker, located at www.mypyramidtracker .gov. You will need to complete the free registration in order to use the site, or log in with the user name and password you created in the Chapter 6 Portfolio activity. The physical activity tracker provides an online assessment tool that will help you evaluate your daily physical activity.

Part 1

Complete the activity log below, noting all your activity over a period of 24 hours, including time spent sleeping, watching TV, and so on.

Day/Date: _____

Activity	Duration

Part 2

Now enter the information from your activity log in the "Assess Your Physical Activity" section of MyPyramid Tracker (go to www.mypyramidtracker.gov, complete the free registration, and click on the Proceed to Physical Activity link). Enter the activities you recorded, select a duration for each, click the Save & Analyze button, and then click the Analyze button, which will take you to the "Analyze Your Physical Activity" section. Review your Physical Activity Analysis to find out your physical activity score and how many calories you expended from physical activity.

CRITICAL THINKING QUESTIONS

1. What was your score for physical activity? What does it say about your current level of physical activity?

2. As mentioned in Chapter 7, walking is an excellent lifestyle physical activity for health. Walking to public transportation, like the bus or the subway, can be an easy way to accumulate the weekly recommended amount of physical activity. How do you get to and from campus (and around your campus itself) and to your job if you have one? What factors affect how much you are or aren't able to incorporate walking into your daily activity? For example, perhaps you are taking this class online and thus don't have to leave the house to attend class. Or perhaps your part-time job as a dog walker means you walk for two hours five days a week.

3. If your score was less than 100, what are some things you can do personally to increase your daily physical activity?

4. Think about your neighborhood or community. Does it facilitate physical activity, or does it present barriers to physical activity? For example, can you and your neighbors walk to the local grocery store? Is there a park nearby where you can walk or play sports? If your community does not encourage physical activities, what needs to change?

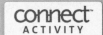
You can *estimate* your daily energy needs by (1) determining your basal metabolic rate (BMR) and (2) determining your energy expenditure above BMR from physical activity. Combining the two numbers gives you an estimate of your total energy requirement. This will require fine-tuning based on your body composition, metabolism, and activity and is intended as a start.

1. First, estimate your BMR, the minimum energy required to maintain your body's functions at rest. Begin by converting your weight in pounds to weight in kilograms. Then multiply by the BMR factor, which is estimated at 1.0 calorie/kg/hour for men and 0.9 for women. Then multiply by 24 hours to get your daily energy needs from BMR.

   • Let's look at Gary, a 30-year-old, 180-pound man.

   $$\frac{180 \text{ lb}}{2.2 \text{ lb/kg}} = 82 \text{ kg}$$

   82 kg × 1 calorie/kg/hour = 82 calories/hour

   82 calories/hour × 24 hours/day = 1,968 calories/day

   Gary's BMR—the energy he uses every day just to stay alive—is 1,968 calories.

   • Now let's look at Lisa, a 24-year-old, 115-pound woman.

   $$\frac{115 \text{ lb}}{2.2 \text{ lb/kg}} = 52 \text{ kg}$$

   52 kg × 0.9 calorie/kg/hour = 47 calories/hour

   47 calories/hour × 24 hours/day = 1,128 calories/day

   Lisa's BMR is 1,128 calories per day.

   • Now calculate your own BMR.

   Your weight in lbs _____ /2.2 lb/kg = _____ kg

   _____ kg × 1 (men) = _____ calories/hour

   _____ kg × 0.9 (women) = _____ calories/hour

   _____ calories/hour × 24 hours/day = _____ calories/day

2. Next, estimate your voluntary muscle activity level. The following table gives approximations according to the amount of muscular work you typically perform in a day. To select the category appropriate for you, think in terms of muscle use, not just activity.

Lifestyle	BMR factor
Sedentary (mostly sitting)	0.4–0.5
Lightly active (such as a student)	0.55–0.65
Moderately active (such as a nurse)	0.65–0.7
Highly active (such as a bicycle messenger or an athlete)	0.75–1

A certain amount of honest guesswork is necessary. If you have a sedentary job but walk or bicycle to work every day, you could change your classification to lightly active (or even higher, depending on distance). If you have a moderately active job but spend all your leisure time on the couch, consider downgrading your classification to lightly active. Competitive athletes in training may actually need to increase the factor above 1.

   • Let's assume that Gary works in an office. He does walk around to talk to coworkers, go to the cafeteria for lunch, make photocopies, and do other everyday activities. We'll assess his lifestyle as sedentary but on the high side of activity for that category, say 0.5. To estimate Gary's energy expenditure above BMR, we multiply his BMR by this factor:

   1,968 calories/day × 0.50 = 984 calories/day

   • Let's assume that Lisa works as a stock clerk in a computer store. She spends a lot of time walking around and sometimes lifts fairly heavy merchandise. She doesn't own a car and rides her bike several miles to and from work each day and also for many errands, so she's at the high end of moderately active, say 0.7. To estimate Lisa's energy expenditure above BMR, we multiply her BMR by this factor:

   1,128 calories/day × 0.70 = 790 calories/day

Note that although Lisa is much more active than Gary, she uses less energy because of her lower body weight.

   • Now calculate your own estimated energy expenditure from physical activity.

   _____ calories/day × BMR factor _____
   = _____ calories/day

3. To find your total daily energy needs, add your BMR and your estimated energy expenditure.

- For Gary, this is

  1,968 calories/day + 984 calories/day
  = 2,952 calories/day

- For Lisa, it is

  1,128 calories/day + 790 calories/day
  = 1,918 calories/day

Because several estimates are used in this method, total daily energy needs should be expressed as a 100-calorie range roughly centered on the final calculated value, which would be about 2,900–3,000 calories/day for Gary and about 1,870–1,970 calories/day for Lisa.

- Now calculate your total daily energy needs.

  BMR calories/day _____
  + physical activity calories/day _____
  = _____ total calories/day

Finally, compare your daily energy needs with your daily calorie intake. You may want to refer to question 2 from the Chapter 6 Portfolio activity, where you recorded your calorie intake for one day.

Your daily energy needs: _____

Your daily calorie intake: _____

Remember, if you want to lose weight, you need to take in less energy than you use up. You can shift the balance by increasing your activity level or decreasing your food intake. Moderate changes in both intake and activity level are the safest way to lose weight.

CRITICAL THINKING QUESTIONS

1. How do your calorie needs and calorie intake match up? Are you balancing your needs with your intake, or is one higher than the other? Do you need to make any changes to your calorie intake and/or your energy expenditure?

2. What factors influence how well you are able to balance your food intake and energy expenditure? Consider your taste in food and its cost and convenience. Also consider the factors that influence your ability to get daily physical activity, such as your available leisure time, your community's walkability and safety, availability of recreation areas, affordability of the campus gym or local gyms, etc.

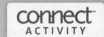

Personal Health Portfolio

Chapter 9
Self-Esteem and Body Image

The goal of this activity is to help you think about your self-esteem and body image. Consider the following statements and then circle the response indicating how strongly you agree or disagree with each of them.

1. On the whole I am satisfied with myself.	Strongly agree	Agree	Neutral	Disagree	Strongly disagree
2. I have a number of good qualities.	Strongly agree	Agree	Neutral	Disagree	Strongly disagree
3. I am able to do things as well as most other people.	Strongly agree	Agree	Neutral	Disagree	Strongly disagree
4. I have done things I am proud of.	Strongly agree	Agree	Neutral	Disagree	Strongly disagree
5. I wish I had more respect for myself.	Strongly agree	Agree	Neutral	Disagree	Strongly disagree
6. I feel more in control when I restrict the food I eat.	Strongly agree	Agree	Neutral	Disagree	Strongly disagree
7. I consistently compare myself to others.	Strongly agree	Agree	Neutral	Disagree	Strongly disagree
8. I make sure to exercise if I have eaten too much.	Strongly agree	Agree	Neutral	Disagree	Strongly disagree
9. I would agree to cosmetic surgery if it were free.	Strongly agree	Agree	Neutral	Disagree	Strongly disagree
10. I am anxious about how people perceive or judge me.	Strongly agree	Agree	Neutral	Disagree	Strongly disagree
11. I eat to make myself feel better when I am sad, upset, or lonely.	Strongly agree	Agree	Neutral	Disagree	Strongly disagree
12. I often skip meals to lose weight.	Strongly agree	Agree	Neutral	Disagree	Strongly disagree

CRITICAL THINKING QUESTIONS

Consider your responses and answer the following questions.

1. Statements 1 through 5 relate to self-esteem. How do you think you do in regard to your self-esteem? What areas do you feel are your strengths? How are you supported in maintaining high self-esteem? Are you supported by family, friends, academics, sports, or other institutions?

2. In areas of lower self-esteem, what are some of the factors that make it difficult or contribute to feelings of self-doubt? Are there areas that you could strengthen or change? Are there ways that family, friends, or community could help you?

3. Statements 6 through 12 relate to body image. Your responses here are probably linked to your responses to the self-esteem statements. What areas appear to be your strengths? What factors support them?

4. Are there areas of concern for you in your body image responses? How might factors in your environment be contributing to these concerns? Is there anything you would like to change or could change in your environment to reduce the impact of these factors?

Note: This activity is not intended to diagnose eating disorders. The intent is to help you think about the factors discussed in the chapter and apply them to your life.

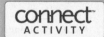
Drinking alcohol is not necessarily bad for you. What does matter is how much you drink and how it affects your life. This Portfolio activity will help you explore the place of alcohol in your life.

Part 1 Track Your Consumption

Recall as best you can your alcohol consumption during the past week (do not include today).

Date	Situation (people, place) or trigger (incident, feelings)	Type of drink(s)	Amount	Consequence (what happened?)

Now track your alcohol consumption for the next week, starting with today.

Date	Situation (people, place) or trigger (incident, feelings)	Type of drink(s)	Amount	Consequence (what happened?)

Part 2 Assess Your Consumption

Using the drink sizes from Figure 10.1 in your textbook or from www.rethinkingdrinking.niaaa.nih.gov, answer the following questions:

1. On any one day in the past two weeks, have you ever had

    Men: more than 4 drinks? Yes _____   No _____

    Women: more than 3 drinks? Yes _____   No _____

2. On average, how many days a week did you drink alcohol?

   _____ Days

3. On average, how many drinks did you have over the past two weeks?

   _____ Drinks

Source: Rethinking Drinking, *National Institute on Alcohol Abuse and Alcoholism, 2009, NIH Publication No. 09-3770.*

CRITICAL THINKING QUESTIONS

1. If you consume alcohol, are you a low-risk drinker or an at-risk drinker? Recall that low-risk drinking means no more than 14 drinks per week and no more than 4 drinks on any one day for men. For women, it means no more than 7 drinks per week and no more than 3 drinks on any one day. Drinks above these levels are considered at risk.

2. What were the situations and triggers that affected your decision to drink or not drink on various days? For example, if you ended up drinking more on one day than you had intended to, what led you to overindulge? If you did not drink at all during the two weeks, were you ever tempted to, or does your environment make the decision not to drink an easy one?

3. What are some reasons why you may want to make a change in your alcohol consumption? What are some of the barriers to making this change? How will you overcome these barriers?

4. What policies are in place at your campus to prevent or control excessive drinking? Are these policies effective?

Personal Health Portfolio

Chapter 11
Assessing Your Drug Use

If you wonder whether you are becoming dependent on a drug, complete the following assessment. These questions refer to your use of drugs other than alcohol. Circle the letters of the answers which best describe your use of the drug(s) you use most. Even if none of the answers seems exactly right, pick the one(s) that come closest to being true. If a question does not apply to you, leave it blank.

1. How often do you use drugs?
   - (0) a. never
   - (2) b. once or twice a year
   - (3) c. once or twice a month
   - (4) d. every weekend
   - (5) e. several times a week
   - (6) f. every day
   - (7) g. several times a day

2. When did you last use drugs?
   - (0) a. never used drugs
   - (2) b. not for over a year
   - (3) c. between 6 months and 1 year ago
   - (4) d. several weeks ago
   - (5) e. last week
   - (6) f. yesterday
   - (7) g. today

3. I usually start to use drugs because:
   (Circle all that are true for you.)
   - (1) a. I like the feeling
   - (2) b. to be like my friends
   - (3) c. to feel like an adult
   - (4) d. I feel nervous, tense, full of worries or problems
   - (5) e. I feel sad, lonely, sorry for myself

4. How do you get your drugs?
   (Circle all that are true for you.)
   - (1) a. use at parties
   - (2) b. get from friends
   - (3) c. get from parents
   - (4) d. buy my own
   - e. other (please explain)

   _____

5. When did you first use drugs?
   - (0) a. never
   - (1) b. recently
   - (2) c. after age 15
   - (3) d. at ages 14 or 15
   - (4) e. between ages 10 and 13
   - (5) f. before age 10

6. What time of day do you use drugs?
   (Circle all that apply to you.)
   - (1) a. at night
   - (2) b. afternoons
   - (3) c. before or during school or work
   - (4) d. in the morning or when I first wake
   - (5) e. I often get up in my sleep to use drugs

7. Why did you first use drugs?
   (Circle all that apply to you.)
   - (1) a. curiosity
   - (2) b. parents or relatives offered
   - (3) c. friends encouraged me
   - (4) d. to feel more like an adult
   - (5) e. to get high

8. Who do you use drugs with?
   (Circle all that are true for you.)
   - (1) a. parents or relatives
   - (2) b. brothers or sisters
   - (3) c. friends own age
   - (4) d. older friends
   - (5) e. alone

9. What effects have you had from drugs?
   (Circle all that apply to you.)
   - (1) a. got high
   - (2) b. got wasted
   - (3) c. became ill
   - (4) d. passed out
   - (5) e. overdosed
   - (6) f. freaked out
   - (7) g. used a lot and next day didn't remember

10. What effect has using drugs had on your life?
    (Circle all that apply.)
    - (0) a. none
    - (2) b. has interfered with talking to someone
    - (3) c. has prevented me from having a good time
    - (4) d. has interfered with my schoolwork
    - (5) e. have lost friends because of drug use
    - (6) f. has gotten me into trouble at home
    - (7) g. was in a fight or destroyed property
    - (8) h. has resulted in an accident, an injury, arrest, or being punished at school for using drugs

11. How do you feel about your use of drugs? (Circle all that apply.)

    (0) a. no problem at all

    (0) b. I can control it and set limits on myself

    (3) c. I can control myself, but my friends easily influence me

    (4) d. I often feel bad about my drug use

    (5) e. I need help to control myself

    (6) f. I have had professional help to control my drug use

12. How do others see you in relation to your drug use? (Circle all that apply to you.)

    (0) a. I can't say or no problem with drug use

    (2) b. when I use drugs, I tend to neglect my family or friends

    (3) c. my family or friends advise me to control or cut down on my drug use

    (4) d. my family or friends tell me to get help for my drug use

    (5) e. my family or friends have already gone for help for my drug use

Source: "The Adolescent Drug Involvement Scale," by D. P. Moberg and L. Hahn, 1991, Journal of Adolescent Chemical Dependency 2(1), pp. 75–88.

Scoring

Add up the point values of your responses. For questions where you circled multiple answers, add the highest point value of your answers.

Score: _____

The higher your score, the more serious your level of drug involvement is. Plot your score on the continuum below.

⟵————————————|————————————|————————————|————————————⟶

0 **No dependence**   **Severe dependence 69**

CRITICAL THINKING QUESTIONS

1. Reflect on your score. What do your responses indicate about your drug use?

2. Is there anything in your environment that makes it easy or difficult to control or limit your drug use?

3. In what direction are you moving on the continuum—toward increased dependence, toward decreased dependence, or holding steady? Do you need to make any changes to your substance use? If so, what?

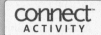

Personal Health Portfolio

Good communication is vital to keeping your relationships healthy. However, bad communication habits—like avoiding discussing difficult subjects—are easy to fall into. This assessment will help you determine how well you are communicating with your partner. If you aren't currently in an intimate relationship, take this assessment with a close friendship in mind. Communication is important in all relationships—intimate or not.

Read each question and choose the response that reflects how you think or respond the majority of the time. Think about what you actually do or believe as opposed to what you "know" you should do or believe.

1. Do you believe that disagreements or arguments are
   a. harmful and negative for a relationship or
   b. helpful and positive for a relationship

2. Do you believe that your partner should
   a. know what you are thinking and feeling or
   b. hear what you are thinking and feeling

3. Do you
   a. drop hints about your concerns in the relationship or
   b. get right to the point when discussing a concern in the relationship

4. Do you tell your partner
   a. what you don't like about him or her and your relationship or
   b. what you like about him or her and your relationship

5. Do you
   a. withdraw from a conflict or conversation with your partner or
   b. stay around until there is a resolution of the conflict or conversation

6. Do you
   a. hint at what you want or don't want from your partner or
   b. state clearly what you want and don't want

7. Do you
   a. interrupt your partner's conversation or
   b. wait until your partner has finished stating his or her thoughts and ideas

8. Do you
   a. blame your partner or others for your relationship problems or
   b. acknowledge and accept your part in your relationship problems

9. Were your parents
   a. poor communicators or
   b. good communicators

Source: "Communication Assessment," by Steven Martin and Catherine Martin, The Positive Way®, from www.positive-way.com/communication.htm.

Turn over the page to score your responses and view feedback for each question.

Scoring

The answer "b" to all questions indicates more effective communication. The more "b's" you have, the better you're doing. The "a's" indicate an opportunity to improve.

Here is why "b" is the better answer for each question:

1. Intimacy and conflict go hand in hand. If you want real intimacy with your mate, then there will be real conflict. People just don't agree on everything at all times. How you handle the resulting disagreements is more important than whether or not you have them. The most successful couples work through their disagreements and conflicts together and develop a stronger relationship as a result of that teamwork.

2. No one is a mind reader, and it is really impossible for your partner to know what you are thinking and feeling no matter how long you have known each other. It is important that you agree to *say* what is important and to *talk* until you both agree that you *understand*.

3. Dropping hints wastes your time and your partner's time, and it usually leads to misunderstanding and disappointment. Get right to the point so your partner won't have to guess what your concerns are in the relationship. State how you feel by using "I" statements instead of "you" statements.

4. Concentrating on what you like about your mate and your relationship will lead to a more positive relationship. If you concentrate on the things you don't like, it's easy to overlook the good things. Negativity breeds negativity, which then makes communication and problem solving more difficult. Use positive elements of the relationship as a foundation upon which to learn and grow.

5. Communication requires two people. Issues will remain unsettled unless you and your partner agree to communicate. We recommend that you agree to communicate with the guidelines of *understanding, kindness, honesty,* and *respect* as ground rules. These guidelines will serve to reduce tension and remind you both that you are on the same team. As a couple, agree to your own discussion rules, which can include such things as *time-outs* for cooling off or thinking.

6. Most of us don't pick up on hints, so don't expect your partner to guess what you do or don't want. Make clear and direct statements. Follow the guidelines of *understanding, kindness, honesty,* and *respect.* These guidelines make it easier to state your desires in a positive way and are more likely to be understood and well received.

7. Successful communication requires good listening. No one wants to be interrupted while speaking. We all want our feelings and thoughts to be heard, valued, and understood. Listen for understanding. Rephrase what you have heard your partner say, and then ask if this is correct. Save your side of the discussion until you have validated your partner's feelings. Validating your partner's feelings and thoughts is the key to success.

8. Blame fuels the fire of disagreement. Most of the time we believe that our position is acceptable and tend to blame the other person for any misunderstanding rather than seeing our own flaws in communicating. Analyze your part in fueling a problem, and avoid blaming others. Be responsible for your role in the relationship.

9. We tend to learn by example. If your parents were poor communicators, more than likely you have learned and now act out some ineffective ways of communicating. These habits may seem quite comfortable to you even if they are not working. It is up to you to learn new positive ways to communicate. Be persistent and practice until they become habit.

CRITICAL THINKING QUESTIONS

1. How did you do on the assessment? Discuss your strengths and any areas for improvement.

2. Think more about your parents' communication. Why did you respond the way you did to question 9? How did they handle conflict? Do you see yourself following any of their habits, good or bad?

Personal Health Portfolio

connect ACTIVITY

As you learned in Chapter 13, many contraception options are available to you. This activity will help you determine which contraceptive method best fits your needs. You may also want to discuss your options and decisions with your primary care physician, especially since many methods require a prescription.

Part 1 Your Partner's and Your Preferences

	Yes	No
1. I am sure I do not want children at this time.		
2. My partner and I are in a monogamous relationship with no concerns about sexually transmitted diseases.		
3. I want a method that I can control myself.		
4. My partner or I am good at remembering to take medication daily.		
5. My partner or I am willing to visit a physician or clinic to get birth control.		
6. My partner or I like sexual spontaneity and don't want to have to worry about contraception right before sex.		
7. Using birth control is not acceptable within my moral and/or religious belief system.		

Part 2 Your Sexual Behavior

	Yes	No
1. I sometimes have sex after using alcohol or drugs.		
2. I sometimes hook up with people I don't know well.		
3. I am in a relatively new relationship or have more than one partner.		
4. I have not discussed with my partner his/her prior sexual history or history of sexually transmitted diseases.		

Part 3 Risk Factors

Do any of the following apply to you (if you are a female) or your partner (if you are a male)?	Yes	No
1. Over age 35 and a smoker		
2. Liver disease, blood clots, breast cancer		
3. Personal history of migraine headaches		
4. Family history of blood clots, stroke, heart attack		

Interpretation

Part 1

Question 1. Yes responses: If you do not want children at any time in the future, permanent sterilization may be the best option. However, if your goal is to delay children for several years, you may want a reliable reversible contraceptive, such as an IUD or birth control pills.

Question 2. Yes responses: You do not need to use condoms or other barrier methods to provide STD protection. Hormonal methods are an option for you.

Question 3. Yes responses: If you are male, the male condom and vasectomy will allow you to take full responsibility for contraception. If you are female, tubal ligation, hormonal contraception, and barrier methods (excluding the male condom) will all allow you to take full responsibility for contraception.

Question 4. Yes responses: Birth control pills would be an effective option for you since they need to be taken daily. The vaginal ring and the transdermal patch, which must be changed every month, are other options.

Question 5. No responses: Contraceptive methods that can be purchased over the counter include male and female condoms and the contraceptive sponge.

Question 6. Yes responses: You may benefit from hormonal contraception such as an IUD or a contraceptive implant that does not require any action at the time of sex. However, if you are at risk for STDs, you will still need to use a barrier method like a condom, even if you would prefer not to.

Question 7. Yes responses: Your options are fertility awareness–based methods if you are sexually active or abstinence. Withdrawal may be another option, but keep in mind that many do not consider this to be a real contraceptive method.

Part 2

If you answered yes to the majority of questions in this section, condom use is an important part of your contraceptive needs. Hooking up and alcohol and drug use all increase the risk for sexually transmitted diseases. However, these behaviors also make it less likely that you will actually use a condom or other barrier method at the time of intercourse, so it is also recommended that women use a reliable contraceptive to prevent pregnancy that does not require action at the time of intercourse (like birth control pills or the vaginal ring).

Part 3

These factors increase the risk of side effects from hormonal contraceptives. If you answered yes to any of these questions, you and your partner may want to consider a barrier contraceptive or permanent contraception, depending on your future plans.

See Table 13.1 for an overview of specific contraceptive methods.

CRITICAL THINKING QUESTIONS

1. Based on your responses, what type of contraception would be best for you? Are you using this method currently? Why or why not?

2. What factors in your environment influence your sexual decision making and contraception use? Consider your partner pattern and your social network.

3. Is there anything you would like to change in this area of your life? If so, consider making a behavior change plan and decide what your first steps would be.

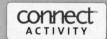
Vaccination, screening, and good hygiene habits are all ways to prevent the spread of infectious disease. Complete the following activity to see how well you are keeping yourself and others from contracting an infectious disease.

Part 1 Immunizations

Collect your immunization records. If you do not have a copy of your records, start by asking your parents or guardians. If they do not have records, check with your doctor. Your state health department may also have a program to track childhood vaccines. Record your immunizations in the table below.

Vaccine	Type of vaccination	Date	Location (doctor's office and doctor name, health clinic, etc.)
Tetanus, diphtheria, pertussis			
Human papillomavirus (HPV)			
Varicella			
Zoster			
Measles, mumps, rubella (MMR)			
Influenza			
Pneumococcal, polysaccharide			
Hepatitis A			
Hepatitis B			
Meningococcal			

Part 2 STD Risk

1. Are you sexually active?

   ☐ Yes   ☐ No

2. If yes, have you ever been tested for sexually transmitted diseases?

   ☐ Yes   ☐ No   ☐ N/A

3. Have you had a new partner since you were last tested?

   ☐ Yes   ☐ No   ☐ N/A

Part 3 Basic Hygiene Practices

1. Do you wash your hands with soap and warm water regularly before preparing food or eating, after using the toilet, and prior to touching your face?

   ☐ Most of the time   ☐ Sometimes   ☐ Rarely

2. Do you shower after exercise?

   ☐ Most of the time   ☐ Sometimes   ☐ Rarely

3. Do you share personal items (clothes, towels, etc.) with others?

   ☐ Often   ☐ Sometimes   ☐ Rarely

CRITICAL THINKING QUESTIONS

1. Compare your vaccine record to the immunization recommendations in the box "Vaccinations: Not Just for Kids" and in Figure 14.5. Are you current on all your vaccination recommendations? If not, which ones do you need to get?

2. Find two sites in your community where you can go to obtain vaccinations. List the name, address, and phone number of each.

3. Based on your responses to Part 2 and based on the recommendations discussed in the section on STDs in Chapter 14, do you need to get tested for STDs?

4. Find two sites in your community where you can get tested for STDs. List the name, address, and phone number of each.

5. Based on your responses to Part 3, evaluate your basic hygiene habits. Is there anything in your environment or community that makes it easier or harder to practice good habits? Where is there room for improvement?

13. McCaffrey, A. M., Eisenberg, D. M., Legedza, A. T. R., Davis, R. B., & Phillips, R. S. (2004). Prayer for health concerns: Results of a national survey on prevalence and patterns of use. *Archives of Internal Medicine, 164*, 858–862.

14. Aten, J. D., & Schenck, J. E. (2007). Reflections on religion and health research: An interview with Dr. Harold G. Koenig. *Journal of Religion and Health, 46* (2), 183–190.

15. Koening, H. G., Larson, D. B., & Larson, S. S. (2001). Religion and coping with serious medical illness. *Annals of Pharmacotherapy, 35*, 352–359.

16. National Center for Complementary and Alternative Medicine. (2010). Funding strategy: Fiscal year 2010. nccam.nih.gov/grants/strategy/2010 .htm#data.

17. Koenig, H. G. (2000). Religion, spirituality, and medicine: Application to clinical practice. *Journal of the American Medical Association, 284*, 1708.

18. Mueller, P. S., Plevak, D. J., & Rummans, T. A. (2001). Religious involvement, spirituality, and medicine: Implications for clinical practice. *Mayo Clinic Proceedings, 76* (12).

19. Benson, H., & Klipper, M. (2000). *The relaxation response.* New York: HarperTorch.

20. Blumenthal, J. A., Babyak, M. A., Ironson, G., et al. (2007). Spirituality, religion and clinical outcomes in patients recovering from an acute myocardial infarction. *Psychosomatic Medicine, 69*, 501–508.

21. Hummer, R. A., Richard, R. G., Charles, N. B., & Christopher, E. G. (1999). Religious participation and U.S. adult mortality. *Demography, 36* (2), 273–285.

22. Strawbridge, W. J., et al. (2001). Religious attendance increases survival by improving and maintaining good health behaviors, mental health, and social relationships. *Annals of Behavioral Medicine, 23*, 68–74.

23. Campaign for Forgiveness Research. (1999–2001). www.forgiving.org.

24. Koenig, H. G., McCullough, M. E., & Larson, D. B. (2001). *Handbook of religion and health.* Oxford, UK: Oxford University Press.

25. Larson, D. B., Swyers, J. P., & McCullough, M. E. (1998). *Scientific research on spirituality and health: A report based on the scientific progress in spirituality conferences.* Rockville, MD: National Institute for Healthcare Research.

26. Seybold, K. S., & Hill, P. C. (2001). The role of religion and spirituality in mental and physical health. *Current Directions in Psychological Science, 10*, 21–24.

27. Chen, Y. Y., & Koenig, H. G. (2006). Do people turn to religion in times of stress? An examination of change in religiousness among elderly, medically ill patients. *Journal of Nervous and Mental Disease, 194*, 114–120.

28. Koenig, H. G. (2007). Religion and depression in older medical inpatients. *American Journal of Geriatric Psychiatry, 15*, 282–291.

29. Koenig, H. G. (2007). Religion and remission of depression in medical inpatients with heart failure/pulmonary disease. *Journal of Nervous and Mental Disease, 195*, 389–395.

30. Brady, M. J., et al. (1999). A case for including spirituality in quality of life measurement in oncology. *Psychooncology, 8*, 417–428.

31. Pargament, K. I. (1997). *The psychology of religion and coping: Theory, research, practice.* New York: Guilford Press.

32. Pargament, K. I., et al. (2001). Religious struggle as a predictor of mortality among medically ill elderly patients. *Archives of Internal Medicine, 161*, 1881–1885.

33. Fitchett, G., et al. (1999). The role of religion in medical rehabilitation outcomes: A longitudinal study. *Rehabilitation Psychology, 44*, 1–22.

34. Koenig, H. G., Pargament, K. I., & Nielsen, J. (1998). Religious coping and health status in medically ill hospitalized older adults. *Journal of Nervous Mental Disorders, 186*, 513–521.

35. Gaudia, G. (2007). About intercessory prayer: The scientific study of miracles. *Medscape General Medicine, 9.* Medscape.com.

36. Kabat-Zinn, J. (1993). Mindfulness meditation: Health benefits of an ancient Buddhist practice. In D. Goleman & J. Gurin (Eds.), *Mind/body medicine.* Yonkers, NY: Consumer Reports Books.

37. Csikszentmihalyi, M. (1998). *Finding flow: The psychology of engagement with everyday life.* New York: Basic Books.

38. Ellsberg, R. (Ed.). (2001). *Thich Nhat Hanh: Essential writings.* Maryknoll, NY: Orbis Books.

39. Pennebaker, J. W. (1997). *Opening up: The healing power of expressing emotion.* New York: Guilford Press.

40. DeSalvo, L. A. (2000). *Writing as a way of healing: How telling our stories transforms our lives.* Boston: Beacon Press.

41. Beckett, W. (1993). *The mystical now: Art and the sacred.* New York: Universe Publishing.

42. Pew Research Center. (2010). Millennials: A portrait of generation next. http://pewsocialtrends.org/assets/pdf/millennials-confident-connected -open-to-change.pdf.

43. Luks, A., (1988, October). Helper's high. *Psychology Today*, 39–42.

44. Farino, L. (n.d.). Do good, feel good. MSN Health & Fitness. www.health .msn.com.

45. Hafen, B. Q., et al. (1996). *Mind/body health: The effects of attitudes, emotions and relationships.* Boston: Allyn and Bacon.

46. Luks, A., & Payne, P. (1992). *The healing power of doing good: The health and spiritual benefits of helping others.* New York: Fawcett Columbine.

47. Howe, N., & Strauss, W. (2000). *Millennials rising: The next great generation.* New York: Vintage Books.

48. House, J. S., Landis, K. R., & Umberson, P. (1988). Social relationships and health. *Science, 241*, 540–545.

49. Skinhauser, K., Christakis, N., Clipp, E., et al. (2000). Factors considered important at the end of life by patients. *Journal of the American Medical Association, 284*, 2476–2482.

50. Kübler-Ross, E. (1997). *On death and dying.* New York: Simon & Schuster Adult Publishing Group.

51. Moss, E., & Dobson, K. (2006). Psychology, spirituality and end of life care: An ethical integration. *Canadian Psychology, 47* (4), 284–299.

52. Can you die of a broken heart? (2002, January). *Harvard Mental Health Letter.*

53. Bonanno, G. A. (2009). *The other side of sadness: What the new science of bereavement tells us about life after loss.* New York: Basic Books.

54. Gesensway, D. (1998, May). Talking about end-of-life issues. *ACP Observer.*

55. U.S. Government Advisory Committee on Organ Transplantation. (2009). 2009 Campus Donation Challenge. www.organdonor.gov.

56. Braude, S. (2003). *Immortal remains: The evidence for life after death.* Lanham, MD: Rowman & Littlefield.

57. Evidence of "life after death" (2000, October 23). BBC News. http://news .bbc.co.uk.

Chapter 5

1. American College Health Association. (2009). National College Health Assessment—Spring 2008. www.acha-ncha.org/docs/ACHA-NCHA _Reference_Group_ExecutiveSummary_Spring2008.pdf.

2. Forquer L. M., Camden, A. E., Gavriau, K. M., et al. (2008). Sleep patterns of college students at a public university. *Journal of American College Health, 56* (5), 563–565.

3. National Sleep Foundation. (2009). 2009 Sleep in America poll, executive report. www.sleepfoundation.org.

4. Endeshaw, Y. W., Bloom, H. L., and Bliwise, D. L. (2008). Sleep-disordered breathing and cardiovascular disease in the Bay area sleep cohort. *Journal of Sleep, 31* (4), 563–568.

5. Institute of Medicine. (2006). *Sleep disorders and sleep deprivation.* Washington, DC: National Academies Press.

6. Gangwisch, J. E., Heymsfield, S. B., Boden-Albala, B., et al. (2006). Short sleep deprivation as a risk factor for hypertension: Analyses of the First National Health and Nutrition Examination Survey. *Hypertension, 47*, 833–839.

7. Schenck, C. H. (2007). *Sleep: The mysteries, the problems and the solutions.* New York: Penguin Books.

8. Zee, P. C., & Turek, F. W. (2006). Sleep and health. *Archives of Internal Medicine, 166* (16), 1686–1688.

9. Klauer, S. G., Dingus, T. A., Neale, V. L., Sudweeks, J. D., & Ramsey, D. J. (2006). *The impact of driver inattention on near-crash/crash risk: An analysis using the 100-car naturalistic driving study data* (Publication No. DOT HS 810594). Washington, DC: U.S. Department of Transportation.

10. Maruff, P., Falleti, M. G., Collie, A., et al. (2005). Fatigue-related impairment in the speed, accuracy and variability of psychomotor performance: Comparison with blood alcohol levels. *Journal of Sleep Research, 14* (1), 21–27.

11. Stickgold, R., and Wehrwein, P. (2009, April 27). Sleep now, remember later. *Newsweek*, pp. 56–57.

12. Epstein, L. J. (2007). *A good night's sleep.* New York: McGraw-Hill.

13. Moore, R. Y. The neurobiology of sleep-wake regulation. www.medscape .com/viewarticle/491041.

14. Roehrs, T., Kapke, A., Roth, T., et al. (2006). Sex differences in the polysomnographic sleep of young adults: A community based study. *Sleep Medicine, 7* (1), 49–53.

15. State of the Science Panel. (2005). National Institutes of Health State of the Science Conference: Manifestations and management of chronic insomnia in adults, June 13–15. *Sleep, 28*, 1049–1057.

16. Kantrowitz, B. (2006, April 24). The quest for rest. *Newsweek*, pp. 51–56.

17. Rosenthal, L. (2005). Excessive daytime sleepiness: From an unknown medical condition to a known public health risk. *Sleep Medicine, 6* (6), 485–486.

18. Rauchs, G., Desgranges, B., Foret, J., et al. (2005). The relationships between memory systems and sleep stages. *Journal of Sleep Research, 14* (2), 123–140.

19. Ferreni, A. F., & Ferreni, R. L. (2008). *Health in the later years.* New York: McGraw-Hill.

References

20. Goldman, S. E., Hall, M., Bourdeau, R., et al. (2008). Association between nighttime sleep and napping in older adults. *Journal of Sleep, 31* (5), 733–740.
21. National Sleep Foundation. (2007). Stressed-out American women have no time for sleep [press release]. www.sleepfoundation.org.
22. Chokroverty, S. (1999). *Sleep disorders medicine: Basic science, technical considerations, and clinical aspects* (2nd ed.). Boston: Butterworth-Heinemann.
23. National Sleep Foundation. Can't sleep? What to know about insomnia. Retrieved March 7, 2010, from www.sleepfoundation.org/article/sleep-related-problems/insomnia-and-sleep.
24. Guilleminault, C., & Robinson, A. (2006). Central sleep apnea, upper airway resistance and sleep. *Sleep Medicine, 7* (2), 189–191.
25. National Sleep Foundation. Obstructive sleep apnea and sleep. Retrieved March 7, 2010, from www.sleepfoundation.org/article/sleep-related-problems/obstructive-sleep-apnea-and-sleep.
26. Hiestand, D. M., Britz, P., Goldman, M., & Phillips, B. (2006). Prevalence of symptoms and risk of sleep apnea in the US population: Results from the National Sleep Foundation Sleep in America poll. *Chest, 130* (3), 780–786.
27. Wang, H., Newton, G. E., Floras, J. S., et al. (2007). Influence of obstructive sleep apnea on mortality in patients with heart failure. *Journal of American Cardiology, 49*, 1625–1631.
28. Artz, M. A., Young, T., Finn, L., et al. (2006). Sleepiness and sleep in patients with both systolic heart failure and obstructive sleep apnea. *Archives of Internal Medicine, 166*, 1716–1722.
29. Practice parameters for the use of laser-assisted uvulopalatoplasty: An update for 2000. (2001). Position paper. *Sleep, 24* (5), 603–619.
30. National Sleep Foundation. Narcolepsy and sleep. Retrieved March 8, 2010, from www.sleepfoundation.org/article/sleep-related-problems/narcolepsy-and-sleep.
31. National Sleep Foundation. Restless legs syndrome (RLS) and sleep. Retrieved March 8, 2010, from www.sleepfoundation.org/article/sleep-related-problems/restless-legs-syndrome-rls-and-sleep.
32. American Academy of Sleep Medicine. (2005). *The international classification of sleep disorders.* Westchester, IL: American Academy of Sleep Medicine.
33. Griefahn, B. Brode, P., Marks, A., et al. (2008). Autonomic arousals related to traffic noise during sleep. *Journal of Sleep, 31* (4), 569–577.
34. National Sleep Foundation. (2006). Sleep aids. www.sleepfoundation.org.
35. Wesenten, N. J., William, D., Kilgore, S., & Balkin, T. J. (2005). Performance and alertness effects of caffeine, dextroamphetamine, and modafinil during sleep deprivation. *Journal of Sleep Research, 14* (3), 255–266.
36. Boggan, B. Alcohol, chemistry and you: Ethanol and sleep. www.chemcases.com/alcohol/alc-09.htm.
37. Wetter, D. W., & Young, T. B. (1994). The relation between cigarette smoking and sleep disturbance. *Preventive Medicine, 23*, 328–334.
38. Maas, J. B. (1998). *Power sleep.* New York: Villard Books/Random House.
39. O'Hanlon, B. (2000). *Overcoming sleep disorders: A natural approach.* Freedom, CA: Crossing Press.

Chapter 6

1. Wardlaw, G. M., & Smith, A. M. (2011). *Contemporary nutrition.* New York: McGraw-Hill.
2. Wardlaw, G. M., Hampl, J. S., & DiSilvestro, R. A. (2009). *Perspectives in nutrition.* New York: McGraw-Hill.
3. Dunford, M. (2010). *Fundamentals of sport and exercise nutrition.* Champaign, IL: Human Kinetics.
4. Johnson, R. K., Appel, L. J., Brands, M., et al. on behalf of the American Heart Association Nutrition Committee of the Council on Nutrition, Physical Activity, and Metabolism and the Council on Epidemiology and Prevention. (2009). Dietary sugars intake and cardiovascular health: A scientific statement from the American Heart Association. *Circulation, 120*, 1011–1020.
5. Willet, D. C. (2005). Diet and cancer. *Journal of the American Medical Association, 293* (12), 233–234.
6. Yeh, M., Moysich, K. B., Jayaprakash V., et al. (2009). Higher intakes of vegetables and vegetable-related nutrients are associated with lower endometrial cancer risk. *Journal of Nutrition, 139*, 317–322.
7. *Dietary reference intakes for energy, carbohydrate, fiber, fat, fatty acids, cholesterol, protein, and amino acids (macronutrients).* (2002). Washington, DC: National Academies Press.
8. Park, Y., Hunter, D. J., Spielgelman, D., et al. (2005). Dietary fiber intake and risk of colorectal cancer. *Journal of the American Medical Association, 294* (2), 2849–2857.
9. Baron, J. A. (2005). Dietary fiber and colorectal cancer: An on-going saga. *Journal of the American Medical Association, 293* (22), 86–89.
10. U.S. Department of Agriculture. (2005). *2005 dietary guidelines for Americans.* www.health.gov/dietaryguidelines.
11. Furtado, J. D., Campos, H., Appel, L. J., et al. (2008, June). Effect of protein, unsaturated fat, and carbohydrate intakes on plasma apolipoprotein B and VLDL and LDL containing apolipoprotein C-III: Results from the Omniheart Trial. *American Journal of Clinical Nutrition, 87* (6), 1623–1630.
12. Klingburg, S., Ellegard, L., Johansson, I., et al. (2008). Inverse relation between dietary intake of naturally occurring plant sterols and serum cholesterol in northern Sweden. *American Journal of Clinical Nutrition, 87* (4), 993–1001.
13. Mozafarrian, D., Katan, M. B., Scherio, A., et al. (2006). Trans fatty acids and cardiovascular disease. *New England Journal of Medicine, 354* (15), 1601–1613.
14. Harvard Medical School. (2007, February 13). The dish on fish. *Health Newsletter.* www.health.harvard.edu.
15. Schumann, K., Borch-Johnsen, B., Hentze, M. W., & Marx, J. M. (2002). Tolerable upper intakes for dietary iron set by the U.S. Food and Nutrition Board. *American Journal of Clinical Nutrition, 76* (3), 499–500.
16. Ribnicky, D. M., Poulev, A., Schmidt, B., et al. (2008). Evaluation of botanicals for improving human health. *American Journal of Clinical Nutrition, 87* (2), 472S–475S.
17. Geleijnse, J. M., & Hollman, P. (2008). Flavanoids and cardiovascular health: Which compounds, which mechanisms. *American Journal of Clinical Nutrition, 87* (7), 12–13.
18. Willett, C. W. (2001). *Eat, drink and be healthy.* New York: Simon & Schuster.
19. Nuovo, J. (1999). AHA statement on antioxidants and coronary disease. *American Family Physician, 59* (10).
20. U.S. Food and Drug Administration. (2007). Final rule promotes safe use of dietary supplements. www.fda.gov/consumer/updates/dietarysupps062207.html.
21. Sabate, J. (2003). The contribution of vegetarian diets to health and disease: A paradigm shift. *American Journal of Clinical Nutrition, 78* (3), 502–507.
22. Borta, S. (2006). Consumer perspectives on food labels. *American Journal of Clinical Nutrition, 83* (5), 1235S.
23. Jacobson, M. F. (2006). *Liquid candy: How soft drinks are harming Americans' health.* Washington, DC: Center for Science in the Public Interest.
24. Popkin, B. M., Armstrong, L. E., Brat, G. M., et al. (2006). A new proposed guidance system for beverage consumption in the United States. *American Journal of Clinical Nutrition, 83* (3), 529–542.
25. Popkin, B. M. (2006). Pour better or pour worse. Center for Science in the Public Interest. *Nutrition Action Healthletter, 33* (5), 1–5.
26. High blood pressure: The end of an epidemic. (2000, December 3–9). *Nutrition Action Newsletter, 33* (5), 1–5.
27. Dahl, R. (2006). Food safety: Allergen labels take effect. *Environmental Health Perspectives, 114* (1), A24.
28. Bostwick, H. (2006). McDonald's french fry lawsuit: More than meets the fry. www.lawsuitsearch.com/product-liability/.
29. Liebman, B., & Schardt, D. (2006). Bar exam: Energy bars flunk. Center for Science in the Public Interest. *Nutrition Action Healthletter, 27* (6), 10–12.
30. Thombs, D. L., O'Mara, R. J., Tsukamoto, M., et al. (2010, April). Event-level analyses of energy drink consumption and alcohol intoxication in bar patrons. *Addictive Behavior, 35* (4), 325–330.
31. Nordqvist, C. (2004, February 8). French ban on Red Bull (drink) upheld by European court. *Medical News Today.* www.medicalnewstoday.com/articles/5753.php.
32. Severson, K. (2006). Energy drinks are fueling concerns. *New York Times,* June 19, p. 9.
33. Barston, S. (2008). *Healthy fast food: Guide to healthy fast food restaurants.* www.helpguide.org/life/fast_food_nutrition.htm.
34. Schardt, D. (2007). Organic food: Worth the price. Center for Science in the Public Interest. *Nutrition Action Healthletter, 34* (6), 1, 2–8.
35. Barrett, J., Jarvis, W. T., Kroger, M., & London, W. M. (2007). *Consumer health: A guide to intelligent decisions.* Dubuque, IA: Brown & Benchmark.
36. Centers for Disease Control and Prevention: Incidence of foodborne illnesses. (1999). Preliminary data from the foodborne disease active surveillance network (food net). *Morbidity and Mortality Weekly Report, 48* (9), 189–194.
37. Centers for Disease Control and Prevention, Division of Bacterial and Mycotic Diseases. *Escherichia coli O157:H7.* www.cdc.gov/nczved/dfbmd/disease_listing/stec_gi.html.
38. Centers for Disease Control and Prevention. (2005). Foodborne illness. www.cdc.gov/ncidod/dbmd/diseaseinfo/foodborneinfections_g.htm.
39. Fox, N. (1999). *It was probably something you ate.* New York: Penguin Books.
40. Greene, L. W., & Ottoson, J. M. (2001). *Community and population health.* Dubuque, IA: WCB/McGraw-Hill.
41. United States Department of Agriculture. (2009, January 19). USDA issues final rule on mandatory country of origin labeling. www.usda.gov.
42. Brown, K. (2001). Seeds of concern. *Scientific American, 284* (4), 60–61.

Chapter 7

1. Department of Health and Human Services. (2008). Physical activity facts. www.fitness.gov/resources/facts/.
2. Sisson, S. B., McClain, J. J., & Tudor-Locke, C. (2008). Campus walkability, pedometer-determined steps, and moderate-to-vigorous physical activity: A comparison of two university campuses. *Journal of American College Health, 56* (5), 585–592.
3. Corbin, C. B., & Pangrazi, R. (2000). *Definitions: Health fitness and physical activity.* President's Council on Physical Fitness and Sports, *3* (9), 1–8.
4. Warburton, D., Nicol, C. W., & Bredin, S. D. (2006). Health benefits of physical activity: The evidence. *Canadian Medical Association Journal, 174,* 801–809.
5. Kodama, S., Saito, K., Tanaka, S., et al. (2009). Cardiorespiratory fitness as a qualitative predictor of all-cause mortality and cardiovascular events in healthy men and women. *Journal of the American Medical Association, 310* (19), 2024–2035.
6. Morey, M. C., Snyder, D. C., Sloane, R., et al. (2009). Effects of home-based diet and exercise on functional outcomes among older, overweight, long-term cancer survivors. *Journal of the American Medical Association, 310* (18), 1883–1891.
7. Friedrich, M. J. (2008). Exercise may boost aging immune system. *Journal of the American Medical Association, 299* (2), 160–161.
8. Flynn, K. E., Pina, I. L., Whellan, D. J., et al. (2009). Effects of exercise training on health status in patients with chronic heart failure. *Journal of the American Medical Association, 310* (14), 1451–1459.
9. Djousse, L., Driver, J. A., & Gaziano, M. (2009). Relation between modifiable lifestyle factors and lifetime risk of heart failure. *Journal of the American Medical Association, 301* (4), 394–400.
10. Bruunsgard, H. (2005). Physical activity modulation of systemic low-level inflammation. *Journal of the American Medical Association, 78,* 819–835.
11. Frontier, W. R. (2006). *Exercise in rehabilitation medicine.* Champaign, IL: Human Kinetics.
12. Chodzko-Zajko, W., Kramer, A. F., & Poon, L. W. (2009). *Enhancing cognitive functioning and brain plasticity.* Champaign, IL: Human Kinetics.
13. Scarmeas, N., Luchsinger, J. A., Schupf, N., et al. (2009). Physical activity, diet, and risk of Alzheimer's disease. *Journal of the American Medical Association, 302* (6), 627–637.
14. Trine, M. R. (1999). Physical activity and quality of life. In J. Rippe (Ed.), *Lifestyle medicine.* Malden, MA: Blackwell Science.
15. American College of Sports Medicine. (2003). *ACSM Fitness Book* (3rd ed.). Champaign, IL: Human Kinetics.
16. Department of Health and Human Services. (2008). 2008 Physical activity guidelines for Americans. www.health.gov/paguidelines/.
17. American College of Sports Medicine. (2010). *ACSM's guidelines for exercise testing and prescription.* Baltimore: Lippincott Williams & Wilkins.
18. Larew, K., Hunter, G. R., Larson-Meyer, D. E., Newcomer, B. R., McCarthy, J. P., & Weinsier, R. L. (2003). Muscle metabolic function, exercise performance, and weight gain. *Medicine and Science in Sports and Exercise, 35* (2), 230–236.
19. American College of Sports Medicine. (1998). Position stand: Exercise and physical activity for older adults. *Medicine and Science in Sports and Exercise, 30,* 992–1008.
20. Baechle, T. R., & Earle, R. W. (2008). *Essentials of strength training and conditioning.* Champaign, IL: Human Kinetics.
21. American College of Sports Medicine. (2009, March). Position stand: Progression models in resistance training for healthy adults. *Medicine & Science in Sports & Exercise, 41* (3), 687–708.
22. Stoppani, J. (2006). *Encyclopedia of muscle and strength.* Champaign, IL: Human Kinetics.
23. Hunter, J. P., & Marshall, R. N. (2002). Effects of power and flexibility training on vertical jump technique. *Medicine and Science in Sports and Exercise, 34* (3), 478–486.
24. Kibler, W. B., Press, J., & Sciascia, A. (2006). The role of core stability in athletic function. *Sports Medicine, 36* (3), 189–198.
25. Benardot, D. (2010). *Advanced sports nutrition.* Champaign, IL: Human Kinetics.
26. Williams, M. H. (2005). *Nutrition for health, fitness and sport* (7th ed.). New York: McGraw-Hill.
27. Cardwell, G. (2006). *Gold medal nutrition.* Champaign, IL: Human Kinetics.
28. Nelson, A. (2007). *Stretching anatomy.* Champaign, IL: Human Kinetics.
29. Sports Fitness Advisor. (2008, July). PNF stretching. www.sport-fitness-advisor.com/pnfstretching.html.
30. Levine, J. A., Lanningham-Foster, L. M., McCrady, S. K., et al. (2005, January 28). "Interindividual variation in posture allocation: Possible role in human obesity." *Science, 307* (5709), 584–586.
31. Brown, W. J., Burton, N. W., & Rowan, P. J. (2007). Updating the evidence of physical activity and walking in women. *American Journal of Preventive Medicine 33* (5), 404–411.
32. 10,000 Steps Program. (2003). Shape Up America. www.shapeup.org.
33. Mestek, M. L., Plaisance, E., & Grandjean, P. (2008). The relationship between pedometer-determined and self-reported physical activity and body composition variables in college-aged men and women. *Journal of American College Health 57* (1), 39–44.
34. Graf, D. L., Pratt, L. V., Hester, C. N., et al. (2009). Playing active video games increases energy expenditure in children. *Pediatrics, 124* (2), 534–540.
35. Harvard Medical School. (2006). A little bit at a time: Eating and exercising in bits and pieces. www.health.harvard.edu/fhg/updates/A-little-at-a-time-Eating-and-exercising-in-bits-and-pieces.shtml.
36. Eberle, S. G. (2000). *Endurance sports nutrition.* Champaign, IL: Human Kinetics.
37. Schnirring, L. (2003). New hydration recommendations: Risk of hyponatremia plays a big role. *Physician and Sports Medicine, 31* (7), 15–18.
38. American College of Sports Medicine. (1996). Position stand: Exercise and fluid replacement. *Medicine & Science in Sports & Exercise, 28* (1), i–vii.
39. American College of Sports Medicine. (2007, February). Position statement: Exercise and fluid replacement. *Medicine & Science in Sports & Exercise, 39* (2), 377–390.
40. Linn, S. W., & Gong, H. (1999). Air pollution exercise, nutrition, and health. In J. Rippe (Ed.), *Lifestyle medicine.* Malden, MA: Blackwell Science.
41. Trost, S. G., & Pate, R. R. (1999). Physical activity in children and youth. In J. Rippe (Ed.), *Lifestyle medicine.* Malden, MA: Blackwell Science.
42. Schnirring, L. (2005). Groups endorse ECG screening for athletes. *Physician and Sports Medicine, 33* (3), 12–15.
43. Spivock M., Gauvin, L., Riva M., et al. (2008). Promoting active living among people with physical disabilities: Evidence for neighborhood-level buoys. *American Journal of Preventive Medicine 34* (4), 291–298.
44. Armitage, C. J. (2005). Can the theory of planned behavior predict the maintenance of physical activity? *Health Psychology, 24* (3), 235–245.
45. Floyd, M. F., Crespo, C. J., & Sallis, J. F. (2008). Active living research in diverse and disadvantaged communities: Stimulating dialogue and policy solutions. *American Journal of Preventive Medicine 34* (4), 271–274.
46. Centers for Disease Control and Prevention. (2005). Creating or improving access to places for physical activity is recommended to increase physical activity. www.thecommunityguide.org/pa/pa-int-create-access.pdf.
47. Sallis, J. F., Bowles, H. R., Bauman, A., et al. (2009). Neighborhood environments and physical activity among adults in 11 countries. *American Journal of Preventive Medicine 36* (6), 484–490.
48. Duany, A. (n.d.). Smartcode: A comprehensive form-based planning ordinance. www.smartcodecentral.com.
49. Mansnerus, L. (2003, May 24). New Jersey is running out of open land it can build on. *New York Times.* www.nytimes.com.
50. Centers for Disease Control and Prevention. (n.d.). Physical activity resources for health professionals: Active environments. www.cdc.gov/nccdphp/dnpa/physical/health_professionals/active_environments/index.htm.

Chapter 8

1. Flegal, K. M., Carroll, M. D., Ogden, C. L., et al. (2010, January 20). Prevalence and trends in obesity among US adults, 1999–2008. *Journal of the American Medical Association, 303* (3), 235–241.
2. Centers for Disease Control and Prevention. (2009). U.S. obesity trends, 1985–2008. www.cdc.gov.
3. World Health Organization. (n.d.). Global strategy on diet, physical activity and health: Obesity and overweight. www.who.int/dietphysicalactivity/publications/facts/obesity/en/.
4. Ogden, C. L., Carroll, M. D., & Flegal, K. M. (2008). High body mass index for age among U.S. children and adolescents, 2003–2006. *Journal of the American Medical Association, 299* (20), 2401–2405.
5. Centers for Disease Control and Prevention. (2009, July 24). Obesity prevalence among low-income, preschool-aged children—United States, 1998–2008. *Morbidity and Mortality Weekly Report, 58* (28), 769–773.
6. Gallagher, D., Heymsfield, S. B., Heo, M., et al. (2000). Healthy percentage body fat ranges: An approach for developing guidelines based on body mass index. *American Journal of Clinical Nutrition, 72* (3), 694–701.
7. Bray, G. A. (2003). *An atlas of obesity and weight control.* New York: Parthenon Publishing Group.
8. Wahrenberg, H., Hertel, K., Leijonhufvud, B., Persson, L.-G., et al. (2005). Use of waist circumference to predict insulin resistance: Retrospective study. *British Medical Journal, 330* (7504), 1363–1364.
9. Waller, D. K., Shaw, G. M., Rasmussen, S. A., et al. (2007). Prepregnancy obesity as a risk factor for structural birth defects. *Archives of Pediatrics and Adolescent Medicine, 161* (8), 725–814.

10. Flegal, K. M., Graubard, B. I., Williamson, D. F., et al. (2005). Excess deaths associated with underweight, overweight and obesity. *Journal of the American Medical Association, 293* (15), 1861–1867.

11. Neary, M. T., & Batterham, R. L. (2009). Gut hormones: Implications for the treatment of obesity. *Pharmacology and Therapeutics, 124* (1), 44–56.

12. Schulz, L. O., Bennett, P. H., Ravussin, E., et al. (2006). Effects of traditional and Western environments on prevalence of Type 2 diabetes in Pima Indians in Mexico and the U.S. *Diabetes Care, 29* (8), 1866–1871.

13. Nelsen, M. C., Neumark-Stzainer, D., Hannan, P. J., et al. (2006). Longitudinal and secular trends in physical activity and sedentary behavior during adolescence. *Pediatrics, 118* (6), e1627–e1634.

14. Gunderson, E., & Abrams, B. (2000). Epidemiology of gestational weight gain and body weight changes after pregnancy. *Epidemiology Reviews, 22* (2), 261–274.

15. Drewnowski, A., & Eichelsdoerfer, P. (2009). Can low-income Americans afford a healthy diet? CPHN Public Health Research Brief. www.cphn.org/reports/brief1.pdf.

16. Darmon, N., & Drewnowski, A. (2008). Does social class predict diet quality? *American Journal of Clinical Nutrition, 87* (5), 1107–1117.

17. French, S. A., Strory, M., & Jeffery, T. W. (2001). Environmental influences on eating and physical activity. *Annual Review of Public Health, 22,* 309–335.

18. Crombie, A. P., Ilich, J. Z., Dutton, G. R., et al. (2009). The freshman weight gain phenomenon revisited. *Nutrition Reviews, 67* (2), 83–94.

19. Wang, Y., & Beydom, M. A. (2007). The obesity epidemic in the United States—Gender, age, socioeconomic, racial/ethnic, and geographic characteristics: A systematic review and meta-regression analysis. *Epidemiologic Review, 29* (1), 6–28.

20. National Center for Chronic Disease Prevention and Health Promotion, Division of Nutrition and Physical Activity. (2006). Do increased portion sizes affect how much we eat? (Research to Practice Series, No. 2.) Centers for Disease Control and Prevention. www.cdc.gov/nccdphp/dnpa/nutrition/pdf/portion_size_research.pdf.

21. Dietz, W. H., & Gortmaker, S. L. (2001). Preventing obesity in children and adolescents. *Annual Review of Public Health, 22,* 337–353.

22. Frank, L. D., Andresen, M. A., & Schmid, T. L. (2004). Obesity relationship with community design, physical activity and time spent in cars. *American Journal of Preventive Medicine, 27* (2), 87–96.

23. Papas, M. A., Alberg, A. J., Ewing, R., et al. (2007). The built environment and obesity. *Epidemiological Reviews, 29,* 129–143.

24. The Nielsen Company. (2009). A2/M2 three screen report: Television, Internet, and mobile phone usage in the United States 5 (2nd quarter). http://blog.nielsen.com/nielsenwire/wp-content/uploads/2009/09/3ScreenQ209_US_rpt_090209.pdf.

25. Christakis, N. A., & Fowler, J. H. (2007). The spread of obesity in a large social network over 32 years. *The New England Journal of Medicine, 357* (4), 370–379.

26. U.S. Department of Health and Human Services. (2010, January). *The surgeon general's vision for a healthy and fit nation.* Rockville, MD: U.S. Department of Health and Human Services, Office of the Surgeon General.

27. Market Data Enterprises, Inc. (2009). *The U.S. weight loss and diet control market* (10th ed.). Tampa, FL: Author.

28. Sacks, F. M., Bray, G. A., Carey, V. J., Smith, S. R., et al. (2009). Comparison of weight-loss diets with different compositions of fat, protein and carbohydrates. *New England Journal of Medicine 360* (9), 859–873.

29. Tsai, A. G., & Wadden, T. A. (2005). Systematic review: An evaluation of major commercial weight loss programs in the United States. *Annals of Internal Medicine, 142* (1), 56–67.

30. Dickerson, L. M., & Carek, P. J. (2009). Pharmacotherapy for the obese patient. *Primary Care: Clinics in Office Practice, 36* (2), 407–415.

31. Bogle, K. E., & Smith, B. H. (2009, May). Illicit methylphenidate use: A review of the prevalence, availability, pharmacology and consequences. *Current Drug Abuse Review 2* (2), 157–176.

32. Wu, L., Pillowsky, D. J., Schlenger, W. E., & Galvin, D. M. (2007). Misuse of methamphetamine and prescription stimulants among youths and young adults in the community. *Drug and Alcohol Dependence, 89* (2–3), 195–205.

33. DeMaria, E. J. (2007). Bariatric surgery for morbid obesity. *New England Journal of Medicine, 356* (21), 2176–2183.

34. Hasani-Ranjbar, S., Nayebi, N., Larijani, B., & Abdollahi, M. (2009). A systematic review of the efficacy and safety of herbal medicines used in the treatment of obesity. *World Journal of Gastroenterology, 15* (25), 3073–3085.

35. National Association to Advance Fat Acceptance. www.naafa.org.

36. Spark, A. (2001). Health at any size: The self-acceptance non-diet movement. *Journal of the American Medical Association, 56* (2), 69–72.

Chapter 9

1. National Eating Disorders Association. (2009). National Eating Disorders Association unveils powerful and provocative ad campaign. www.nationaleatingdisorders.org.

2. Morris, A. M., & Katzman, D. K. (2003). The impact of the media on eating disorders in children and adolescents. *Adolescent Medicine, 14* (1), 109–118.

3. Derenne, J. L., & Beresin, E. V. (2006). Body image, media, and eating disorders. *Academic Psychiatry, 30* (3), 181–198.

4. Striegel-Moore, R. H., & Bulik, C. M. (2007). Risk factors for eating disorders. *American Psychologist, 62* (3), 181–198.

5. Rodgers, R., & Chabrol, H. (2009). Parental attitudes, body image disturbance and disordered eating amongst adolescents and young adults: A review. *European Eating Disorders Review, 17* (2), 137–151.

6. Hogan M. J., & Strasburger, V. C. (2008). Body image, eating disorders, and the media. *Adolescent Medicine State of the Art Review, 19* (3), 521–546.

7. Barlett, C. P., Vowels, C. L., & Saucier, D. A. (2008). Meta-analysis of the effects of media images on men's body-image concerns. *Journal of Social and Clinical Psychology, 27* (3), 279–310.

8. Grieve, F. G. (2007). A conceptual model of factors contributing to the development of muscle dysmorhpia. *Eating Disorders, 15,* 63–80.

9. Cafri, G., Thompson, J. K., Ricciardell, L., & McCabe, M. (2005). Pursuit of the muscular ideal: Physical and psychological consequences and putative risk factors. *Clinical Psychology Review, 25* (2), 215–239.

10. Hudson, J. I., Hiripi, E., Pope, H. G., & Kessler, R. C. (2007). The prevalence and correlates of eating disorders in the National Comorbidity Survey Replication. *Biological Psychiatry, 61,* 348–358.

11. Hautala, L. A., Junnila, J., Helenius, H., et al. (2008). Towards understanding gender differences in disordered eating among adolescents. *Journal of Clinical Nursing, 17* (3), 1803–1813.

12. Shaw, H., Ramirez, L., Trost, A., et al. (2004). Body image and eating disturbances across ethnic groups: More similarities than differences. *Psychology of Addictive Behaviors, 18* (1), 12–18.

13. Ricciardelli, L. A., McCabe, M. P., Williams, R. J., & Thompson, J. K. (2007). The role of ethnicity and culture in body image and disordered eating among males. *Clinical Psychology Review, 27,* 582–606.

14. Becker, A. E. (2007). Culture and eating disorders classification. *International Journal of Eating Disorders, 40* (Suppl. 3), S111–S116.

15. Bonci, C. M., Bonci, L. J., et al. (2008). National Athletic Trainers' Association position statement on preventing, detecting and managing disordered eating. *Journal of Athletic Training, 43* (1), 80–108.

16. Neumark-Sztainer, D. (2005). *I'm, like, SO fat!* New York: Guilford.

17. Klump, K. L., Bulik, C. M., Kaye, W. H., et al. (2009). Academy for Eating Disorders position paper: Eating disorders are serious mental illnesses. *International Journal of Eating Disorders, 42* (2), 97–103.

18. Feldman, M. B., & Meyer, I. H. (2007). Eating disorders in diverse lesbian, gay and bisexual populations. *International Journal of Eating Disorders, 40* (3), 218–226.

19. Costin, C. (1999). *The eating disorder sourcebook: A comprehensive guide to causes, treatments and prevention of eating disorders.* Lincolnwood, IL: Lowell House.

20. American Psychiatric Association. (2000). *Diagnostic and statistical manual of mental disorders* (4th ed., Text Revision [DSM-IV-TR]). Washington, DC: American Psychiatric Association.

21. Yager, Y. (2008). Binge eating disorder: The search for better treatments. *American Journal of Psychiatry, 165,* 4–6.

22. Wilfley, D. E., Bishop, M. E., Wilson, G. T., & Agras, A. S. (2007). Classification of eating disorders: Toward DSM-V. *International Journal of Eating Disorders, 40* (Suppl. 3), S123–S129.

23. Zipfel, S., Lowe, B., Reas, D. L., et al. (2000). Long-term prognosis in anorexia nervosa: Lessons from a 21-year follow up study. *Lancet, 355,* 721.

24. Ecklund, K., Vajapeyam, S., Feldman, H. A., et al. (2010). Bone marrow changes in adolescent girls with anorexia nervosa. *Journal of Bone and Mineral Research, 25* (2), 298–304.

25. Steinhausen, H. C., & Weber, S. (2009). The outcome of bulimia nervosa: Findings from one-quarter century of research. *American Journal of Psychiatry, 166* (12), 1331–1341.

26. Steinhausen, H. C. (2009). Outcome of eating disorders. *Child and Adolescent Psychiatric Clinics of North America, 18* (1), 225–242.

27. Chavez, M., & Insel, T. R. (2007). Eating disorders: National Institute of Mental Health's perspective. *American Psychologist, 62* (3), 159–166.

28. Pavan, C., Simonato, P., Marini, M., et al. (2008). Psychopathologic aspects of body dysmorphic disorder: A literature review. *Aesthetic Plastic Surgery, 32,* 473–484.

29. National Institute on Drug Abuse. NIDA InfoFacts: Steroids (anabolic-androgenic). National Institute of Health. www.drugabuse.gov/infofacts/steroids.html.

30. National Clearinghouse of Plastic Surgery Statistics. 2009 report of the 2008 statistics. American Society of Plastic Surgeons. www.plasticsurgery.org.

31. Armstrong, M. L., Roberts, A. E., Koch, J. R., et al. (2008). Motivation for contemporary tattoo removal. *Archives of Dermatology, 144* (7).

32. Burris, K., & Kim, K. (2007). Tattoo removal. *Clinics in Dermatology, 25* (4), 388–392.

3. Centers for Disease Control. Fruits and veggies—more matters. (n.d.). www.fruitsandveggiesmatter.gov.

4. Kushi, L. H., Byers, T., Doyle, C., et al. (2006). American Cancer Society guidelines on nutrition and physical activity for cancer prevention: Reducing the risk of cancer with healthy food choices and physical activity. *CA: A Cancer Journal for Clinicians, 56,* 254–281.

5. Zheng, W., & Lee, S. A. (2009). Well-done meat intake, heteroxyclic amine exposure and cancer risk. *Nutrition and Cancer, 61* (4), 437–446.

6. World Cancer Research Fund/American Institute for Cancer Research. (2007). *Food, nutrition, physical activity, and the prevention of cancer: A global perspective.* Washington, DC: Author.

7. Percik, R., & Stumvoll, M. (2009). Obesity and cancer. *Experimental Clinics of Endocrinology and Diabetes, 117* (10), 563–566.

8. Chen, L., Gallicchio, L., Boyd-Lindsey, K., Tao, X. G., et al. (2009). Alcohol consumption and the risk of nasopharyngeal carcinoma: A systematic review. *Nutrition and Cancer, 61* (1), 1–15.

9. The Cancer Council Australia. (n.d.). SunSmart. www.cancer.org.au/cancersmartlifestyle/sunsmart.htm.

10. Gallagher, R. P., & Lee, T. K. (2006). Adverse effects of ultraviolet radiation: A brief review. *Progress in Biophysics and Molecular Biology, 92* (1), 119–131.

11. Board on Radiation Effects Research, Committee to Assess Health Risks from Exposure to Low Levels of Ionizing Radiation, National Research Council. (2006). *Health risks from exposure to low levels of ionizing radiation: BEIR VII phase 2.* Washington, DC: National Academies Press.

12. Gilbert, E. S. (2009). Ionizing radiation and cancer risks: What have we learned from epidemiology? *International Journal of Radiation Biology, 85* (6), 467–482.

13. Clapp, R. W., Jacobs, M. M., & Loechler, E. L. (2008). Environmental and occupational causes of cancer: New evidence, 2005–2007. *Review of Environmental Health, 23* (1), 1–37.

14. Fontham, E. T. H., Thun, M. J., Ward, E., Balch, A. J., et al. (2009). American Cancer Society perspectives on environmental factors and cancer. *CA: A Cancer Journal for Clinicians, 59* (6), 343–351.

15. Clapp, R. W., Howe, G. K., & Jacobs, M. M. (2007). Environmental and occupational causes of cancer: A call to act on what we know. *Biomedicine and Pharmacotherapy, 61* (10), 631–639.

16. Burk, R. D., Chen, Z., & Van Doorslaer, K. (2009). Human papillomaviruses: Genetic basis of carcinogenicity. *Public Health Genomics, 12* (5–6), 281–290.

17. Shah, K. M., & Young, L. S. (2009). Epstein-Barr virus and carcinogenesis: Beyond Burkitt's lymphoma. *Clinical Microbiology and Infection, 15* (11), 982–988.

18. Herrera, V., & Parsonnet, J. (2009). Helicobacter pylori and gastric adenocarcinoma. *Clinical Microbiology and Infection, 15* (11), 971–976.

19. Fung, J., Lai, C.L., & Yuen, M. F. (2009). Hepatitis B and C virus-related carcinogenesis. *Clinical Microbiology and Infection, 15* (11), 964–970.

20. Jung, R. J., McKay, J. D., Gaborieau, V., et al. (2008). A susceptibility locus for lung cancer maps to nicotinic acetylcholine receptor subunit genes on 15q25. *Nature, 452,* 633–637.

21. Thorgeirsson, T. E., Geller, F., Sulem, P., et al. (2008). A variant associated with nicotine dependence, lung cancer and peripheral arterial disease. *Nature, 452,* 638–642.

22. National Cancer Institute. (2009). Lung cancer screening (PDQ) health professional version. www.cancer.gov/cancertopics/pdq/screening/lung/healthprofessional/allpages/print#section_16.

23. American Cancer Society. (2010). Colorectal cancer facts and figures 2008–2010. www.cancer.org/docroot/stt/stt_0.asp?from-fast.

24. U.S. Preventative Task Force. (2009, November). Screening for breast cancer. www.ahrq.gov/clinic/uspstf/uspsbrca.htm.

25. Nossov, V., Amneus, M., Su, F., Lang, J., et al. (2008). The early detection of ovarian cancer: From traditional methods to proteomics: Can we really do better than serum CA-125? *American Journal of Obstetrics and Gynecology, 199* (3), 215–223.

26. National Cancer Institute. (n.d.). Ovarian cancer. www.cancer.gov/cancertopics/types/ovarian/.

27. Runger, T. M., & Kappes, U. P. (2008). Mechanisms of mutation formation with long-wave ultraviolet light (UVA). *Photodermatology, Photoimmunology, and Photomedicine, 24* (1), 2–10.

28. National Cancer Institute. (n.d.). Types of treatment. www.cancer.gov/cancertopics/treatment/types-of-treatment.

29. Hayes-Lattin, B., & Nichols, C. R. (2009). Testicular cancer: A prototypic tumor of young adults. *Seminars in Oncology, 36* (5), 432–438.

30. National Center for Complementary and Alternative Medicine. (n.d.). Get the facts: Cancer and CAM. http://nccam.nih.gov/health/camcancer/.

31. Velicer, C. M., & Ulrich, C. M. (2008). Vitamin and mineral supplement use among US adults after cancer diagnosis: A systematic review. *Journal of Clinical Oncology, 26* (4), 665–673.

32. Menfee Pujol, L. A., & Monti, D. A. (2007). Managing cancer pain with nonpharmocologic and complementary therapies. *Journal of the American Osteopathic Association, 107* (7), 15–21.

Chapter 17

1. Bever, D. L. (1998). *Safety: A personal focus.* New York: WCB and McGraw-Hill.

2. Centers for Disease Control and Prevention, National Center for Injury Prevention and Control. (2009). *CDC injury fact book.* www.cdc.gov/injury/publications/factbook/.

3. U.S. Department of Transportation. (2009). *An analysis of speeding-related crashes: Definitions and the effects of road environments.* (Publication No. DOT HS 811090). Washington, DC: National Highway Traffic Safety Administration.

4. National Highway Traffic Safety Administration. (2006). *The impact of driver inattention on near crash/crash risk: An analysis using the 100-Car Naturalistic Driving Study data* (Publication No. DOT HS 810594). Washington, DC: U.S. Department of Transportation.

5. Centers for Disease Control and Prevention. *Preventing injuries in America: Public health in action.* www.cdc.gov.

6. Larson, J. (1999). *Road rage.* Tom Doherty Associates.

7. U.S. Department of Transportation. (2009). *Alcohol-impaired drivers involved in fatal crashes, by gender and state: 2007–2008* (Publication No. DOT HS 811195). Washington, DC: National Highway Traffic Safety Administration.

8. U.S. Department of Transportation. (2004). *U.S. DOT proposes tougher standard to protect occupants in side-impact crashes.* Washington, DC: National Highway Traffic Safety Administration.

9. Decker, M. D., Rice, T. M., & Anderson C. L. (2009). The use and efficacy of child restraint devices. *American Journal of Public Health, 99* (7), 1161–1162.

10. Rosenberg, J. (2008). Electronic stability control. www.cars.com/go/advice/Story.jsp?section=safe&story=techStability&subject=safe_tech&referer=.

11. Homer, J., & French, M. (2009). Motorcycle helmet laws in the United States from 1990 to 2005: Politics and public health. *American Journal of Public Health, 99* (3), 408–415.

12. Insurance Institute for Highway Safety, Highway Loss Data Institute. (2008). Current U.S. motorcycle and bicycle helmet laws. www.iihs.org/laws/helmetusecurrent.aspx.

13. Retting, R. A., Ferguson, S. A., & McCarthy, A. T. (2003). A review of evidence-based traffic engineering measures to reduce pedestrian–motor vehicle crashes. *American Journal of Public Health, 93* (9), 1456–1462.

14. Praderelli, M. (2005). As ATV usage soars, safety needs to take a front seat. *Midwest Injury Prevention Control, 7* (1), 1.

15. Crispi, K. (n.d.). Pocket bikes. *FindLaw.* htpp://injury.findlaw.com/personal-injury-a-z/pocket-bikes.html.

16. Saluja, G., Brenner, R. A., Trumble, A., et al. (2006). Swimming pool drownings among U.S. residents aged 5–24 years: Understanding racial/ethnic disparities. *American Journal of Public Health, 96* (4), 778–783.

17. Centers for Disease Control and Prevention. (2008). Water-related injury: Fact sheet. www.cdc.gov/ncipc/factsheets/drown.htm.

18. Fiore, K. (2009). Rock climbing injuries going up. ABC News. http://abcnews.go.com/print?id=8165004.

19. Centers for Disease Control and Prevention. (2006). *Injury surveillance training manual.* www.ihs.gov/medicalprograms/portlandinjury/pdfs/injurysurveillancetrainingmanual.pdf.

20. Kannus, P., Parkkari, J., Niemi, S., et al. (2005). Induced deaths among elderly people. *American Journal of Public Health, 95* (3), 422–424.

21. Centers for Disease Control and Prevention. (2009). Fire deaths and injuries: Fact sheet. www.cdc.gov/ncipc/factsheets/fire.htm.

22. Eisler, P., & Levin, A. (2007, March 6). Batteries can pose risk to planes. *USA Today,* p. 3A.

23. National Fire Protection Agency. (2006). *Fire in your home.* Washington, DC: Author.

24. Centers for Disease Control and Prevention. (2008). Poisoning in the United States: Fact sheet. www.cdc.gov/ncipc/factsheets/poisoning.htm.

25. Centers for Disease Control and Prevention. (2008). Tips to prevent poisoning. www.cdc.gov/ncipc/factsheets/poisonprevention.htm.

26. Null, J., & Quinn, J. (2005). Heat stress from enclosed vehicles: Moderate ambient temperatures cause significant temperature rise in enclosed vehicles. *Pediatrics, 116* (1), e109–e112.

27. Park, A. (2009). iPod safety: Preventing hearing loss in teens. *Time.* http://time.com/time/printout/0,8816,1881130,00.html.

28. Gupta, S. (2009, September 20). New ways to survive cardiac arrest. *Parade,* 8, 9.

29. Lynch, J. (2002). Crime in international perspective. In J. Q. Wilson & J. Petersilia (Eds.), *Crime: Public policies for crime control* (pp. 5–42). San Francisco: ICS Press.

30. Bureau of Justice Statistics. (2007). Firearms and crime statistics. www.ojp .usdoj.gov/bjs/guns.htm.

31. Potter, L. B. (2006). Violence prevention. In S. S. Gorin & J. Arnold (Eds.), *Health promotion practice.* San Francisco: Jossey-Bass.

32. Barnett, O. W., Miller-Perrin, C. L., & Perrin, R. D. (2004). *Family violence across the lifespan: An introduction* (2nd ed.). Thousand Oaks, CA: Sage Publications.

33. Bureau of Justice Statistics. (2007). Homicide trends in the U.S. www.ojp .usdoj.gov/bjs/homicide/homtrnd.htm.

34. Rosenfeld, R. (2004, February). The case of the unsolved crime decline. *Scientific American.*

35. Centers for Disease Control and Prevention. (2007). Youth violence: Fact sheet. www.cdc.gov/ncipc/factsheets/yvfacts.htm.

36. Goodson, B., & Muncie, J. (2006). *Youth crime and justice.* Newbury Park, CA: Sage.

37. Security on Campus, Inc. (2006). College university campus crime statistics. www.securityoncampus.org/crimestats/.

38. Newer, H. (2003). *The hazing reader: Examining rites gone wrong in fraternities, professional and amateur athletics, high schools, and the military.* Auckland, New Zealand: Reid Publishing.

39. Hudson, D. L. (2007). Hate speech and campus speech codes. www .firstamendmentcenter.org/speech/pubcollege/topic.aspx?topic=campus _speech_codes.

40. Carr, J. L. (2005). *Campus violence white paper.* Baltimore, MD: American College Health Association.

41. Rapoza, K. A., & Drake, J. E. (2009). Relationships of hazardous alcohol use, alcohol expectancies, and emotional commitments to male sexual coercion and aggression in dating. *Journal of the Study of Alcohol and Drugs, 70* (1), 55–63.

42. Fisher, B. S., Cullen, F. T., & Turner, M. G. (2000, December). The sexual victimization of college women. *National Institute of Justice Research Report.* Rockville, MD: National Criminal Justice Reference Center.

43. Tjaden, P., & Thoennes, N. (2000). Full report of the prevalence, incidence, and consequences of violence against women: Findings from the National Violence Against Women Survey. Report NCJ 183781. Washington, DC: National Institute of Justice.

44. Bureau of Justice Statistics. (2009). National Crime Victimization Survey, 2009. www.ojp.usdoj.gov/bjs.

45. Male Survivor Organization. (2007). Myths about male sexual victimization. www.malesurvivor.org/myths.html.

46. American College Health Association. (2008). *Shifting the paradigm: Primary prevention of sexual violence.* Baltimore, MD: Author.

47. Center for Public Integrity. (2009). Sexual assault on campus shrouded in secrecy. www.publicintegrity.org/investigations/campus_assault/articles/ entry/1838/.

48. Center for Public Integrity. (2009). Campus sexual assault statistics don't add up. www.publicintegrity.org/investigations/campus_assault/articles/ entry/1841/.

49. Center for Public Integrity. (2009). Barriers curb reporting on campus sexual assault. www.publicintegrity.org/investigations/campus_assault/articles/ entry/1822/.

50. Wallace, H. (2005). *Family violence: Legal, medical and social perspectives.* Boston: Allyn & Bacon.

51. McCarty, C. (2007). New Jersey attorney general subpoenas Facebook over sex offender data. http://news.cnet.com/8301-13577_3-9790064-36.html.

52. U.S. Equal Employment Opportunity Commission. (2008). Sexual harassment. www.eeoc.gov/types/sexual_harassment.html.

53. Rospenda, K. M., Richman, J. A., & Shannon, C. A. (2009). Prevalence and mental health correlates of harassment and discrimination in the workplace. *Journal of Interpersonal Violence, 24* (50), 819–843.

54. National Center for Victims of Crime. (n.d.). Stalking. www.ncvc.org.

55. Crime Library. (n.d.). Cyber-stalking: Risk management. www.crimelibrary .com/criminal_mind/psychology/cyberstalking/6.html.

56. U.S. Department of Health and Human Services. (2007). *Child maltreatment.* Washington, DC: Administration for Children and Families.

57. Centers for Disease Control and Prevention, National Center for Injury Prevention and Control. (2004). Child maltreatment: Fact sheet. www.cdc.gov.

58. Theo, A. (2006). *Deviant behaviors.* Boston: Allyn & Bacon.

59. Gross, M. N., & Graham-Berman, S. A. (2006). Gender, categories, and science-as-usual: A critical review of gender and PTSD. *Violence Against Women, 12* (4), 393–406.

60. Centers for Disease Control and Prevention. (2006). Intimate partner violence: Fact sheet. www.cdc.gov/ncipc/dvp/ipv_factsheet.pdf.

61. Cornelius, T. L., Sullivan K. T., Wyngarden. N., et al. (2009). Participation in prevention programs for dating violence. *Journal of Interpersonal Violence, 24* (6), 1057–1078.

62. Murphy, C. M., Winters, J., O'Farrell, T. J., et al. (2005). Alcohol consumption and intimate partner violence by alcoholic men: Comparing violent and non-violent conflicts. *Psychology of Addictive Behaviors, 19,* 35–42.

63. Perry, B. (2001). *In the name of hate: Understanding hate crimes.* New York: Routledge.

64. Fenske, R. H., & Gordon, L. (1998). Reducing race and ethnic hate crimes on campus: The need for community. In A. M. Hoffman, J. H. Schuh, & R. H. Fenske (Eds.), *Violence on campus: Defining the problems, strategies for action.* Gaithersburg, MD: Aspen Publishers.

65. McPhail, B. A., & Dinitto, D. M. (2006). Prosecutorial perspectives on gender bias and hate crimes. *Violence Against Women, 11* (19), 1162–1185.

66. Cole, T. B., & Johnson, R. M. (2005). Storing guns safely in homes with children and adolescents. *Journal of the American Medical Association, 293* (6), 740–744.

67. Teret, S. P., & Culross, P. L. (2000). Product-oriented approaches to reducing youth gun violence. *The Future of Children, 12* (2), 119.

68. Kelly, C. (2004). *Blown away: American women and guns.* New York: Simon & Schuster.

69. Minnebo, J. (2006). The relation between psychological distress, television exposure, and television-viewing motives in crime victims. *Media Psychology, 8* (2), 61–63.

70. Bok, S. (1999). *Mayhem: Violence as public entertainment.* New York: Basic Books.

71. Murray, C. (2002). The physical environment. In J. Q. Wilson & J. Petersilia (Eds.), *Crime: Public policies for crime control* (pp. 349–361). San Francisco: ICS Press.

72. Furedi, F. (2005). *The culture of fear: Why Americans are afraid of the wrong things.* New York: Continuum Intermediate Publishing Group.

73. Stephens, K. A. (2009). Rape prevention with college men. *Journal of Interpersonal Violence, 24* (6), 996–1013.

74. Samson, R. J. (2002). The community. In J. Q. Wilson & J. Petersilia (Eds.), *Crime: Public policies for crime control* (pp. 225–252). San Francisco: ICS Press.

Chapter 1

p.1: © Comstock/PhotoLibrary; p.2 (top): istockphoto.com/giuseppe perrone; p.2 (bottom): istockphoto.com/Mark Evans; p.3 (top): © JupiterImages; p.3 (bottom): RubberBall Productions; p.5: American Red Cross/Virginia Hart; p.6: © RF/Corbis; p.7 (top): © Flickr/Getty Images; p.7 (bottom): © Jemal Countess/Getty Images; p.8: ©Rachel Epstein/The Image Works; p.9: Photodisc Collection/Getty Images; p.10: The McGraw-Hill Companies, Inc./ John Flournoy, photographer; p.11: PRNewsFoto/Dynakor Pharmacal/AP Wide World Photos; p.12: D. Hurst/Alamy; p.13 © Angelo Cavalli/Getty Images; p.14: © Javier Pierini/Getty Images; p.15: RubberBall Productions

Chapter 2

p.19: © Don Mason/Blend Images/Getty Images; p.20: IMAGEMORE Co, Ltd./Getty Images; p.23: © Jerritt Clark/WireImage/Getty Images; p.25 (left): © Beyond/SuperStock; p.25 (right): © Custom Medical Stock Photo/ Alamy; p.26: © TLC Photographer: Daniel Hennessy/Photofest; p.27: © Tim Defrisco/Getty Images; p.30: The McGraw-Hill Companies, Inc./Roger Loewenberg, photographer; p.31 (top): © NBC/AP Wide World Photos; p.31 (bottom): Photodisc/Getty Images; p.32: Stockbyte/Alamy; p.33: © Michael Newman/PhotoEdit; p.35: © AP Wide World Photos; p.36: C Squared Studios/Getty Images

Chapter 3

p.39: Rubberball Productions/Getty Images; p.40: © Photodisc/Punchstock; p.41: S. MeltzerPhotoLink/Getty Images; p.43: Brand X Pictures/Jupiter Images; p.44: Royalty-Free/Corbis; p.47: © MICHAEL REYNOLDS/epa/ Corbis; p.48 © Stockdisc/Stockbyte/Getty Images; p.49 (top to bottom): Burke/Triolo Productions/Getty Images; Courtesy of U.S. Drug Enforcement Agency; Photodisc Collection/Getty Images; © Ingram Publishing/ Fotosearch; © Comstock/PunchStock; © RF/Corbis; © Janis Christie/Getty Images; © RF/Corbis; © RF/Corbis; p.51: Photodisc Collection/Getty Images; p.54: © Galen Rowell/Corbis; p.56: Photo by U.S. Army Pfc. Andrya Hill, 4th Brigade Combat Team, 25th Infantry Division Public Affairs; p.58: © AP Wide World Photos; p.59: ©Peter Hvizdak/The Image Works; p.60: Comstock Images/Alamy; p.61: © AP Wide World Photos; p.62: JEWEL SAMAD/AFP/Getty Images; p.63: C Squared Studios/Getty Images; p.64: © Simon Jarratt/Corbis; p.65: blue jean images/Getty Images; p.66: Mike Powell/Digital Vision/Getty Images

Chapter 4

p.69: © Tim Platt/Getty Images; p.70: © Kayte Deioma/PhotoEdit; p.71: © James Marshall/The Image Works; p.72: Tinette Reed/Brand X Pictures/ JupiterImages; p.73: © Anna Pena/Stone/Getty Images; p.74: © Frances Roberts/Alamy; p.75: © Photodisc/Getty Images; p.76: © Stockbyte; p.77: © Fly Fernandez/Corbis; p.78: Michael Hitoshi/Taxi Japan/Getty Images; p.79: Corporation for National & Community Service; p.80: © John Kelly/ Getty Images; p.81: © Spencer Grant/PhotoEdit

Chapter 5

p.86: © Kane Skennar/Photodisc/Getty Images; p.87: © Koichi Kamoshida/ Getty Images; p.89: © PhotoAlto/PunchStock; p.90: © Hammo 2008/Getty Images; p.92: © Digital Vision/PunchStock; p.94: © Win McNamee/Getty Images; p.95: PhotoAlto/Alix Minde/Getty Images; p.96: Plush Studios/ Getty Images; p.97: © Marco Cristofori/age fotostock/PhotoLibrary; p.98: © Photodisc; p.99 (left to right): Photo by Eric Erbe/United States Department of Agriculture; Department of Health and Human Services; Centers for Disease Control and Prevention; p.100: Tim Boyle/Getty Images; p.101: © Elizabeth Whiting & Associates/Alamy; p.102: Courtesy of Carole McDonnell

Chapter 6

p.105: Todd Pearson/Getty Images; p.106: © Pixtal/age fotostock; p.107 (top): Jupiterimages/Getty Images; p.107 (bottom): Ingram Publishing/ Alamy; p.108: © Ingram Publishing/Fotosearch; p.109: Tooga/Getty Images; p.110: Tooga/Getty Images; p.111: Getty Images/Jonelle Weaver; p.113: Jana Leon/Stone/Getty Images; p.116: Source: MyPyramid, 2005, U.S. Department of Agriculture, Center for Nutrition Policy and Promotion; p.118: Lew Robertson/Getty Images; p.119: The McGraw-Hill Companies, Inc./Jill Braaten, photographer; p.122: Burke/Triolo Productions/Getty Images; p.123: Eddie Mejia/Splash News/Newscom; p.125 (top): Banana Stock/JupiterImages; p.125 (bottom): C Squared Studios/Getty Images; p.127 (clockwise): © iStockphoto.com/Romas Bercic; © istockPhoto.com/ webking; © iStockPhoto.com/Roberto Adrian; © iStockphoto.com/orix3; © iStockPhoto.com/Rebecca Ellis; © iStockPhoto.com/Pam R; © iStockPhoto.com/ Graca; p.128: © Photodisc/Getty Images; p.129: McDonald's Corporation

Chapter 7

p.131: Tim Platt/Iconica/Getty Images; p.133 (top): mlorenzphotography/ Flickr/Getty Images; p.133 (bottom): Photodisc/Getty Images; p.134 (top): C Squared Studios/Getty Images; p.134 (bottom): © iStockphoto.com/James Phelps; p.136 (top): © RF/Corbis; p.136 (bottom): Stockdisc/PunchStock; p.138: © RF/Corbis; p.139: Ingram Publishing/Alamy; p.141: © Stockbyte/PunchStock; p.142: © Ryan McVay/Getty Images; p.143: Mark Hamel/ Getty Images; p.145 (top): Ryan Collerd/The New York Times/Redux Pictures; p.145 (bottom): Pete Saloutos/Getty Images; p.146: © Rubberball Productions; p.147: Stockbyte/Getty Images; p.148: Adam Pretty/Getty Images; p.151: © Barry Lewis/In Pictures/Corbis

Chapter 8

p.154: © Image Source/Alamy; p.156: © Isaac Baldizon/NBAE/Getty Images; p.157: © Brand X Pictures/PunchStock; p.159: © Big Cheese Photo/PunchStock; p.161: Scott Olson/Getty Images; p.162 (top): Image Source/Getty Images; p.162 (fig 8.1): © Photodisc/Getty Images; © Pixtal/ SuperStock; istockphoto.com/Andrzej Burak; istockphoto.com/Victor Burnside; © Image Source/PunchStock; C Squared Studios/Getty Images; p.163: Image Source/Getty Images; p.164: Vstock/Getty Images; p.166: © Stockbyte; p.167: © F. Seefried/WireImage; p.168: Comstock Images; p.169: Doug Menuez/Getty Images; p.170: Paul Burns/Getty Images; p.171: © AP Wide World Photos

Chapter 9

p.173: Mike Kemp/Getty Images; p.174: © David J. Green - Lifestyle/ Alamy; p.175 (left): © AP Wide World Photos; p.175 (right): © Bill Aron/ PhotoEdit; p.176 (top right): © JG Photography/Alamy; p.176 (bottom left): COLUMBIA/THE KOBAL COLLECTION/MORTON, MERRICK; p.177: © Kevin Winter/Getty Images; p.180: Jeff Kravitz/FilmMagic/Getty Images; p.182: photosindia/Getty Images; p.183: © BananaStock/PunchStock; p.185: Photodisc/Getty Images; p.186: © Digital Vision/Alamy; p.189: PRNewsFoto/Iconix/AP Wide World Photos

Chapter 10

p.192: Jay B Sauceda/Getty Images; p.193 (left to right): © iStockphoto.com Bjorn Heller; © iStockphoto.com/Plainview; © iStockphoto.com/Chris Hutchinson; © iStockphoto/Rebecca Ellis; p.194: © Rudi Von Briel/ PhotoEdit; p.196: © Mark Peterson 2009/Redux Pictures; p.197: George Doyle/Getty Images; p.198: © AP Wide World Photos; p.201: © Getty Images; p.202: Courtesy of National Institute on Alcohol Abuse and Alcoholism of the National Institute of Health; p.203: C Squared Studios/Getty Images; p.204: © Newscom; p.205: © Janine Wiedel/Photolibrary/Alamy; p.206: Blend Images/Alamy; p.208: © Newscom; p.209: Photo by Bob Nichols, USDA Natural Resources Conservation Service; p.210 (top): simon de glanville/Alamy; p.210 (bottom): © Fuse/Getty Images; p.211: © Vehbi Koca/Alamy; p.213: © Image Source; p.214: California Department of Health Services and CDC/Office on Smoking and Health (OSH) Media Campaign Resource Center (MCRC); p.215: © Kayte M. Deioma/ PhotoEdit; p.216: © Newscom; p.217: © Brooks Kraft/Corbis; p.220: BS/Photofest

Chapter 11

p.224: © Matthew Staver/Landov; p.225: © Brand X Pictures/PunchStock; p.227: © RF/Corbis; p.228: Courtesy of U.S. Drug Enforcement Agency; p.229: © RF/Corbis; p.230 (top): ER Productions/Getty Images; p.230 (bottom): © David Hoffman Photo Library/Alamy; p.231: Danny Moloshok/ Landov; p.234: Multnomah County Sheriff's Office, www.facesofmeth.us; p.235: Courtesy of U.S. Drug Enforcement Agency; p.236: © AP Wide World Photos; p.237: Darren McCollester/Getty Images; p.238: © Reuters/ Landov; p.239: Courtesy of U.S. Drug Enforcement Agency; p.241: Partnership for a Drug Free America/www.theantidrug.com

Credits

Boldface numbers indicate pages on which glossary definitions appear. Page numbers followed by *f* indicate figures. Page numbers followed by *t* indicate tables.

Index

Index

Index

quackery, medical, 424
quarantine, for infectious diseases, 331
Quinlan, Karen Ann, 84

R

race, **7**. *See also* ethnicity
racism, as source of stress, 7–8, 62
radiation
  as cancer treatment, 374
  ionizing, 363–364
  radioactive waste, 441
  ultraviolet, 362–363, 370–371
radioactive waste, 441
radon exposure, 363, **438**
Rahe, Richard, 59
random variation in traits, 22
rape, 202, 286, 286*f*, 395–398
Rape, Abuse, Incest National Network (RAINN), 397, 398
Rape Victim Advocacy Program (RVAP), 397, 398
rapid eye movement (REM) sleep, 90–92, 91*f*
Rational Recovery, 206
Real ID Act, 402
rebound effect, **235**
rebound insomnia, 100
Recommended Dietary Allowance (RDA), **106,** 114*t*
recycling, **441**
  community programs, 441
  of e-waste, 440
  individual actions, 441–443, 442*f*
  water conservation, 431
reductionist thinking, 409
red zone, 396, 397
refractory period, **261**
Reiki, **421**
relapse, **9,** 206, 218
relationships, 247–258
  attraction in, 249–250
  blended families, 258
  cohabitation, 256–257
  cohesion and flexibility in, 258
  communication in, 251–253, 253*t*, 271
  divorce, 257–258
  friendships, 247
  gay and lesbian partnerships, 256
  gender roles in, 253–254
  healthy *vs.* unhealthy, 247–248, 249
  hooking up, 248, 271, 272
  Internet dating, 250
  love and intimacy, 248–251, 251*f*, 265
  marriage, 255–256, 255*t*, 256*t*, 273–274, 400–401
  partnership characteristics, 247–248
  singlehood, 258
relaxation response, **53**
relaxation techniques, 64–66
religion. *See* spirituality
REM rebound effect, 91
REM (rapid eye movement) sleep, 90–92, 91*f*
REM sleep paralysis, 90
repetitive strain injuries, **389**–390, 390*f*
reproductive choices, 276–300. *See also* contraception
  abstinence, 265, 269, 270, 278*t*, 280, 313
  choosing a contraceptive method, 277, 280
  choosing adoption for the child, 288–289
  communicating about contraception, 277
  deciding to become a parent, 288
  egg and sperm donation, 298–299
  elective abortion, 289–290
  infertility and, 290–291
  pregnancy signs, 287
  supporting fathers, 289
  teen pregnancies and, 276
  unintended pregnancy, 276–277, 287–290
reservoirs, of pathogens, 302
resilience, **42,** 58
resistance training, 138–141
restless legs syndrome (RLS), 95
retreats, 77
retroviruses. *See* HIV/AIDS
reverse anorexia (muscle dysmorphia), **176,** 185, 187
rheumatic fever, **342**
rheumatic heart disease, **342**–343

R-I-C-E principle, 145
rickets, 378
right-to-die questions, 84
Ritalin, 88, 167, 233, 241
RLS (restless legs syndrome), 95
road rage, 382
rock climbing safety, 385
Roe v. Wade, 289
Rohypnol, 232*t*–233*t*, 235
Rolfing, 420
Rowling, J. K., 47*f*
RU486, 290
rubella (German measles), 292
running shoes, 147
RVAP (Rape Victim Advocacy Program), 397, 398

S

SADD (Students Against Destructive Decisions), 208
safer sex, **269**–271
safety. *See* injuries
safety belts, 383
salmonella enteritis, 126, 310
salt. *See* sodium
SAMHSA (Substance Abuse and Mental Health Services Administration), 46
samnoplasty, 94
sanitary landfills, **439,** 441
SA (sinoatrial) node, **335**
sarcomas, **359**
SARS (severe acute respiratory syndrome), 311
saturated fats, 111, 114*t*
scabies, 329
SCCC (Students for Concealed Carry on Campus), 405
Schiavo, Terri, 84
schizophrenia, 30, 48–49
school shootings, 392, 393–394
SCN (suprachiasmic nuclei), 89, 89*f*
screening tests, **374,** 375
secondary prevention, 5, 242
second-growth forests, 443
secondhand smoke, **215**–216
Security on Campus (SOC), 393–394
self-actualization, 40–42, 42*f*
self-care, medical, 421–422
self-efficacy, 8, 42
self-esteem, 40, 247
self-hypnosis, 416
self-injury, 50
self-stimulation, 265–266
septal defect, **343**
September 11, 2001 attacks, 401–402, 402*f*
serotonin, 44, 419
serotonin syndrome, 419
service learning, **79**
serving sizes, 119, 119*f*, 162, 162*f*
set point, for happiness, 72–73
severe acute respiratory syndrome (SARS), 311
sex, **253**
sex addiction, 271
sex drive, **261**
sex games, 266
sex-linked chromosomes, **26**
sex offenders, 398–399
sexsomnia, 96
sexting, 270, 272, 272*f*
sexual anatomy, 259–261, 259*f*, 260*f*
sexual arousal, 261, 262*f*
sexual assault, **395**
  on campus, 393, 395
  child sexual abuse, 398–399
  rape, 202, 286, 286*f*, 395–398
  red zone, 396, 397
  sexual coercion, 395
  sexual harassment, 399
  statutory rape, 395
sexual coercion, **395**
sexual desire, 263, 267, 268
sexual desire disorders, 267, 268
sexual dysfunction, **267**
  in men, 268–269
  tobacco use and, 214
  in women, 267–268
sexual harassment, **399**

sexual intercourse, 266
sexuality
  across the lifespan, 263–264
  alcohol and, 269
  atypical sexual behaviors, 266–267
  culture and, 271–272
  gender, 253–254
  intersex, 253
  safer sex, 269–271
  sexual anatomy, 259–261, 259*f*, 260*f*
  sexual dysfunction, 214, 267–269
  sexual response, 261–263, 262*f*
  typical forms of sexual expression, 264–266
sexually transmitted diseases (STDs), 317–329
  bacterial, 324–325, 326*t*
  bacterial vaginosis, 325
  birth control pills and, 280
  candidiasis, 304, 329
  chlamydia, 268, 324–325, 326*t*, 348
  genital herpes, 327*t*, 328–329
  gonorrhea, 268, 325, 326*t*
  hepatitis, 292, 313, 327*t*, 329, 354
  HIV/AIDS, 316, 320–324, 320*f*, 321*f*, 326*t*
  human papillomavirus, 325, 327*t*, 328, 364, 369
  infection risk in, 311–312
  overview of common diseases, 326*t*–327*t*
  pain during intercourse in, 268
  pelvic inflammatory disease, 325
  prevention of, 313
  pubic lice and scabies, 329
  syphilis, 325, 326*t*
  telling a partner you have, 330
  trichomoniasis, 327*t*, 329
  viral, 325–329, 326*t*–327*t*
sexually transmitted infections (STIs), 317. *See also* sexually transmitted diseases
sexual orientation, **254**
  continuum of, 254–255
  eating disorders and, 178
  gay and lesbian partnerships, 256
  genetic influences in, 31
  hate crimes and, 401
  same-sex marriage, 273–274
  stress from, 63
sexual response, 261–263, 262*f*
Shape Up America! program, 143
shisah, 210
shoes, running, 147
sibutramine, 166
sickle cell disease, 27–28, 29
SIDS (sudden infant death syndrome), 214, 216, **292**
signature strengths, 71
simian immunodeficiency virus, 320
similarity theory, 250
simple carbohydrates, **109**
single-gene disorders, **26**–28
singlehood, 258
sinoatrial (SA) node, **335**
sinus node, **335,** 338
size acceptance movement, 167–168
skill-related fitness, **133**
skin, as defense system, 305
skin cancer, 362–363, 370–372, 371*f*
skinfold measurement, 156
skin wetting, in hot weather, 146
sleep, 86–104
  controls for, 89, 89*f*
  driving and, 94, 102–103
  dust mites and other pests, 99, 99*f*
  dyssomnias, 92–95, 95*f*
  establishing good habits, 97–100
  evaluating, 96
  health effects of, 87
  napping, 98–99
  parasomnias, 95–96
  short *vs.* long, 87
  sleep aids, 100–101
  sleep deprivation, 87–89
  structure of, 90–92, 91*f*
sleep apnea, 92, 93–94, 95*f*, 98
sleep cycles, 91–92, 91*f*
sleep debt, 88
sleep latency, 96
sleep medication, 100–101